PDR®

PHYSICIANS' DESK REFERENCE®

ADDENDUM

Dear Doctor,

Thomson PDR and Wellness International would like to provide you with the complete product information for three Wellness International products that missed the publication deadline for the *2007 PDR for Nonprescription Drugs, Dietary Supplements, and Herbs (NPD)*.

Enclosed you'll find the information for BioLean II, Stephan Elixir, and Winomeg3Complex. Please insert these in the Dietary Supplement section of your 2007 NPD.

Cordially,

Michael J. DeLuca, PharmD, MBA
Manager, Professional Services
Physicians' Desk Reference®

BIOLEAN II®
(Wellness International)
Herbal & Amino Acid Dietary Supplement

Description: BioLean II® is an ephedra-free dietary supplement for weight loss, appetite suppression and increased energy without the harmful side effects found in many supplements of this nature. BioLean II® has a proprietary synergistic blend of natural herbal extracts and pharmaceutical grade amino acids that promote a multifaceted approach to fat loss. Key ingredients such as Advantra Z®, guarana seed extract, green tea leaf extract and L-carnitine work together to increase the metabolic rate and encourage fat loss by elevating rates of thermogenesis and lipolysis.

Uses: BioLean II® may:
• Enhance weight loss
• Aid weight maintenance
• Suppress appetite
• Increase energy and alertness
• Increase lipolysis or fat breakdown
• Increase ratio of lean muscle mass to total body mass
• Increase metabolic rate or thermogenesis

Directions: Recommended Use: AM Serving - As a dietary supplement, take one white tablet and two green tablets with low calorie food. PM Serving - Take one green tablet with low calorie food. If using BioLean II® for the first time, limit daily intake to one white tablet and one green tablet on days one and two and one white tablet and two green tablets on day three. Needs may vary with each individual.

Warnings: CAUTION PHENYLKETONURICS: Contains 196 mg phenylalanine per AM serving. Not for use by children under the age of 18, pregnant or lactating women. If you have heart disease, thyroid disease, diabetes, high blood pressure, depression or other psychiatric condition, glaucoma, difficulty urinating, prostate enlargement, or seizure disorder, if you are using a monoamine oxidase inhibitor (MAOI), consult a health professional before using this product. Exceeding recommended serving may cause serious adverse effects. Discontinue use and consult your health professional if dizziness, sleeplessness, severe headache, heart palpitations or other similar symptoms occur. The recommended dose of this product contains about as much caffeine as a cup of coffee.

Limit the use of caffeine-containing medications, food, or beverages while taking this product because too much caffeine may cause nervousness, irritability, sleeplessness, and occasionally, rapid heart beat. If allergic symptoms develop, discontinue use immediately.

Ingredients: Calcium (as calcium carbonate, calcium phosphate dibasic), Proprietary Blend: [Caffeine (as Guarana Seed 50% Extract, Yerba Mate Leaf 10% Extract, Green Tea Leaf 40% Extract), Citrus Aurantium Fruit 30% Extract (Advantra Z®), Schizandra Berry, Gymnema Sylvestre Leaf 25% Extract, Rehmannia Root, Hawthorne Root, Jujube Seed, Alisma Root, Angelicae dahuricae Radix, Epemidium grandiflorum Radix, Poria Cocos Mushroom, Rhubarb Root, Angelicae sinensis Radix, Codonopsis Root, Eucommia Bark, Panax notoginseng Radi], L-Tyrosine, L-Phenylalanine, L-Carnitine (as L-Car nitine Bitartrate), Calcium Carbonate, Starch, Stearic Acid, Cellulose, Hydroxypropylcellulose, Croscarmellose Sodium, Magnesium Stearate, Silicon Dioxide, Calcium Phosphate Dibasic, Stearic acid, Silicon Dioxide, Croscarmelose Sodium, Hydroxypropylcellulose, Magnesium Stearate, Ethylcellulose.

Advantra Z® - registered trademark of Nutratech, Inc./Zhishin, LLC licensor of U.S. Patents.

How Supplied: One box contains 28 packets, with one white tablet and three green tablets per packet.

Additional Information: For additional information on ingredients or uses, please visit www.winltd.com.

Supplement Facts

[See table below]

Other Ingredients (Herbal Blend): Calcium carbonate, starch, stearic acid, cellulose, hydroxypropylcellulose, croscarmelose, sodium, magnesium stearate, silicon dioxide.

Other Ingredients (Amino Acid): Calcium phosphate dibasic, stearic acid, silicon dioxide, croscarmelose sodium, hydroxypropylcellulose, magnesium stearate, ethylcellulose.

These statements have not been evaluated by the Food & Drug Administration. This product is not intended to diagnose, treat, cure or prevent any disease.

BioLean II®
AM Serving Size 2 green tablets, 1 white tablet
PM Serving Size 1 green tablet
Servings Per Container 56 (28 Daily Servings)

	Amount per AM Serving	Amount per PM Serving	% Daily Value
Calcium (as calcium carbonate, calcium phosphate dibasic)	206.76 mg	91.88 mg	AM = 20% PM = 9%
BIOLEAN II Proprietary Blend	1661.68 mg	830.34 mg	†
Caffeine (as Guarana Seed 50% Extract, Yerba Mate Leaf 10% Extract Green Tea Leaf 40% Extract)	167 mg	83.5 mg	†
Citrus Aurantium Fruit 30% Extract (Advantra Z®)			†
Schizandrae Berry			†
Gymnema Sylvestre Leaf 25% Extract			†
Rehmannia Root			†
Hawthorne Root			†
Jujube Seed			†
Alisma Root			†
Angelicae dahuricae Radix			†
Epemidium grandiflorum Radix			†
Poria Cocos Mushroom			†
Rhubarb Root			†
Angelicae sinensis Radix			†
Codonopsis Root			†
Euconium Bark			†
Panax notoginseng Radix			†
L-Tyrosine	196 mg		†
L-Phenylalanine	196 mg		†
L-Camitine (as L-Carnitine Bitartrate)	8 mg		†

†Daily Value not established

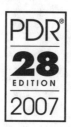

PDR
28
EDITION
2007

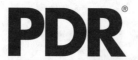

PDR®

for Nonprescription Drugs,
Dietary Supplements, and Herbs

Executive Vice President, PDR: Kevin D. Sanborn
Senior Vice President, PDR Sales: Roseanne McCauley
Vice President, Product Management: William T. Hicks
Vice President, Regulatory Affairs: Mukesh Mehta, RPh
Vice President, PDR Services: Brian Holland
Senior Director, Pharmaceutical Solutions Sales:
Anthony Sorce
National Solutions Managers: Frank Karkowsky,
Marion Reid, RPh
Senior Solutions Managers: Debra Goldman,
Elaine Musco, Warner Stuart, Suzanne E. Yarrow, RN
Solutions Managers: Eileen Bruno, Cory Coleman,
Marjorie A. Jaxel, Lois Smith, Richard Zwickel
Sales Coordinators: Dawn McPartland, Janet Wallendal

Senior Director, New Business Development:
Michael Bennett
Director of Trade Sales: Bill Gaffney
Senior Manager, Direct Marketing: Amy Cheong
Promotion Manager: Linda Levine

**Senior Director of Product Management, Electronic
Solutions:** Valerie E. Berger
Director of Product Management, Monographs:
Jeffrey D. Schaefer
Director of Product Management, Pharma Promotions:
Swan Oey
Associate Director, Practitioners Database: Jennifer M.
Fronzaglia
Senior Marketing Manager: Kim Marich

Senior Director, Client Services: Stephanie Struble
Director of Operations: Robert Klein

Director of Finance: Mark S. Ritchin
Director, Editorial Services: Bette LaGow
Manager, Professional Services: Michael DeLuca,
PharmD, MBA
Drug Information Specialists: Majid Kerolous, PharmD;
Nermin Shenouda, PharmD; Greg Tallis, RPh
Senior Editor: Lori Murray
Production Editor: Elise Philippi
Manager, Client Services: Travis Northern
Customer Service Supervisor: Todd Taccetta
Vendor Management Specialist: Gary Lew

Manager, Production Purchasing: Thomas Westburgh
PDR Production Manager: Steven Maher
PDR Index Supervisor: Shannon R. Spare
Index Editor: Allison O'Hare
Production Specialist: Christina Klinger
Senior Production Coordinators: Gianna Caradonna,
Yasmin Hernández
Production Coordinator: Nick W. Clark
Format Editor: Michelle G. Auffant
Traffic Assistant: Kim Condon

Production Design Supervisor: Adeline Rich
Senior Electronic Publishing Designer: Livio Udina
Electronic Publishing Designers: Deana DiVizio,
Carrie Faeth, Monika Popowitz
Production Associate: Joan K. Akerlind
Digital Imaging Manager: Christopher Husted
Digital Imaging Coordinator: Michael Labruyere

ISBN: 1-56363-570-4

FOREWORD TO THE 28TH EDITION

Over-the-counter (OTC) medications play an important role in national healthcare, with consumers buying around 5 billion OTC drug products a year. The choices are staggering: More than 100,000 OTC drugs are available, including over 800 active ingredients and 100 therapeutic classes or categories. Factor in the millions of Americans taking prescription medications—not to mention dietary supplements and herbs—and the risk for side effects or drug interactions increases rapidly.

To aid healthcare professionals in providing safe drug management, we've redesigned the format for this latest edition of the *PDR® for Nonprescription Drugs, Dietary Supplements, and Herbs.* In the main section, *Nonprescription Drug Information,* manufacturer-supplied labeling is now organized by therapeutic category according to the product's primary indication. When applicable, products with secondary indications are cross-referenced in those therapeutic categories as well. Within each category, products are listed alphabetically by brand name. The labeling in this section covers products marketed in compliance with the Code of Federal Regulations labeling requirements for OTC drugs.

The book's other product information sections, *Dietary Supplement Information* and *Herbal Medicine Information,* contain manufacturer-supplied labeling for nutritional supplements and herbal remedies arranged alphabetically by brand name. Please note that these products are marketed under the Dietary Supplement Health and Education Act of 1994 and therefore have not been evaluated by the Food and Drug Administration. Such products are not intended to diagnose, treat, cure, or prevent any disease.

As in past editions, the book also features five color-coded indices and a full-color Product Identification Guide. The indices contain manufacturer contact information, product names, prescribing categories, active ingredients, and a listing of "companion" OTC drugs that may be recommended to relieve symptoms caused by prescription drug therapy.

About This Book
PDR® for Nonprescription Drugs, Dietary Supplements, and Herbs is published annually by Thomson PDR. The book is made possible through the courtesy of the manufacturers whose products appear in it. The information on each product described in the book has been prepared by the manufacturer and edited and approved by the manufacturer's medical department, medical director, or medical counsel. The function of the publisher is the compilation, organization, and distribution of this information. During compilation of this information, the publisher has emphasized the necessity of describing products comprehensively in order to provide all the facts necessary for sound and intelligent decision-making.

Descriptions seen here include all information made available by the manufacturer.

In organizing and presenting the material in *PDR® for Nonprescription Drugs, Dietary Supplements, and Herbs,* the publisher does not warrant or guarantee any of the products described, or perform any independent analysis in connection with any of the product information contained herein. *Physicians' Desk Reference®* does not assume, and expressly disclaims, any obligation to obtain and include any information other than that provided to it by the manufacturer. It should be understood that by making this material available the publisher is not advocating the use of any product described herein, nor is the publisher responsible for misuse of a product due to typographical error. Additional information on any product may be obtained from the manufacturer.

Other Prescribing Aids from PDR
For complicated cases and special patient problems, there is no substitute for the in-depth data contained in *Physicians' Desk Reference.* But for those times when you need quick access to critical prescribing information, you may want to consult the **PDR® Monthly Prescribing Guide™**, the essential drug reference designed specifically for use at the point of care. Distilled from the pages of *PDR,* this digest-sized reference presents the key facts on more than 1,500 drug formulations, including therapeutic class, indications and contraindications, warnings and precautions, pregnancy rating, drug interactions and side effects, and adult and pediatric dosages. The guide is intended to supplement full prescribing information for Rx medications, although in certain instances OTC products are included as well. When applicable, each drug entry also gives the *PDR* page number to turn to for further information. In addition, a full-color insert of pill images allows you to correctly identify each product. Issued monthly, the guide is regularly updated with detailed descriptions of new drugs soon to receive FDA approval, as well as FDA-approved revisions to existing product information. You'll also find bulletins about major new developments in the pharmaceutical industry, an overview of important new agents nearing approval, and recent clinical findings on common nutritional supplements. To learn more about this useful publication and to inquire about subscription rates, call 800-232-7379.

If you prefer to carry drug information with you on a handheld device like a Palm® or Pocket PC, consider **mobilePDR®**. This easy-to-use software allows you to retrieve in an instant concise summaries of the FDA-approved and other manufacturer-supplied labeling for 2,000 of the most frequently used Rx medications, although in certain instances OTC products are included as well. In addition, *mobilePDR* lets you run automatic interaction checks on multidrug regimens and even alerts you to significant changes in drug

labeling, usually within 24 to 48 hours of announcements. You can look up drugs by brand or generic name, by indication, and by therapeutic class. The drug interaction checker allows you to screen for interactions among as many as 32 drugs. The What's New feature provides daily alerts about such things as drug recalls, labeling changes, and new drug introductions. Our auto-update feature updates the content and the software, so upgrades are easy to manage. *mobilePDR* works with both the Palm and Pocket PC operating systems, and it's free for U.S.-based MDs, DOs, dentists, NPs, and PAs in full-time patient practice, as well as for medical students, residents, and other select prescribing allied health professionals. Check it out today at www.pdr.net.

For those who prefer to access drug information on the Internet, **PDR.net** is an excellent online source for FDA-approved and other manufacturer-supplied labeling information, as found in *PDR*. Updated monthly, this incredible resource allows you to look up drugs by brand or generic name, by keyword, or by indication, side effect, contraindication, or manufacturer. The drug interaction checker allows you to screen for interactions among as many as 32 different drugs. The site provides an index that can be searched to find comparable drugs, and images of all products are included for easy identification. As an added benefit, *PDR.net* also gives users the option to order drug samples online. In addition, the site offers Resource Centers for a variety of medical specialties. Each one includes clinical news, disease information, important drug updates, patient education handouts, and other valuable features.

Finally, *PDR.net* hosts the download for *mobilePDR*. At this one website you get two great *PDR* products. In addition to this, *PDR.net* provides links to such useful information as *Stedman's Medical Dictionary*, MEDLINE, online CME programs, clinical trials registries, evidence-based treatment decision tools, medical newsletters, Internet directories, practice-specific resource centers, online formularies, and the FDA's Medwatch. A wealth of information all in one place! Registration for *PDR.net* is free for U.S.-based MDs, DOs, dentists, NPs, and PAs in full-time patient practice, as well as for medical students, residents, and other select prescribing allied health professionals. Visit *www.pdr.net* today to register.

For more information on these or any other members of the growing family of *PDR* products, please call, toll-free, 1-800-232-7379 or fax 201-722-2680.

HOW TO USE THIS BOOK

The 2007 edition of *PDR® for Nonprescription Drugs, Dietary Supplements, and Herbs* features a new format designed to help you find the information you need as quickly and easily as possible. Now, in addition to consulting the five color-coded indices, you can go directly to a specific therapeutic category to find the relevant OTC products for a particular condition. Details of this new organization are outlined below.

NONPRESCRIPTION DRUG INFORMATION

Organized by therapeutic category and indication. The product labeling in this section is now grouped into 10 therapeutic categories according to the product's main indication. For ease of use, products are listed alphabetically by brand name rather than by manufacturer. When applicable, products that have secondary indications are cross-referenced in those therapeutic categories as well.

For example, all products primarily indicated for headache appear under the "Headache/Migraine" section in the "Central Nervous System" category. If one of these products has a secondary indication for backache, it would be cross-referenced under the "Aches and Pains" section in the "Musculoskeletal System" category. The cross-reference would direct you to the page number where the product labeling appears. **Please keep in mind that the product information included herein is valid as of press time (July 2006).** Additional information, as well as updates to the product labeling, can be obtained from the manufacturer.

DIETARY SUPPLEMENT INFORMATION

Organized by brand name. This section contains product labeling for dietary and nutritional supplements marketed under the Dietary Supplement Health and Education Act of 1994. The listings are arranged alphabetically by brand name. Be aware that these products are not federally regulated and are not intended to diagnose, treat, cure, or prevent any disease.

HERBAL MEDICINE INFORMATION

Organized by brand name. Similar to dietary supplements, this section contains labeling for herbal products marketed under the Dietary Supplement Health and Education Act of 1994. The listings are arranged alphabetically by brand name. Again, these products are not federally regulated and are not intended to diagnose, treat, cure, or prevent any disease.

COLOR-CODED INDICES

- **Manufacturers' Index** (white pages) lists all pharmaceutical manufacturers that provided OTC drug labeling for this edition. Each entry contains addresses, phone numbers, and emergency contacts, as well as a listing of that manufacturer's products and the corresponding page numbers for labeling information.

- **Product Name Index** (pink pages) provides the page number of each product description in the Nonprescription Drug, Dietary Supplement, and Herbal Medicine sections. Listings appear alphabetically by brand name.

- **Product Category Index** (blue pages) lists all fully described products according to therapeutic or pharmaceutical drug category (e.g., acetaminophen combinations).

- **Active Ingredients Index** (yellow pages) contains product cross-references by generic ingredient.

- **Companion Drug Index** (white pages) lists OTC products that may be used in conjunction with prescription drug therapy to relieve symptoms of a particular condition or drug-induced side effects.

PRODUCT IDENTIFICATION GUIDE

Organized alphabetically by manufacturer name. This section shows full-color, actual-sized photos of tablets and capsules, plus a variety of other dosage forms and packages. As in previous editions, product photos are arranged alphabetically by manufacturer name.

CONTENTS

Dietary Supplement Information (White Pages)   **805**
Section 8

Includes manufacturers' descriptions of a variety of natural remedies and nutritional supplements marketed under the Dietary Supplement Health and Education Act of 1994. Entries are organized alphabetically by brand name.

Herbal Medicine Information (White Pages)   **825**
Section 9

Includes manufacturers' descriptions of a variety of herbal remedies marketed under the Dietary Supplement Health and Education Act of 1994. Entries are organized alphabetically by brand name.

SECTION 1

MANUFACTURERS' DIRECTORY

This index lists manufacturers that have supplied information for this edition. Each company's entry includes the address, phone, and fax number of its headquarters and regional offices, as well as company contacts for inquiries, orders, and emergency information.

Products with entries in the Nonprescription Drug Information section are listed with their page numbers under the heading "OTC Products Described." Products with entries in the Dietary Supplement Information section are listed with their page numbers under the heading "Dietary Supplements Described." Other OTC products and dietary supplements available from the manufacturer follow these two sections.

A bold page number next to the manufacturer's name shows where to find product photographs, when available.

- The ◆ symbol marks drugs shown in the Product Identification Guide.

- *Italic page numbers* signify partial information.

A & Z PHARMACEUTICAL INC.

180 Oser Avenue, Suite 300
Hauppauge, NY 11788
Direct Inquiries to:
(631) 952-3800

Dietary Supplements Described:
D-Cal Chewable Caplets **812**

ACTAVIS, INC.

7205 Windsor Boulevard
Baltimore, MD 21244
Direct Inquiries to:
Customer Service
(800) 432-8534

OTC Products Described:
Permethrin Lotion **641**

ADAMS RESPIRATORY THERAPEUTICS   **503**

14841 Sovereign Road
Fort Worth, TX 76155
Direct Inquiries to:
(866) Mucinex

OTC Products Described:
◆ Humibid Extended-Release
    Bi-Layer Tablets **503, 720**
◆ Mucinex Extended-Release
    Bi-Layer Tablets **503, 720**
◆ Mucinex D Extended-Release
    Bi-Layer Tablets **503, 776**
◆ Mucinex DM Extended-Release
    Bi-Layer Tablets **503, 720**

ALTO PHARMACEUTICALS, INC.

P.O. Box 271150
Tampa, FL 33688-1150
3172 Lake Ellen Drive
Tampa, FL 33618
Direct Inquiries to:
John J. Cullaro
Customer Service
www.altopharm.com
(800) 330-2891
(813) 968-0527

Dietary Supplements Described:
Zinc-220 Capsules **824**

Other Products Available:
Amino-G Tablets
Tri-Enz Tablets

AWARENESS CORPORATION/dba AWARENESSLIFE   **503**

25 South Arizona Place, Suite 500
Chandler, AZ 85225
Direct Inquiries to:
1-800-69AWARE
www.awarenesslife.net

Dietary Supplements Described:
Awareness Clear Capsules **827**
◆ Daily Complete Liquid **503, 827**
◆ Experience Capsules **503, 828**
◆ Female Balance *503*
◆ Pure Gardens Cream **832**
◆ PureTrim Mediterranean
    Wellness Shake **503, 818**
◆ SynergyDefense Capsules **503, 833**

BAUSCH & LOMB   **503**

1400 North Goodman Street
Rochester, NY 14609
Direct Inquiries to:
Main Office
(585) 338-6000
Consumer Affairs
(800) 553-5340

Dietary Supplements Described:
◆ Bausch & Lomb Ocuvite Adult
    Eye Vitamin and Mineral
    Supplement Soft Gels **503, 706**
◆ Bausch & Lomb Ocuvite Adult
    50+ Eye Vitamin and
    Mineral Supplement Soft
    Gels **503, 706**
◆ Bausch & Lomb PreserVision
    Eye Vitamin and Mineral
    Supplement Original
    Tablets **503, 806**
◆ Bausch & Lomb PreserVision
    AREDS Eye Vitamin and
    Mineral Supplement Soft
    Gels **503, 806**
◆ Bausch & Lomb PreserVision
    Lutein Eye Vitamin and
    Mineral Supplement Soft
    Gels **503, 807**
◆ Ocuvite Lutein Vitamin and
    Mineral Supplement **503, 707**

BAYER HEALTHCARE LLC CONSUMER CARE DIVISION   **503**

36 Columbia Road
P.O. Box 1910
Morristown, NJ 07962-1910

BAYER HEALTHCARE LLC CONSUMER CARE DIVISION—cont.

Direct Inquiries to:
Consumer Relations
(800) 331-4536
www.bayercare.com

For Medical Emergencies Contact:
Bayer Healthcare LLC Consumer Care Division
(800) 331-4536

OTC Products Described:

Dietary Supplements Described:

Other Products Available:
Alka-Seltzer Effervescent Original and Lemon-Lime, Gold, Extra-Strength, Morning Relief, Heartburn Relief and PM
Alka-Seltzer Plus Effervescent Cold Original, Cold Day-Time, Cold Night-Time, Cold & Cough and Cold & Sinus
Alka-Seltzer Plus Liquid-Gels Cold Day-Time, Cold Night-Time and Cold & Cough
Alka-Seltzer Plus Effervescent Flu
Bactine Original First Aid Liquid and Pain Relieving Cleansing Spray
Campho-Phenique Antiseptic Gel and Liquid
Campho-Phenique Cold Sore Treatment with Drying Action and Cold Sore Treatment for Scab Relief
Domeboro Astringent Solution
Midol Menstrual Complete, Extended Relief, Teen Formula and Cramps & Body Aches
Neo-Synephrine Medicated Drops
Neo-Synephrine Nasal Saline Moisturizer
Neo-Synephrine Nasal Spray 12 Hour, Extra/Regular/Mild Strength
Phillips' Milk of Magnesia (MOM) Liquid, Concentrated MOM Liquid, Caplets, Chewable Tablets, Stool Softener Liquid-Gels, Phillips' M-O Liquid
RID Shampoo, Egg & Nit Comb-out Gel, Home Lice Control Spray, No Drip Mousse, Dual Comb and Complete Elimination Kit
Vanquish Extra-Strength Pain Reliever

BEACH PHARMACEUTICALS

Division of Beach Products, Inc.
EXECUTIVE OFFICE:
5220 South Manhattan Avenue
Tampa, FL 33611
(813) 839-6565
Direct Inquiries to:
Richard Stephen Jenkins, Exec. V.P.:
(813) 839-6565
Clete Harmon, Sr. V.P., Regulatory and Business Affairs:
(864) 277-7282
Manufacturing and Distribution:
1700 Perimeter Road
Greenville, SC 29605
(800) 845-8210
Dietary Supplements Described:

BEUTLICH LP, PHARMACEUTICALS

1541 Shields Drive
Waukegan, IL 60085-8304
Direct Inquiries to:
(847) 473-1100
(800) 238-8542 in the U.S. and Canada
M-Th: 7:30 a.m. - 5:00 p.m.,
F: 7:30 a.m. - 4:00 p.m. CT
FAX: (847) 473-1122
www.beutlich.com
E-mail: beutlich@beutlich.com

OTC Products Described:

Dietary Supplements Described:

BOEHRINGER INGELHEIM CONSUMER HEALTHCARE PRODUCTS   504

Division of Boehringer Ingelheim Pharmaceuticals, Inc.
900 Ridgebury Road
P.O. Box 368
Ridgefield, CT 06877
Direct Inquiries to:
(888) 285-9159

OTC Products Described:

DANNMARIE, LLC.

2005 Palmer Avenue, #200
Larchmont, New York 10538
Direct Inquiries to:
(877) 425-8767
www.premcal.com
E-mail: info@premcal.com
Dietary Supplements Described:

ENIVA NUTRACEUTICS   504

Minneapolis, MN 55449
Direct Inquiries to:
www.enivaquality.com
Dietary Supplements Described:

4LIFE RESEARCH

9850 South 300 West
Sandy, UT 84070
Direct Inquiries to:
(801) 562-3600
FAX: (801) 562-3699
E-mail: productsupport@4life.com
www.4life.com

Dietary Supplements Described:

Other Products Available:
4Life Transfer Factor Advanced Formula
4Life Transfer Factor Age-Defying Effects
4Life Transfer Factor Belle Vie
4Life Transfer Factor Cardio
4Life Transfer Factor Chewable
4Life Transfer Factor énummi
4Life Transfer Factor GluCoach
4Life Transfer Factor Go Stix
4Life Transfer Factor Immune Spray
4Life Transfer Factor Kids
4Life Transfer Factor MalePro
4Life Transfer Factor ReCall
4Life Transfer Factor RenewAll
4Life Transfer Factor RioVida
4Life Transfer Factor Toothpaste

GLAXOSMITHKLINE CONSUMER HEALTHCARE, L.P.   504

Post Office Box 1467
Pittsburgh, PA 15230
Direct Inquiries to:
Consumer Affairs
(800) 245-1040
For Medical Emergencies Contact:
Consumer Affairs
(800) 245-1040

OTC Products Described:

GREEK ISLAND LABS

7620 E. McKellips Road
Suite 4 PMB 86
Scottsdale, AZ 85257
Direct Inquiries to:
www.greekislandlabs.com
(888) 841-7363

**JOHNSON & JOHNSON –
MERCK CONSUMER
PHARMACEUTICALS CO.**   **506**

7050 Camp Hill Road
Fort Washington, PA 19034
Direct Inquiries to:
Consumer Relationship Center
Fort Washington, PA 19034
(800) 755-4008

LEGACY FOR LIFE, LLC

P.O. Box 410376
Melbourne, FL 32941-0376
Direct Inquiries to:
(800) 557-8477
(321) 951-8815
info@legacyforlife.net
www.legacyforlife.net

MANNATECH, INC.   **507**

600 S. Royal Lane
Suite 200
Coppell, TX 75019
Direct Inquiries to:
Customer Service
(972) 471-8111
For Medical Information Contact:
Stephen Boyd, MD, PhD
(972) 471-7400
E-mail: Sboyd@mannatech.com
www.mannatech.com
(for product information)
www.glycoscience.org
(for ingredient information)

MATRIXX INITIATIVES, INC.   **507**

4742 North 24th Street
Suite 455
Phoenix, AZ 85016
Direct Inquiries to:
(602) 385-8888
FAX: (602) 385-8850
www.zicam.com

PERFORMANCE HEALTH

1017 Boyd Road
Export, PA 15632-8997
Direct Inquiries to:
(724) 733-9500
FAX: (724) 733-4266
E-mail: PDR@Biofreeze.com
OTC Products Described:
Biofreeze Pain Relieving Roll on/Gel

PFIZER CONSUMER HEALTHCARE, PFIZER INC.

201 Tabor Road
Morris Plains, NJ 07950
Address Questions & Comments to:
Consumer Affairs, Pfizer Consumer
Healthcare
182 Tabor Road
Morris Plains, NJ 07950
**For Medical Emergencies or Information
Contact:**
(800) 223-0182
(800) 524-2624
(800) 378-1783 (e.p.t.)
(800) 337-7266 (e.p.t.)

OTC Products Described:

Other Products Available:
Actifed Cold & Allergy Tablets
Actifed Cold & Sinus Caplets
Benadryl Allergy Kapseal Capsules
Benadryl Allergy Ultratab Tablets
Benadryl Dye-Free Allergy Liqui-Gels
    Softgels
Benadryl Allergy & Cold Caplets
Benadryl Allergy & Sinus Headache
    Caplets & Gelcaps
Benadryl Maximum Strength Severe
    Allergy & Sinus Headache
    Caplets
Benadryl D Allergy and Sinus
    Tablets
Benadryl D Allergy and Sinus
    Fastmelt Tablets
Benadryl Itch Relief Stick Extra
    Strength
Benadryl Itch Stopping Cream Extra
    Strength
Benadryl Itch Stopping Cream
    Original Strength
Benadryl Itch Stopping Gel Extra
    Strength
Benadryl Itch Stopping Spray Extra
    Strength
Children's Benadryl Allergy Liquid
Children's Benadryl Dye-Free Allergy
    Liquid
Children's Benadryl Allergy & Cold
    Fastmelt Tablets
Children's Benadryl Allergy Fastmelt
    Tablets
Children's Benadryl D Allergy &
    Sinus Fastmelt Tablets
Children's Benadryl D Allergy and
    Sinus Liquid
BenGay External Analgesic
    Ointments and Creams
BenGay Pain Relieving Patch
BenGay Ultra Strength Pain
    Relieving Patch
Benylin

PFIZER CONSUMER HEALTHCARE, PFIZER INC.—cont.

Caladryl Anti-Itch Lotion
Caladryl Clear Anti-Itch Lotion
Corn Huskers Lotion
Cortizone 5 Ointment
Cortizone 10 Creme
Cortizone 10 Plus Creme
Cortizone 10 External Anal Itch
     Cream
Cortizone 10 Ointment
Cortizone 10 Maximum Strength
     Quick Shot Spray
Desitin Creamy Diaper Rash
     Ointment
Desitin Diaper Rash Ointment
Doxidan Stimulant Laxative
Dramamine
Efferdent Original Denture Cleanser
Efferdent Plus (Mint and Gold)
     Denture Cleanser
Effergrip Denture Adhesive Cream
Emetrol for Nausea
e.p.t. Certainty Digital Home
     Pregnancy Tests
e.p.t. +/- Home Pregnancy Tests
Fresh n' Brite Denture Toothpaste
Gelusil Antacid/Anti-Gas Tablets
Hemorid Hemorrhoidal (Cream and
     Ointment)
Kaopectate Anti-Diarrheal/Upset
     Stomach Reliever Liquid
Extra Strength Kaopectate Anti-
     Diarrheal Liquid
Kaopectate Stool Softener
Lavacol Rubbing Alcohol
Listerine Antiseptic
Advance Listerine with Tartar
     Protection Antiseptic
Listerine Agent Cool Blue Plaque-
     Detecting Rinse (Bubbleblast
     and Glacier Mint)
Cool Mint Listerine Antiseptic
Listerine Essential Care Toothpaste
Fresh Burst Listerine Antiseptic
Natural Citrus Listerine Antiseptic
Listerine PocketMist (Cool Mint and
     Fresh Citrus)
Listerine PocketPaks (Cool Mint,
     Fresh Burst, Fresh Citrus and
     Cinnamon)
Vanilla Mint Listerine Antiseptic
Listerine Whitening Pre-Brush Rinse
Listermint Mouthwash
Lubriderm Advanced Therapy
     Moisturizing Lotion
Lubriderm Body Bar
Lubriderm Daily Moisture Lotions
     (Scented and Fragrance Free)
Lubriderm Daily Moisture with SPF
     15 Lotion
Lubriderm Sensitive Skin Therapy
     Moisturizing Lotion
Lubriderm Skin Nourishing
     Moisturizing Lotions (Premium
     Oat Extract, Sea Kelp Extract
     and Shea & Cocoa Butters)
Micatin Antifungal Cream, Spray
     Liquid and Spray Powder
Myadec Multivitamin-Multimineral
     Supplement
Nasal Crom Nasal Spray
Neosporin AF Antifungal Cream,
     Spray Liquid and Spray Powder
Neosporin LT Lip Treatment
Neosporin Scar Solution Silicone
     Scar Sheets
Pacquin Plus with Aloe, Dry Skin
     Pacquin, Medicated Pacquin

PediaCare Multi-Symptom Cold
     Liquid
PediaCare Freezer Pops Long-Acting
     Cough - Glacier Grape and Polar
     Berry Blue
PediaCare Long-Acting Cough Plus
     Cold Liquid
PediaCare Long-Acting Cough Infant
     Drops
PediaCare Decongestant & Cough
     Infant Drops
PediaCare Decongestant Infant
     Drops
PediaCare NightRest Cough & Cold
     Liquid
Plax Pre-Brushing Rinse
Polysporin First Aid Antibiotic
     Powder
Progaine Shampoos (2 in 1, Deep
     Cleansing and Volumizing)
Progaine Volumizing Foam
Progaine Weightless Conditioner
Proxacol Hydrogen Peroxide First Aid
     Antiseptic
Purell Instant Hand Sanitizers
Rolaids Antacid Tablets
Extra Strength Rolaids Antacid
     Softchews
Extra Strength Rolaids Antacid
     Tablets
Rolaids Multi-Symptom Antacid &
     Antigas Tablets
Sinutab Sinus Caplets
Sinutab Maximum Strength Sinus
     Allergy Caplets
Sinutab Nondrying Liquid Caps
Sudafed 12 Hour Caplets - Nasal
     Decongestant
Sudafed 24 Hour Tablets - Nasal
     Decongestant
Sudafed Nasal Decongestant
     Tablets
Sudafed Non-Drowsy Severe Cold
     Caplets
Sudafed Non-Drowsy Severe Cold
     Tablets
Sudafed Non-Drying Sinus Liquid
     Caps
Sudafed PE Nasal Decongestant
     Tablets
Sudafed PE Sinus Headache
     Caplets
Sudafed Sinus & Allergy Tablets
Sudafed Sinus Headache Caplets
     and Tablets
Surfak Stool Softener
Three Flowers Brillantine Liquid and
     Solid Hair Tonic
Tucks Hemorrhoidal Ointment
Tucks Hemorrhoidal Suppositories
Tucks Anti-Itch Ointment
Tucks TakeAlongs Medicated
     Towelettes
Tucks Witch Hazel Hemorrhoidal
     Pad
Unicap Dietary Supplement
Unisom Maximum Strength
     SleepGels Gelcaps
Unisom Sleep Tabs Tablets
Visine Original Eye Drops
Visine A.C. Eye Drops
Visine Advanced Relief Eye Drops
Visine for Contacts
Visine L.R. Eye Drops
Visine Pure Tears (Single Drop
     Dispenser)
Visine Tears Eye Drops
Visine Tears Pure Portables
     Preservative Free Eye Drops
     (vials)

Visine-A Eye Drops
Wart-Off Wart Remover
Zantac 75 Tablets Acid Reducer
Zantac 150 Maximum Strength
     Tablets Acid Reducer

PROCTER & GAMBLE   516

P.O. Box 559
Cincinnati, OH 45201
Direct Inquiries to:
Consumer Relations
(800) 832-3064

REESE PHARMACEUTICAL COMPANY 517

10617 Frank Avenue
Cleveland, OH 44106
Direct Inquiries to:
Voice: (800) 321-7178
FAX: (216) 231-6444
www.reesepharmaceutical.com

OTC Products Described:
◆ Reese's Pinworm
  Treatments **517, 670**
Refenesen 400 Caplets **721**
Refenesen DM Caplets **721**
Refenesen PE Caplets **721**

Other Products Available:
Dentapaine Oral Pain Reliever
Double Tussin DM Intense Strength
  Cough Reliever

SCHERING-PLOUGH HEALTHCARE PRODUCTS 517

556 Morris Avenue
Summit, NJ 07901-1330
Direct Product Requests to:
Schering-Plough HealthCare Products
556 Morris Avenue
Summit, NJ 07901-1330
For Medical Emergencies Contact:
Consumer Relations Department
P.O. Box 377
Memphis, TN 38151
(901) 320-2988 (Business Hours)
(901) 320-2364 (After Hours)

OTC Products Described:
◆ Children's Claritin Allergy Oral
  Solution **517, 771**
◆ Claritin Non-Drowsy 24 Hour
  Tablets **517, 772**
◆ Claritin Reditabs 24 Hour Non-
  Drowsy Tablets **517, 772**
◆ Claritin-D Non-Drowsy 12 Hour
  Tablets **517, 772**
◆ Claritin-D Non-Drowsy 24 Hour
  Tablets **517, 772**

STANDARD HOMEOPATHIC COMPANY

210 West 131st Street
Box 61067
Los Angeles, CA 90061
Direct Inquiries to:
Jay Borneman
(800) 624-9659, Ext. 20

OTC Products Described:
Hyland's BackAche with Arnica
  Caplets **828**
Hyland's Calm Forté 4 Kids
  Tablets **828**
Hyland's Calms Forté Tablets and
  Caplets **828**
Hyland's Complete Flu Care
  Tablets **828**
Hyland's Complete Flu Care 4 Kids
  Tablets **732**
Hyland's Earache Drops **828**
Hyland's Earache Tablets **829**
Hyland's Leg Cramps with Quinine
  Tablets and Caplets **829**
Hyland's Nerve Tonic Tablets and
  Caplets **829**
Hyland's Restful Legs Tablets **829**
Hyland's Sniffles 'N Sneezes 4 Kids
  Tablets **732**

Hyland's Teething Gel **830**
Hyland's Teething Tablets **830**
Smile's Prid Salve **833**

TAHITIAN NONI INTERNATIONAL 517

333 West River Park Drive
Provo, UT 84604
Direct Inquiries to:
(801) 234-1000
www.tahitiannoni.com

Dietary Supplements Described:
◆ Tahitian Noni Leaf Serum
  Soothing Gel **517, 833**
◆ Tahitian Noni Liquid **517, 834**
◆ Tahitian Noni Seed Oil **517, 834**

UAS LABORATORIES

9953 Valley View Road
Eden Prairie, MN 55344
Direct Inquiries to:
Dr. S.K. Dash
(952) 935-1707
FAX: (952) 935-1650
For Medical Emergencies Contact:
Dr. S.K. Dash
(952) 935-1707
FAX: (952) 935-1650

OTC Products Described:
DDS-Acidophilus Capsules, Tablets,
  and Powder **812**

UCB, INC. 517

1950 Lake Park Drive
Smyrna, GA 30080
Direct Inquiries to:
(888) 963-3382

OTC Products Described:
◆ Delsym Extended-Release
  Suspension 12 Hour
  Cough Suppressant **517, 730**

UPSHER-SMITH LABORATORIES, INC.

6701 Evenstad Drive
Maple Grove, MN 55369
Direct Inquiries to:
Professional Services
(800) 654-2299
FAX: (763) 315-2001
For Medical Emergencies Contact:
Professional Services
(800) 654-2299
FAX: (763) 315-2001
Branch Offices:
14905 23rd Avenue N.
Plymouth, MN 55447
(763) 473-4412
FAX: (800) 328-3344
301 South Cherokee Street
Denver, CO 80223
(800) 445-8091
(303) 607-4500
FAX (303) 607-4503

OTC Products Described:
Amlactin AP Anti-Itch Moisturizing
  Cream *639*
Amlactin Moisturizing Lotion and
  Cream *639*
Amlactin XL Moisturizing Lotion *639*

VEMMA NUTRITION COMPANY 517

8322 E. Hartford Drive
Scottsdale, AZ 85255
Direct Inquiries to:
Product Knowledge Department
(800) 577-0777
E-mail: ms@vemma.com
www.vemma.com

Dietary Supplements Described:
◆ Vemma Nutrition Program -
  Essential Minerals **517, 835**
◆ Vemma Nutrition Program -
  Mangosteen Plus **517, 835**

WELLNESS INTERNATIONAL NETWORK, LTD.

5800 Democracy Drive
Plano, TX 75024
Direct Inquiries to:
Product Inquiries
(972) 312-1100
E-mail: products@winltd.com
Branch Office:
WIN Worldwide BV
Kruisweg 583-2132 NA Hoofddorp,
Nederland
Tel: 31-20-446-46-46
FAX: 31-20-446-4647

Dietary Supplements Described:
BioLean Accelerator Tablets **631**
BioLean Free Tablets **631**
BioLean LipoTrim Capsules **631**
BioLean ProXtreme Dietary
  Supplement **808**
DHEA Plus Capsules **827**
Food for Thought Dietary
  Supplement **814**
Mass Appeal Tablets **830**
Phyto-Vite Tablets **831**
Satiete Tablets **832**
Sleep-Tite Caplets **832**
StePHan Clarity Capsules **819**
StePHan Elasticity Capsules **819**
StePHan Essential Capsules **820**
StePHan Feminine Capsules **833**
StePHan Flexibility Capsules **820**
StePHan Lovpil Capsules **820**
StePHan Masculine Capsules **821**
StePHan Protector Capsules **821**
StePHan Relief Capsules **821**
StePHan Tranquility Capsules **821**
Sure2Endure Tablets **821**
Winrgy Dietary Supplement **823**

Other Products Available:
WINSalon Collection
WINSpa Collection

WYETH CONSUMER HEALTHCARE

Wyeth
Five Giralda Farms
Madison, NJ 07940-0871
Direct Inquiries to:
Wyeth Consumer Healthcare
(800) 322-3129 (9-5 E.S.T.)

OTC Products Described:
Advil Allergy Sinus Caplets **770**
Advil Caplets **674**
Children's Advil Oral Suspension ... **603**
Children's Advil Chewable
  Tablets **603**
Advil Cold & Sinus Caplets **723**

ZAVITA　　　　　　　　　　　　**517**

1430 Bradley Lane
Suite 196
Carrollton, TX 75007
Direct Inquiries to:
Customer Service
(888) 492-8482

SECTION 2

PRODUCT NAME INDEX

This index includes all entries in the Product Information sections. Products are listed alphabetically by brand name.

If an entry in the index lists multiple page numbers, the first one shown refers to the photograph of the product, the last one to its prescribing information.

- **Bold page numbers** indicate that the entry contains full product information.

- *Italic page numbers* signify partial information.

SECTION 3

PRODUCT CATEGORY INDEX

This index cross-references each brand by pharmaceutical category. All fully described products in the Product Information sections are included.

If an entry in the index lists multiple page numbers, the first one shown refers to the photograph of the product,

the last one to its prescribing information.

The classification of each product is determined by the publisher in cooperation with the product's manufacturer or, when necessary, by the publisher alone.

SECTION 4

ACTIVE INGREDIENTS INDEX

This index cross-references each brand by its generic ingredients. All entries in the Product Information sections are included. Under each generic heading, all fully described products are listed first, followed by those with only partial descriptions.

If an entry in the index lists multiple page numbers, the first one shown refers to the photograph of the

product, the last one to its prescribing information.

- **Bold page numbers** indicate full product information.

- *Italic page numbers* signify partial information.

Classification of products under these headings has been determined in cooperation with the products' manufacturers or, if necessary, by the publisher alone.

COMPANION DRUG INDEX

This index is a quick-reference guide to OTC products that may be used in conjunction with prescription drug therapy to reverse drug-induced side effects, relieve symptoms of the illness itself, or treat sequelae of the initial disease. All entries are derived from the FDA-approved prescribing information published by *PDR*.

The products listed are generally considered effective for temporary symptomatic relief. They may not, however, be appropriate for sustained therapy, and each case must be approached on an individual basis. Certain common side effects may be harbingers of more serious reactions. When making a recommendation, be sure to adjust for the patient's age, concurrent medical conditions, and complete drug regimen.

Consider timing as well, since simultaneous ingestion may not be recommended in all instances.

Please note that only products fully described in *Physicians' Desk Reference* and its companion volumes are included in this index. The publisher therefore cannot guarantee that all entries are totally accurate or complete. Keep in mind, too, that although a given OTC product is usually an appropriate companion for an entire class of prescription medications, certain drugs within the class may be exceptions. If you have any doubt about the suitability of a particular OTC product in a given situation, be sure to check the underlying *PDR* prescribing information and the relevant medical literature.

CONSTIPATION

May result from the use of ace inhibitors, hmg-coa reductase inhibitors, anticholinergics, anticonvulsants, antidepressants, beta blockers, bile acid sequestrants, butyrophenones, calcium and aluminum-containing antacids, calcium channel blockers, ganglionic blockers, hematinics, monoamine oxidase inhibitors, narcotic analgesics, nonsteroidal anti-inflammatory drugs or phenothiazines. The following products may be recommended:

CYSTIC FIBROSIS, NUTRIENTS DEFICIENCY SECONDARY TO

Cystic fibrosis may be treated with dornase alfa. The following products may be recommended for relief of nutrients deficiency:

DENTAL CARIES

May be treated with fluoride preparations or vitamin and fluoride supplements. The following products may be recommended for relief of symptoms:

DIABETES MELLITUS, CONSTIPATION SECONDARY TO

Diabetes mellitus may be treated with insulins or oral hypoglycemic agents. The following products may be recommended for relief of constipation:

DIABETES MELLITUS, POORLY CONTROLLED, CANDIDAL VULVOVAGINITIS SECONDARY TO

Diabetes mellitus may be treated with insulins or oral hypoglycemic agents. The following products may be recommended for relief of candidal vulvovaginitis:

DIABETES MELLITUS, POORLY CONTROLLED, GINGIVITIS SECONDARY TO

Diabetes mellitus may be treated with insulins or oral hypoglycemic agents. The following products may be recommended for relief of gingivitis:

DIABETES MELLITUS, POORLY CONTROLLED, VITAMINS AND MINERALS DEFICIENCY SECONDARY TO

Diabetes mellitus may be treated with insulins or oral hypoglycemic agents. The following products may be recommended for relief of vitamins and minerals deficiency:

DIARRHEA

May result from the use of ace inhibitors, beta blockers, cardiac glycosides, chemotherapeutic agents, diuretics, magnesium-containing antacids, nonsteroidal anti-inflammatory drugs, potassium supplements, acarbose, alprazolam, colchicine, divalproex sodium, ethosuximide, fluoxetine hydrochloride, guanethidine monosulfate, hydralazine hydrochloride, levodopa, lithium carbonate, lithium citrate, mesna, metformin hydrochloride, misoprostol, olsalazine sodium, pancrelipase, procainamide hydrochloride, reserpine, succimer, ticlopidine hydrochloride or valproic acid. The following products may be recommended:

DIARRHEA, ANTIBIOTIC-INDUCED

May result from the use of cephalosporins, erythromycin, erythromycin-sulfisoxazole, ampicillin or clindamycin palmitate hydrochloride. The following products may be recommended:

DIARRHEA, INFECTIOUS

May be treated with sulfamethoxazole-trimethoprim, ciprofloxacin or furazolidone. The following products may be recommended for relief of symptoms:

DYSPEPSIA

May result from the use of chronic systemic corticosteroid therapy, nonsteroidal anti-inflammatory drugs, ulcerogenic medications or mexiletine hydrochloride. The following products may be recommended:

ENTEROBIASIS, PERIANAL PRURITUS SECONDARY TO

Enterobiasis may be treated with mebendazole. The following products may be recommended for relief of perianal pruritus:

FEVER

May result from the use of immunization. The following products may be recommended:

FLATULENCE

May result from the use of nonsteroidal anti-inflammatory drugs, potassium supplements, acarbose, cisapride, guanadrel sulfate, mesalamine, metformin hydrochloride, methyldopa, octreotide acetate or ursodiol. The following products may be recommended:

INFECTIONS, SKIN AND SKIN STRUCTURE

May be treated with aminoglycosides, amoxicillin, amoxicillin-clavulanate, cephalosporins, doxycycline, erythromycin, macrolide antibiotics, penicillins or quinolones. The following products may be recommended for relief of symptoms:

IRRITABLE BOWEL SYNDROME

May be treated with anticholinergic combinations, dicyclomine hydrochloride or hyoscyamine sulfate. The following products may be recommended for relief of symptoms:

ISCHEMIC HEART DISEASE

May be treated with beta blockers, calcium channel blockers, isosorbide dinitrate, isosorbide mononitrate or nitroglycerin. The following products may be recommended for relief of symptoms:

KERATOCONJUNCTIVITIS, VERNAL

May be treated with ophthalmic mast cell stabilizers. The following products may be recommended for relief of symptoms:

MYOCARDIAL INFARCTION, ACUTE

May be treated with ace inhibitors, anticoagulants, beta blockers, thrombolytic agents or nitroglycerin. The following products may be recommended for relief of symptoms:

NASAL POLYPS, RHINORRHEA SECONDARY TO

Nasal polyps may be treated with nasal steroidal anti-inflammatory agents. The following products may be recommended for relief of rhinorrhea:

NECATORIASIS, IRON-DEFICIENCY ANEMIA SECONDARY TO

Necatoriasis may be treated with mebendazole or thiabendazole. The following products may be recommended for relief of iron-deficiency anemia:

OSTEOPOROSIS

May be treated with biphosphonates, calcitonin or estrogens. The following products may be recommended for relief of symptoms:

OSTEOPOROSIS, SECONDARY

May result from the use of chemotherapeutic agents, phenytoin, prolonged glucocorticoid therapy, thyroid hormones, carbamazepine or methotrexate sodium. The following products may be recommended:

PRURITUS, PERIANAL

May result from the use of broad-spectrum antibiotics. The following products may be recommended:

RENAL OSTEODYSTROPHY, HYPOCALCEMIA SECONDARY TO

Renal osteodystrophy may be treated with vitamin d sterols. The following products may be recommended for relief of hypocalcemia:

RESPIRATORY TRACT ILLNESS, INFLUENZA A VIRUS-INDUCED

May be treated with amantadine hydrochloride or rimantadine hydrochloride. The following products may be recommended for relief of symptoms:

RHEUMATOID ARTHRITIS, KERATOCONJUNCTIVITIS SICCA SECONDARY TO

Rheumatoid arthritis may be treated with corticosteroids, nonsteroidal anti-inflammatory drugs or azathioprine. The following products may be recommended for relief of keratoconjunctivitis sicca:

RHINITIS, NONALLERGIC

May be treated with nasal steroids or ipratropium bromide. The following products may be recommended for relief of symptoms:

SKIN IRRITATION

May result from the use of transdermal drug delivery systems. The following products may be recommended:

STOMATITIS, APHTHOUS

May result from the use of selective serotonin reuptake inhibitors, aldesleukin, clomipramine hydrochloride, didanosine, foscarnet sodium, indinavir sulfate, indomethacin, interferon alfa-2b, recombinant, methotrexate sodium, naproxen, naproxen sodium, nicotine polacrilex or stavudine. The following products may be recommended:

TUBERCULOSIS, NUTRIENTS DEFICIENCY SECONDARY TO

Tuberculosis may be treated with capreomycin sulfate, ethambutol hydrochloride, ethionamide, isoniazid, pyrazinamide, rifampin or streptomycin sulfate. The following products may be recommended for relief of nutrients deficiency:

VAGINOSIS, BACTERIAL

May be treated with sulfabenzamide/sulfacetamide/sulfathiozole or metronidazole. The following products may be recommended for relief of symptoms:

VULVOVAGINITIS, CANDIDAL

May result from the use of estrogen-containing oral contraceptives, immunosuppressants or recent broad-spectrum antibiotic therapy. The following products may be recommended:

XERODERMA

May result from the use of aldesleukin, protease inhibitors, retinoids, topical acne preparations, topical corticosteroids, topical retinoids, benzoyl peroxide, clofazimine, interferon alfa-2a, recombinant, interferon alfa-2b, recombinant or pentostatin. The following products may be recommended:

XEROMYCTERIA

May result from the use of anticholinergics, antihistamines, retinoids, apraclonidine hydrochloride, clonidine, etretinate, ipratropium bromide, isotretinoin or lodoxamide tromethamine. The following products may be recommended:

VERIFIED HERBAL INDICATIONS

Claims made for herbs in the popular press often outdistance their actual benefits. Which indications should be taken seriously and which dismissed? The most authoritative answers come from Germany, where the efficacy of medicinal herbs undergoes official scrutiny by the German Regulatory Authority's "Commission E." This agency has conducted an intensive analysis of the peer-reviewed literature on some 300 common botanicals, weighing the quality of the clinical evidence and identifying the uses for which the herb can reasonably be considered effective. The results of this effort are summarized in the table below.

Herb	Indications	Herb	Indications
Adonis (Adonis vernalis)	Arrhythmias Anxiety disorders, management of	**Asparagus** (Asparagus officinalis)	Infections, urinary tract Renal calculi
Agrimony (Agrimonia eupatoria)	Diarrhea, symptomatic relief of Skin, inflammatory conditions Stomatitis	**Bean Pod** (Phaseolus vulgaris)	Infections, urinary tract Renal calculi
Aloe Vera (Aloe barbadensis)	Constipation	**Belladonna** (Atropa belladonna)	Liver and gallbladder complaints
Angelica (Angelica archangelica)	Appetite, stimulation of Digestive disorders, symptomatic relief of Cold, common, symptomatic relief of Fever associated with common cold Infections, urinary tract	**Bilberry** (Vaccinium myrtillus)	Diarrhea, symptomatic relief of Stomatitis
		Birch (Betula species)	Infections, urinary tract Renal calculi Rheumatic disorders, unspecified
Anise (Pimpinella anisum)	Appetite, stimulation of Bronchitis, acute Cold, common, symptomatic relief of Cough, symptomatic relief of Digestive disorders, symptomatic relief of Fever associated with common cold Stomatitis	**Bitter Orange** (Citrus aurantium)	Appetite, stimulation of Digestive disorders, symptomatic relief of
		Bittersweet Nightshade (Solanum dulcamara)	Acne, unspecified Furunculosis Dermatitis, eczematoid Warts
Arnica (Arnica montana)	Bronchitis, acute Cold, common, symptomatic relief of Cough, symptomatic relief of Fever associated with common cold Infection, tendency to Rheumatic disorders, unspecified Skin, inflammatory conditions Stomatitis Trauma, blunt	**Black Cohosh** (Cimicifuga racemosa)	Menopause, climacteric complaints Premenstrual syndrome, management of
		Blackberry (Rubus fruticosus)	Diarrhea, symptomatic relief of Stomatitis
		Blessed Thistle (Cnicus benedictus)	Appetite, stimulation of Digestive disorders, symptomatic relief of
		Bog Bean (Menyanthes trifoliata)	Appetite, stimulation of Digestive disorders, symptomatic relief of
Artichoke (Cynara scolymus)	Appetite, stimulation of Liver and gallbladder complaints	**Boldo** (Peumus boldus)	Digestive disorders, symptomatic relief of

Herb	Indications	Herb	Indications
Brewer's Yeast (*Saccharomyces cerevisiae*)	Acne vulgaris Appetite, stimulation of Digestive disorders, symptomatic relief of Furunculosis Skin, inflammatory conditions	**Chaste Tree** (*Vitex agnus-castus*)	Premenstrual syndrome, management of Menopause, climacteric complaints
Buckthorn (*Rhamnus catharticus*)	Constipation	**Chicory** (*Cichorium intybus*)	Appetite, stimulation of Digestive disorders, symptomatic relief of
Bugleweed (*Lycopus virginicus*)	Anxiety disorders, management of Premenstrual syndrome, management of Sleep, induction of	**Chinese Cinnamon** (*Cinnamomum aromaticum*)	Appetite, stimulation of Digestive disorders, symptomatic relief of
		Chinese Rhubarb (*Rheum palmatum*)	Constipation
Butcher's Broom (*Ruscus aculeatus*)	Hemorrhoids, symptomatic relief of Venous conditions	**Cinnamon** (*Cinnamomum verum*)	Appetite, stimulation of Digestive disorders, symptomatic relief of
Cajuput (*Melaleuca leucadendra*)	Rheumatic disorders, unspecified Infection, tendency to Pain, muscular, temporary relief of Pain, neurogenic Wound care, adjunctive therapy in	**Cinquefoil** (*Potentilla erecta*)	Diarrhea, symptomatic relief of Stomatitis
		Clove (*Syzygium aromaticum*)	Pain, dental Stomatitis
Camphor Tree (*Cinnamomum camphora*)	Anxiety disorders, management of Arrhythmias Bronchitis, acute Cough, symptomatic relief of Hypotension Rheumatic disorders, unspecified	**Coffee** (*Coffea arabica*)	Diarrhea, symptomatic relief of Stomatitis
		Cola (*Cola acuminata*)	Lack of stamina
Canadian Golden Rod (*Solidago canadensis*)	Infections, urinary tract Renal calculi	**Colchicum** (*Colchicum autumnale*)	Brucellosis Gout, management of signs and symptoms
Caraway (*Carum carvi*)	Digestive disorders, symptomatic relief of	**Colt's Foot** (*Tussilago farfara*)	Bronchitis, acute Cough, symptomatic relief of Stomatitis
Cardamom (*Elettaria cardamomum*)	Digestive disorders, symptomatic relief of	**Comfrey** (*Symphytum officinale*)	Trauma, blunt
Cascara Sagrada (*Rhamnus purshianus*)	Constipation	**Condurango** (*Marsdenia condurango*)	Appetite, stimulation of Digestive disorders, symptomatic relief of
Cayenne (*Capsicum annuum*)	Muscle tension Rheumatic disorders, unspecified	**Coriander** (*Coriandrum sativum*)	Appetite, stimulation of Digestive disorders, symptomatic relief of
Celandine (*Chelidonium majus*)	Liver and gallbladder complaints	**Cowslip** (*Primula veris*)	Bronchitis, acute Cough, symptomatic relief of
Centaury (*Centaurium erythraea*)	Appetite, stimulation of Digestive disorders, symptomatic relief of	**Curcuma** (*Curcuma xanthorrhizia*)	Appetite, stimulation of Digestive disorders, symptomatic relief of

Herb	Indications	Herb	Indications
Dandelion (*Taraxacum officinale*)	Appetite, stimulation of Digestive disorders, symptomatic relief of Infections, urinary tract Liver and gallbladder complaints	**European Mistletoe** (*Viscum album*)	Rheumatic disorders, unspecified Tumor therapy adjuvant
		European Sanicle (*Sanicula europaea*)	Bronchitis, acute Cough, symptomatic relief of
Devil's Claw (*Harpagophytum procumbens*)	Appetite, stimulation of Digestive disorders, symptomatic relief of Rheumatic disorders, unspecified	**Fennel** (*Foeniculum vulgare*)	Bronchitis, acute Cough, symptomatic relief of Digestive disorders, symptomatic relief of
Dill (*Anethum graveolens*)	Digestive disorders, symptomatic relief of	**Fenugreek** (*Trigonella foenum-graecum*)	Appetite, stimulation of Skin, inflammatory conditions
Echinacea Pallida (*Echinacea pallida*)	Cold, common, symptomatic relief of Fever associated with common cold	**Flax** (*Linum usitatissimum*)	Constipation Skin, inflammatory conditions
Echinacea Purpurea (*Echinacea purpurea*)	Bronchitis, acute Cold, common, symptomatic relief of Cough, symptomatic relief of Fever associated with common cold Infections, tendency to Infections, urinary tract Stomatitis Wound care, adjunctive therapy in	**Frangula** (*Rhamnus frangula*)	Constipation
		Fumitory (*Fumaria officinalis*)	Liver and gallbladder complaints
English Hawthorn (*Crataegus laevigata*)	Cardiac output, low	**Garlic** (*Allium sativum*)	Arteriosclerosis Hypercholesterolemia Hypertension
English Ivy (*Hedera helix*)	Bronchitis, acute Cough, symptomatic relief of	**German Chamomile** (*Matricaria recutita*)	Bronchitis, acute Cold, common, symptomatic relief of Cough, symptomatic relief of Fever associated with common cold Infection, tendency to Skin, inflammatory conditions Stomatitis Wound care, adjunctive therapy in
English Lavender (*Lavandula angustifolia*)	Anxiety disorders, management of Appetite, stimulation of Circulatory disorders Digestive disorders, symptomatic relief of Sleep, induction of		
English Plantain (*Plantago lanceolata*)	Bronchitis, acute Cold, common, symptomatic relief of Cough, symptomatic relief of Fever associated with common cold Skin, inflammatory conditions Stomatitis	**Ginger** (*Zingiber officinale*)	Appetite, stimulation of Digestive disorders, symptomatic relief of Motion sickness
		Ginkgo (*Ginkgo biloba*)	Claudication, intermittent Organic brain dysfunction, symptomatic relief of Tinnitus Vertigo
Eucalyptus (*Eucalyptus globulus*)	Bronchitis, acute Cough, symptomatic relief of Rheumatic disorders, unspecified	**Ginseng** (*Panax ginseng*)	Lack of stamina
European Elder (*Sambucus nigra*)	Bronchitis, acute Cold, common, symptomatic relief of Cough, symptomatic relief of Fever associated with common cold	**Guaiac** (*Guaiacum officinale*)	Rheumatic disorders, unspecified

Herb	Indications	Herb	Indications
Gumweed (*Grindelia* species)	Bronchitis, acute Cough, symptomatic relief of	**Japanese Mint** (*Mentha arvensis piperascens*)	Bronchitis, acute Cold, common, symptomatic relief of Cough, symptomatic relief of Fever associated with common cold Infection, tendency to Liver and gallbladder complaints Pain, unspecified Stomatitis
Haronga (*Haronga madagascariensis*)	Digestive disorders, symptomatic relief of		
Heartsease (*Viola tricolor*)	Skin, inflammatory conditions		
Hempnettle (*Galeopsis segetum*)	Bronchitis, acute Cough, symptomatic relief of	**Java Tea** (*Orthosiphon spicatus*)	Infections, urinary tract Renal calculi
Henbane (*Hyoscyamus niger*)	Digestive disorders, symptomatic relief of	**Juniper** (*Juniperus communis*)	Appetite, stimulation of Digestive disorders, symptomatic relief of
High Mallow (*Malva sylvestris*)	Bronchitis, acute Cough, symptomatic relief of Stomatitis	**Kava-Kava** (*Piper methysticum*)	Anxiety disorders, management of Sleep, induction of
Hops (*Humulus lupulus*)	Anxiety disorders, management of Sleep, induction of	**Knotweed** (*Polygonum aviculare*)	Bronchitis, acute Cough, symptomatic relief of Stomatitis
Horehound (*Marrubium vulgare*)	Appetite, stimulation of Digestive disorders, symptomatic relief of	**Lady's Mantle** (*Alchemilla vulgaris*)	Diarrhea, symptomatic relief of
Horse Chestnut (*Aesculus hippocastanum*)	Venous conditions	**Larch** (*Larix decidua*)	Blood pressure problems Bronchitis, acute Cold, common, symptomatic relief of Cough, symptomatic relief of Fever associated with common cold Infection, tendency to Rheumatic disorders, unspecified Stomatitis
Horseradish (*Armoracia rusticana*)	Bronchitis, acute Cough, symptomatic relief of Infections, urinary tract		
Horsetail (*Equisetum arvense*)	Infections, urinary tract Renal calculi Wound care, adjunctive therapy in	**Lemon Balm** (*Melissa officinalis*)	Anxiety disorders, management of Sleep, induction of
Iceland Moss (*Cetraria islandica*)	Appetite, stimulation of Bronchitis, acute Cough, symptomatic relief of Digestive disorders, symptomatic relief of Stomatitis	**Lesser Galangal** (*Alpinia officinarum*)	Appetite, stimulation of Digestive disorders, symptomatic relief of Stomatitis
Immortelle (*Helichrysum arenarium*)	Digestive disorders, symptomatic relief of	**Licorice** (*Glycyrrhiza glabra*)	Bronchitis, acute Cough, symptomatic relief of Gastritis
		Lily-of-the-Valley (*Convallaria majalis*)	Anxiety disorders, management of Arrhythmias Cardiac output, low
Jambolan (*Syzygium cumini*)	Diarrhea, symptomatic relief of Skin, inflammatory conditions Stomatitis	**Linden** (*Tilia* species)	Bronchitis, acute Cough, symptomatic relief of

Herb	Indications	Herb	Indications
Lovage (*Levisticum officinale*)	Infections, urinary tract Renal calculi	**Oak** (*Quercus robur*)	Bronchitis, acute Cough, symptomatic relief of Diarrhea, symptomatic relief of Skin, inflammatory conditions Stomatitis
Ma-Huang (*Ephedra sinica*)	Bronchitis (acute), cough **Note:** The FDA banned ephedra products in Feb. 2004.	**Oats** (*Avena sativa*)	Skin, inflammatory conditions Warts
Manna (*Fraxinus ornus*)	Constipation	**Onion** (*Allium cepa*)	Appetite, stimulation of Arteriosclerosis Bronchitis, acute Cold, common, symptomatic relief of Cough, symptomatic relief of Digestive disorders, symptomatic relief of Fever associated with common cold Hypertension Infection, tendency to Stomatitis
Marigold (*Calendula officinalis*)	Stomatitis Wound care, adjunctive therapy in		
Marshmallow (*Althaea officinalis*)	Bronchitis, acute Cough, symptomatic relief of		
Maté (*Ilex paraguariensis*)	Lack of stamina		
Mayapple (*Podophyllum peltatum*)	Warts	**Parsley** (*Petroselinum crispum*)	Infections, urinary tract Renal calculi
Meadowsweet (*Filipendula ulmaria*)	Bronchitis, acute Cold, common, symptomatic relief of Cough, symptomatic relief of Fever associated with common cold	**Passion Flower** (*Passiflora incarnata*)	Anxiety disorders, management of Sleep, induction of
Milk Thistle (*Silybum marianum*)	Digestive disorders, symptomatic relief of Liver and gallbladder complaints	**Peppermint** (*Mentha piperita*)	Bronchitis, acute Cold, common, symptomatic relief of Cough, symptomatic relief of Digestive disorders, symptomatic relief of Fever associated with common cold Infection, tendency to Liver and gallbladder complaints Stomatitis
Motherwort (*Leonurus cardiaca*)	Anxiety disorders, management of		
Mullein (*Verbascum densiflorum*)	Bronchitis, acute Cough, symptomatic relief of	**Petasites** (*Petasites hybridus*)	Renal calculi
Myrrh (*Commiphora molmol*)	Stomatitis	**Pimpinella** (*Pimpinella major*)	Cough, symptomatic relief of Bronchitis, acute
Nasturtium (*Tropaeolum majus*)	Bronchitis, acute Cough, symptomatic relief of Infections, urinary tract	**Pineapple** (*Ananas comosus*)	Wound care, adjunctive therapy in
Niauli (*Melaleucea viridiflora*)	Bronchitis, acute Cough, symptomatic relief of	**Poplar** (*Populus* species)	Hemorrhoids, symptomatic relief of Wound care, adjunctive therapy in

Herb	Indications	Herb	Indications
Potentilla (*Potentilla anserina*)	Diarrhea, symptomatic relief of Premenstrual syndrome, management of Stomatitis	**Scopolia** (*Scopolia carniolica*)	Liver and gallbladder complaints
		Scotch Broom (*Cytisus scoparius*)	Hypertension Circulatory disorders
Psyllium (*Plantago ovata*)	Constipation Diarrhea, symptomatic relief of Hemorrhoids Hypercholesterolemia, primary, adjunct to diet	**Scotch Pine** (*Pinus* species)	Blood pressure problems Bronchitis, acute Cold, common, symptomatic relief of Cough, symptomatic relief of Fever associated with common cold Infection, tendency to Pain, neurogenic Rheumatic disorders, unspecified Stomatitis
Psyllium Seed (*Plantago afra*)	Constipation Diarrhea, symptomatic relief of		
Pumpkin (*Cucurbita pepo*)	Urinary frequency, symptomatic relief of Prostatic hyperplasia, benign, symptomatic treatment of		
		Seneca Snakeroot (*Polygala senega*)	Bronchitis, acute Cough, symptomatic relief of
Quinine (*Cinchona pubescens*)	Appetite, stimulation of Digestive disorders, symptomatic relief of	**Senna** (*Cassia senna*)	Constipation
Radish (*Raphanus sativus*)	Bronchitis, acute Cough, symptomatic relief of Digestive disorders, symptomatic relief of	**Shepherd's Purse** (*Capsella bursa-pastoris*)	Hemorrhage, nasal Premenstrual syndrome, management of Wound care, adjunctive therapy in
Rauwolfia			
(*Rauwolfia serpentina*)	Anxiety disorders, management of Hypertension Sleep, induction of	**Siberian Ginseng** (*Eleutherococcus senticosus*)	Infection, tendency to Lack of stamina
Rhatany (*Krameria triandra*)	Stomatitis	**Sloe** (*Prunus spinosa*)	Stomatitis
Rose (*Rosa centifolia*)	Stomatitis	**Soapwort** (*Saponaria officinalis*)	Bronchitis, acute Cough, symptomatic relief of
Rosemary (*Rosmarinus officinalis*)	Appetite, stimulation of Blood pressure problems Digestive disorders, symptomatic relief of Rheumatic disorders, unspecified	**Soybean** (*Glycine soja*)	Hypercholesterolemia, primary, adjunct to diet
		Spiny Rest Harrow (*Ononis spinosa*)	Infections, urinary tract Renal calculi
Sage (*Salvia officinalis*)	Appetite, stimulation of Hyperhidrosis Stomatitis	**Spruce** (*Picea* species)	Bronchitis, acute Cold, common, symptomatic relief of Cough, symptomatic relief of Fever associated with common cold Infection, tendency to Pain, neurogenic Rheumatic disorders, unspecified Stomatitis
Sandalwood (*Santalum album*)	Infections, urinary tract		
Saw Palmetto (*Serenoa repens*)	Urinary frequency, symptomatic relief of Prostatic hyperplasia, benign, symptomatic treatment of		

Herb	Indications
Squill (*Drimia maritima*)	Anxiety disorders, management of Arrhythmias Cardiac output, low
St. John's Wort (*Hypericum perforatum*)	Anxiety disorders, management of Depression, relief of symptoms Skin, inflammatory conditions Trauma, blunt Wound care, adjunctive therapy in
Star Anise (*Illicium verum*)	Appetite, stimulation of Bronchitis, acute Cough, symptomatic relief of
Stinging Nettle (*Urtica dioica*)	Infections, urinary tract Renal calculi Rheumatic disorders, unspecified Prostatic hyperplasia, benign, symptomatic treatment of Urinary frequency, symptomatic relief of
Sundew (*Drosera rotundifolia*)	Bronchitis, acute Cough, symptomatic relief of
Sweet Clover (*Melilotus officinalis*)	Hemorrhoids, symptomatic relief of Trauma, blunt Venous conditions
Sweet Orange (*Citrus sinensis*)	Appetite, stimulation of Digestive disorders, symptomatic relief of
Thyme (*Thymus vulgaris*)	Bronchitis, acute Cough, symptomatic relief of
Tolu Balsam (*Myroxylon balsamum*)	Bronchitis, acute Cough, symptomatic relief of Hemorrhoids, symptomatic relief of Wound care, adjunctive therapy in
Triticum (*Agropyron repens*)	Infections, urinary tract Renal calculi
Turmeric (*Curcuma domestica*)	Appetite, stimulation of Digestive disorders, symptomatic relief of
Usnea (*Usnea species*)	Stomatitis
Uva-Ursi (*Arctostaphylos uva-ursi*)	Infections, urinary tract

Herb	Indications
Uzara (*Xysmalobium undulatum*)	Diarrhea, symptomatic relief of
Valerian (*Valeriana officinalis*)	Anxiety disorders, management of Sleep, induction of
Walnut (*Juglans regia*)	Hyperhidrosis Skin, inflammatory conditions
Watercress (*Nasturtium officinale*)	Bronchitis, acute Cough, symptomatic relief of
White Fir (*Abies alba*)	Pain, neurogenic Rheumatic disorders, unspecified
White Mustard (*Sinapis alba*)	Bronchitis, acute Cold, common, symptomatic relief of Cough, symptomatic relief of Rheumatic disorders, unspecified
White Nettle (*Lamium album*)	Bronchitis, acute Cough, symptomatic relief of Skin, inflammatory conditions Stomatitis
White Willow (*Salix species*)	Pain, unspecified Rheumatic disorders, unspecified
Wild Thyme (*Thymus serpyllum*)	Bronchitis, acute Cough, symptomatic relief of
Witch Hazel (*Hamamelis virginiana*)	Hemorrhoids, symptomatic relief of Skin disorders Skin, inflammatory conditions Venous conditions Wound care, adjunctive therapy in
Wormwood (*Artemisia absinthium*)	Appetite, stimulation of Digestive disorders, symptomatic relief of Liver and gallbladder complaints
Yarrow (*Achillea millefolium*)	Appetite, stimulation of Digestive disorders, symptomatic relief of Liver and gallbladder complaints
Yellow Gentian (*Gentiana lutea*)	Appetite, stimulation of Digestive disorders, symptomatic relief of

PRODUCT IDENTIFICATION GUIDE

For quick identification, this section provides full-color reproductions of product packaging, as well as some actual-sized photographs of tablets and capsules. In all, the section contains over 350 photos.

Products in this section are arranged alphabetically by manufacturer. In some instances, not all dosage forms and sizes are pictured. For more information on any of the products in this section, please turn to the page indicated above the product's photo or check directly with the product's manufacturer.

While every effort has been made to guarantee faithful reproduction of the photos in this section, changes in size, color, and design are always a possibility. Be sure to confirm a product's identity with the manufacturer or your pharmacist.

MANUFACTURER'S INDEX

ADAMS RESPIRATORY THERAPEUTICS

OTC   ADAMS RESPIRATORY   P. 720
THERAPEUTICS

600 mg

Mucinex®
(guaifenesin)
extended-release bi-layer tablets

OTC   ADAMS RESPIRATORY   P. 777
THERAPEUTICS

600 mg/60 mg

Mucinex® D
(guaifenesin/pseudoephedrine HCl)
extended-release bi-layer tablets

OTC   ADAMS RESPIRATORY   P. 720
THERAPEUTICS

600 mg/30 mg

Mucinex® DM
(guaifenesin/dextromethorphan HBr)
extended-release bi-layer tablets

OTC   ADAMS RESPIRATORY   P. 720
THERAPEUTICS

1200 mg

Humibid®
(guaifenesin)
extended-release bi-layer tablets

AWARENESS CORPORATION

OTC   AWARENESS   P. 828, 831, 833
CORPORATION/AWARENESSLIFE

Daily Complete®   Experience®
Liquid Vitamins/   Regularity/Colon
Minerals   Cleanse

SynergyDefense®   Female Balance®
Enzyme/Probiotic/   Menopause/PMS
Antioxidant

Awareness Natural Dietary Supplements

OTC   AWARENESS CORPORATION/   P.818
AWARENESSLIFE

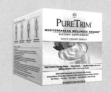

Puretrim®
Mediterranean
Wellness Shakes

Dietary Supplement

PureTrim® Weight Management System

FACED WITH AN
Rx SIDE EFFECT?

Turn to the
Companion Drug Index
(Green Pages)
for products that provide
symptomatic relief.

BAUSCH & LOMB

OTC   BAUSCH & LOMB INCORPORATED   P. 707

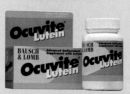

Vitamin and Mineral Supplement

Ocuvite® Lutein

OTC   BAUSCH & LOMB INCORPORATED   P. 706

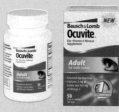

Adult Formula
Eye Vitamin and Mineral Supplement

Ocuvite® Adult Formula

OTC   BAUSCH & LOMB INCORPORATED   P. 706

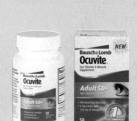

Adult 50+ Formula
Eye Vitamin and Mineral Supplement

Ocuvite® Adult 50+ Formula

OTC   BAUSCH & LOMB INCORPORATED   P. 806

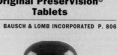

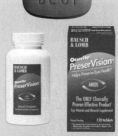

Eye Vitamin and Mineral Supplement

Original PreserVision® Tablets

OTC   BAUSCH & LOMB INCORPORATED   P. 806

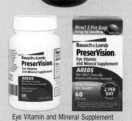

Eye Vitamin and Mineral Supplement

PreserVision® AREDS Soft Gels

OTC   BAUSCH & LOMB INCORPORATED   P. 807

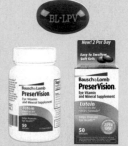

Eye Vitamin and Mineral Supplement

PreserVision® Lutein Soft Gels

BAYER HEALTHCARE LLC

OTC   BAYER HEALTHCARE LLC   P. 675

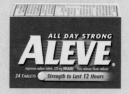

Easy-open Arthritis cap available.

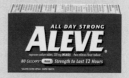

Easy-open Arthritis cap available.

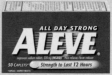

Tablets and Caplets available in
24, 50, 100, 150 and 200 count.

Gelcaps available in 20, 40
and 80 count.
Easy-open Arthritis cap available.

Aleve®

OTC   BAYER HEALTHCARE LLC   P. 724

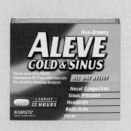

Aleve® Cold & Sinus

OTC   BAYER HEALTHCARE LLC

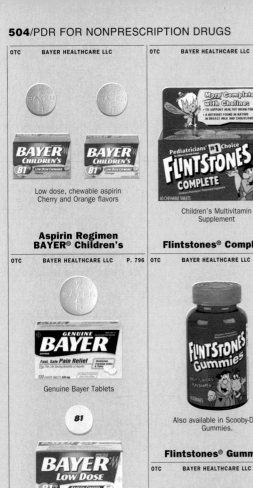

Low dose, chewable aspirin
Cherry and Orange flavors

**Aspirin Regimen
BAYER® Children's**

OTC   BAYER HEALTHCARE LLC   P. 796

Genuine Bayer Tablets

Aspirin Regimen 81 mg

Aspirin Regimen 325 mg

BAYER® Aspirin

OTC   BAYER HEALTHCARE LLC   P. 814

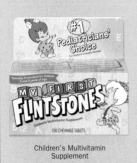

Children's Multivitamin
Supplement

My First Flintstones®

OTC   BAYER HEALTHCARE LLC   P. 813

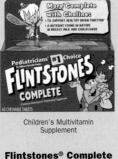

Children's Multivitamin
Supplement

Flintstones® Complete

OTC   BAYER HEALTHCARE LLC   P. 813

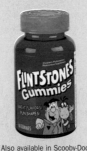

Also available in Scooby-Doo
Gummies.

Flintstones® Gummies

OTC   BAYER HEALTHCARE LLC   P. 815

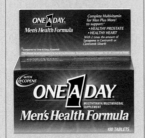

**One-A-Day®
Men's Health Formula**

OTC   BAYER HEALTHCARE LLC   P. 816

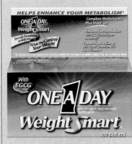

**One-A-Day®
Weight Smart®**

OTC   BAYER HEALTHCARE LLC   P. 816

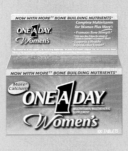

One-A-Day® Women's

OTC   BAYER HEALTHCARE LLC   P. 815

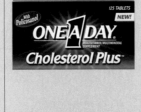

**One-A-Day®
Cholesterol Plus™**

BOEHRINGER INGELHEIM

OTC   BOEHRINGER INGELHEIM
CONSUMER H.C.   P. 648

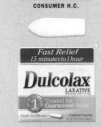

4 Comfort Shaped Suppositories
Also available in packages of 8, 16
and 28 suppositories

Dulcolax® Laxative

OTC   BOEHRINGER INGELHEIM
CONSUMER H.C.   P. 649

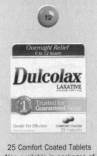

25 Comfort Coated Tablets
Also available in packages of
10, 50, 100 and 150 tablets

Dulcolax® Laxative

OTC   BOEHRINGER INGELHEIM   P. 648
CONSUMER H.C.

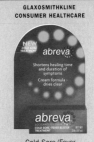

25 Liquid Gels
Also available in packages of
50, 100 and 180 liquid gels

Dulcolax® Stool Softener

ENIVA

OTC   ENIVA NUTRACEUTICS   P. 822

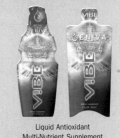

Liquid Antioxidant
Multi-Nutrient Supplement
32 fl. oz. bottle and 1 fl. oz. packet

VIBE™

GLAXOSMITHKLINE
CONSUMER HEALTHCARE, L. P.

OTC   GLAXOSMITHKLINE   P. 710
CONSUMER HEALTHCARE

Cold Sore/Fever
Blister Treatment Cream

Abreva®

OTC   GLAXOSMITHKLINE   P. 648
CONSUMER HEALTHCARE

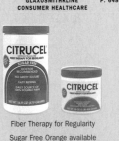

Fiber Therapy for Regularity

Sugar Free Orange available
in 8.6 oz., 16.9 oz.,
and 32 oz. containers.

Regular Orange available in
16 oz., 30 oz., and 50 oz. containers.

Citrucel®

SEEKING AN ALTERNATIVE?

Check the Product Category Index, where you'll find alphabetical listings of all the products in each therapeutic class.

OTC   GLAXOSMITHKLINE   P. 681
CONSUMER HEALTHCARE

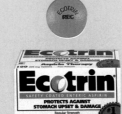

Regular Strength Tablets in bottles of 100 and 250.
Ecotrin®

OTC   GLAXOSMITHKLINE   P. 658
CONSUMER HEALTHCARE

12 fl. oz.
Gaviscon® Regular Strength Liquid Antacid

OTC   GLAXOSMITHKLINE   P. 709
CONSUMER HEALTHCARE

1/2 fl. oz.   2 fl. oz.
Gly-Oxide® Liquid

OTC   GLAXOSMITHKLINE   P. 728, 729
CONSUMER HEALTHCARE

Multisymptom Cold & Flu Relief Maximum Strength Formula in packages of 16 and 30 caplets. Non-Drowsy Formula in packages of 16 caplets.
Contac® Severe Cold & Flu

OTC   GLAXOSMITHKLINE   P. 681
CONSUMER HEALTHCARE

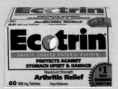

Maximum Strength Tablets in bottles of 60 and 150.
Ecotrin®

OTC   GLAXOSMITHKLINE   P. 658
CONSUMER HEALTHCARE

Available in 100-tablet bottles and 30-tablet boxes.
Gaviscon® Regular Strength Antacid

LOOKING FOR A PARTICULAR COMPOUND?

In the Active Ingredients Index (Yellow Pages), you'll find all the brands that contain it.

OTC   GLAXOSMITHKLINE   P. 715
CONSUMER HEALTHCARE

Drops Available in 1/2 fl. oz. and 1 fl. oz.
Debrox®

OTC   GLAXOSMITHKLINE   P. 812
CONSUMER HEALTHCARE

Packages of 30 caplets

OTC   GLAXOSMITHKLINE   P. 658
CONSUMER HEALTHCARE

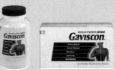

Extra Strength Formula 12 fl. oz.
Gaviscon® Extra Strength Liquid Antacid

OTC   GLAXOSMITHKLINE   P. 618
CONSUMER HEALTHCARE

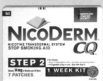

Step 1
Also available in 2 week kit.

Step 2
Also available in 2 week kit.

Step 3
Also available in 2 week kit.
Includes User's Guide, Audio Tape and Child-Resistant Disposal Tray
Stop Smoking Aid
Nicotine Transdermal System
NicoDerm® CQ®

OTC   GLAXOSMITHKLINE   P. 681
CONSUMER HEALTHCARE

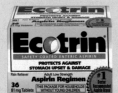

Adult Low Strength Tablets in bottles of 36 and 120.
Ecotrin®

OTC   GLAXOSMITHKLINE   P. 658
CONSUMER HEALTHCARE

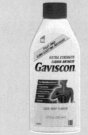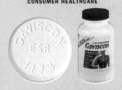

Extra Strength Formula Available in 100-tablet bottles and 6 and 30-tablet boxes.
Gaviscon® Extra Strength Antacid

Packages of 100 tablets Iron Supplement
Feosol®

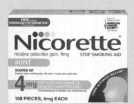

4 mg

Stop Smoking Aid in mint flavor
Nicotine Polacrilex Gum

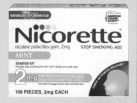

2 mg

Stop Smoking Aid in mint flavor
Nicotine Polacrilex Gum

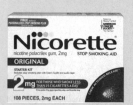

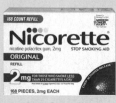

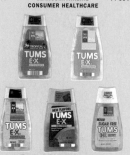

2 mg

Stop Smoking Aid in Original flavor
Nicotine Polacrilex Gum

Nicorette®

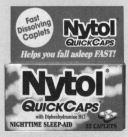

QuickCaps®

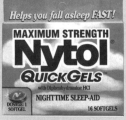

QuickGels™

Nytol®

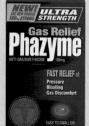

Calcium Supplement

Os-Cal®

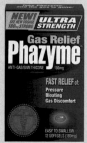

180 mg softgels

Gas Relief Phazyme®

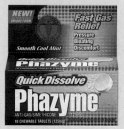

125 mg chewable tablets

**Quick Dissolve
Phazyme®**

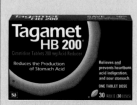

Acid Reducer
Packages of 6, 12, 18,
30, 50, 70 and 80 tablets.

Tagamet HB 200®

Peppermint and
Assorted flavors

Tums®

Tropical Fruit, Wintergreen,
Assorted Flavors, Assorted Berry
and Sugar Free Orange Cream flavors

Tums E-X®

Assorted Mint and Fruit Flavors
Also available in Tropical Fruit,
Assorted Berries and
Spearmint flavors.

Tums® Ultra™

Alertness Aid with Caffeine
Available in tablets and caplets.

Vivarin®

J&J-MERCK CONSUMER

Available in blister packs of 30 ct.
and bottles of 60 and 90 ct.

Pepcid® AC Tablets

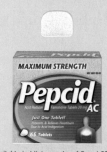

Available in blister packs of 8 and 25 ct.;
bottles of 50 and 60 ct.

**Maximum Strength
Pepcid® AC Tablets**

OTC	J&J-MERCK CONSUMER	P. 661

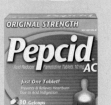

Available in blister packs of 30 ct.

Pepcid® AC Gelcaps

OTC	J&J-MERCK CONSUMER	P. 662

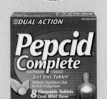

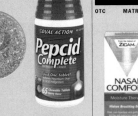

Mint available in 8 ct. individual pouches
and 25 and 50 ct. bottles
Berry available in 2, 8, and 15 ct.
individual pouches
and 25, 50, and 65 ct. bottles

**Pepcid® Complete
Chewable Tablets**

MANNATECH, INC.

OTC	MANNATECH, INC.	P. 826

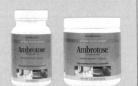

A Glyconutritional Dietary Supplement

Ambrotose®

OTC	MANNATECH, INC.	P. 826

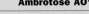

A Glyconutritional Antioxidant Supplement

Ambrotose AO™

OTC	MANNATECH, INC.	P. 831

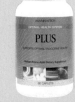

Herbal-Amino Acid Dietary Supplement

**PLUS with
Ambrotose® complex**

MATRIXX INITIATIVES

OTC	MATRIXX INITIATIVES, INC.	P. 733

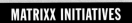

Scented   Unscented

**Nasal Comfort®
Moisture Therapy**

OTC	MATRIXX INITIATIVES, INC.

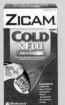 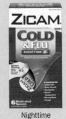

Daytime   Nighttime

**Zicam®
Cold & Flu**

OTC	MATRIXX INITIATIVES, INC.	P. 768

 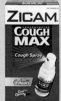

Daytime   Nighttime

**Zicam®
Maximum Strength Flu**

OTC	MATRIXX INITIATIVES, INC.	P. 766

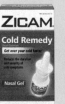 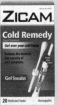

Nasal Gel™   Gel Swabs™

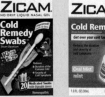

Cold Remedy Swabs™   Oral Mist™

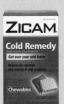

RapidMelts®   Chewables™

OTC	MATRIXX INITIATIVES, INC.

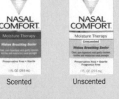

RapidMelts® with   ChewCaps™
Vitamin C

**Zicam®
Cold Remedy**

OTC	MATRIXX INITIATIVES, INC.	P. 767

Cough Spray   Cough Melts

**Zicam®
Cough Spray/   Cough Spray plus
Nighttime   Nasal Decongestant**

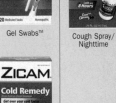

Cough Spray/   Cough Spray plus
Nighttime   Nasal Decongestant

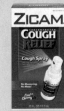

Cough Spray
Available in Cool Cherry and
Honey Lemon Flavors

Zicam® Cough

OTC	MATRIXX INITIATIVES, INC.	P. 774

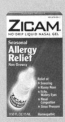

**Zicam® No-Drip
Liquid Nasal Gel
Allergy Relief**

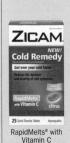

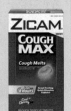

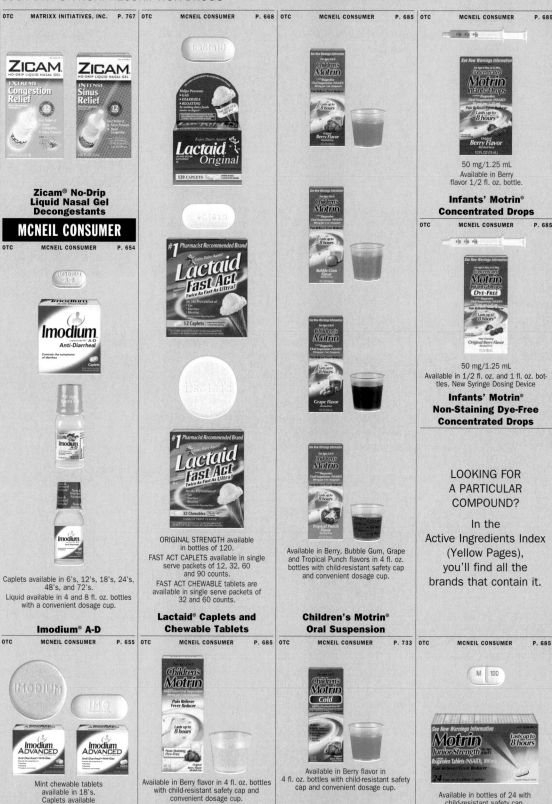

OTC   MATRIXX INITIATIVES, INC.   P. 767

Zicam® No-Drip Liquid Nasal Gel Decongestants

MCNEIL CONSUMER

OTC   MCNEIL CONSUMER   P. 654

Caplets available in 6's, 12's, 18's, 24's, 48's, and 72's.
Liquid available in 4 and 8 fl. oz. bottles with a convenient dosage cup.

Imodium® A-D

OTC   MCNEIL CONSUMER   P. 655

Mint chewable tablets available in 18's.
Caplets available in 12's, 18's and bottles of 30 and 42.

Imodium® Advanced

OTC   MCNEIL CONSUMER   P. 668

Helps Prevent:
• GAS
• DIARRHEA
• BLOATING
by making dairy foods easier to digest*

Enjoy Dairy Again!
Lactaid Original
LACTASE ENZYME SUPPLEMENT
120 CAPLETS

#1 Pharmacist Recommended Brand
Enjoy Dairy Again!
Lactaid Fast Act
Twice As Fast As Ultra!
for the Prevention of
• Gas
• Diarrhea
• Bloating
12 Caplets

#1 Pharmacist Recommended Brand
Enjoy Dairy Again!
Lactaid Fast Act
Twice As Fast As Ultra!
for the Prevention of
• Gas
• Diarrhea
• Bloating
32 Chewables
VANILLA TWIST FLAVOR

ORIGINAL STRENGTH available in bottles of 120.
FAST ACT CAPLETS available in single serve packets of 12, 32, 60 and 90 counts.
FAST ACT CHEWABLE tablets are available in single serve packets of 32 and 60 counts.

Lactaid® Caplets and Chewable Tablets

OTC   MCNEIL CONSUMER   P. 685

Children's **Motrin**
Pain Reliever Fever Reducer
Lasts up to 8 hours
Non-Staining Dye-Free
Original Berry Flavor
Alcohol Free

Available in Berry flavor in 4 fl. oz. bottles with child-resistant safety cap and convenient dosage cup.

Children's Motrin® Non-Staining Dye-Free Oral Suspension

OTC   MCNEIL CONSUMER   P. 685

Available in Berry, Bubble Gum, Grape and Tropical Punch flavors in 4 fl. oz. bottles with child-resistant safety cap and convenient dosage cup.

Children's Motrin® Oral Suspension

OTC   MCNEIL CONSUMER   P. 733

Children's **Motrin Cold**
Pain Reliever/Fever Reducer

Available in Berry flavor in 4 fl. oz. bottles with child-resistant safety cap and convenient dosage cup.

Children's Motrin® Cold Oral Suspension

OTC   MCNEIL CONSUMER   P. 685

50 mg/1.25 mL
Available in Berry flavor 1/2 fl. oz. bottle.

Infants' Motrin® Concentrated Drops

OTC   MCNEIL CONSUMER   P. 685

50 mg/1.25 mL
Available in 1/2 fl. oz. and 1 fl. oz. bottles. New Syringe Dosing Device

Infants' Motrin® Non-Staining Dye-Free Concentrated Drops

LOOKING FOR
A PARTICULAR
COMPOUND?

In the
Active Ingredients Index
(Yellow Pages),
you'll find all the
brands that contain it.

OTC   MCNEIL CONSUMER   P. 685

Motrin Junior Strength
Ibuprofen Tablets (NSAID), 100mg
Pain Reliever/Fever Reducer
24

Available in bottles of 24 with child-resistant safety cap.

Junior Strength Motrin® Caplets

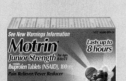

Available in Orange and Grape-flavored
chewable tablets of 100 mg.
Available in bottles of 24 with child-
resistant safety cap.

Junior Strength Motrin® Chewable Tablets

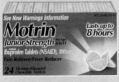

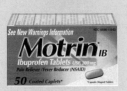

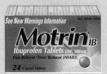

Caplets available in
tamper evident packaging
of 24, 50, 100,,165,
250 and 300.
Tablets available in
tamper evident packaging
of 24, 50, 100 and 165.

Motrin® IB

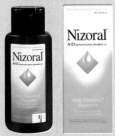

Available in 4 and 7 fl. oz. bottles.

Nizoral® A-D

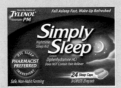

Mini-caplets available in blister packs
of 24, 48, 100 and 130.

Simply Sleep™

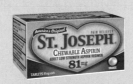

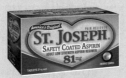

Available in enteric coated tablets
and adult chewable tablets.

St. Joseph®

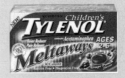

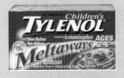

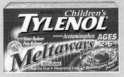

Grape Punch and Wacky
Watermelon bottles of 30 with
child-resistant safety cap.
Bubblegum Burst bottles of
30 with child resistant safety
cap and blister packs of 48.

Children's TYLENOL® Meltaways

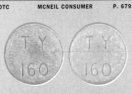

Available in blister packs of 24
chewable tablets. Grape Punch and
Bubblegum Burst.

Jr. TYLENOL® Meltaways

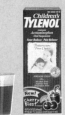

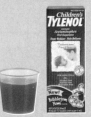

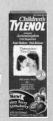

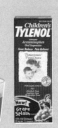

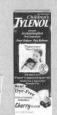

Available in Cherry Blast flavor
in 2 and 4 fl. oz. bottles.
Bubble Gum Yum, Very Berry Strawberry,
Grape Splash, and Dye-Free Cherry
flavors in 4 fl. oz bottles
with child-resistant safety cap
and convenient dosage cup.
Alcohol Free.
80 mg per $1/_2$ teaspoon

Children's TYLENOL® Suspension Liquid

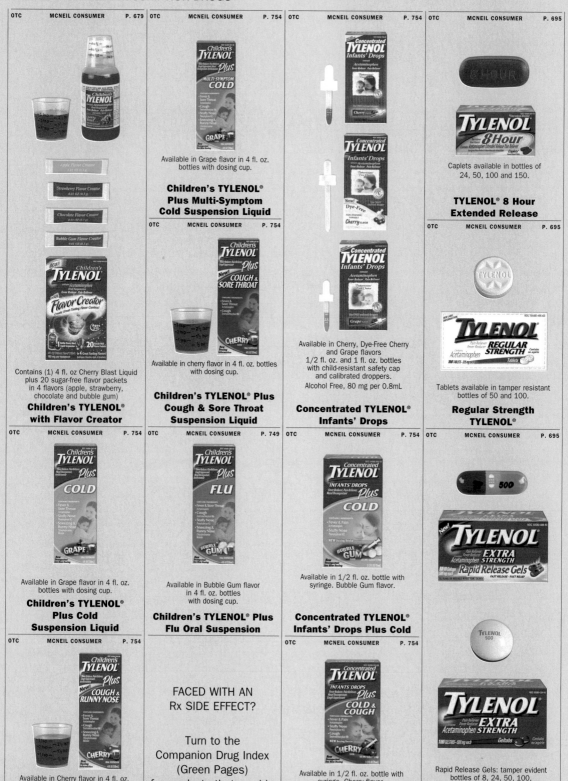

OTC   MCNEIL CONSUMER   P. 679

Contains (1) 4 fl. oz Cherry Blast Liquid plus 20 sugar-free flavor packets in 4 flavors (apple, strawberry, chocolate and bubble gum)

**Children's TYLENOL®
with Flavor Creator**

OTC   MCNEIL CONSUMER   P. 754

Available in Grape flavor in 4 fl. oz. bottles with dosing cup.

**Children's TYLENOL®
Plus Multi-Symptom
Cold Suspension Liquid**

OTC   MCNEIL CONSUMER   P. 754

Available in cherry flavor in 4 fl. oz. bottles with dosing cup.

**Children's TYLENOL® Plus
Cough & Sore Throat
Suspension Liquid**

OTC   MCNEIL CONSUMER   P. 754

Available in Cherry, Dye-Free Cherry and Grape flavors
1/2 fl. oz. and 1 fl. oz. bottles with child-resistant safety cap and calibrated droppers.
Alcohol Free, 80 mg per 0.8mL

**Concentrated TYLENOL®
Infants' Drops**

OTC   MCNEIL CONSUMER   P. 695

Caplets available in bottles of 24, 50, 100 and 150.

**TYLENOL® 8 Hour
Extended Release**

OTC   MCNEIL CONSUMER   P. 695

Tablets available in tamper resistant bottles of 50 and 100.

**Regular Strength
TYLENOL®**

OTC   MCNEIL CONSUMER   P. 754

Available in Grape flavor in 4 fl. oz. bottles with dosing cup.

**Children's TYLENOL®
Plus Cold
Suspension Liquid**

OTC   MCNEIL CONSUMER   P. 754

Available in Cherry flavor in 4 fl. oz. bottles with dosing cup.

**Children's TYLENOL® Plus
Cough & Runny Nose
Suspension Liquid**

OTC   MCNEIL CONSUMER   P. 749

Available in Bubble Gum flavor in 4 fl. oz. bottles with dosing cup.

**Children's TYLENOL® Plus
Flu Oral Suspension**

FACED WITH AN
Rx SIDE EFFECT?

Turn to the
Companion Drug Index
(Green Pages)
for products that provide
symptomatic relief.

OTC   MCNEIL CONSUMER   P. 754

Available in 1/2 fl. oz. bottle with syringe. Bubble Gum flavor.

**Concentrated TYLENOL®
Infants' Drops Plus Cold**

OTC   MCNEIL CONSUMER   P. 754

Available in 1/2 fl. oz. bottle with syringe. Cherry flavor.

**Concentrated TYLENOL®
Infants' Drops Plus
Cold & Cough**

Rapid Release Gels: tamper evident bottles of 8, 24, 50, 100, 150, 225 and 290.

Geltabs available in tamper-resistant bottles of 50 and 100.

Extra Strength TYLENOL®

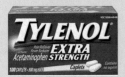

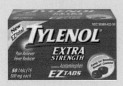
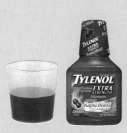

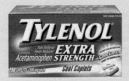

Caplets: tamper-resistant vials
of 10 and bottles of 24, 50, 100,
150, 225 and 325.
EZ Tabs: tamper-evident bottles of
24, 50, 100, 150, and 225.
Liquid: tamper-evident
8 fl. oz. bottles.
Cool Caplets: 8, 24, 50, 100
and 150.

Extra Strength TYLENOL®

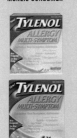

Caplets available in
blister packs of 24 and 48.
Gelcaps available in blister packs of 24.

**TYLENOL® Allergy
Multi-Symptom**

Caplets available in
blister packs of 24.

**TYLENOL® Allergy
Multi-Symptom Nighttime**

Caplets available in
blister packs of 24.

TYLENOL® Severe Allergy

Caplets and Gelcaps available in
blister packs of 24.

**TYLENOL®
Cold Multi-Symptom
Daytime**

Caplets available in
blister packs of 24.

**TYLENOL®
Cold Multi-Symptom
Nighttime**

Caplets available in
blister packs of 24 and 48.

**TYLENOL® Cold
Multi-Symptom Severe**

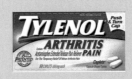

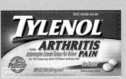

Caplets available in 24's, 50's,
100's, 150's, and 225's.
Geltabs available in
20's, 40's, and 80's.

**TYLENOL® Arthritis Pain
Extended Release**

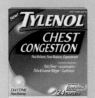

Caplets available in
blister packs of 24.

**TYLENOL® Chest
Congestion**

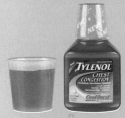

Liquid available in
8 fl. oz. bottles.

**TYLENOL® Chest
Congestion**

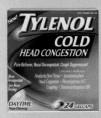

Gelcaps available in
blister packs of 24.

**TYLENOL® Cold
Head Congestion Daytime**

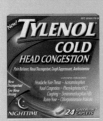

Caplets available in
blister packs of 24.

**TYLENOL® Cold Head
Congestion Nighttime**

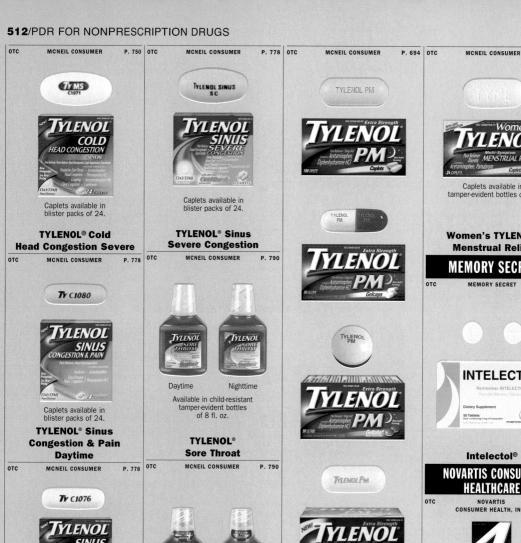

Caplets available in
blister packs of 24.

**TYLENOL® Cold
Head Congestion Severe**

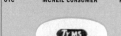

Caplets available in
blister packs of 24.

**TYLENOL® Sinus
Congestion & Pain
Daytime**

Caplets available in
blister packs of 24.

**TYLENOL® Sinus
Congestion & Pain
Nighttime**

Caplets available in
blister packs of 24.

**TYLENOL® Sinus
Congestion &
Pain Severe**

Caplets available in
blister packs of 24.

**TYLENOL® Sinus
Severe Congestion**

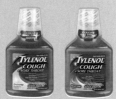

Daytime   Nighttime
Available in child-resistant
tamper-evident bottles
of 8 fl. oz.

**TYLENOL®
Sore Throat**

Daytime   Nighttime
Available in 8 fl. oz. bottles.

**TYLENOL® Cough &
Sore Throat**

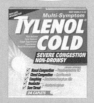

Caplets available in blister
packs of 24.

**TYLENOL® Cold Severe
Congestion Non-Drowsy**

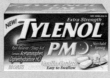

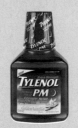

Caplets available in tamper-resistant
bottles of 24, 50, 100,
150 and 225.
Gelcaps available in tamper-resistant
bottles of 24 and 50.
Geltabs available in tamper-resistant
bottles of 24, 50, 100 and 150.
Geltabs, Caplets and Gelcaps
available in bottles of 50
for households without children.
Vanilla Caplets available in tamper
evident bottles of 6, 24, 100
and 225; liquid available in 1 fl. oz.
and 8 fl. oz. bottles.

**Extra Strength
TYLENOL® PM**

Caplets available in
tamper-evident bottles of 24.

**Women's TYLENOL®
Menstrual Relief**

MEMORY SECRET

INTELECTOL®

Intelectol®

NOVARTIS CONSUMER HEALTHCARE

Fast Acting
Available in 1/2 oz. and 1 oz. atomizers.
Mentholated: available in 1/2 oz. atomizer.
Also available: 12 Hour and Saline
Moisturizing Mist.

4 Way® Nasal Spray

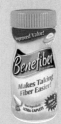

Available in 72 ct. (24 servings) and
114 ct. (38 servings).

**Benefiber®
Fiber Supplement Caplets**

OTC	NOVARTIS	P. 807
	CONSUMER HEALTH, INC.	

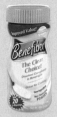

Available in 20 servings, 38 servings,
62 servings, 90 servings,
and 125 servings bottles.
Non-Thickening Powder

**Benefiber®
Fiber Supplement Powder**

OTC	NOVARTIS	P. 725
	CONSUMER HEALTH, INC.	

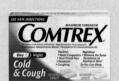

Available in cartons of 10 ct.
and 20 ct. caplets.

**Comtrex® Cold & Cough
Non-Drowsy**

OTC	NOVARTIS	P. 635
	CONSUMER HEALTH, INC.	

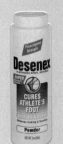

Powder	Spray Powder
Available in	Available in
1.5 & 3.0 oz	4.0 oz cans.
bottles.	

OTC	NOVARTIS	P. 609
	CONSUMER HEALTH, INC.	

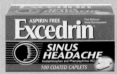

Caplets and tablets available in 24 ct.,
50 ct., 100 ct., and 250 ct., cartons.
Geltabs in 24 ct., 50 ct.,
and 100 ct. cartons.

Excedrin® Migraine

OTC	NOVARTIS	P. 808
	CONSUMER HEALTH, INC.	

Available in 90 ct. bottles
Wild Berry chewable tablets.

**Benefiber® Plus
Calcium Chewable Tablets**

OTC	NOVARTIS	P. 726
	CONSUMER HEALTH, INC.	

Available in cartons
of 20 ct. caplets.

**Comtrex® Cold & Cough
Day/Night**

OTC	NOVARTIS	P. 609
	CONSUMER HEALTH, INC.	

Antifungal Cream
Available in 15 g.

Desenex®

OTC	NOVARTIS	P. 609
	CONSUMER HEALTH, INC.	

Caplets available in 2 ct., 24 ct., 50 ct.,
100 ct., and 250 ct., cartons.
Tablets in 10 ct., 24 ct., 50 ct.,
and 100 ct. cartons.

Excedrin® Sinus Headache

OTC	NOVARTIS	P. 725
	CONSUMER HEALTH, INC.	

Orange creme available in
36 ct. and 100 ct. bottles.

**Benefiber®
Fiber Supplement
Chewable Tablets**

OTC	NOVARTIS	P. 725
	CONSUMER HEALTH, INC.	

Available in cartons
of 20 ct. caplets.

**Comtrex® Severe
Cold & Sinus Day/Night**

OTC	NOVARTIS	P. 609
	CONSUMER HEALTH, INC.	

Caplets and Geltabs available in
24 ct., 50 ct., and 100 ct. cartons.
Tablets available in 2 ct., 10 ct.,
24 ct., 50 ct., and 100 ct. cartons.

Excedrin PM®

LOOKING FOR
A PARTICULAR
COMPOUND?

In the
Active Ingredients Index
(Yellow Pages),
you'll find all the
brands that contain it.

OTC	NOVARTIS	P. 678
	CONSUMER HEALTH, INC.	

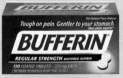

Regular Strength available in
cartons of 39 ct., 65 ct.,
and 130 ct. tablets.
Also available in
Extra Strength.

Bufferin®

SEEKING AN
ALTERNATIVE?

Check the
Product Category Index,
where you'll find
alphabetical listings of
all the products in each
therapeutic class.

OTC	NOVARTIS	P. 684
	CONSUMER HEALTH, INC.	

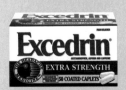

Caplets available in 24 ct., 50 ct.,
100 ct., and 250 ct. cartons.
Tablets in 10 ct., 24 ct., 50 ct., 100 ct.,
and 250 ct. cartons.
Geltabs in 24 ct., 50 ct.,
and 100 ct. cartons.

Excedrin® Extra Strength

OTC	NOVARTIS	P. 611
	CONSUMER HEALTH, INC.	

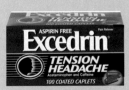

Caplets availabe in 2 ct., 24 ct., 50 ct.,
100 ct., and 250 ct. cartons.
Tablets in 10 ct., 24 ct., 50 ct.,
100 ct., and 250 ct. cartons.
Geltabs in 24 ct., 50 ct.,
and 100 ct. cartons.

**Excedrin® Tension
Headache**

OTC	NOVARTIS CONSUMER HEALTH, INC.	P. 649

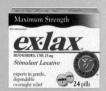

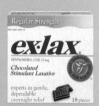

Available in Regular Strength 8's
and 30's, Maximum Strength 24's,
48's, and 90's, and Regular Strength
Chocolated Laxative
12's, 18's and 48's.

Ex•Lax®

OTC	NOVARTIS CONSUMER HEALTH, INC.	

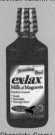

Chocolate Creme
12 fl. oz.
Also available in Mint and
Raspberry Creme flavors.

**Ex•Lax®
Milk of Magnesia**

OTC	NOVARTIS CONSUMER HEALTH, INC.	P. 656

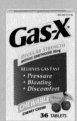

Available in
Cherry 36 ct. cartons.
Also available in
Peppermint 36 ct. cartons.

Gas-X®

OTC	NOVARTIS CONSUMER HEALTH, INC.	P. 656

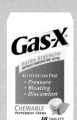

Available in Extra Strength Cherry
18 ct. and 48 ct. cartons.
Extra Strength Peppermint available in
18 ct. and 48 ct. cartons.

Gas-X®

OTC	NOVARTIS CONSUMER HEALTH, INC.	P. 656

Extra Strength Softgels
in cartons of 10's, 30's, 50's, and 72's.

Gas-X®

OTC	NOVARTIS CONSUMER HEALTH, INC.	P. 656

Maximum Strength Softgels
in cartons of 50's.

Gas-X®

OTC	NOVARTIS CONSUMER HEALTH, INC.	P. 657

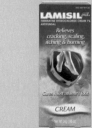

Available in cartons of 18 ct.,
in Cinnamon and Peppermint flavors.

Gas-X® Thin Strips™

OTC	NOVARTIS CONSUMER HEALTH, INC.	P. 656

Available in Extra Strength
Wild Berry, 8's, 24's and
Extra Strength Orange 8's and 24's.

Gas-X® with Maalox®

OTC	NOVARTIS CONSUMER HEALTH, INC.	P. 656

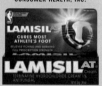

Extra Strength Softgels
in cartons of 24's and 48's.

**Gas-X® with
Maalox® Softgels**

OTC	NOVARTIS CONSUMER HEALTH, INC.	P. 636

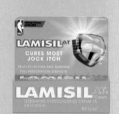

Athlete's Foot Cream available in
12 g and 24 g.
Jock Itch Cream available in 12 g.

LamisilAT® Cream

OTC	NOVARTIS CONSUMER HEALTH, INC.	P. 636

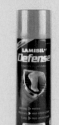

Also availabe in shake powder.

**LamisilAT® Defense
Spray Powder**

OTC	NOVARTIS CONSUMER HEALTH, INC.	

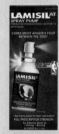

30 mL (1 fl. oz.)

**LamisilAT®
Athlete's Foot
Spray Pump**

OTC	NOVARTIS CONSUMER HEALTH, INC.	

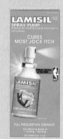

30 mL (1 fl. oz.)

**LamisilAT® Jock Itch
Spray Pump**

OTC	NOVARTIS CONSUMER HEALTH, INC.	P. 660

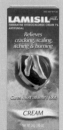
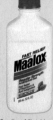

Cooling Mint Liquid
Also available in Smooth Cherry
12 fl. oz., 26 fl. oz.,
and bottles of 5 fl. oz. (Mint Only).

**Maalox® Antacid/Anti-Gas
Regular Strength**

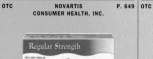

OTC | NOVARTIS CONSUMER HEALTH, INC. | P. 659

Also available in assorted and lemon 85 ct.

Maalox® Quick Dissolve Regular Strength Tablets Antacid/Calcium Supplement

OTC | NOVARTIS CONSUMER HEALTH, INC. | P. 659

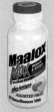

Assorted 35, 65, 90 ct.
Also available in Wild Berry and Lemon 35, 65 ct.

Maalox® Max Quick Dissolve Maximum Strength Tablets Antacid/AntiGas

OTC | NOVARTIS CONSUMER HEALTH, INC. | P. 660

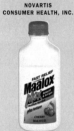

Cherry Liquid
Also available in Lemon (12 & 26 fl. oz.),
Mint, Vanilla Creme, and Wild Berry (12 fl. oz.).

Maalox® Antacid/Anti-Gas Maximum Strength

OTC | NOVARTIS CONSUMER HEALTH, INC. | P. 672

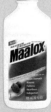

12 fl. oz.
Available in Strawberry & Mint Flavor

Maalox® TOTAL Stomach Relief™ Maximum Strength

OTC | NOVARTIS CONSUMER HEALTH, INC. | P. 819

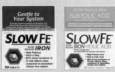

Slow Release Iron available in 30, 60 and 90 ct. tablets.
Slow Release Iron & Folic Acid available in 20 ct. tablets.

Slow Fe®

OTC | NOVARTIS CONSUMER HEALTH, INC. | P. 744, 745

Multi Symptom and Long Acting Cough
Available in 12 ct. cartons.

Theraflu® Thin Strips®

OTC | NOVARTIS CONSUMER HEALTH, INC. | P. 740, 742

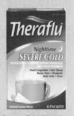

Severe Cold Nighttime available in 6 ct. cartons.
Also available in Flu & Chest Congestion, Flu & Sore Throat, Daytime Severe Cold, Cold & Sore Throat, and Cold & Cough, in 6 ct. cartons.

TheraFlu®

OTC | NOVARTIS CONSUMER HEALTH, INC. | P. 743

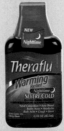

Cherry Flavor available in 8.3 fl. oz. bottles.
Also available Daytime Severe Cold Warming Relief in 8.3 fl. oz. bottles.

TheraFlu® Warming Relief

OTC | NOVARTIS CONSUMER HEALTH, INC. | P. 685

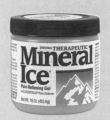

Available in 3.5 oz., 8 oz. and 16 oz. jars.
Pain Relieving Gel

Therapeutic Mineral Ice®

OTC | NOVARTIS CONSUMER HEALTH, INC. | P. 749, 778

Cough and Runny Nose

Long Acting Cough

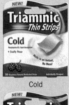

Cold

Cold & Cough
Available in 16 ct. cartons.

Triaminic Thin Strips®

OTC | NOVARTIS CONSUMER HEALTH, INC. | P. 747

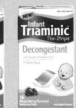

Decongestant Plus Cough | Decongestant
Available in 16 ct. cartons.

Infant Triaminic® Thin Strips™

OTC | NOVARTIS CONSUMER HEALTH, INC. | P. 745, 746

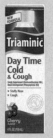 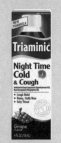

Day Time Cold & Cough | Night Time Cold & Cough

Triaminic®

FACED WITH AN Rx SIDE EFFECT?

Turn to the Companion Drug Index (Green Pages) for products that provide symptomatic relief.

OTC | NOVARTIS CONSUMER HEALTH, INC. | P. 804

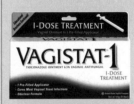

Anti-fungal Vaginal Ointment

Vagistat®-1

SEEKING AN ALTERNATIVE?

Check the Product Category Index, where you'll find alphabetical listings of all the products in each therapeutic class.

PROCTER & GAMBLE

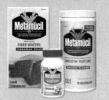

Available in 30, 48, 72, 114 and
180 dose canisters and cartons of
30 one-dose packets.
Also available in sugar free.
Capsules available in 100 ct and 160 ct.
Cinnamon Spice and Apple Crisp Wafers
available in 12-dose cartons.

Metamucil®

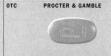

Also available in Maximum Strength
Liquid, Chewable Tablets and
Swallowable Caplets

Pepto-Bismol®

LOOKING FOR
A PARTICULAR
COMPOUND?

In the
Active Ingredients Index
(Yellow Pages),
you'll find all the
brands that contain it.

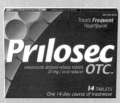

20 mg

Prilosec OTC™

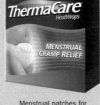

Back/Hip Wrap for Pain Relief
and Muscle Relaxation

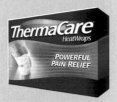

Menstrual patches for
Menstrual Cramp Relief

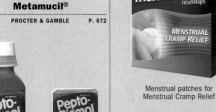

Knee & Elbow Wrap for Pain Relief
and Reduced Stiffness

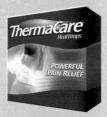

Neck, Shoulder & Wrist Wrap
for Pain Relief
and Muscle Relaxation

Air-Activated Heat Wraps

ThermaCare®

Multi-Symptom
Cold/Flu Relief
Also available as DayQuil Liquid.

**VICKS® DayQuil®
LiquiCaps®**

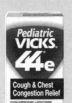

44®e
Cough & Chest Congestion Relief

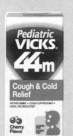

44®m
Cough & Cold Relief

Pediatric VICKS®

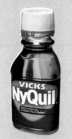

Multi-Symptom
Cold/Flu Relief
Also available as NyQuil LiquiCaps.

**VICKS® NyQuil®
Liquid**

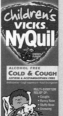

Cherry Flavor
Cold & Cough Relief

**Children's VICKS®
NyQuil®**

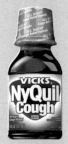

Cough Relief

**VICKS® NyQuil®
Cough**

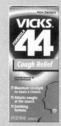

VICKS® 44® Cough Relief

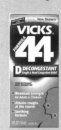

VICKS® 44®D
Cough & Head Congestion Relief

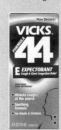

VICKS® 44® E
Cough & Chest Congestion Relief

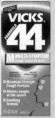

VICKS® 44® M
Cough, Cold & Flu Relief

VICKS®

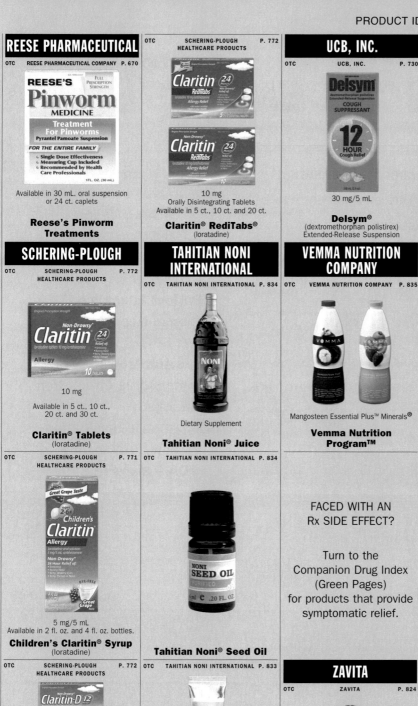

REESE PHARMACEUTICAL

OTC   REESE PHARMACEUTICAL COMPANY   P. 670

Available in 30 mL. oral suspension
or 24 ct. caplets

**Reese's Pinworm
Treatments**

SCHERING-PLOUGH

OTC   SCHERING-PLOUGH   P. 772
HEALTHCARE PRODUCTS

10 mg

Available in 5 ct., 10 ct.,
20 ct. and 30 ct.

Claritin® Tablets
(loratadine)

OTC   SCHERING-PLOUGH   P. 771
HEALTHCARE PRODUCTS

5 mg/5 mL
Available in 2 fl. oz. and 4 fl. oz. bottles.

Children's Claritin® Syrup
(loratadine)

OTC   SCHERING-PLOUGH   P. 772
HEALTHCARE PRODUCTS

5 mg/120 mg
Available in 10 ct., 20 ct. and 30 ct.

10 mg/240 mg
Available in 5 ct., 10 ct. and 15 ct.
Available in 12 hour and
24 hour extended release tablets.

Claritin-D®
(loratadine/pseudoephedrine sulfate)

OTC   SCHERING-PLOUGH   P. 772
HEALTHCARE PRODUCTS

10 mg
Orally Disintegrating Tablets
Available in 5 ct., 10 ct. and 20 ct.

Claritin® RediTabs®
(loratadine)

TAHITIAN NONI INTERNATIONAL

OTC   TAHITIAN NONI INTERNATIONAL   P. 834

Dietary Supplement

Tahitian Noni® Juice

OTC   TAHITIAN NONI INTERNATIONAL   P. 834

Tahitian Noni® Seed Oil

OTC   TAHITIAN NONI INTERNATIONAL   P. 833

Tahitian Noni® Leaf Serum

UCB, INC.

OTC   UCB, INC.   P. 730

30 mg/5 mL

Delsym®
(dextromethorphan polistirex)
Extended-Release Suspension

VEMMA NUTRITION COMPANY

OTC   VEMMA NUTRITION COMPANY   P. 835

Mangosteen Essential Plus™ Minerals®

**Vemma Nutrition
Program™**

FACED WITH AN
Rx SIDE EFFECT?

Turn to the
Companion Drug Index
(Green Pages)
for products that provide
symptomatic relief.

ZAVITA

OTC   ZAVITA   P. 824

Liquid Herbal Supplement

Zavita®

PDR® for Herbal Medicines, *3rd Edition*.

The most authoritative resource on herbal medicines.

Patients who use herbals — prescribed or otherwise — are a daily reality for virtually every physician. But the herbal's contribution to a patient's health can be unclear and hard to assess. To make the best call for your patient, you need an authoritative, trustworthy reference that answers all your questions. It's here — the new updated *PDR® for Herbal Medicines, 3rd Edition*.

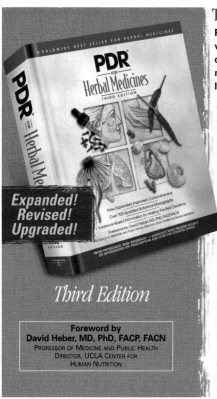

Expanded! Revised! Upgraded!

Third Edition

**Foreword by
David Heber, MD, PhD, FACP, FACN**
PROFESSOR OF MEDICINE AND PUBLIC HEALTH
DIRECTOR, UCLA CENTER FOR
HUMAN NUTRITION

Respected, comprehensive and current!

This *3rd Edition* is the definitive guide to current herbal practices. With more than 700 monographs, a new section on the most popular nutritional supplements, and new information on clinical management of interactions, this edition is the ultimate source for accurate, evidence-based, trustworthy herbal information.

New interactions added

When herbal mixes with prescription, concerns over interactions are paramount. This edition offers the most current, exhaustive interaction data available for the most extensive list of herbals assembled in one reference.

The most popular nutritional supplements added

Consumption of nutritional supplements has increased in the last decade as well. Therefore monographs of some of the most popular supplements make a logical addition to this guide.

New clinical management of interactions

At last, there's evidence-based guidance for managing herbal medicines with the most frequently prescribed drugs. This important section helps you make thoroughly informed decisions.

An herbal guide you can trust

In a field where scientific standards are not always applicable, a guide's source information is even more important. Here are three reasons why the *PDR® for Herbal Medicines, 3rd Edition* is the world's most authoritative herbal reference:

1 The foundation for this edition continues to be the extensive herbal database of the **PhytoPharm U.S. Institute of Phytopharmaceuticals.** This resource provides extensive pharmacological and indication details that are generally not available from other sources.

2 The findings of the **German Regulatory Authority (Commission E)** are recognized for their expert consensus in the herbal field. Their widely accepted conclusions add an additional valuable dimension for physicians looking for the best counsel.

3 Finally, this edition is assembled by the same **PDR®** Editorial Team that produces all the PDR® reference guides. Only after their standards had been met was the *PDR® for Herbal Medicines, 3rd Edition* ready for publication.

A typical monograph covers these critical aspects:

- herbs are listed by common name followed by its scientific name
- a thorough description of the herb is provided, including its medicinal parts (e.g., flower and fruit, etc.); unique characteristics, and additional common names and synonyms
- a detailed summary of the active compounds and the herb's clinical effects
- indications and usage — where applicable — under five categories: Commission E Approved; Chinese Medicine; Indian Medicine; Homeopathic; Unproven
- clinical studies are cited for many monographs
- drug/herb interactions and clinical management of those interactions
- precautions, adverse reactions, and dosage information provide a comprehensive overview
- a unique bibliography of the literature

ARNICA / 41

HERBAL MONOGRAPHS

Arnica
Arnica montana

DESCRIPTION

Medicinal Parts: The medicinal parts of Arnica are the ethereal oil of the flowers, the dried flowers, the leaves collected before flowering and dried, the roots, and the dried rhizome and roots.

Flower and Fruit: The terminal composite flower is found in the leaf axils of the upper pair of leaves. They have a diameter of 6 to 8 cm, are usually egg yolk-yellow to orange-yellow, but occasionally light yellow. The receptacle and epicalyx are hairy. The 10 to 20 female ray flowers are lingui-form. In addition, there are about 100 disc flowers, which are tubular. The 5-ribbed fruit is black-brown and has a bristly tuft of hair.

Leaves, Stem and Root: Arnica is a herbaceous plant growing 20 to 50 cm high. The brownish rhizome is 0.5 cm thick by 10 cm long, usually unbranched, 3-sectioned and sympodial. The rhizome may also be 3-headed with many yellow-brown secondary roots. Leaves are in basal rosettes. They are in 2 to 3 crossed opposite pairs and are obovate and entire-margined with 5 protruding vertical ribs. The glandular-haired stem has 2 to 6 smaller leaves, which are ovate to lanceolate, entire-margined or somewhat dentate.

Characteristics: The flower heads are aromatic; the taste is bitter and irritating.

Habitat: Arnica is found in Europe from Scandinavia to southern Europe. It is also found in southern Russia and

Not to be Confused With: Other yellow-flowering ...

Other Names: Arnica Flowers, Arnica Root, Leopard's Bane, Mountain Tobacco, Wolfsbane

ACTIONS AND PHARMACOLOGY

Caffeic acid derivatives: including chlorogenic acid, 1,5-dicaffeoyl quinic acid

Flavonoids: numerous flavone and flavonol glycosides and their aglycones

EFFECTS

Arnica preparations have an antiphlogistic, analgesic and antiseptic effect when applied topically, due to the sesquiterpene lactone component. The flavonoid bonds, essential oils and polyynes may also be involved. In cases of inflammation, Arnica preparations also show analgesic and antiseptic activity. The sesquiterpenes (helenalin) in the drug have an antimicrobial effect in vitro and an antiphlogistic effect in animal tests. A respiratory-analeptic, uterine tonic and cardiovascular effect (increase of contraction amplitude with simultaneous increase in frequency, i.e. positive inotropic effect) was demonstrated.

INDICATIONS AND USAGE

Approved by Commission E:

- Fever and colds
- Inflammation of the skin
- Cough/bronchitis
- Inflammation of the mouth and pharynx
- Rheumatism
- Common cold
- Blunt injuries
- Tendency to infection

Unproven Uses: External folk medicine uses include consequences of injury such as traumatic edema, hematoma, contusions, as well as rheumatic muscle and joint problems. Other applications are inflammation of the oral and throat region, furunculosis, inflammation caused by insect bites and ... drug is used to treat ... due to psychological causes. ... most are unproven.

PRECAUTIONS AND ADVERSE REACTIONS

General: The risks connected with the external, appropriate administration of therapeutic dosages of the drug a ... administration, in particular of the und...

G-14/PDR FOR HERBAL MEDICINES

HENBANE	HIBISCUS	HOLLY
	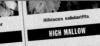	HO...
Hyoscyamus niger	Hibiscus sabdariffa	Alcea
HENNA	HIGH MALLOW	HO...

See other side for ordering information

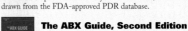

SECTION 7

NONPRESCRIPTION DRUG INFORMATION

This section presents information on nonprescription drugs and other medical products marketed for home use by consumers. It is made possible through the courtesy of the manufacturers whose products appear on the following pages. The information concerning each product has been prepared, edited, and approved by the manufacturer's professional staff.

Pharmaceutical product descriptions in this section must be in compliance with the Code of Federal Regulations labeling requirements for over-the-counter drugs. The descriptions are designed to provide all information necessary for informed use, including, when applicable, active ingredients, inactive ingredients, indications, actions, warnings, cautions, drug interactions, symptoms and treatment of oral overdosage, dosage and directions for use, professional labeling, and how supplied. In some cases, additional information has been supplied to complement the standard labeling.

In compiling this section, the publisher has emphasized the necessity of describing products comprehensively. The descriptions seen here include all information made available by the manufacturer. The publisher does not warrant or guarantee any product described here, and does not perform any independent analysis of the information provided. Inclusion of a product in this book does not represent an endorsement, and the publisher does not necessarily advocate the use of any product listed.

Central Nervous System:
Drowsiness/Fatigue

VIVARIN Tablets & Caplets
(GlaxoSmithKline Consumer)
Alertness Aid with Caffeine
Maximum Strength

Each Tablet or Caplet Contains 200 mg. Caffeine, Equal to About Two Cups of Coffee

Take Vivarin for a safe, fast pick up anytime you feel drowsy and need to be alert. The caffeine in Vivarin is less irritating to your stomach than coffee, according to a government appointed panel of experts.

> **FDA APPROVED USES:** Helps restore mental alertness or wakefulness when experiencing fatigue or drowsiness.

Active Ingredients: Caffeine 200 mg.

Inactive Ingredients: Tablet: Colloidal Silicon Dioxide, D&C Yellow #10 Al. Lake, Dextrose, FD&C Yellow #6 Al. Lake, Magnesium Stearate, Microcrystalline Cellulose, Starch.

Caplet: Carnauba Wax, Colloidal Silicon Dioxide, D&C Yellow #10 Al Lake, Dextrose, FD&C Yellow #6 Al Lake, Hypromellose, Magnesium Stearate, Microcrystalline Cellulose, Polyethylene Glycol, Polysorbate 80, Starch, Titanium Dioxide.

Directions: Adults and children 12 years and over: Take 1 tablet (200 mg) not more often than every 3 to 4 hours.

Warnings: The recommended dose of this product contains about as much caffeine as two cups of coffee. Limit the use of caffeine containing medications, foods, or beverages while taking this product because too much caffeine may cause nervousness, irritability, sleeplessness, and occasionally, rapid heartbeat. For occasional use only. Not intended for use as a substitute for sleep. If fatigue or drowsiness persists or continues to recur, consult a doctor. Do not give to children under 12 years of age. As with any drug, if you are pregnant or nursing a baby, seek the advice of a health professional before using this product. In case of accidental overdose, seek professional assistance or contact a poison control center immediately. Keep this and all drugs out of the reach of children.

Tamper Evident Feature: Individually sealed in foil for your protection. Do not use if foil or plastic bubble is torn or punctured.

Store at room temperature, avoid excessive heat (greater than 100°F) or humidity.

How Supplied:
Tablets: Consumer packages of 16, 40 and 80 tablets
Caplets: Consumer packages of 24 and 48 caplets
Comments or Questions? Call Toll-Free 1-800-245-1040 Weekdays.
GlaxoSmithKline Consumer Healthcare, L.P.
Moon Township, PA 15108. Made in U.S.A.
©2004 GlaxoSmithKline, L.P.

Shown in Product Identification
Guide, page 506

Central Nervous System:
Fever

ADVIL® (Wyeth Consumer)
Ibuprofen Tablets, USP
Ibuprofen Caplets (Oval-Shaped Tablets)
Ibuprofen Gel Caplets (Oval-Shaped Gelatin Coated Tablets)
Ibuprofen Liqui-Gel Capsules
Pain reliever/Fever Reducer (NSAID)

For full product information see page 674.

ADVIL® ALLERGY SINUS CAPLETS (Wyeth Consumer)
ADVIL® MULTI-SYMPTOM COLD CAPLETS
Pain Reliever/Fever Reducer (NSAID)
Nasal Decongestant
Antihistamine

For full product information see page 770.

ADVIL® COLD & SINUS
Caplets, and Liqui-Gels
Pain Reliever/Fever Reducer/(NSAID)
Nasal Decongestant

For full product information see page 723.

CHILDREN'S ADVIL CHEWABLE TABLETS (Wyeth Consumer)
Fever Reducer/Pain Reliever (NSAID)

Active Ingredient:
(in each tablet)
Ibuprofen 50 mg (NSAID)*
*nonsteroidal anti-inflammatory drug

Uses: temporarily:
• reduces fever
• relieves minor aches and pains due to the common cold, flu, sore throat, headaches and toothaches

Warnings:
Allergy alert: Ibuprofen may cause a severe allergic reaction, especially in people allergic to aspirin. Symptoms may include:
• hives
• facial swelling
• asthma (wheezing)
• shock
• skin reddening
• rash
• blisters
If an allergic reaction occurs, stop use and seek medical help right away.

Stomach bleeding warning: This product contains a nonsteroidal anti-inflammatory drug (NSAID), which may cause stomach bleeding. The chance is higher if the child:

• has had stomach ulcers or bleeding problems
• takes a blood thinning (anticoagulant) or steroid drug
• takes other drugs containing an NSAID [aspirin, ibuprofen, naproxen, or others]
• takes more or for a longer time than directed

Sore throat warning: Severe or persistent sore throat or sore throat accompanied by high fever, headache, nausea, and vomiting may be serious. Consult doctor promptly. Do not use more than 2 days or administer to children under 3 years of age unless directed by doctor.

Do not use
• if the child has ever had an allergic reaction to any other pain reliever/fever reducer
• right before or after heart surgery

Ask a doctor before use if the child has
• problems or serious side effects from taking pain relievers or fever reducers
• stomach problems that last or come back, such as heartburn, upset stomach, or stomach pain
• ulcers
• bleeding problems
• not been drinking fluids
• lost a lot of fluid due to vomiting or diarrhea
• high blood pressure
• heart or kidney disease
• taken a diuretic

Ask a doctor or pharmacist before use if the child is
• taking any other drug containing an NSAID (prescription or nonprescription)
• taking a blood thinning (anticoagulant) or steroid drug
• under a doctor's care for any serious condition
• taking any other drug

When using this product
• take with food or milk if stomach upset occurs
• long term continuous use may increase the risk of heart attack or stroke

Stop use and ask a doctor if
• the child feels faint, vomits blood, or has bloody or black stools. These are signs of stomach bleeding.

• stomach pain or upset gets worse or lasts
• the child does not get any relief within first day (24 hours) of treatment
• fever or pain gets worse or lasts more than 3 days
• redness or swelling is present in the painful area
• any new symptoms appear

Keep out of reach of children. In case of overdose, get medical help or contact a Poison Control Center right away.

Directions:
• **this product does not contain directions or complete warnings for adult use**
• **do not give more than directed**
• do not give longer than 10 days, unless directed by a doctor (see Warnings)
• find right dose on chart below. If possible, use weight to dose; otherwise use age
• repeat dose every **6–8 hours**, if needed
• do not use more than **4 times a day**

[See table below]

Other Information:
• **Phenylketonurics:** contains phenylalanine 2.1 mg per tablet
• one dose lasts 6–8 hours
• store in a dry place at 20–25°C (68–77°F)

Inactive Ingredients: aspartame, cellacefate, colloidal silicon dioxide, D&C red no. 30 aluminum lake, FD&C blue no. 2 aluminum lake, gelatin, magnesium stearate, mannitol, microcrystalline cellulose, natural and artificial flavors, sodium starch glycolate

How Supplied: Blister of 24 (grape flavor).

CHILDREN'S ADVIL SUSPENSION (Wyeth Consumer)
Fever Reducer/Pain Reliever (NSAID)

Active Ingredient:
(in each 5 mL)
Ibuprofen 100 mg (NSAID)*
*nonsteroidal anti-inflammatory drug

Dosing Chart		
Weight (lb)	Age (yr)	Dose (tablets)
under 24 lb	under 2 yr	ask a doctor
24–35 lb	2–3 yr	2 tablets
36–47 lb	4–5 yr	3 tablets
48–59 lb	6–8 yr	4 tablets
60–71 lb	9–10 yr	5 tablets
72–95 lb	11 yr	6 tablets

Children's Advil Susp.—Cont.

Uses: temporarily:
- reduces fever
- relieves minor aches and pains due to the common cold, flu, sore throat, headaches and toothaches

Warnings:

Allergy alert: Ibuprofen may cause a severe allergic reaction, especially in people allergic to aspirin. Symptoms may include:
- hives
- facial swelling
- asthma (wheezing)
- shock
- skin reddening
- rash
- blisters

If an allergic reaction occurs, stop use and seek medical help right away.

Stomach bleeding warning: This product contains a nonsteroidal antiinflammatory drug (NSAID), which may cause stomach bleeding. The chance is higher if the child:
- has had stomach ulcers or bleeding problems
- takes a blood thinning (anticoagulant) or steroid drug
- takes other drugs containing an NSAID [aspirin, ibuprofen, naproxen, or others]
- takes more or for a longer time than directed

Sore throat warning: Severe or persistent sore throat or sore throat accompanied by high fever, headache, nausea, and vomiting may be serious. Consult doctor promptly. Do not use more than 2 days or administer to children under 3 years of age unless directed by doctor.

Do not use
- if the child has ever had an allergic reaction to any other pain reliever/fever reducer
- right before or after heart surgery

Ask a doctor before use if the child has
- problems or serious side effects from taking pain relievers or fever reducers
- stomach problems that last or come back, such as heartburn, upset stomach, or stomach pain
- ulcers
- bleeding problems
- not been drinking fluids
- lost a lot of fluid due to vomiting or diarrhea
- high blood pressure

- heart or kidney disease
- taken a diuretic

Ask a doctor or pharmacist before use if the child is
- taking any other drug containing an NSAID (prescription or nonprescription)
- taking a blood thinning (anticoagulant) or steroid drug
- under a doctor's care for any serious condition
- taking any other drug

When using this product
- take with food or milk if stomach upset occurs
- long term continuous use may increase the risk of heart attack or stroke

Stop use and ask a doctor if
- the child feels faint, vomits blood, or has bloody or black stools. These are signs of stomach bleeding.
- stomach pain or upset gets worse or lasts
- the child does not get any relief within first day (24 hours) of treatment
- fever or pain gets worse or lasts more than 3 days
- redness or swelling is present in the painful area
- any new symptoms appear

Keep out of reach of children. In case of overdose, get medical help or contact a Poison Control Center right away.

Directions:
- **this product does not contain directions or complete warnings for adult use**
- **do not give more than directed**
- do not give longer than 10 days, unless directed by a doctor (see Warnings)
- **shake well before using**
- find right dose on chart below. If possible, use weight to dose; otherwise use age.
- repeat dose every **6–8 hours**, if needed
- do not use more than **4 times a day**
- measure only with the blue dosing cup provided. Blue dosing cup to be used with Children's Advil Suspension only. Do not use with other products. Dose lines account for product remaining in cup due to thickness of suspension.

[See table below]

Other Information:
- one dose lasts 6–8 hours
- store at 20–25°C (68–77°F)

Inactive Ingredients: (FRUIT FLAVOR) artificial flavors, carboxymethylcellulose sodium, citric acid, edetate disodium, FD&C red no. 40, glycerin, microcrystalline cellulose, polysorbate 80, purified water, sodium benzoate, sorbitol solution, sucrose, xanthan gum
Each teaspoon contains: sodium 3 mg

Inactive Ingredients: (GRAPE FLAVOR) acetic acid, artificial flavor, butylated hydroxytoluene, carboxymethylcellulose sodium, citric acid, edetate disodium, FD&C blue no. 1, FD&C red no. 40, glycerin, microcrystalline cellulose, polysorbate 80, propylene glycol, purified water, sodium benzoate, sorbitol solution, sucrose, xanthan gum
Each teaspoon contains: sodium 3 mg

Inactive Ingredients: (BLUE RASPBERRY FLAVOR) carboxymethylcellulose sodium, citric acid, edetate disodium, FD&C blue no. 1, glycerin, microcrystalline cellulose, natural and artificial flavors, polysorbate 80, propylene glycol, purified water, sodium benzoate, sodium citrate, sorbitol solution, sucrose, xanthan gum
Each teaspoon contains: sodium 10 mg

How Supplied: Bottles of 4 fl. oz. in grape, fruit, and blue raspberry flavors.

INFANTS' ADVIL CONCENTRATED DROPS
(Wyeth Consumer)
INFANT'S ADVIL WHITE GRAPE CONCENTRATED DROPS
(DYE-FREE)
Fever Reducer/Pain Reliever (NSAID)

Active Ingredient:
(in each 1.25 mL)
Ibuprofen 50 mg (NSAID)*
*nonsteroidal anti-inflammatory drug

Uses: temporarily:
- reduces fever
- relieves minor aches and pains due to the common cold, flu, headaches and toothaches

Warnings:

Allergy alert: Ibuprofen may cause a severe allergic reaction, especially in people allergic to aspirin. Symptoms may include:
- hives • facial swelling • asthma (wheezing)
- shock • skin reddening • rash • blisters

If an allergic reaction occurs, stop use and seek medical help right away.

Stomach bleeding warning: This product contains a nonsteroidal antiinflammatory drug (NSAID), which may cause stomach bleeding. The chance is higher if the child:
- has had stomach ulcers or bleeding problems
- takes a blood thinning (anticoagulant) or steroid drug
- takes other drugs containing an NSAID [aspirin, ibuprofen, naproxen, or others]

Dosing Chart		
Weight (lb)	Age (yr)	Dose (tsp)
under 24 lb	under 2yr	ask a doctor
24–35 lb	2–3 yr	1 tsp
36–47 lb	4–5 yr	1½ tsp
48–59 lb	6–8 yr	2 tsp
60–71 lb	9–10 yr	2½ tsp
72–95 lb	11 yr	3 tsp

Dosing Chart		
Weight (lb)	Age (mos)	Dose (mL)
under 6 mos		ask a doctor
12–17 lb	6–11 mos	1.25 mL
18–23 lb	12–23 mos	1.875 mL

• takes more or for a longer time than directed

Do not use

• if the child has ever had an allergic reaction to any other pain reliever/fever reducer
• right before or after heart surgery

Ask a doctor before use if the child has

• problems or serious side effects from taking pain relievers or fever reducers
• stomach problems that last or come back, such as heartburn, upset stomach, or stomach pain
• ulcers
• bleeding problems
• not been drinking fluids
• lost a lot of fluid due to vomiting or diarrhea
• high blood pressure
• heart or kidney disease
• taken a diuretic

Ask a doctor or pharmacist before use if the child is

• taking any other drug containing an NSAID (prescription or nonprescription)
• taking a blood thinning (anticoagulant) or steroid drug
• under a doctor's care for any serious condition
• taking any other drug

When using this product

• take with food or milk if stomach upset occurs
• long term continuous use may increase the risk of heart attack or stroke

Stop use and ask a doctor if

• the child feels faint, vomits blood, or has bloody or black stools. These are signs of stomach bleeding.
• stomach pain or upset gets worse or lasts
• the child does not get any relief within first day (24 hours) of treatment
• fever or pain gets worse or lasts more than 3 days
• redness or swelling is present in the painful area
• any new symptoms appear

Keep out of reach of children. In case of overdose, get medical help or contact a Poison Control Center right away.

Directions:

• **this product does not contain directions or complete warnings for adult use**
• **do not give more than directed**
• do not give longer than 10 days, unless directed by a doctor (see Warnings)
• **shake well before using**
• find right dose on chart below. If possible, use weight to dose; otherwise use age.
• repeat dose every **6–8 hours,** if needed

• do not use more than **4 times a day**
• measure with the dosing device provided. Do not use with any other device. [See table above]

Other Information:

• one dose lasts 6–8 hours
• store at 20–25°C (68–77°F)

Inactive Ingredients: (WHITE GRAPE FLAVOR) artificial flavor, carboxymethylcellulose sodium, citric acid, edetate disodium, glycerin, microcrystalline cellulose, polysorbate 80, propylene glycol, purified water, sodium benzoate, sorbitol solution, sucrose, xanthan gum

Inactive Ingredients: (GRAPE FLAVOR) artificial flavor, carboxymethylcellulose sodium, citric acid, edetate disodium, FD&C blue no. 1, FD&C red no. 40, glycerin, microcrystalline cellulose, polysorbate 80, purified water, sodium benzoate, sorbitol solution, sucrose, xanthan gum

How Supplied: Bottles of ½ fl. oz. in grape and white grape flavors.

**JUNIOR STRENGTH ADVIL®
SWALLOW TABLETS (Wyeth
Consumer)
Fever Reducer/Pain Reliever (NSAID)**

**Active Ingredient:
(in each tablet)**
Ibuprofen 100 mg (NSAID)*
*nonsteroidal anti-inflammatory drug

Uses:
temporarily:
• reduces fever
• relieves minor aches and pains due to the common cold, flu, sore throat, headaches and toothaches

Warnings:

Allergy alert: Ibuprofen may cause a severe allergic reaction, especially in people allergic to aspirin. Symptoms may include:
• hives
• facial swelling
• asthma (wheezing)
• shock
• skin reddening
• rash
• blisters
If an allergic reaction occurs, stop use and seek medical help right away.

Stomach bleeding warning: This product contains a nonsteroidal anti-inflammatory drug (NSAID), which may

cause stomach bleeding. The chance is higher if the child:
• has had stomach ulcers or bleeding problems
• takes a blood thinning (anticoagulant) or steroid drug
• takes other drugs containing an NSAID [aspirin, ibuprofen, naproxen, or others]
• takes more or for a longer time than directed

Sore throat warning: Severe or persistent sore throat or sore throat accompanied by high fever, headache, nausea, and vomiting may be serious. Consult doctor promptly. Do not use more than 2 days or administer to children under 3 years of age unless directed by doctor.

Do not use

• if the child has ever had an allergic reaction to any other pain reliever/fever reducer
• right before or after heart surgery

Ask a doctor before use if the child has

• problems or serious side effects from taking pain relievers or fever reducers
• stomach problems that last or come back, such as heartburn, upset stomach, or stomach pain
• ulcers
• bleeding problems
• not been drinking fluids
• lost a lot of fluid due to vomiting or diarrhea
• high blood pressure
• heart or kidney disease
• taken a diuretic

Ask a doctor or pharmacist before use if the child is

• taking any other drug containing an NSAID (prescription or nonprescription)
• taking a blood thinning (anticoagulant) or steroid drug
• under a doctor's care for any serious condition
• taking any other drug

When using this product

• take with food or milk if stomach upset occurs
• long term continuous use may increase the risk of heart attack or stroke

Stop use and ask a doctor if

• the child feels faint, vomits blood, or has bloody or black stools. These are signs of stomach bleeding.
• stomach pain or upset gets worse or lasts
• the child does not get any relief within first day (24 hours) of treatment
• fever or pain gets worse or lasts more than 3 days
• redness or swelling is present in the painful area
• any new symptoms appear

Keep out of reach of children. In case of overdose, get medical help or contact a Poison Control Center right away.

Continued on next page

Junior Strength Advil—Cont.

Directions:
- **this product does not contain directions or complete warnings for adult use**
- **do not give more than directed**
- do not give longer than 10 days, unless directed by a doctor (see Warnings)
- find right dose on chart below. If possible, use weight to dose; otherwise use age.
- repeat dose every **6–8 hours,** if needed
- do not use more than **4 times a day**

Dosing Chart		
Weight (lb)	**Age (yr)**	**Dose (tablets)**
under 48 lb	under 6 yr	ask a doctor
48–71 lb	6–10 yr	2 tablets
72–95 lb	11 yr	3 tablets

Other Information:
- one dose lasts 6–8 hours
- store at 20–25°C (68–77°F)

Inactive Ingredients:
acetylated monoglycerides, carnauba wax, colloidal silicon dioxide, croscarmellose sodium, iron oxides, methylparaben, microcrystalline cellulose, povidone, pregelatinized starch, propylene glycol, propylparaben, shellac, sodium benzoate, starch, stearic acid, sucrose, titanium dioxide

How Supplied:
Coated Tablets in bottles of 24.

ALEVE CAPLETS (Bayer Healthcare)
(NSAID Labeling)
[a-lēv]

For full product information see page 675.

ALEVE COLD & SINUS CAPLETS
(Bayer Healthcare)
(NSAID Labeling)
[a-lēv]

For full product information see page 724.

ALEVE GELCAPS
(Bayer Healthcare)
(NSAID Labeling)
[a-lēv]

For full product information see page 675.

ALEVE TABLETS (Bayer Healthcare)
(NSAID Labeling)
[a-lēv]

For full product information see page 676.

BC® POWDER
(GlaxoSmithKline Consumer)
ARTHRITIS STRENGTH BC®
POWDER
BC® COLD POWDER LINE

For full product information see page 677.

BUFFERIN®
(Novartis Consumer Health, Inc.)
Regular/Extra Strength
Pain Reliever/Fever Reducer

For full product information see page 678.

COMTREX®
(Novartis Consumer Health, Inc.)
MAXIMUM STRENGTH
Pain Reliever/Fever Reducer, Cough Suppressant, Nasal Decongestant
Acetaminophon, Dextromethorphan HBr, Phenylephrine HCl
Non-Drowsy Cold & Cough

For full product information see page 726.

COMTREX® Cold & Cough Day/Night
(Novartis Consumer Health, Inc.)
Pain Reliever/Fever Reducer

For full product information see page 725.

CONTAC® COLD AND FLU DAY AND NIGHT
(GlaxoSmithKline Consumer)

For full product information see page 727.

CONTAC COLD AND FLU NON-DROWSY MAXIMUM STRENGTH
(GlaxoSmithKline Consumer)

For full product information see page 728.

CONTAC® COLD AND FLU MAXIMUM STRENGTH
(GlaxoSmithKline Consumer)

For full product information see page 728.

GOODY'S®
(GlaxoSmithKline Consumer)
Extra Strength Headache Powder

For full product information see page 611.

GOODY'S®
(GlaxoSmithKline Consumer)
Extra Strength Pain Relief Tablets

For full product information see page 685.

CHILDREN'S MOTRIN® Cold
(McNeil Consumer)
ibuprofen/pseudoephedrine HCl
Oral Suspension

For full product information see page 733.

INFANTS' MOTRIN® ibuprofen
Concentrated Drops
(McNeil Consumer)
CHILDREN'S MOTRIN® ibuprofen
Oral Suspension
JUNIOR STRENGTH MOTRIN®
ibuprofen Caplets and Chewable Tablets
Product information for all dosages of Children's MOTRIN have been combined under this heading

For full product information see page 685.

MOTRIN® IB (Ibuprofen)
Pain Reliever/Fever Reducer
Tablets and Caplets
(McNeil Consumer)

For full product information see page 687.

THERAFLU® Nighttime Severe Cold
(Novartis Consumer Health, Inc.)
Pain Reliever-Fever Reducer
(Acetaminophen)
Antihistamine (Pheniramine maleate)
Nasal Decongestant
(Phenylephrine HCl)

For full product information see page 740.

THERAFLU® Cold & Cough
(Novartis Consumer Health, Inc.)
Cough Suppressant
(Dextromethorphan HBr)
Antihistamine (Pheniramine maleate)
Nasal Decongestant
(Phenylephrine HCl)

For full product information see page 740.

THERAFLU® Cold & Sore Throat
(Novartis Consumer Health, Inc.)
Pain Reliever-Fever Reducer
(Acetaminophen)
Antihistamine (Pheniramine maleate)
Nasal Decongestant (Phenylephrine HCl)

For full product information see page 742.

THERAFLU® Flu & Chest Congestion
(Novartis Consumer Health, Inc.)
Pain Reliever-Fever Reducer
(Acetaminophen)
Expectorant (Guaifenesin)

For full product information see page 741.

**THERAFLU® Flu & Sore Throat
(Novartis Consumer Health, Inc.)
Pain Reliever-Fever Reducer
(Acetaminophen)
Antihistamine (Pheniramine maleate)
Nasal Decongestant (Phenylephrine
HCl)**

For full product information see page 741.

**THERAFLU® Daytime Severe Cold
(Novartis Consumer Health, Inc.)
Pain Reliever-Fever Reducer
(Acetaminophen)
Nasal Decongestant (Phenylephrine
HCl)**

For full product information see page 742.

**THERAFLU® DAYTIME WARMING
RELIEF
(Novartis Consumer Health, Inc.)
Pain Reliever/Fever Reducer/Cough
Suppressant/Nasal Decongestant**

For full product information see page 743.

**THERAFLU® NIGHTTIME WARMING
RELIEF
(Novartis Consumer Health, Inc.)
Cough Suppressant/Antihistamine/Pain
Reliever/Fever Reducer/Nasal
Decongestant**

For full product information see page 743.

**TRIAMINIC® COUGH & SORE
THROAT
(Novartis Consumer Health, Inc.)
Pain Reliever/Fever Reducer/Cough
Suppressant**

For full product information see page 747.

**CHILDREN'S TYLENOL® Plus Cold
& Allergy (McNeil Consumer)**

For full product information see page 716.

**CHILDREN'S TYLENOL® Plus Flu
(McNeil Consumer)**

For full product information see page 749.

**CONCENTRATED TYLENOL®
acetaminophen Infants' Drops
(McNeil Consumer)**

**CHILDREN'S TYLENOL®
acetaminophen Suspension Liquid
and Meltaways**

**JR. TYLENOL®
acetaminophen Meltaways**

**CHILDREN'S TYLENOL®
Suspension with Flavor Creator**

**Product information for all dosages
of Children's TYLENOL have been
combined under this heading**

For full product information see page 754.

**REGULAR STRENGTH TYLENOL®
acetaminophen Tablets
(McNeil Consumer)**

**EXTRA STRENGTH TYLENOL®
acetaminophen Geltabs, Caplets,
Cool Caplets, and EZ Tabs**

**EXTRA STRENGTH TYLENOL®
acetaminophen Rapid Release Gels**

**EXTRA STRENGTH TYLENOL®
acetaminophen Adult Liquid Pain
Reliever**

**TYLENOL® Arthritis Pain
Acetaminophen Extended Release
Geltabs/Caplets**

**TYLENOL® 8 Hour Acetaminophen
Extended Release Caplets**

**Product information for all dosage
forms of Adult TYLENOL
acetaminophen have been combined
under this heading.**

For full product information see page 695.

**TYLENOL® Chest Congestion
Caplets with Cool Burst™
(McNeil Consumer)**

**TYLENOL® Chest Congestion
Liquid with Cool Burst™**

For full product information see page 722.

**TYLENOL® Cold Head Congestion
Daytime Caplets with Cool Burst™
and Gelcaps (McNeil Consumer)**

**TYLENOL® Cold Head Congestion
Nighttime Caplets with Cool
Burst™**

**TYLENOL® Cold Head Congestion
Severe Caplets with Cool Burst™**

For full product information see page 750.

**TYLENOL® COLD
Severe Congestion Non-Drowsy
Caplets with Cool Burst™
(McNeil Consumer)**

For full product information see page 751.

**TYLENOL® Cold Multi-Symptom
Daytime Caplets with Cool Burst™
and Gelcaps (McNeil Consumer)**

**TYLENOL® Cold Multi-Symptom
Nighttime Caplets with Cool
Burst™**

**TYLENOL® Cold Multi-Symptom
Severe Caplets with Cool Burst™**

**TYLENOL® Cold Multi-Symptom
Daytime Liquid**

**TYLENOL® Cold Multi-Symptom
Nighttime Liquid with Cool Burst™**

**TYLENOL® Cold Multi-Symptom
Severe Daytime Liquid**

For full product information see page 752.

**TYLENOL® Sore Throat Daytime
Liquid with Cool Burst™
(McNeil Consumer)**

**TYLENOL® Sore Throat Nighttime
Liquid with Cool Burst™**

**TYLENOL® Cough & Sore Throat
Daytime Liquid with Cool Burst™**

**TYLENOL® Cough & Sore Throat
Nighttime Liquid with Cool Burst™**

For full product information see page 790.

**CONCENTRATED TYLENOL®
Infants' Drops Plus Cold Nasal
Decongestant, Fever Reducer &
Pain Reliever (McNeil Consumer)**

**CONCENTRATED TYLENOL®
Infants' Drops Plus Cold & Cough
Nasal Decongestant, Fever Reducer
& Pain Reliever, Cough
Suppressant**

**CHILDREN'S TYLENOL® Plus
Cough & Sore Throat Suspension
Liquid**

**CHILDREN'S TYLENOL® Plus
Cough & Runny Nose Suspension
Liquid**

**CHILDREN'S TYLENOL® Plus Multi-
Symptom Cold Suspension Liquid**

**CHILDREN'S TYLENOL® Plus
Cold Suspension Liquid**

For full product information see page 754.

**VICKS® 44M® (Procter & Gamble)
COUGH, COLD & FLU RELIEF
Cough Suppressant/Antihistamine/Pain
Reliever–Fever Reducer Alcohol 10%
Maximum strength cough formula**

For full product information see page 760.

**VICKS® DAYQUIL® LIQUID
(Procter & Gamble)**

**VICKS® DAYQUIL® LIQUICAPS®
Multi-Symptom Cold/Flu Relief
Nasal Decongestant/Pain Reliever/
Cough Suppressant/Fever Reducer
Non-drowsy**

For full product information see page 761.

**VICKS® NYQUIL® LIQUICAPS®/
LIQUID MULTI-SYMPTOM COLD/
FLU RELIEF (Proctor & Gamble)**

For full product information see page 763.

ZICAM® Flu Daytime (Matrixx)

ZICAM® Nighttime

For full product information see page 768.

Central Nervous System:
Headache/Migraine

ADVIL® (Wyeth Consumer)
Ibuprofen Tablets, USP
Ibuprofen Caplets (Oval-Shaped Tablets)
Ibuprofen Gel Caplets (Oval-Shaped Gelatin Coated Tablets)
Ibuprofen Liqui-Gel Capsules
Pain reliever/Fever Reducer (NSAID)

For full product information see page 674.

ADVIL® ALLERGY SINUS CAPLETS (Wyeth Consumer)
ADVIL® MULTI-SYMPTOM COLD CAPLETS
Pain Reliever/Fever Reducer (NSAID)
Nasal Decongestant
Antihistamine

For full product information see page 770.

ADVIL® COLD & SINUS
Caplets, and Liqui-Gels
Pain Reliever/Fever Reducer/(NSAID)
Nasal Decongestant

For full product information see page 723.

ADVIL® MIGRAINE Liquigels (Wyeth Consumer)
Pain reliever (NSAID)

Active Ingredient:
Each brown, oval capsule contains solubilized ibuprofen, a pain reliever, equal to 200 mg ibuprofen (NSAID)* (present as the free acid and potassium salt)
*nonsteroidal anti-inflammatory drug

Use: Treats migraine

Warnings:
Allergy alert: Ibuprofen may cause a severe allergic reaction, especially in people allergic to aspirin. Symptoms may include:
• hives
• facial swelling
• asthma (wheezing)
• shock
• skin reddening
• rash
• blisters
If an allergic reaction occurs, stop use and seek medical help right away.
Stomach bleeding warning: This product contains a nonsteroidal anti-inflammatory drug (NSAID), which may cause stomach bleeding. The chance is higher if you:
• are age 60 or older

• have had stomach ulcers or bleeding problems
• take a blood thinning (anticoagulant) or steroid drug
• take other drugs containing an NSAID [aspirin, ibuprofen, naproxen, or others]
• have 3 or more alcoholic drinks every day while using this product
• take more or for a longer time than directed
Do not use
• if you have ever had an allergic reaction to any other pain reliever/fever reducer
• right before or after heart surgery
Ask a doctor before use if you have
• never had migraines diagnosed by a health professional
• a headache that is different from your usual migraines
• the worst headache of your life
• fever and stiff neck
• headaches beginning after or caused by head injury, exertion, coughing or bending
• experienced your first headache after the age of 50
• daily headaches
• a migraine so severe as to require bed rest
• problems or serious side effects from taking pain relievers or fever reducers
• stomach problems that last or come back, such as heartburn, upset stomach, or stomach pain
• ulcers
• bleeding problems
• high blood pressure
• heart or kidney disease
• taken a diuretic
• reached age 60 or older
Ask a doctor or pharmacist before use if you are
• taking any other drug containing an NSAID (prescription or nonprescription)
• taking a blood thinning (anticoagulant) or steroid drug
• under a doctor's care for any serious condition
• taking aspirin to prevent heart attack or stroke, because ibuprofen may decrease this benefit of aspirin
• taking any other drug
When using this product
• take with food or milk if stomach upset occurs
• long term continuous use may increase the risk of heart attack or stroke
Stop use and ask a doctor if
• you feel faint, vomit blood, or have bloody or black stools. These are signs of stomach bleeding.
• migraine headache pain is not relieved or gets worse after first dose

• stomach pain or upset gets worse or lasts
• any new symptoms appear
If pregnant or breast-feeding, ask a health professional before use. It is especially important not to use ibuprofen during the last 3 months of pregnancy unless definitely directed to do so by a doctor because it may cause problems in the unborn child or complications during delivery.
Keep out of reach of children. In case of overdose, get medical help or contact a Poison Control Center right away.

Directions:
• **do not take more than directed**
• **the smallest effective dose should be used**

Adults:	• take 2 capsules with a glass of water • if symptoms persist or worsen, ask your doctor • do not take more than 2 capsules in 24 hours, unless directed by a doctor
Under 18 years of age:	• ask a doctor

Other Information:
• **each capsule contains:**
potassium 20 mg
• read all directions and warnings before use. Keep carton.
• store at 20–25°C (68–77°F)
• avoid excessive heat 40°C (above 104°F)

Inactive Ingredients:
D&C yellow no. 10, FD&C green no. 3, FD&C red no. 40, gelatin, light mineral oil, pharmaceutical ink, polyethylene glycol, potassium hydroxide, purified water, sorbitan, sorbitol

How Supplied: Bottles of 20, & 40 liquigels.

CHILDREN'S ADVIL CHEWABLE TABLETS (Wyeth Consumer)
Fever Reducer/Pain Reliever (NSAID)

For full product information see page 603.

CHILDREN'S ADVIL SUSPENSION (Wyeth Consumer)
Fever Reducer/Pain Reliever (NSAID)

For full product information see page 603.

INFANTS' ADVIL CONCENTRATED DROPS
(Wyeth Consumer)
INFANT'S ADVIL WHITE GRAPE CONCENTRATED DROPS
(DYE-FREE)
Fever Reducer/Pain Reliever (NSAID)

For full product information see page 604.

JUNIOR STRENGTH ADVIL® SWALLOW TABLETS
(Wyeth Consumer)
Fever Reducer/Pain Reliever (NSAID)

For full product information see page 605.

ALEVE CAPLETS (Bayer Healthcare)
(NSAID Labeling)
[a-lēv]

For full product information see page 675.

ALEVE COLD & SINUS CAPLETS
(Bayer Healthcare)
(NSAID Labeling)
[a-lēv]

For full product information see page 672.

ALEVE GELCAPS
(Bayer Healthcare)
(NSAID Labeling)
[a-lēv]

For full product information see page 675.

ALEVE TABLETS (Bayer Healthcare)
(NSAID Labeling)
[a-lēv]

For full product information see page 676.

BC® POWDER
(GlaxoSmithKline Consumer)
ARTHRITIS STRENGTH BC® POWDER
BC® COLD POWDER LINE

For full product information see page 677.

BUFFERIN®
(Novartis Consumer Health, Inc.)
Regular/Extra Strength
Pain Reliever/Fever Reducer

For full product information see page 678.

COMTREX®
(Novartis Consumer Health, Inc.)
MAXIMUM STRENGTH
Pain Reliever/Fever Reducer, Cough Suppressant, Nasal Decongestant
Acetaminophon, Dextromethorphan HBr, Phenylephrine HCI
Non-Drowsy Cold & Cough

For full product information see page 726.

COMTREX®
(Novartis Consumer Health, Inc.)
MAXIMUM STRENGTH
Day/Night Severe Cold & Sinus
Pain Reliever/Fever Reducer – Nasal Decongestant – Antihistamine*
Acetaminophen, Phenylephrine HCI, Chlorpheniramine Maleate*

For full product information see page 725.

COMTREX® Cold & Cough Day/Night (Novartis Consumer Health, Inc.)
Pain Reliever/Fever Reducer

For full product information see page 726.

CONTAC® COLD AND FLU DAY AND NIGHT
(GlaxoSmithKline Consumer)

For full product information see page 727.

CONTAC COLD AND FLU NON-DROWSY MAXIMUM STRENGTH
(GlaxoSmithKline Consumer)

For full product information see page 728.

CONTAC® COLD AND FLU MAXIMUM STRENGTH
(GlaxoSmithKline Consumer)

For full product information see page 728.

EXCEDRIN® MIGRAINE
PAIN RELIEVER/PAIN RELIEVER AID
(Novartis Consumer Health, Inc.)

Drug Facts

Active Ingredients   Purposes:
(in each caplet/tablet/geltab):
Acetaminophen
  250 mg .... Pain reliever
Aspirin 250 mg .... Pain reliever
Caffeine 65 mg .... Pain reliever aid

Use:
• treats migraine

Warnings:

Reye's syndrome: Children and teenagers who have or are recovering from chicken pox or flu-like symptoms should not use this product. When using this product, if changes in behavior with nausea and vomiting occur, consult a doctor because these symptoms could be an early sign of Reye's syndrome, a rare but serious illness.

Allergy alert: Aspirin may cause a severe allergic reaction, which may include:
• hives • facial swelling
• asthma (wheezing) • shock

Alcohol warning: If you consume 3 or more alcoholic drinks every day, ask your doctor whether you should take acetaminophen and aspirin or other pain relievers/fever reducers. Acetaminophen and aspirin may cause liver damage and stomach bleeding.

Caffeine warning: The recommended dose of this product contains about as much caffeine as a cup of coffee. Limit the use of caffeine-containing medications, foods, or beverages while taking this product because too much caffeine may cause nervousness, irritability, sleeplessness, and, occasionally, rapid heartbeat.

Do not use
• if you have ever had an allergic reaction to any other pain reliever/fever reducer
• with any other products containing acetaminophen. Taking more than directed may cause liver damage.

Ask a doctor before use if you have
• never had migraines diagnosed by a health professional
• a headache that is different from your usual migraines
• the worst headache of your life
• fever and stiff neck
• headaches beginning after or caused by head injury, exertion, coughing or bending
• experienced your first headache after the age of 50
• daily headaches
• a migraine so severe as to require bed rest
• asthma • bleeding problems
• ulcers
• stomach problems such as heartburn, upset stomach, or stomach pain that do not go away or recur
• problems or serious side effects from taking pain relievers or fever reducers
• vomiting with your migraine headache

Ask a doctor or pharmacist before use if you are
• taking a prescription drug for:
  • anticoagulation (thinning of the blood)
  • diabetes • gout • arthritis
• under a doctor's care for any serious condition
• taking any other drug
• taking any other product that contains aspirin, acetaminophen, or any other pain reliever/fever reducer

Stop use and ask a doctor if
• an allergic reaction occurs. Seek medical help right away.
• your migraine is not relieved or worsens after first dose
• new or unexpected symptoms occur
• stomach pain or upset gets worse or lasts
• ringing in the ears or loss of hearing occurs

If pregnant or breast-feeding, ask a health professional before use. It is espe-

Continued on next page

Excedrin Migraine—Cont.

cially important not to use aspirin during the last 3 months of pregnancy unless definitely directed to do so by a doctor because it may cause problems in the unborn child or complications during delivery.

Keep out of reach of children.

Overdose warning: Taking more than the recommended dose can cause serious health problems. In case of overdose, get medical help or contact a Poison Control Center right away. Quick medical attention is critical for adults as well as for children even if you do not notice any signs or symptoms.

Directions:

- do not use more than directed
- adults: take 2 tablets, caplets or geltabs with a glass of water
- if symptoms persist or worsen, ask your doctor
- do not take more than 2 tablets, caplets or geltabs in 24 hours, unless directed by a doctor
- under 18 years of age: ask a doctor

Other Information:

- store at 20°-25°C (68°-77F)
- read all product information before using. Keep the box for important information.

Inactive Ingredients:

Tablets

benzoic acid, carnauba wax, FD&C blue #1*, hydroxypropylcellulose, hypromellose, microcrystalline cellulose, mineral oil, polysorbate 20, povidone, propylene glycol, simethicone emulsion, sorbitan monolaurate, stearic acid, titanium dioxide*

Geltabs

benzoic acid, D&C yellow #10 lake, disodium EDTA, FD&C blue #1 lake, FD&C red #40 lake, ferric oxide, gelatin, glycerin, hydroxypropylcellulose, hypromellose, maltitol solution, microcrystalline cellulose, mineral oil, pepsin, polysorbate 20, povidone, propylene glycol, propyl gallate, simethicone emulsion, sorbitan monolaurate, stearic acid, titanium dioxide*

Caplets

benzoic acid, carnauba wax, FD&C blue #1*, hydroxypropylcellulose, hypromellose, microcrystalline cellulose, mineral oil, polysorbate 20, povidone, propylene glycol, simethicone emulsion, sorbitan monolaurate, stearic acid, titanium dioxide*

---

*may contain these ingredients

Questions or comments?
1-800-468-7746

How Supplied: Tablets in 24 ct., 50 ct., 100 ct. and 250 ct. cartons. Caplets in 24 ct., 50 ct., 100 ct. and 250 ct. cartons. Geltabs in 24 ct., 50 ct., and 100 ct. cartons.

Shown in Product Identification Guide, page 513

EXCEDRIN PM®
(Novartis Consumer Health, Inc.)
PAIN RELIEVER/NIGHTTIME SLEEP AID

Drug Facts
Active Ingredients: **Purpose:**
(in each caplets/tablets/geltabs)

Acetaminophen 500 mg ..... Pain reliever
Diphenhydramine
citrate 38 mg .... Nighttime sleep aid

Uses: for the temporary relief of occasional headaches and minor aches and pains with accompanying sleeplessness.

Warnings:

Alcohol warning: If you consume 3 or more alcoholic drinks every day, ask your doctor whether you should take acetaminophen or other pain relievers/fever reducers. Acetaminophen may cause liver damage.

Do not use

- in children under 12 years of age
- with any other product containing diphenhydramine, even one used on skin
- with any other products containing acetaminophen. Taking more than directed may cause liver damage.

Ask a doctor before use if you have

- glaucoma
- a breathing problem such as emphysema or chronic bronchitis
- trouble urinating due to an enlarged prostate gland

Ask a doctor or pharmacist before use if you are taking sedatives or tranquilizers.

When using this product

- avoid alcoholic drinks
- drowsiness may occur
- be careful when driving a motor vehicle or operating machinery

Stop use and ask a doctor if

- new symptoms occur
- sleeplessness lasts continuously for more than 2 weeks. Insomnia may be a symptom of serious underlying medical illness.
- pain gets worse or lasts for more than 10 days
- painful area is red or swollen
- fever gets worse or lasts for more than 3 days

If pregnant or breast-feeding, ask a health professional before use.

Keep out of reach of children.

Overdose warning: Taking more than the recommended dose can cause serious health problems. In case of overdose, get medical help or contact a Poison Control Center right away. Quick medical attention is critical for adults as well as for children even if you do not notice any signs or symptoms.

Directions:

- do not use more than directed **(see overdose warning)**
- children under 12 years of age: consult a doctor
- adults and children 12 years and over:

take 2 caplets, tablets or geltabs at bedtime, if needed, or as directed by a doctor

Other Information:

- store at room temperature
- read all product information before using.

Inactive Ingredients:
Caplets/Tablets

benzoic acid, carnauba wax, croscarmellose sodium*, crospovidone*, D&C yellow #10 lake, FD&C blue #1 lake, hypromellose, magnesium stearate, methylparaben*, microcrystalline cellulose, mineral oil, polysorbate 20, povidone, pregelatinized starch, propylene glycol, propylparaben*, simethicone emulsion, sodium citrate, sorbitan monolaurate, stearic acid, titanium dioxide

---

*may contain these ingredients

Inactive Ingredients:
Geltabs

benzoic acid, croscarmellose sodium, crospovidone*, D&C red #33 lake, edetate disodium, FD&C blue #1, FD&C blue #1 lake, gelatin, glycerin, hypromellose, magnesium stearate, methylparaben*, microcrystalline cellulose, mineral oil, polysorbate 20, povidone, pregelatinized starch, propylene glycol, propylparaben*, simethicone emulsion, sorbitan monolaurate, stearic acid, titanium dioxide

---

*may contain these ingredients

Questions or comments?
1-800-468-7746

How Supplied: Caplets available in 24 ct., 50 ct. and 100 ct. cartons. Tablets available in 2 ct., 10 ct., 24 ct., 50 ct. and 100 ct. cartons. Geltabs available in 24 ct., 50 ct., and 100 ct. cartons.

Shown in Product Identification Guide, page 513

EXCEDRIN® SINUS HEADACHE
(Novartis Consumer Health, Inc.)
Acetaminophen and Phenylephrine HCl

Drug Facts
Active Ingredients:
(in each caplet/tablet)   **Purposes:**

Acetaminophen
   325 mg .... Pain reliever
Phenylephrine HCl
   5 mg .... Nasal decongestant

Uses:

- temporarily relieves:
  - headache • minor aches and pains
  - nasal congestion • sinus congestion and pressure
  - helps clear nasal passages; shrinks swollen membranes

Warnings:

Alcohol warning: If you consume 3 or more alcoholic drinks every day, ask your doctor whether you should take acetaminophen or other pain relievers/fever re-

ducers. Acetaminophen may cause liver damage.

Do not use
- with any other products containing acetaminophen. Taking more than directed may cause liver damage.
- if you are now taking a prescription monoamine oxidase inhibitor (MAOI) (certain drugs for depression, psychiatric or emotional conditions, or Parkinson's disease), or for 2 weeks after stopping the MAOI drug. If you do not know if your prescription drug contains an MAOI, ask a doctor or pharmacist before taking this product.

Ask a doctor before use if you have
- trouble urinating due to an enlarged prostate gland
- heart disease • high blood pressure
- thyroid disease • diabetes

When using this product
- do not use more than directed

Stop use and ask a doctor if
- new symptoms occur
- you get nervous, dizzy, or sleepless
- redness or swelling is present
- pain or nasal congestion gets worse or lasts more than 7 days
- fever gets worse or lasts more than 3 days

If pregnant or breast-feeding, ask a health professional before use.

Keep out of reach of children.

Overdose warning:

Taking more than the recommended dose can cause serious health problems. In case of overdose, get medical help or contact a Poison Control Center right away. Quick medical attention is critical for adults as well as for children even if you do not notice any signs or symptoms.

Directions:
- do not use more than directed (see overdose warning)
- children under 12 years of age: ask a doctor
- adults and children 12 years of age and over: take 2 caplets or tablets, every 4 hours
- do not take more than 12 caplets or tablets in 24 hours

Other Information:
- store at room temperature
- read all product information before using.

Inactive Ingredients: benzoic acid, carnauba wax, corn starch, FD&C blue # 1, hypromellose, magnesium stearate, microcrystalline cellulose, mineral oil, polysorbate 20, povidone, propylene glycol, simethicone emulsion, sorbitan monolaurate, stearic acid, titanium dioxide

Questions or comments?
1–800–468–7746

How Supplied:
Caplets available in 2 ct., 24 ct., 50 ct., 100 ct. & 250 ct. cartons.

Tablets available in 10 ct., 24 ct., 50 ct. & 100 ct. cartons.

EXCEDRIN® TENSION HEADACHE (Novartis Consumer Health, Inc.)
PAIN RELIEVER

Drug Facts

Active Ingredients   Purpose:
(in each geltab/tablets/caplets):
Acetaminophen
   500 mg .... Pain reliever
(formulated with 65 mg caffeine)

Uses:
- temporarily relieves minor aches and pains due to:
  - headache • muscular aches

Warnings:

Alcohol warning: If you consume 3 or more alcoholic drinks every day, ask your doctor whether you should take acetaminophen or other pain relievers/fever reducers. Acetaminophen may cause liver damage.

Caffeine warning: The recommended dose of this product contains about as much caffeine as a cup of coffee. Limit the use of caffeine-containing medications, foods, or beverages while taking this product because too much caffeine may cause nervousness, irritability, sleeplessness, and, occasionally, rapid heartbeat.

Do not use
- with any other products containing acetaminophen. Taking more than directed may cause liver damage.

Stop use and ask a doctor if
- new symptoms occur
- symptoms do not get better or worsen
- painful area is red or swollen
- pain gets worse or lasts for more than 10 days
- fever gets worse or lasts for more than 3 days

If pregnant or breast-feeding, ask a health professional before use.

Keep out of reach of children.

Overdose warning: Taking more than the recommended dose can cause serious health problems. In case of overdose, get medical help or contact a Poison Control Center right away. Quick medical attention is critical for adults as well as for children even if you do not notice any signs or symptoms.

Directions:
- do not use more than directed (see overdose warning)
- adults and children 12 years of age and over: take 2 geltabs, tablets or caplets every 6 hours; not more than 8 geltabs, tablets or caplets in 24 hours
- children under 12 years of age: ask a doctor

Other Information:
- store at room temperature

Inactive Ingredients:
Tablets/Caplets
benzoic acid, corn starch, croscarmellose sodium*, FD&C blue #1, FD&C red #40, FD&C yellow #6, gelatin, hypromellose, magnesium stearate, methylparaben*, microcrystalline cellulose, mineral oil, polysorbate 20, povidone, pregelatinized starch, propylene glycol, propylparaben*, simethicone emulsion, sorbitan monolaurate, stearic acid, titanium dioxide
Geltabs
benzoic acid, corn starch, croscarmellose sodium*, FD&C blue #1, FD&C red #40, FD&C yellow #6, gelatin, glycerin, hypromellose, magnesium stearate, methylparaben*, microcrystalline cellulose, mineral oil, polysorbate 20, povidone, pregelatinized starch, propylene glycol, propylparaben*, simethicone emulsion, sorbitan monolaurate, stearic acid, titanium dioxide

---

*may contain these ingredients

Questions or comments?
1-800-468-7746

How Supplied: Tablets in 24 ct., 50 ct., 100 ct. and 250 ct. cartons. Caplets in 24 ct., 50 ct., 100 ct. and 250 ct. cartons. Geltabs in 24 ct., 50 ct., and 100 ct. cartons.
Shown in Product Identification Guide, page 513

EXCEDRIN® EXTRA STRENGTH (Novartis Consumer Health, Inc.)
PAIN RELIEVER

For full product information see page 684.

**GOODY'S
(GlaxoSmithKline Consumer)
Body Pain Formula Powder**

For full product information see page 684.

**GOODY'S®
(GlaxoSmithKline Consumer)
Extra Strength Headache Powder**

Indications: For Temporary Relief of Minor Aches & Pains Due to Headaches, Arthritis, Colds & Fever

Directions: Adults: Place one powder on tongue and follow with liquid or stir powder into a glass of water or other liquid. May be repeated in 4 to 6 hours. Do not take more than 4 powders in any 24-hour period. Children under 12 years of age: Consult a doctor.

Warnings: Children and teenagers should not use this medicine for chicken pox or flu symptoms before a doctor is consulted about Reye's Syndrome, a

Continued on next page

Goody's Headache—Cont.

rare but serious illness reported to be associated with aspirin. **Do not use** with any other product containing acetaminophen. **Ask a doctor before use if you have** asthma, ulcers, a bleeding problem, stomach problems that last or come back such as heartburn, upset stomach or pain. **Ask a doctor or pharmacist before use if** you are taking a prescription drug for gout, diabetes, arthritis or anticoagulation (blood thinning). **When using this product** limit the use of caffeine containing drugs, foods, or drinks, because too much caffeine may cause nervousness, irritability, sleeplessness, and occasionally, rapid heartbeat. **Stop use and ask a doctor if** an allergic reaction occurs, ringing in ears or loss of hearing occurs, pain gets worse or persists for more than 10 days, fever lasts for more than 3 days, redness or swelling is present, or new symptoms occur. As with any drug, if you are pregnant, or nursing a baby, seek the advice of a health professional before using this product. **IT IS ESPECIALLY IMPORTANT NOT TO USE ASPIRIN DURING THE LAST 3 MONTHS OF PREGNANCY UNLESS SPECIFICALLY DIRECTED TO DO SO BY A DOCTOR BECAUSE IT MAY CAUSE PROBLEMS IN THE UNBORN CHILD OR COMPLICATIONS DURING DELIVERY. Alcohol Warning:** If you consume 3 or more alcoholic drinks every day, ask your doctor whether you should take acetaminophen and aspirin or other pain relievers/fever reducers. Acetaminophen and aspirin may cause liver damage and stomach bleeding. **Keep this and all medicines out of the reach of children. Overdose warning:** Taking more than the recommended dose can cause serious health problems. In case of overdose, contact a doctor or poison control center immediately.

Active Ingredients: Each Powder contains 520 mg. aspirin in combination with 260 mg. acetaminophen and 32.5 mg. caffeine.

Inactive Ingredients: Lactose Monohydrate and Potassium Chloride.

GOODY'S®
(GlaxoSmithKline Consumer)
Extra Strength Pain Relief Tablets

For full product information see page 685.

GOODY'S PM® POWDER
(GlaxoSmithKline Consumer)
For Pain with Sleeplessness

Indications: For temporary relief of occasional headaches and minor aches and pains with accompanying sleeplessness.

Directions: Adults and children 12 years of age and older: One dose (2 pow-

ders). Take both powders at bedtime, if needed, or as directed by a doctor. Place powders on tongue and follow with liquid. If you prefer, stir powders into glass of water or other liquid.

Warnings: Keep this and all medicines out of the reach of children. Overdose Warning: Taking more than the recommended dose can cause serious health problems. In case of accidental overdose, contact a doctor or poison control center immediately. Prompt medical attention is critical for adults as well as for children even if you do not notice any signs or symptoms.
As with any drug, if you are pregnant or nursing a baby, seek the advice of a health professional before using this product. Do not give this product to children under 12 years of age. Do not use for more than 10 days or for fever for more than 3 days unless directed by a doctor. Consult your doctor if redness or swelling is present, symptoms persist or get worse or new ones occur. If sleeplessness persists continuously for more than 2 weeks consult your doctor. Insomnia may be a symptom of serious underlying medical illness. Do not take this product, unless directed by a doctor, if you have a breathing problem such as emphysema or chronic bronchitis or if you have glaucoma or diffiiculty in urination due to enlargement of the prostate gland. **Do Not Use** with any other product containing diphenhydramine, including one applied topically, or with any other product containing acetaminophen. Avoid alcoholic beverages while taking this product. Do not use this product if you are taking sedatives or tranquilizers without first consulting your doctor. **Alcohol Warning:** If you consume 3 or more alcoholic drinks every day, ask your doctor whether you should take acetaminophen or other pain relievers/ fever reducers. Acetaminophen may cause liver damage.

Caution: This product will cause drowsiness. Do not drive a motor vehicle or operate machinery after use.

Active Ingredients: Each powder contains 500 mg. Acetaminophen and 38 mg. Diphenhydramine Citrate.

Inactive Ingredients: Citric Acid, Docusate Sodium, Fumaric Acid, Glycine, Lactose Monohydrate, Magnesium Stearate, Potassium Chloride, Silica Gel, Sodium Citrate Dihydrate.

CHILDREN'S MOTRIN® Cold
(McNeil Consumer)
ibuprofen/pseudoephedrine HCl
Oral Suspension

For full product information see page 733.

INFANTS' MOTRIN® ibuprofen Concentrated Drops (McNeil Consumer)

CHILDREN'S MOTRIN® ibuprofen Oral Suspension

JUNIOR STRENGTH MOTRIN® ibuprofen Caplets and Chewable Tablets
Product information for all dosages of Children's MOTRIN have been combined under this heading

For full product information see page 685.

MOTRIN® IB (Ibuprofen)
Pain Reliever/Fever Reducer
Tablets and Caplets (McNeil Consumer)

For full product information see page 687.

THERAFLU® Nighttime Severe Cold
(Novartis Consumer Health, Inc.)
Pain Reliever-Fever Reducer (Acetaminophen)
Antihistamine (Pheniramine maleate)
Nasal Decongestant (Phenylephrine HCl)

For full product information see page 740.

THERAFLU® Cold & Cough
(Novartis Consumer Health, Inc.)
Cough Suppressant (Dextromethorphan HBr)
Antihistamine (Pheniramine maleate)
Nasal Decongestant (Phenylephrine HCl)

For full product information see page 740.

THERAFLU® Cold & Sore Throat
(Novartis Consumer Health, Inc.)
Pain Reliever-Fever Reducer (Acetaminophen)
Antihistamine (Pheniramine maleate)
Nasal Decongestant (Phenylephrine HCl)

For full product information see page 742.

THERAFLU® Flu & Chest Congestion
(Novartis Consumer Health, Inc.)
Pain Reliever-Fever Reducer (Acetaminophen)
Expectorant (Guaifenesin)

For full product information see page 741.

THERAFLU® Flu & Sore Throat
(Novartis Consumer Health, Inc.)
Pain Reliever-Fever Reducer (Acetaminophen)
Antihistamine (Pheniramine maleate)
Nasal Decongestant (Phenylephrine HCl)

For full product information see page 741.

THERAFLU® Daytime Severe Cold (Novartis Consumer Health, Inc.)
Pain Reliever-Fever Reducer (Acetaminophen)
Nasal Decongestant (Phenylephrine HCl)

For full product information see page 742.

THERAFLU® DAYTIME WARMING RELIEF
(Novartis Consumer Health, Inc.)
Pain Reliever/Fever Reducer/Cough Suppressant/Nasal Decongestant

For full product information see page 743.

THERAFLU® NIGHTTIME WARMING RELIEF
(Novartis Consumer Health, Inc.)
Cough Suppressant/Antihistamine/Pain Reliever/Fever Reducer/Nasal Decongestant

For full product information see page 743.

TRIAMINIC® COUGH & SORE THROAT
(Novartis Consumer Health, Inc.)
Pain Reliever/Fever Reducer/Cough Suppressant

For full product information see page 747.

CHILDREN'S TYLENOL® Plus Cold & Allergy (McNeil Consumer)

For full product information see page 716.

CHILDREN'S TYLENOL® Plus Flu (McNeil Consumer)

For full product information see page 749.

CONCENTRATED TYLENOL®
acetaminophen Infants' Drops
(McNeil Consumer)

CHILDREN'S TYLENOL®
acetaminophen Suspension Liquid and Meltaways

JR. TYLENOL®
acetaminophen Meltaways

CHILDREN'S TYLENOL®
Suspension with Flavor Creator

Product information for all dosages of Children's TYLENOL have been combined under this heading

For full product information see page 754.

REGULAR STRENGTH TYLENOL®
acetaminophen Tablets (McNeil Consumer)

EXTRA STRENGTH TYLENOL®
acetaminophen Geltabs, Caplets, Cool Caplets, and EZ Tabs

EXTRA STRENGTH TYLENOL®
acetaminophen Rapid Release Gels

EXTRA STRENGTH TYLENOL®
acetaminophen Adult Liquid Pain Reliever

TYLENOL® Arthritis Pain Acetaminophen Extended Release Geltabs/Caplets

TYLENOL® 8 Hour Acetaminophen Extended Release Caplets

Product information for all dosage forms of Adult TYLENOL acetaminophen have been combined under this heading.

For full product information see page 695.

TYLENOL® Severe Allergy Caplets (McNeil Consumer)

TYLENOL® Allergy Multi-Symptom Caplets with Cool Burst™ and Gelcaps

TYLENOL® Allergy Multi-Symptom Nighttime Caplets with Cool Burst™

For full product information see page 717.

TYLENOL® Chest Congestion Caplets with Cool Burst™ (McNeil Consumer)

TYLENOL® Chest Congestion Liquid with Cool Burst™

For full product information see page 722.

TYLENOL® Cold Head Congestion Daytime Caplets with Cool Burst™ and Gelcaps (McNeil Consumer)

TYLENOL® Cold Head Congestion Nighttime Caplets with Cool Burst™

TYLENOL® Cold Head Congestion Severe Caplets with Cool Burst™

For full product information see page 750.

TYLENOL® COLD
Severe Congestion Non-Drowsy Caplets with Cool Burst™ (McNeil Consumer)

For full product information see page 751.

TYLENOL® Cold Multi-Symptom Daytime Caplets with Cool Burst™ and Gelcaps (McNeil Consumer)

TYLENOL® Cold Multi-Symptom Nighttime Caplets with Cool Burst™

TYLENOL® Cold Multi-Symptom Severe Caplets with Cool Burst™

TYLENOL® Cold Multi-Symptom Daytime Liquid

TYLENOL® Cold Multi-Symptom Nighttime Liquid with Cool Burst™

TYLENOL® Cold Multi-Symptom Severe Daytime Liquid

For full product information see page 752.

TYLENOL® Sinus Congestion & Pain Daytime Caplets with Cool Burst™ and Gelcaps (McNeil Consumer)

TYLENOL® Sinus Congestion & Pain Nighttime Caplets with Cool Burst™

TYLENOL® Sinus Congestion & Pain Severe Caplets with Cool Burst™

TYLENOL® Sinus Severe Congestion Caplets with Cool Burst™
Product information for all dosage forms of TYLENOL Sinus have been combined under this heading.

For full product information see page 778.

TYLENOL® Sore Throat Daytime Liquid with Cool Burst™ (McNeil Consumer)

TYLENOL® Sore Throat Nighttime Liquid with Cool Burst™

TYLENOL® Cough & Sore Throat Daytime Liquid with Cool Burst™

TYLENOL® Cough & Sore Throat Nighttime Liquid with Cool Burst™

For full product information see page 790.

CONCENTRATED TYLENOL®
Infants' Drops Plus Cold Nasal Decongestant, Fever Reducer & Pain Reliever (McNeil Consumer)

CONCENTRATED TYLENOL®
Infants' Drops Plus Cold & Cough Nasal Decongestant, Fever Reducer & Pain Reliever, Cough Suppressant

Continued on next page

Tylenol—Cont.

CHILDREN'S TYLENOL® Plus Cough & Sore Throat Suspension Liquid

CHILDREN'S TYLENOL® Plus Cough & Runny Nose Suspension Liquid

CHILDREN'S TYLENOL® Plus Multi-Symptom Cold Suspension Liquid

CHILDREN'S TYLENOL® Plus Cold Suspension Liquid

For full product information see page 754.

**VICKS® 44M® (Procter & Gamble)
COUGH, COLD & FLU RELIEF**
Cough Suppressant/Antihistamine/Pain Reliever–Fever Reducer Alcohol 10%
Maximum strength cough formula
For full product information see page 760.

VICKS® DAYQUIL® LIQUID (Procter & Gamble)

**VICKS® DAYQUIL® LIQUICAPS®
Multi-Symptom Cold/Flu Relief
Nasal Decongestant/Pain Reliever/
Cough Suppressant/Fever Reducer
Non-drowsy**

For full product information see page 761.

**VICKS® NYQUIL® LIQUICAPS®/
LIQUID MULTI-SYMPTOM COLD/
FLU RELIEF (Proctor & Gamble)**

For full product information see page 763.

ZICAM® Flu Daytime (Matrixx)

ZICAM® Nighttime

For full product information see page 768.

Central Nervous System:
Sleeplessness

ADVIL PM CAPLETS (Wyeth Consumer)
Pain reliever (NSAID)/Nighttime sleep-aid

Active Ingredients (in each caplet):
Diphenhydramine citrate 38 mg
Ibuprofen 200 mg (NSAID)*

*nonsteroidal anti-inflammatory drug

Uses:
- for relief of occasional sleeplessness when associated with minor aches and pains
- helps you fall asleep and stay asleep

Warnings:
Allergy alert: Ibuprofen may cause a severe allergic reaction, especially in people allergic to aspirin. Symptoms may include:
- hives
- facial swelling
- asthma (wheezing)
- shock
- skin reddening
- rash
- blisters

If an allergic reaction occurs, stop use and seek medical help right away.

Stomach bleeding warning: This product contains a nonsteroidal anti-inflammatory drug (NSAID), which may cause stomach bleeding. The chance is higher if you:
- are age 60 or older
- have had stomach ulcers or bleeding problems
- take a blood thinning (anticoagulant) or steroid drug
- take other drugs containing an NSAID [aspirin, ibuprofen, naproxen, or others]
- have 3 or more alcoholic drinks every day while using this product
- take more or for a longer time than directed

Do not use
- if you have ever had an allergic reaction to any other pain reliever/fever reducer
- unless you have time for a full night's sleep
- in children under 12 years of age
- right before or after heart surgery
- with any other product containing diphenhydramine, even one used on skin
- if you have sleeplessness without pain

Ask a doctor before use if you have
- a breathing problem such as emphysema or chronic bronchitis
- problems or serious side effects from taking pain relievers or fever reducers

- stomach problems that last or come back, such as heartburn, upset stomach or stomach pain
- ulcers
- bleeding problems
- high blood pressure
- heart or kidney disease
- taken a diuretic
- reached age 60 or older
- glaucoma
- trouble urinating due to an enlarged prostate gland

Ask a doctor or pharmacist before use if you are
- taking sedatives or tranquilizers, or any other sleep-aid
- taking any other drug containing an NSAID (prescription or nonprescription)
- under a doctor's care for any continuing medical illness
- taking any other antihistamines
- taking a blood thinning (anticoagulant) or steroid drug
- taking aspirin to prevent heart attack or stroke, because ibuprofen may decrease this benefit of aspirin
- taking any other drug

When using this product
- drowsiness will occur
- avoid alcoholic drinks
- do not drive a motor vehicle or operate machinery
- take with food or milk if stomach upset occurs
- long term continuous use may increase the risk of heart attack or stroke

Stop use and ask a doctor if
- you feel faint, vomit blood, or have bloody or black stools. These are signs of stomach bleeding.
- pain gets worse or lasts more than 10 days
- sleeplessness persists continuously for more than 2 weeks. Insomnia may be a symptom of a serious underlying medical illness.
- stomach pain or upset gets worse or lasts
- redness or swelling is present in the painful area
- any new symptoms appear

If pregnant or breast-feeding, ask a health professional before use. It is especially important not to use ibuprofen during the last 3 months of pregnancy unless definitely directed to do so by a doctor because it may cause problems in the unborn child or complications during delivery.

Keep out of the reach of children. In case of overdose, get medical help or contact a Poison Control Center right away.

Directions:
- **do not take more than directed**
- do not take longer than 10 days, unless directed by a doctor (see Warnings)
- adults and children 12 years and over: take 2 caplets at bedtime
- do not take more than 2 caplets in 24 hours

Other Information:
- read all warnings and directions before use. Keep carton.
- store at 20–25°C (68–77°F)
- avoid excessive heat above 40°C (104°F)

Inactive Ingredients:
calcium stearate, carnauba wax, colloidal silicon dioxide, croscarmellose sodium, FD&C blue no. 2, FD&C blue no. 2 aluminum lake, glyceryl behenate, hypromellose, lactose monohydrate, microcrystalline cellulose, polydextrose, polyethylene glycol, pregelatinized starch, propylene glycol, sodium lauryl sulfate, sodium starch glycolate, starch, stearic acid, titanium dioxide

How Supplied:
Bottle of 20, 40, 80 and 180 caplets

EXCEDRIN PM®
(Novartis Consumer Health, Inc.)
PAIN RELIEVER/NIGHTTIME SLEEP AID

For full product information see page 610.

NYTOL® QUICKCAPS® CAPLETS
(GlaxoSmithKline Consumer)

Indication: For relief of occasional sleeplessness.

Directions: Adults and children 12 years of age and over: oral dosage is two caplets (50 mg) at bedtime if needed, or as directed by a doctor.

Warnings: Do not give to children under 12 years of age. If sleeplessness persists continuously for more than two weeks, consult your doctor. Insomnia may be a symptom of serious underlying medical illness. **Do not take this product, unless directed by a doctor, if you have a breathing problem such as emphysema or chronic bronchitis, or if you have glaucoma or difficulty in urination due to enlargement of the prostate gland. Do not use** with any other product containing diphenhydramine, including one applied topically. Avoid alcoholic beverages while taking this product. Do not take this product if you are taking seda-

Continued on next page

Nytol Caplets—Cont.

tives or tranquilizers, without first consulting your doctor. In case of accidental overdose, seek professional assistance or contact a Poison Control Center immediately. As with any drug, if you are pregnant or nursing a baby, seek the advice of a health professional before using this product. Keep out of reach of children.

Drug Interactions: Alcohol and other drugs which cause CNS depression will heighten the depressant effect of this product. Monoamine oxidase (MAO) inhibitors will prolong and intensify the anticholinergic effects of antihistamines.

Symptoms and Treatment of Oral Overdosage: In adults, overdose may cause CNS depression resulting in hypnosis and coma. In children, CNS hyperexcitability may follow sedation; the stimulant phase may bring tremor, delirium and convulsions. Gastrointestinal reactions may include dry mouth, appetite loss, nausea and/or vomiting. Respiratory distress and cardiovascular complications (hypotension) may be evident. Treatment includes inducing emesis and controlling symptoms.

Active Ingredient: Diphenhydramine Hydrochloride 25 mg per caplet.

Inactive Ingredients: Corn Starch, Lactose, Microcrystalline Cellulose, Silica, Stearic Acid.

How Supplied: Available in tamper-evident packages of 16, 32 and 72 caplets.
Shown in Product Identification Guide, page 506

MAXIMUM STRENGTH

NYTOL® QUICKGELS® SOFTGELS
(GlaxoSmithKline Consumer)

Indication: For relief of occasional sleeplessness.

Directions: Adults and children 12 years of age and over: oral dosage is one softgel (50 mg) at bedtime if needed, or as directed by a doctor.

Warnings: Do not give to children under 12 years of age. If sleeplessness persists continuously for more than two weeks, consult your doctor. Insomnia may be a symptom of serious underlying medical illness. **Do not take this product, unless directed by a doctor, if you have a breathing problem such as emphysema or chronic bronchitis, or if you have glaucoma or difficulty in urination due to enlargement of the prostate gland. Do not use** with any other product containing diphenhydramine, including one applied topically. Avoid alcoholic beverages while taking this product. Do not take this product if you are taking sedatives or tranquilizers, without first consulting your doctor. In case of accidental overdose, seek professional assistance or

contact a Poison Control Center immediately. As with any drug, if you are pregnant or nursing a baby, seek the advice of a health professional before using this product. Keep out of reach of children.

Drug Interactions: Alcohol and other drugs which cause CNS depression will heighten the depressant effect of this product. Monoamine oxidase (MAO) inhibitors will prolong and intensify the anticholinergic effects of antihistamines.

Symptoms and Treatment of Oral Overdosage: In adults overdose may cause CNS depression resulting in hypnosis and coma. In children CNS hyperexcitability may follow sedation; the stimulant phase may bring tremor, delirium and convulsions. Gastrointestinal reactions may include dry mouth, appetite loss, nausea and/or vomiting. Respiratory distress and cardiovascular complications (hypotension) may be evident. Treatment includes inducing emesis and controlling symptoms.

Active Ingredient: Diphenhydramine Hydrochloride 50 mg per softgel.

Inactive Ingredients: Edible Ink, Gelatin, Glycerin, Polyethylene Glycol, Purified Water, Sorbitol.

How Supplied: Available in packages of 8 and 16 softgels.
Shown in Product Identification Guide, page 506

SIMPLY SLEEP™
Nighttime Sleep Aid
(McNeil Consumer)

Description:
SIMPLY SLEEP™ is a non habit-forming nighttime sleep aid. Each *SIMPLY SLEEP*™ Caplet contains diphenhydramine HCl 25 mg.

Actions:
SIMPLY SLEEP™ contains an antihistamine (diphenhydramine HCl) which has sedative properties.

Use:
relief of occasional sleeplessness

Directions:
• **do not take more than directed (see overdose warning)**

adults and children 12 years and over	take 2 caplets at bedtime if needed or as directed by a doctor
children under 12 years	do not use

Warnings:
Do not use
• with any other product containing diphenhydramine, even one used on skin
• in children under 12 years of age

Ask a doctor before use if you have
• a breathing problem such as emphysema or chronic bronchitis
• trouble urinating due to an enlarged prostate gland
• glaucoma

Ask a doctor or pharmacist before use if you are taking sedatives or tranquilizers
When using this product
• drowsiness may occur
• avoid alcoholic drinks

Stop use and ask a doctor if
• sleeplessness persists continuously for more than 2 weeks. Insomnia may be a symptom of serious underlying medical illness.

If pregnant or breast-feeding, ask a health professional before use.
Keep out of reach of children. In case of overdose, get medical help or contact a Poison Control Center (1-800-222-1222) right away.

Other Information:
• one caplet contains: **calcium 20 mg**
• store between 20–25°C (68–77°F)

Inactive Ingredients: carnauba wax, cellulose, croscarmellose sodium, dibasic calcium phosphate, FD&C Blue #1, hypromellose, magnesium stearate, polyethylene glycol, polysorbate 80, titanium dioxide

How Supplied:
Light blue mini-caplets embossed with "SL" on one side in blister packs of 24 and 48, 100 & 130 count bottles.
Shown in Product Identification Guide, page 509

SOMINEX Original Formula
(GlaxoSmithKline Consumer)
Nighttime Sleep Aid
Doctor-preferred sleep ingredient

Indications: Helps to reduce difficulty falling asleep.

Directions: Adults and children 12 years and over: Take 2 tablets at bedtime if needed, or as directed by a doctor. For best results, take recommended dose. This will provide approximately six to eight hours of restful sleep.

Warnings: Do not give to children under 12 years of age. If sleeplessness persists continually for more than 2 weeks, consult your doctor. Insomnia may be a symptom of serious underlying medical illness. Do not take this product, unless directed by a doctor, if you have a breathing problem such as emphysema or chronic bronchitis, or if you have glaucoma or difficulty in urination due to enlargement of the prostate gland. Avoid alcoholic beverages while taking this product. Do not take this product if you are taking sedatives or tranquilizers, without first consulting your doctor. As with any drug, if you are pregnant or nursing a baby, seek the advice of a health professional before using this product.

Keep this and all drugs out of the reach of children. In case of accidental overdose, seek professional assistance or contact a poison control center immediately.

Active Ingredients: Each tablet contains 25 mg Diphenhydramine HCl.

Inactive Ingredients: Dibasic Calcium Phosphate, FD&C Blue #1, Magnesium Stearate, Microcrystalline Cellulose, Silicon Dioxide, Starch.

Tamper Evident Feature: Individually sealed in foil for your protection. Do not use if foil or plastic bubble is torn or punctured.

Store at room temperature, avoid excessive heat (greater than 100°F) or humidity.

How Supplied: Consumer Packages of 16, 32 and 72 tablets

Also Available in Maximum Strength Formula.

Comments or Questions? Call Toll-Free 1-800-245-1040 Weekdays.

GlaxoSmithKline Consumer Healthcare, L.P.

Moon Township, PA 15108. Made in U.S.A.

**EXTRA STRENGTH
TYLENOL® PM
(McNeil Consumer)**

Pain Reliever/Sleep Aid Caplets, Vanilla Caplets, Geltabs, Gelcaps, and Liquid

For full product information see page 694.

Central Nervous System:
Smoking Cessation

NICODERM® CQ®
(GlaxoSmithKline Consumer)
Nicotine Transdermal System/Stop Smoking Aid

Formerly available only by prescription. Available as:

> Step 1 - 21 mg/24 hours
> Step 2 - 14 mg/24 hours
> Step 3 - 7 mg/24 hours

If you smoke:
More than 10 Cigarettes per Day: Start with Step 1
10 Cigarettes a Day or Less: Start with Step 2
WHAT IS THE NICODERM CQ PATCH AND HOW IS IT USED?
NicoDerm CQ is a small, nicotine containing patch. When you put on a NicoDerm CQ patch, nicotine passes through the skin and into your body. NicoDerm CQ is very thin and uses special material to control how fast nicotine passes through the skin. Unlike the sudden jolts of nicotine delivered by cigarettes, the amount of nicotine you receive remains relatively smooth throughout the 24 or 16 hours period you wear the NicoDerm CQ patch. This helps to reduce cravings you may have for nicotine.

Active Ingredient: Nicotine

Purpose: Stop Smoking Aid

Use: reduces withdrawal symptoms, including nicotine craving, associated with quitting smoking

Directions:
- **if you are under 18 years of age, ask a doctor before use**
- before using this product, read the enclosed user's guide for complete directions and other information
- stop smoking completely when you begin using the patch
- **if you smoke more than 10 cigarettes per day,** use according to the following 10 week schedule:

STEP 1	STEP 2	STEP 3
Use one 21 mg patch/day	Use one 14 mg patch/day	Use one 7 mg patch/day
Weeks 1–6	Weeks 7–8	Weeks 9–10

- if you smoke **10 or less cigarettes per day,** do not use **STEP 1 (21 mg)**. Start with **STEP 2 (14 mg)** for 6 weeks, then **STEP 3 (7 mg)** for two weeks and then stop.
- steps 2 and 3 allow you to gradually reduce your level of nicotine. Completing the full program will increase your chances of quitting successfully.
- apply one new patch every 24 hours on skin that is dry, clean and hairless
- remove backing from patch and immediately press onto skin. Hold for 10 seconds.
- wash hands after applying or removing patch. Throw away the patch in the enclosed disposal tray. See enclosed user's guide for safety and handling.
- you may wear the patch for 16 or 24 hours
- if you crave cigarettes when you wake up, wear the patch for 24 hours
- if you have vivid dreams or other sleep disturbances, you may remove the patch at bedtime and apply a new one in the morning
- the used patch should be removed and a new one applied to a different skin site at the same time each day
- do not wear more than one patch at a time
- do not cut patch in half or into smaller pieces
- do not leave patch on for more than 24 hours because it may irritate your skin and loses strength after 24 hours
- stop using the patch at the end of 10 weeks. If you started with **STEP 2**, stop using the patch at the end of 8 weeks. If you still feel the need to use the patch talk to your doctor.

Warnings:
If you are pregnant or breast-feeding, only use this medicine on the advice of your health care provider. Smoking can seriously harm your child. Try to stop smoking without using any nicotine replacement medicine. This medicine is believed to be safer than smoking. However, the risks to your child from this medicine are not fully known.
Do Not Use
- if you continue to smoke, chew tobacco, use snuff, or use a nicotine gum or other nicotine containing products
Ask a doctor before use if you have
- heart disease, recent heart attack, or irregular heartbeat. Nicotine can increase your heart rate.
- high blood pressure not controlled with medication. Nicotine can increase your blood pressure.
- an allergy to adhesive tape or skin problems because you are more likely to get rashes
Ask a doctor or pharmacist before use if you are
- using a non-nicotine stop smoking drug
- taking a prescription medication for depression or asthma. Your prescription dose may need to be adjusted.
When using this product

- do not smoke even when not wearing the patch. The nicotine in your skin will still be entering your blood stream for several hours after you take off the patch.
- if you have vivid dreams or other sleep disturbances remove this patch at bedtime
Stop use and ask a doctor if
- skin redness caused by the patch does not go away after four days, or if skin swells, or you get a rash
- irregular heartbeat or palpitations occur
- you get symptoms of nicotine overdose such as nausea, vomiting, dizziness, weakness and rapid heartbeat
Keep out of reach of children and pets. Used patches have enough nicotine to poison children and pets. If swallowed, get medical help or contact a Poison Control Center right away. Dispose of the used patches by folding sticky ends together and inserting in disposal tray in this box.
READ THE LABEL
Read the carton and the User's Guide before using this product. Keep the carton and User's Guide. They contain important information.

Inactive Ingredients: Ethylene vinyl acetate-copolymer, polyisobutylene and high density polyethylene between pigmented and clear polyester backings. Store at 20–25°C (68–77°F)
TO INCREASE YOUR SUCCESS IN QUITTING:
1. You must be motivated to quit.
2. Complete the full treatment program, applying a new patch every day.
3. Use with a support program as described in the Users Guide.
NicoDerm CQ User's Guide
KEYS TO SUCCESS
1) You must really want to quit smoking for **NicoDerm® CQ®** to help you.
2) Complete the full program, applying a new patch every day.
3) **NicoDerm CQ** works best when used together with a support program: See page3 for details.
4) If you have trouble using **NicoDerm CQ**, ask your doctor or pharmacist or call GlaxoSmithKline 1-800-834-5895 weekdays (10:00 am 4:30 pm EST).
SO, YOU'VE DECIDED TO QUIT.
Congratulations. Your decision to stop smoking is one of the most important things you can do to improve your health. Quitting smoking is a two-part process that involves:
1) overcoming your physical need for nicotine, and
2) breaking your smoking habit.
NicoDerm CQ helps smokers quit by reducing nicotine withdrawal symptoms.

Many NicoDerm CQ users will be able to stop smoking for a few days but often will start smoking again. Most smokers have to try to quit several times before they completely stop.

Your own chances of quitting smoking depend on how strongly you are addicted to nicotine, how much you want to quit, and how closely you follow a quitting plan like the one that comes with NicoDerm CQ.

QUITTING SMOKING IS HARD!

If you find you cannot stop or if you start smoking again after using NicoDerm CQ please talk to a health care professional who can help you find a program that may work better for you. Breaking this addiction doesn't happen overnight.

Because NicoDerm CQ provides some nicotine, the NicoDerm CQ patch will help you stop smoking by reducing nicotine withdrawal symptoms such as nicotine craving, nervousness and irritability.

This User's Guide will give you support as you become a non-smoker. It will answer common questions about NicoDerm CQ and give tips to help you stop smoking, and should be referred to often.

WHERE TO GET HELP.

You are more likely to stop smoking by using NicoDerm CQ with a support program that helps you break your smoking habit. There may be support groups in your area for people trying to quit. Call your local chapter of the American Lung Association, American Cancer Society or American Heart Association for further information. Toll free phone numbers are printed on the wallet card on the back cover of this User's Guide.

If you find you cannot stop smoking or if you start smoking again after using NicoDerm CQ, remember breaking this addiction doesn't happen overnight. You may want to talk to a health care professional who can help you improve your chances of quitting the next time you try NicoDerm CQ or another method.

LET'S GET ORGANIZED.

Your reason for quitting may be a combination of concerns about health, the effect of smoking on your appearance, and pressure from your family and friends to stop smoking. Or maybe you're concerned about the dangerous effect of second-hand smoke on the people you care about.

All of these are good reasons. You probably have others. Decide your most important reasons, and write them down on the wallet card inside the back cover of this User's Guide. Carry this card with you. In difficult moments, when you want to smoke, the card will remind you why you are quitting.

WHAT YOU'RE UP AGAINST.

Smoking is addictive in two ways. Your need for nicotine has become both physical and mental. You must overcome both addictions to stop smoking. So while NicoDerm CQ will lessen your body's craving for nicotine, you've got to want to quit smoking to overcome the mental dependence on cigarettes. Once you've decided that you're going to quit, it's time

to get started. But first, there are some important cautions you should consider.

SOME IMPORTANT WARNINGS.

This product is only for those who want to stop smoking.

If you are pregnant or breast-feeding, only use this medicine on the advice of your health care provider. Smoking can seriously harm your child. Try to stop smoking without using any nicotine replacement medicine. This medicine is believed to be safer than smoking. However, the risks to your child from this medicine are not fully known.

Do not use
• if you continue to smoke, chew tobacco, use snuff or use a nicotine gum or other nicotine products.

Ask a doctor before use if you have:
• heart disease, recent heart attack, or irregular heartbeat. Nicotine can increase your heart rate.
• high blood pressure not controlled with medication. Nicotine can increase your blood pressure.
• an allergy to adhesive tape or have skin problems because you are more likely to get rashes.

Ask a doctor or pharmacist before use if you are
• using a non-nicotine stop smoking drug
• taking a prescription medication for asthma or depression. Your prescription dose may need to be adjusted.

When using this product:
• do not smoke even when not wearing the patch. The nicotine in your skin will still be entering your bloodstream for several hours after you take off the patch.
• you have vivid dreams or other sleep disturbances remove this patch at bedtime.

Stop use and ask a doctor if:
• skin redness caused by the patch does not go away after four days, or if your skin swells or you get a rash.
• irregular heartbeat or palpitations occur
• you get symptoms of nicotine overdose, such as nausea, vomiting, dizziness, weakness and rapid heartbeat.

Keep out of reach of children and pets. Used patches have enough nicotine to poison children and pets. If swallowed, get medical help or contact a Poison Control Center right away. Dispose of the used patches by folding sticky ends together and inserting in the disposal tray in this box.

LET'S GET STARTED.

If you are under 18 years of age, ask a doctor before use.

Becoming a non-smoker starts today. Your first step is to read through this entire User's Guide carefully.

First, check that you bought the right starting dose.

If you smoke more than 10 cigarettes a day, begin with Step 1 (21 mg). As the carton indicates, people who smoke 10 or less cigarettes per day should not use Step 1 (21 mg). They should start with Step 2 (14 mg). Throughout this User's Guide we

will give specific instructions for people who smoke 10 or less cigarettes per day.

Next, set your personalized quitting schedule.

Take out a calendar that you can use to track your progress. Pick a quit date, and mark this on your calendar using the stickers in the middle of this User's Guide, as described below.

DIRECTIONS: FOR PEOPLE WHO SMOKE MORE THAN 10 CIGARETTES PER DAY

STEP 1. (Weeks 1–6). Your quit date (and the day you'll start using NicoDerm CQ patch).

Choose your quit date (it should be soon). This is the day you will quit smoking cigarettes entirely and begin using NicoDerm CQ to reduce your cravings for nicotine. Place the Step 1 sticker on this date. For the first six weeks, you'll use the highest-strength (21 mg) NicoDerm CQ patches. Be sure to follow the directions on page 10.

Completing the full program will increase your chances of quitting successfully. This is done by changing over to the Step 2 (14mg) patch for 2 weeks followed by a final 2 weeks with the Step 3 (7mg) patch. The Step 2 and Step 3 treatment periods allow you to gradually reduce the amount of nicotine you get, rather than stopping suddenly, and will increase your chances of quitting.

STEP 2. (Weeks 7–8). The day you'll start reducing your use of NicoDerm CQ patch.

Switching to Step 2 (14mg) patches after 6 weeks begins to gradually reduce your nicotine usage. Place the Step 2 sticker on this date (the first day of week seven). Use the 14mg patches for two weeks.

STEP 3. (Weeks 9–10). The day you'll further start reducing your use of NicoDerm CQ patch.

After eight weeks, nicotine intake is further reduced by moving down to Step 3 (7mg) patches. Place the Step 3 sticker on this date (the first day of week nine). Use the 7 mg patches for two weeks.

THE NICODERM CQ PROGRAM

STEP 1	STEP 2	STEP 3
Use one	Use one	Use one
21 mg	14 mg	7 mg
patch/day	patch/day	patch/day
Weeks 1–6	Weeks 7–8	Weeks 9–10

STOP USING NICODERM CQ AT THE END OF WEEK 10. If you still feel the need to use the patch after Week 10, talk with your doctor or health professional.

DIRECTIONS: FOR PEOPLE WHO SMOKE 10 OR LESS CIGARETTES PER DAY

Do not use Step 1 (21 mg).

Begin with STEP 2 – Initial Treatment Period (Weeks 1–6): 14mg patches.

Continued on next page

Nicoderm CQ—Cont.

Choose our quit date (it should be soon). This is the Day you will quit smoking cigarettes entirely and begin using NicoDerm CQ to reduce your cravings for nicotine. Place the Step 2 sticker on this date. For the first six weeks, you'll use the Step 2 (14mg) NicoDerm CQ patches. Be sure to follow the directions on page 10.

Continue with STEP 3 – Step Down Treatment Period (Weeks 7–8): 7mg patches.

Completing the full program will increase your chances of quitting successfully. This is done by changing over to the Step 3 (7mg) patches for 2 weeks. The two week step down treatment period allows you to gradually reduce the amount of nicotine you get, rather than stopping suddenly, and will increase your chances of quitting. Place the Step 3 sticker on the first day of week seven. Use the 7mg patches for two weeks.

People who smoke 10 or less cigarettes per day should not use NicoDerm CQ for longer than 8 weeks. If you still feel the need to use NicoDerm CQ after 8 weeks, talk with your doctor.

PLAN AHEAD.

Because smoking is an addiction, it is not easy to stop. After you've given up nicotine, you may still have a strong urge to smoke. Plan ahead NOW for these times, so you're not tempted to start smoking again in a moment of weakness. The following tips may help:

- Keep the phone numbers of supportive friends and family members handy.
- Keep a record of your quitting process. In the event that you slip, immediately stop smoking and resume your quit attempt with the NicoDerm CQ patch. If you smoke at all, write down what you think caused the slip.
- Put together an Emergency Kit that includes items that will help take your mind off occasional urges to smoke. You might include cinnamon gum or lemon drops to suck on, a relaxing cassette tape, and something for your hands to play with, like a smooth rock, rubber band or small metal balls.
- Set aside some small rewards, like a new magazine or a gift certificate from your favorite store, which you'll "give" yourself after passing difficult hurdles.
- Think now about the times when you most often want a cigarette, and then plan what else you might do instead of smoking. For instance, you might plan to take your coffee break in a new location, or take a walk right after dinner, so you won't be tempted to smoke.

HOW NICODERM CQ WORKS.

NicoDerm CQ patches provide nicotine to your system. They work as a temporary aid to help you quit smoking by reducing nicotine withdrawal symptoms, including nicotine craving. NicoDerm CQ provides a lower level of nicotine to your blood than cigarettes, and allows you to gradually do away with your body's need for nicotine.

Because NicoDerm CQ does not contain the tar or carbon monoxide of cigarette smoke, it does not have the same health dangers as tobacco. However, it still delivers nicotine, the addictive part of cigarette smoke. Nicotine can cause side effects such as headache, nausea, upset stomach, and dizziness.

HOW TO USE NICODERM CQ PATCHES.

Read all the following instructions, and the instructions on the outer carton, before using NicoDerm CQ. Refer to them often to make sure you're using NicoDerm CQ correctly. Please refer to the CD for additional help.

1) Stop smoking completely before you start using NicoDerm CQ.
2) To reduce nicotine craving and other withdrawal symptoms, use NicoDerm CQ according to the directions on pages 6–8.
3) Insert used NicoDerm CQ patches in the child resistant disposal tray provided in the box – safely away from children and pets.

When to apply and remove NicoDerm CQ patches.

Each day apply a new patch to a different place on skin that is dry, clean and hairless. **You can wear a NicoDerm CQ patch for either 16 or 24 hours.** If you crave cigarettes when you wake up, wear the patch for 24 hours. If you begin to have vivid dreams or other disruptions of your sleep while wearing the patch 24 hours, try taking the patch off at bedtime (after about 16 hours) and putting on a new one when you get up the next day.

PLACE THESE STICKERS ON YOUR CALENDAR

STEP 1	STEP 2
A new 21 mg patch every day AT THE BEGINNING OF WEEK #1 (QUIT DAY)	A new 14 mg patch every day AT THE BEGINNING OF WEEK #7

For people who smoke 10 or less cigarettes per day: Do not use STEP 1 (21 mg). Use STEP 2 (14 mg) at the beginning of week #1 and STEP 3 (7 mg) at the beginning of week #7.

PLACE THESE STICKERS ON YOUR CALENDAR

STEP 3	EX-SMOKER
A new 7 mg patch every day AT THE BEGINNING OF WEEK #9	WHEN YOU HAVE COMPLETED YOUR QUITTING PROGRAM

Do not smoke even when you are not wearing the patch.

Remove the used patch and put on a new patch at the same time every day. Applying the patch at about the same time each day (first thing in the morning, for instance) will help you remember when to

put on a new patch. Do not leave the same NicoDerm CQ patch on for more than 24 hours because it may irritate your skin and because it loses strength after 24 hours.

Do not use NicoDerm CQ continuously for more than 10 weeks (8 weeks for people who smoke 10 or less cigarettes per day).

How to apply a NicoDerm CQ patch.

1. Do not remove the NicoDerm CQ patch from its sealed protective pouch until you are ready to use it. NicoDerm CQ patches will lose nicotine to the air if you store them out of the pouch.
2. Choose a non-hairy, clean, dry area of skin. Do not put a NicoDerm CQ patch on skin that is burned, broken out, cut, or irritated in any way. Make sure your skin is free of lotion and soap before applying a patch.
3. A clear, protective liner covers the sticky back side of the NicoDerm CQ patch—the side that will be put on your skin. The liner has a slit down the middle to help you remove it from the patch. With the sticky back side facing you, pull half the liner away from the NicoDerm CQ patch starting at the middle slit, as shown in the illustration above. Hold the NicoDerm CQ patch at one of the outside edges (touch the sticky side as little as possible), and pull off the other half of the protective liner.

Place this liner in the slot in the disposable tray provided in the NicoDerm CQ package where it will be out of reach of children and pets.

4. Immediately apply the sticky side of the NicoDerm CQ patch to your skin. **Press the patch firmly on your skin with the heel of your hand for at least 10 seconds.** Make sure it sticks well to your skin, especially around the edges.

5. Wash your hands when you have finished applying the NicoDerm CQ patch. Nicotine on your hands could get into your eyes and nose, and cause stinging, redness, or more serious problems.

6. After 24 or 16 hours, remove the patch you have been wearing. Fold the used NicoDerm CQ patch in half with the sticky side together. Carefully dispose of the used patch in the slot of the disposal tray provided in the NicoDerm CQ package where it will be out of the reach of children and pets. Even used patches have enough nicotine to poison children and pets. Wash your hands.

7. Choose a different place on your skin to apply the next NicoDerm CQ patch and repeat Steps 1 to 6. Do not apply a new patch to a previously used skin site for at least one week.

If your NicoDerm CQ patch gets wet during wearing.

Water will not harm the NicoDerm CQ patch you are wearing if applied properly. You can bathe, swim, or shower for short periods while you are wearing the NicoDerm CQ patch.

If your NicoDerm CQ patch comes off while wearing.

NicoDerm CQ patches generally stick well to most people's skin. However, a patch may occasionally come off. If your NicoDerm CQ patch falls off during the day, put on a new patch, making sure you select a non-hairy, non-irritated area of the skin that is clean and dry.

If the soap you use has lanolin or moisturizers, the patch may not stick well. Using a different soap may help. Body creams, lotions and sunscreens can also cause problems with keeping your patch on. Do not apply creams or lotions to the place on your skin where you will put the patch.

If you have followed the directions and the patch still does not stick to you, try using medical adhesive tape over the patch.

Disposing of NicoDerm CQ patches.

Fold the used patch in half with the sticky side together.

Carefully dispose of the patch in the disposal slot of the tray provided in the NicoDerm CQ package where it will be out of the reach of children and pets. Small amounts of nicotine, even from a used patch, can poison children and pets. **Keep all nicotine patches away from children and pets.** Wash your hands after disposing of the patch.

If your skin reacts to the NicoDerm CQ patch.

When you first put on a NicoDerm CQ patch, mild itching, burning, or tingling is normal and should go away within an hour. After you remove a NicoDerm CQ patch, the skin under the patch might be somewhat red. Your skin should not stay red for more than a day after removing the patch. **Stop use and ask a doctor if skin redness caused by the patch does not go away after four days, or if your skin swells, or you get a rash. Do not put on a new patch.**

Storage Instructions

Keep each NicoDerm CQ patch in its protective pouch, unopened, until you are ready to use it, because the patch will lose nicotine to the air if it's outside the pouch. Store NicoDerm CQ patches at 20–25 C (68–77 F) because they are sensitive to heat. Remember, the inside of your car can reach temperatures much higher than this. A slight yellowing of the sticky side of the patch is normal. Do not use NicoDerm CQ patches stored in pouches that are open or torn.

TIPS TO MAKE QUITTING EASIER.

Within the first few weeks of giving up smoking, you may be tempted to smoke for pleasure, particularly after completing a difficult task, or at a party or bar. Hear are some tips to help get you through the important first stages of becoming a non-smoker:

On Your Quit Date:

• Ask your family, friends and co-workers to support you in your efforts to stop smoking.
• Throw away all your cigarettes, matches, lighters, ashtrays, etc.
• Keep busy on your quit day. Exercise.

Go to a movie. Take a walk. Get together with friends.
• Figure out how much money you'll save by not smoking. Most ex-smokers can save more than $1,000 a year on the price of cigarettes alone.
• Write down what you will do with the money you save.
• Know your high risk situations and plan ahead how you will deal with them.
• Visit your dentist and have your teeth cleaned to get rid of the tobacco stains.

Right after Quitting:

• During the first few days after you've stopped smoking, spend as much time as possible at places where smoking is not allowed.
• Drink large quantities of water and fruit juices.
• Try to avoid alcohol, coffee and other beverages you associate with smoking.
• Remember that temporary urges to smoke will pass, even if you don't smoke a cigarette.
• Keep your hands busy with something like a pencil or a paper clip.
• Find other activities that help you relax without cigarettes. Swim, jog, take a walk, play basketball.
• Don't worry too much about gaining weight. Watch what you eat, take time for daily exercise, and change your eating habits if you need to.
• Laughter helps. Watch or read something funny

WHAT TO EXPECT.

The First Few Days.

Your body is now coming back into balance. During the first few days after you stop smoking, you might feel edgy and nervous and have trouble concentrating. You might get headaches, feel dizzy and a little out of sorts, feel sweaty or have stomach upsets. You might even have trouble sleeping at first. These are typical nicotine withdrawal symptoms that will go away with time. Your smoker's cough will get worse before it gets better. But don't worry, that's a good sign. Coughing helps clear the tar deposits out of your lungs.

After A Week Or Two.

By now you should be feeling more confident that you can handle those smoking urges. Many of your nicotine withdrawal symptoms have left by now, and you should be noticing some positive signs: less coughing, better breathing and an improved sense of taste and smell, to name a few.

After A Month.

You probably have the urge to smoke much less often now. But urges may still occur, and when they do, they are likely to be powerful ones that come out of nowhere. Don't let them catch you off guard. Plan ahead for these difficult times.

Concentrate on the ways non-smokers are more attractive than smokers. Their skin is less likely to wrinkle. Their teeth are whiter, cleaner. Their breath is fresher. Their hair and clothes smell better. That cough that seems to make even a laugh sound more like a rattle is a thing of the

past. Their children and others around them are healthier, too.

What To Do About Relapse.

What should you do if you slip and start smoking again? The answer is simple. A lapse of one or two or even a few cigarettes should not spoil your efforts! Throw away your cigarettes, forgive yourself and continue with the program. Listen to the Compact Disc again and re-read the User's Guide to ensure that you're using NicoDerm CQ correctly and following the other important tips for dealing with the mental and social dependence on nicotine. Your doctor, pharmacist or other health professional can also provide useful counseling on the importance of stopping smoking. You should consider them partners in your quit attempt.

What To Do About Relapse After a Successful Quit Attempt.

If you have taken up regular smoking again, don't be discouraged. Research shows that the best thing you can do is try again, since several quitting attempts may be needed before you're successful. And your chances of quitting successfully increase with each quit attempt.

The important thing is to learn from your last attempt.
• Admit that you've slipped, but don't treat yourself as a failure.
• Try to identify the "trigger" that caused you to slip, and prepare a better plan for dealing with this problem next time.
• Talk positively to yourself – tell yourself that you have learned something from this experience.
• Make sure you used NicoDerm CQ patches correctly
• Remember that it takes practice to do anything, and quitting smoking is no exception.

WHEN THE STRUGGLE IS OVER.

Once you've stopped smoking, take a second and pat yourself on your back. Now do it again. You deserve it. Remember now why you decided to stop smoking in the first place. Look at your list of reasons. Read them again. And smile.

Now think about all the money you are saving and what you'll do with it. All the non-smoking places you can go, and what you might do there. All those years you may have added to your life, and what you'll do with them. Remember that temptation may not be gone forever. However, the hard part is behind you so look forward with a positive attitude, and enjoy your new life as a non-smoker.

QUESTIONS & ANSWERS

1. How will I feel when I stop smoking and start using NicoDerm CQ?

You'll need to prepare yourself for some nicotine withdrawal symptoms. These begin almost immediately after you stop smoking, and are usually at their worst during the first three or four days. Understand that any of the following is possible:
• craving for nicotine
• anxiety, irritability, restlessness, mood changes, nervousness

Continued on next page

Nicoderm CQ—Cont.

- disruptions of your sleep
- drowsiness
- trouble concentrating
- increased appetite and weight gain
- headaches, muscular pain, constipation, fatigue.

NicoDerm CQ reduces nicotine withdrawal symptoms such as irritability and nervousness, as well as the craving for nicotine you used to satisfy by having a cigarette.

2. Is NicoDerm CQ just substituting one form of nicotine for another?

NicoDerm CQ does contain nicotine. The purpose of NicoDerm CQ is to provide you with enough nicotine to reduce the physical withdrawal symptoms so you can deal with the mental aspects of quitting.

3. Can I be hurt by using NicoDerm CQ?

For most adults, the amount of nicotine delivered from the patch is less than from smoking. If you believe you may be sensitive to even this amount of nicotine, you should not use this product without advice from your doctor. There are also some important warnings in this User's Guide (See page 4).

4. Will I gain weight?

Many people do tend to gain a few pounds the first 8–10 weeks after they stop smoking. This is a very small price to pay for the enormous gains that you will make in your overall health and attractiveness. If you continue to gain weight after the first two months, try to analyze what you're doing differently. Reduce your fat intake, choose healthy snacks, and increase your physical activity to burn off the extra calories. Drink lots of water. This is good for your body and skin, and also helps to reduce the amount you eat.

5. Is NicoDerm CQ more expensive than smoking?

The total cost of NicoDerm CQ program is similar to what a person who smokes one and a half packs of cigarettes a day would spend on cigarettes for the same period of time. Also, use of NicoDerm CQ is only a short-term cost, while the cost of smoking is a long-term cost, including the health problems smoking causes.

6. What if I slip up?

Discard your cigarettes, forgive yourself and then get back on track. Don't consider yourself a failure or punish yourself. In fact, people who have already tried to quit are more likely to be successful the next time.

GOOD LUCK!
WALLET CARD

My most important reasons to quit smoking are:

WALLET CARD

Where to call for Help:

American Lung Association	American Cancer Society	American Heart Association
800-586-4872	800-227-2345	800-242-8721

For people who smoke more than 10 cigarettes per day:

STEP 1	STEP 2	STEP 3
Use one 21 mg patch/day Weeks 1–6	Use one 14 mg patch/day Weeks 7–8	Use one 7 mg patch/day Weeks 9–10

People who smoke 10 or less cigarettes per day. Do not use STEP 1 (21 mg). Use STEP 2 (14 mg) for six weeks and STEP 3 (7 mg) for two weeks and then stop. Copyright © 2002 GlaxoSmithKline

For your family's protection, NicoDerm CQ patches are supplied in child resistant pouches. Do not use if individual pouch is open or torn.

Manufactured by ALZA Corporation, Mountain View, CA 94043 for GlaxoSmithKline Consumer Healthcare, L.P. Comments or Questions? Call 1–800–834–5895 Weekdays. (10 a.m.–4:30 p.m. EST).

- **Not for sale to those under 18 years of age.**
- **Proof of age required.**
- **Not for sale in vending machines or from any source where proof of age cannot be verified.**

Available as

NicoDerm CQ Step 1 (21 mg/24 hours)–7 Patches*

NicoDerm CQ Step 1 (21 mg/24 hours)–14 Patches*

NicoDerm CQ Step 2 (14 mg/24 hours)–14 Patches*

NicoDerm CQ Step 3 (7 mg/24 hours)–14 Patches*

NicoDerm CQ Clear Step 1 (21 mg/24 hours)–7 Patches*

NicoDerm CQ Clear Step 1 (21 mg/24 hours)–14 Patches*

NicoDerm CQ Clear Step 1 (21 mg/24 hours)–21 Patches*

NicoDerm CQ Clear Step 2 (14 mg/24 hours)–14 Patches*

NicoDerm CQ Clear Step 3 (7 mg/24 hours)–14 Patches**

* User's Guide, CD & Child Resistant Disposal Tray

** User's Guide, & Child Resistant Disposal Tray

Shown in Product Identification Guide, page 505

NICODERM® CQ® CLEAR
(GlaxoSmithKline Consumer)
Nicotine Transdermal System/Stop Smoking Aid

Formerly available only by prescription Available as:

Step 1 - 21 mg/24 hours
Step 2 - 14 mg/24 hours
Step 3 - 7 mg/24 hours

If you smoke:
More than 10 Cigarettes per Day:
Start with Step 1
10 Cigarettes a Day or Less:
Start with Step 2

WHAT IS THE NICODERM CQ PATCH AND HOW IS IT USED?

NicoDerm CQ is a small, nicotine containing patch. When you put on a NicoDerm CQ patch, nicotine passes through the skin and into your body. NicoDerm CQ is very thin and uses special material to control how fast nicotine passes through the skin. Unlike the sudden jolts of nicotine delivered by cigarettes, the amount of nicotine you receive remains relatively smooth throughout the 24 or 16 hours period you wear the NicoDerm CQ patch. This helps to reduce cravings you may have for nicotine.

Active Ingredient: Nicotine

Purpose: Stop Smoking Aid

Use: reduces withdrawal symptoms, including nicotine craving, associated with quitting smoking

Directions:

- if you are under 18 years of age, ask a doctor before use
- before using this product, read the enclosed user's guide for complete directions and other information
- stop smoking completely when you begin using the patch
- **if you smoke more than 10 cigarettes per day,** use according to the following 10 week schedule:

STEP 1	STEP 2	STEP 3
Use one 21 mg patch/day	Use one 14 mg patch/day	Use one 7 mg patch/day
Weeks 1–6	Weeks 7–8	Weeks 9–10

- if you smoke **10 or less cigarettes per day,** do not use **STEP 1 (21 mg)**. Start with **STEP 2 (14 mg)** for 6 weeks, then **STEP 3 (7 mg)** for two weeks and then stop.
- steps 2 and 3 allow you to gradually reduce your level of nicotine. Completing the full program will increase your chances of quitting successfully.
- apply one new patch every 24 hours on skin that is dry, clean and hairless
- remove backing from patch and immediately press onto skin. Hold for 10 seconds.
- wash hands after applying or removing patch. Throw away the patch in the enclosed disposal tray. See enclosed user's guide for safety and handling.
- you may wear the patch for 16 or 24 hours
- if you crave cigarettes when you wake up, wear the patch for 24 hours
- if you have vivid dreams or other sleep disturbances, you may remove the patch at bedtime and apply a new one in the morning
- the used patch should be removed and a new one applied to a different skin site at the same time each day
- do not wear more than one patch at a time
- do not cut patch in half or into smaller pieces
- do not leave patch on for more than 24 hours because it may irritate your skin and loses strength after 24 hours
- stop using the patch at the end of 10 weeks. If you started with **STEP 2**, stop

using the patch at the end of 8 weeks. If you still feel the need to use the patch talk to your doctor.

Warnings:

If you are pregnant or breast-feeding, only use this medicine on the advice of your health care provider. Smoking can seriously harm your child. Try to stop smoking without using any nicotine replacement medicine. This medicine is believed to be safer than smoking. However, the risks to your child from this medicine are not fully known.

Do Not Use

• if you continue to smoke, chew tobacco, use snuff, or use a nicotine gum or other nicotine containing products

Ask a doctor before use if you have

• heart disease, recent heart attack, or irregular heartbeat. Nicotine can increase your heart rate.
• high blood pressure not controlled with medication. Nicotine can increase your blood pressure.
• an allergy to adhesive tape or skin problems because you are more likely to get rashes

Ask a doctor or pharmacist before use if you are

• using a non-nicotine stop smoking drug
• taking a prescription medication for depression or asthma. Your prescription dose may need to be adjusted.

When using this product

• do not smoke even when not wearing the patch. The nicotine in your skin will still be entering your blood stream for several hours after you take off the patch.
• if you have vivid dreams or other sleep disturbances remove this patch at bedtime

Stop use and ask a doctor if

• skin redness caused by the patch does not go away after four days, or if skin swells, or you get a rash
• irregular heartbeat or palpitations occur
• you get symptoms of nicotine overdose such as nausea, vomiting, dizziness, weakness and rapid heartbeat

Keep out of reach of children and pets. Used patches have enough nicotine to poison children and pets. If swallowed, get medical help or contact a Poison Control Center right away. Dispose of the used patches by folding sticky ends together and inserting in disposal tray in this box.

READ THE LABEL

Read the carton and the User's Guide before using this product. Keep the carton and User's Guide. They contain important information.

Inactive Ingredients: Ethylene vinyl acetate-copolymer, polyisobutylene and high density polyethylene between clear polyester backings.

Store at 20–25°C (68–77°F)

TO INCREASE YOUR SUCCESS IN QUITTING:

1. You must be motivated to quit.
2. Complete the full treatment program, applying a new patch every day.

3. Use with a support program as described in the Users Guide.

NicoDerm CQ User's Guide
KEYS TO SUCCESS

1) You must really want to quit smoking for **NicoDerm® CQ®** to help you.
2) Complete the full program, applying a new patch every day.
3) **NicoDerm CQ** works best when used together with a support program: See page 3 for details.
4) If you have trouble using **NicoDerm CQ**, ask your doctor or pharmacist or call GlaxoSmithKline 1-800-834-5895 weekdays (10:00 am 4:30 pm EST).

SO, YOU'VE DECIDED TO QUIT.

Congratulations. Your decision to stop smoking is one of the most important things you can do to improve your health. Quitting smoking is a two-part process that involves:
1) overcoming your physical need for nicotine, and
2) breaking your smoking habit.
NicoDerm CQ helps smokers quit by reducing nicotine withdrawal symptoms.
Many NicoDerm CQ users will be able to stop smoking for a few days but often will start smoking again. Most smokers have to try to quit several times before they completely stop.
Your own chances of quitting smoking depend on how strongly you are addicted to nicotine, how much you want to quit, and how closely you follow a quitting plan like the one that comes with NicoDerm CQ.

QUITTING SMOKING IS HARD!

If you find you cannot stop or if you start smoking again after using NicoDerm CQ please talk to a health care professional who can help you find a program that may work better for you. Breaking this addiction doesn't happen overnight.
Because NicoDerm CQ provides some nicotine, the NicoDerm CQ patch will help you stop smoking by reducing nicotine withdrawal symptoms such as nicotine craving, nervousness and irritability.
This User's Guide will give you support as you become a non-smoker. It will answer common questions about NicoDerm CQ and give tips to help you stop smoking, and should be referred to often.

WHERE TO GET HELP.

You are more likely to stop smoking by using NicoDerm CQ with a support program that helps you break your smoking habit. There may be support groups in your area for people trying to quit. Call your local chapter of the American Lung Association, American Cancer Society or American Heart Association for further information. Toll free phone numbers are printed on the wallet card on the back cover of this User's Guide.
If you find you cannot stop smoking or if you start smoking again after using NicoDerm CQ, remember breaking this addiction doesn't happen overnight. You may want to talk to a health care professional who can help you improve your chances of quitting the next time you try NicoDerm CQ or another method.

LET'S GET ORGANIZED.

Your reason for quitting may be a combination of concerns about health, the effect of smoking on your appearance, and pressure from your family and friends to stop smoking. Or maybe you're concerned about the dangerous effect of second-hand smoke on the people you care about.
All of these are good reasons. You probably have others. Decide your most important reasons, and write them down on the wallet card inside the back cover of this User's Guide. Carry this card with you. In difficult moments, when you want to smoke, the card will remind you why you are quitting.

WHAT YOU'RE UP AGAINST.

Smoking is addictive in two ways. Your need for nicotine has become both physical and mental. You must overcome both addictions to stop smoking. So while NicoDerm CQ will lessen your body's craving for nicotine, you've got to want to quit smoking to overcome the mental dependence on cigarettes. Once you've decided that you're going to quit, it's time to get started. But first, there are some important cautions you should consider.

SOME IMPORTANT WARNINGS.

This product is only for those who want to stop smoking.

If you are pregnant or breast-feeding, only use this medicine on the advice of your health care provider. Smoking can seriously harm your child. Try to stop smoking without using any nicotine replacement medicine. This medicine is believed to be safer than smoking. However, the risks to your child from this medicine are not fully known.

Do not use

• if you continue to smoke, chew tobacco, use snuff or use a nicotine gum or other nicotine products.

Ask a doctor before use if you have:

• heart disease, recent heart attack, or irregular heartbeat, Nicotine can increase your heart rate.
• high blood pressure not controlled with medication. Nicotinea can increase your blood pressure.
• an allergy to adhesive tape or have skin problems because you are more likely to get rashes.

Ask a doctor or pharmacist before use if you are

• using a non-nicotine stop smoking drug
• taking a prescription medication for asthma or depression. Your prescription dose may need to be adjusted.

When using this product:

• do not smoke even when not wearing the patch. The nicotine in your skin will still be entering your bloodstream for several hours after you take off the patch.
• you have vivid dreams or other sleep disturbances remove this patch at bedtime.

Stop use and ask a doctor if:

• skin redness caused by the patch does

Continued on next page

Nicoderm CQ Clear—Cont.

not go away after four days, or if your skin swells or you get a rash.

- irregular heartbeat or palpitations occur
- you get symptoms of nicotine overdose, such as nausea, vomiting, dizziness, weakness and rapid heartbeat.

Keep out of reach of children and pets. Used patches have enough nicotine to poison children and pets. If swallowed, get medical help or contact a Poison Control Center right away. Dispose of the used patches by folding sticky ends together and inserting in the disposal tray in this box.

LET'S GET STARTED.

If you are under 18 years of age, ask a doctor before use.

Becoming a non-smoker starts today. Your first step is to read through this entire User's Guide carefully.

First, check that you bought the right starting dose.

If you smoke more than 10 cigarettes a day, begin with Step 1 (21 mg). As the carton indicates, people who smoke 10 or less cigarettes per day should not use Step 1 (21 mg). They should start with Step 2 (14 mg). Throughout this User's Guide we will give specific instructions for people who smoke 10 or less cigarettes per day.

Next, set your personalized quitting schedule.

Take out a calendar that you can use to track your progress. Pick a quit date, and mark this on your calendar using the stickers in the middle of this User's Guide, as described below.

DIRECTIONS: FOR PEOPLE WHO SMOKE MORE THAN 10 CIGARETTES PER DAY

STEP 1. (Weeks 1–6). Your quit date (and the day you'll start using NicoDerm CQ patch).

Choose your quit date (it should be soon). This is the day you will quit smoking cigarettes entirely and begin using NicoDerm CQ to reduce your cravings for nicotine. Place the Step 1 sticker on this date. For the first six weeks, you'll use the highest-strength (21 mg) NicoDerm CQ patches. Be sure to follow the directions on page 10.

Completing the full program will increase your chances of quitting successfully. This is done by changing over to the Step 2 (14mg) patch for 2 weeks followed by a final 2 weeks with the Step 3 (7mg) patch. The Step 2 and Step 3 treatment periods allow you to gradually reduce the amount of nicotine you get, rather than stopping suddenly, and will increase your chances of quitting.

STEP 2. (Weeks 7–8). The day you'll start reducing your use of NicoDerm CQ patch.

Switching to Step 2 (14mg) patches after 6 weeks begins to gradually reduce your nicotine usage. Place the Step 2 sticker on this date (the first day of week seven). Use the 14mg patches for two weeks.

STEP 3. (Weeks 9–10). The day you'll further start reducing your use of NicoDerm CQ patch.

After eight weeks, nicotine intake is further reduced by moving down to Step 3 (7mg) patches. Place the Step 3 sticker on this date (the first day of week nine). Use the 7 mg patches for two weeks.

THE NICODERM CQ PROGRAM

STEP 1	STEP 2	STEP 3
Use one	Use one	Use one
21 mg	14 mg	7 mg
patch/day	patch/day	patch/day
Weeks 1–6	Weeks 7–8	Weeks 9–10

STOP USING NICODERM CQ AT THE END OF WEEK 10. If you still feel the need to use the patch after Week 10, talk with your doctor or health professional.

DIRECTIONS: FOR PEOPLE WHO SMOKE 10 OR LESS CIGARETTES PER DAY

Do not use Step 1 (21 mg).

Begin with STEP 2 – Initial Treatment Period (Weeks 1–6): 14mg patches.

Choose our quit date (it should be soon). This is the Day you will quit smoking cigarettes entirely and begin using NicoDerm CQ to reduce your cravings for nicotine. Place the Step 2 sticker on this date. For the first six weeks, you'll use the Step 2 (14mg) NicoDerm CQ patches. Be sure to follow the directions on page 10.

Continue with STEP 3 – Step Down Treatment Period (Weeks 7–8): 7mg patches.

Completing the full program will increase your chances of quitting successfully. This is done by changing over to the Step 3 (7mg) patches for 2 weeks. The two week step down treatment period allows you to gradually reduce the amount of nicotine you get, rather than stopping suddenly, and will increase your chances of quitting. Place the Step 3 sticker on the first day of week seven. Use the 7mg patches for two weeks.

People who smoke 10 or less cigarettes per day should not use NicoDerm CQ for longer than 8 weeks. If you still feel the need to use NicoDerm CQ after 8 weeks, talk with your doctor.

PLAN AHEAD.

Because smoking is an addiction, it is not easy to stop. After you've given up nicotine, you may still have a strong urge to smoke. Plan ahead NOW for these times, so you're not tempted to start smoking again in a moment of weakness. The following tips may help:

- Keep the phone numbers of supportive friends and family members handy.
- Keep a record of your quitting process. In the event that you slip, immediately stop smoking and resume your quit attempt with the NicoDerm CQ patch. If you smoke at all, write down what you think caused the slip.
- Put together an Emergency Kit that includes items that will help take your mind off occasional urges to smoke. You might include cinnamon gum or lemon drops to suck on, a relaxing cassette tape, and something for your hands to

play with, like a smooth rock, rubber band or small metal balls.

- Set aside some small rewards, like a new magazine or a gift certificate from your favorite store, which you'll "give" yourself after passing difficult hurdles.
- Think now about the times when you most often want a cigarette, and then plan what else you might do instead of smoking. For instance, you might plan to take your coffee break in a new location, or take a walk right after dinner, so you won't be tempted to smoke.

HOW NICODERM CQ WORKS.

NicoDerm CQ patches provide nicotine to your system. They work as a temporary aid to help you quit smoking by reducing nicotine withdrawal symptoms, including nicotine craving. NicoDerm CQ provides a lower level of nicotine to your blood than cigarettes, and allows you to gradually do away with your body's need for nicotine. Because NicoDerm CQ does not contain the tar or carbon monoxide of cigarette smoke, it does not have the same health dangers as tobacco. However, it still delivers nicotine, the addictive part of cigarette smoke. Nicotine can cause side effects such as headache, nausea, upset stomach, and dizziness.

HOW TO USE NICODERM CQ PATCHES.

Read all the following instructions, and the instructions on the outer carton, before using NicoDerm CQ. Refer to them often to make sure you're using NicoDerm CQ correctly. Please refer to the CD for additional help.

1) Stop smoking completely before you start using NicoDerm CQ.

2) To reduce nicotine craving and other withdrawal symptoms, use NicoDerm CQ according to the directions on pages 6–8.

3) Insert used NicoDerm CQ patches in the child resistant disposal tray provided in the box – safely away from children and pets.

When to apply and remove NicoDerm CQ patches.

Each day apply a new patch to a different place on skin that is dry, clean and hairless. **You can wear a NicoDerm CQ patch for either 16 or 24 hours.** If you crave cigarettes when you wake up, wear the patch for 24 hours. If you begin to have vivid dreams or other disruptions of your sleep while wearing the patch 24 hours, try taking the patch off at bedtime (after about 16 hours) and putting on a new one when you get up the next day.

PLACE THESE STICKERS ON YOUR CALENDAR

STEP 1	STEP 2
A new 21 mg patch every day AT THE BEGINNING OF WEEK #1 (QUIT DAY)	A new 14 mg patch every day AT THE BEGINNING OF WEEK #7

For people who smoke 10 or less cigarettes per day: Do not use STEP 1 (21 mg). Use STEP 2 (14 mg) at the beginning

of week #1 and STEP 3 (7 mg) at the beginning of week #7.

PLACE THESE STICKERS ON YOUR CALENDAR

STEP 3	EX-SMOKER
A new 7 mg patch every day AT THE BEGINNING OF WEEK #9	WHEN YOU HAVE COMPLETED YOUR QUITTING PROGRAM

Do not smoke even when you are not wearing the patch.

Remove the used patch and put on a new patch at the same time every day. Applying the patch at about the same time each day (first thing in the morning, for instance) will help you remember when to put on a new patch. Do not leave the same NicoDerm CQ patch on for more than 24 hours because it may irritate your skin and because it loses strength after 24 hours.

Do not use NicoDerm CQ continuously for more than 10 weeks (8 weeks for people who smoke 10 or less cigarettes per day).

How to apply a NicoDerm CQ patch.

1. Do not remove the NicoDerm CQ patch from its sealed protective pouch until you are ready to use it. NicoDerm CQ patches will lose nicotine to the air if you store them out of the pouch.
2. Choose a non-hairy, clean, dry area of skin. Do not put a NicoDerm CQ patch on skin that is burned, broken out, cut, or irritated in any way. Make sure your skin is free of lotion and soap before applying a patch.
3. A clear, protective liner covers the sticky back side of the NicoDerm CQ patch—the side that will be put on your skin. The liner has a slit down the middle to help you remove it from the patch. With the sticky back side facing you, pull half the liner away from the NicoDerm CQ patch starting at the middle slit, as shown in the illustration above. Hold the NicoDerm CQ patch at one of the outside edges (touch the sticky side as little as possible), and pull off the other half of the protective liner.
Place this liner in the slot in the disposable tray provided in the NicoDerm CQ package where it will be out of reach of children and pets.
4. Immediately apply the sticky side of the NicoDerm CQ patch to your skin. **Press the patch firmly on your skin with the heel of your hand for at least 10 seconds.** Make sure it sticks well to your skin, especially around the edges.
5. Wash your hands when you have finished applying the NicoDerm CQ patch. Nicotine on your hands could get into your eyes and nose, and cause stinging, redness, or more serious problems.
6. After 24 or 16 hours, remove the patch you have been wearing. Fold the used NicoDerm CQ patch in half with the sticky side together. Carefully dispose of the used patch in the slot of the disposal

tray provided in the NicoDerm CQ package where it will be out of the reach of children and pets. Even used patches have enough nicotine to poison children and pets. Wash your hands.
7. Choose a different place on your skin to apply the next NicoDerm CQ patch and repeat Steps 1 to 6. Do not apply a new patch to a previously used skin site for at least one week.

If your NicoDerm CQ patch gets wet during wearing.

Water will not harm the NicoDerm CQ patch you are wearing if applied properly. You can bathe, swim, or shower for short periods while you are wearing the NicoDerm CQ patch.

If your NicoDerm CQ patch comes off while wearing.

NicoDerm CQ patches generally stick well to most people's skin. However, a patch may occasionally come off. If your NicoDerm CQ patch falls off during the day, put on a new patch, making sure you select a non-hairy, non-irritated area of the skin that is clean and dry.
If the soap you use has lanolin or moisturizers, the patch may not stick well. Using a different soap may help. Body creams, lotions and sunscreens can also cause problems with keeping your patch on. Do not apply creams or lotions to the place on your skin where you will put the patch.
If you have followed the directions and the patch still does not stick to you, try using medical adhesive tape over the patch.

Disposing of NicoDerm CQ patches.

Fold the used patch in half with the sticky side together.
Carefully dispose of the patch in the disposal slot of the tray provided in the NicoDerm CQ package where it will be out of the reach of children and pets. Small amounts of nicotine, even from a used patch, can poison children and pets.
Keep all nicotine patches away from children and pets. Wash your hands after disposing of the patch.

If your skin reacts to the NicoDerm CQ patch.

When you first put on a NicoDerm CQ patch, mild itching, burning, or tingling is normal and should go away within an hour. After you remove a NicoDerm CQ patch, the skin under the patch might be somewhat red. Your skin should not stay red for more than a day after removing the patch. **Stop use and ask a doctor if skin redness caused by the patch does not go away after four days, or if your skin swells, or you get a rash. Do not put on a new patch.**

Storage Instructions

Keep each NicoDerm CQ patch in its protective pouch, unopened, until you are ready to use it, because the patch will lose nicotine to the air if it's outside the pouch. Store NicoDerm CQ patches at 20–25 C (68–77 F) because they are sensitive to heat. Remember, the inside of your car can reach temperatures much higher than this. A slight yellowing of the sticky side of the patch is normal. Do not use

NicoDerm CQ patches stored in pouches that are open or torn.

TIPS TO MAKE QUITTING EASIER.

Within the first few weeks of giving up smoking, you may be tempted to smoke for pleasure, particularly after completing a difficult task, or at a party or bar. Hear are some tips to help get you through the important first stages of becoming a non-smoker.

On Your Quit Date:

- Ask your family, friends and co-workers to support you in your efforts to stop smoking.
- Throw away all your cigarettes, matches, lighters, ashtrays, etc.
- Keep busy on your quit day. Exercise. Go to a movie. Take a walk. Get together with friends.
- Figure out how much money you'll save by not smoking. Most ex-smokers can save more than $1,000 a year on the price of cigarettes alone.
- Write down what you will do with the money you save.
- Know your high risk situations and plan ahead how you will deal with them.
- Visit your dentist and have your teeth cleaned to get rid of the tobacco stains.

Right after Quitting:

- During the first few days after you've stopped smoking, spend as much time as possible at places where smoking is not allowed.
- Drink large quantities of water and fruit juices.
- Try to avoid alcohol, coffee and other beverages you associate with smoking.
- Remember that temporary urges to smoke will pass, even if you don't smoke a cigarette.
- Keep your hands busy with something like a pencil or a paper clip.
- Find other activities that help you relax without cigarettes. Swim, jog, take a walk, play basketball.
- Don't worry too much about gaining weight. Watch what you eat, take time for daily exercise, and change your eating habits if you need to.
- Laughter helps. Watch or read something funny

WHAT TO EXPECT.

The First Few Days.

Your body is now coming back into balance. During the first few days after you stop smoking, you might feel edgy and nervous and have trouble concentrating. You might get headaches, feel dizzy and a little out of sorts, feel sweaty or have stomach upsets. You might even have trouble sleeping at first. These are typical nicotine withdrawal symptoms that will go away with time. Your smoker's cough will get worse before it gets better. But don't worry, that's a good sign. Coughing helps clear the tar deposits out of your lungs.

After A Week Or Two.

By now you should be feeling more confident that you can handle those smoking urges. Many of your nicotine withdrawal symptoms have left by now, and you

Continued on next page

Nicoderm CQ Clear—Cont.

should be noticing some positive signs: less coughing, better breathing and an improved sense of taste and smell, to name a few.

After A Month.

You probably have the urge to smoke much less often now. But urges may still occur, and when they do, they are likely to be powerful ones that come out of nowhere. Don't let them catch you off guard. Plan ahead for these difficult times. Concentrate on the ways non-smokers are more attractive than smokers. Their skin is less likely to wrinkle. Their teeth are whiter, cleaner. Their breath is fresher. Their hair and clothes smell better. That cough that seems to make even a laugh sound more like a rattle is a thing of the past. Their children and others around them are healthier, too.

What To Do About Relapse.

What should you do if you slip and start smoking again? The answer is simple. A lapse of one or two or even a few cigarettes should not spoil your efforts! Throw away your cigarettes, forgive yourself and continue with the program. Listen to the Compact Disc again and re-read the User's Guide to ensure that you're using NicoDerm CQ correctly and following the other important tips for dealing with the mental and social dependence on nicotine. Your doctor, pharmacist or other health professional can also provide useful counseling on the importance of stopping smoking. You should consider them partners in your quit attempt.

What To Do About Relapse After a Successful Quit Attempt.

If you have taken up regular smoking again, don't be discouraged. Research shows that the best thing you can do is try again, since several quitting attempts may be needed before you're successful. And your chances of quitting successfully increase with each quit attempt.

The important thing is to learn from your last attempt.

- Admit that you've slipped, but don't treat yourself as a failure.
- Try to identify the "trigger" that caused you to slip, and prepare a better plan for dealing with this problem next time.
- Talk positively to yourself – tell yourself that you have learned something from this experience.
- Make sure you used NicoDerm CQ patches correctly
- Remember that it takes practice to do anything, and quitting smoking is no exception.

WHEN THE STRUGGLE IS OVER.

Once you've stopped smoking, take a second and pat yourself on your back. Now do it again. You deserve it. Remember now why you decided to stop smoking in the first place. Look at your list of reasons. Read them again. And smile.

Now think about all the money you are saving and what you'll do with it. All the non-smoking places you can go, and what you might do there. All those years you

may have added to your life, and what you'll do with them. Remember that temptation may not be gone forever. However, the hard part is behind you so look forward with a positive attitude, and enjoy your new life as a non-smoker.

QUESTIONS & ANSWERS

1. How will I feel when I stop smoking and start using NicoDerm CQ?

You'll need to prepare yourself for some nicotine withdrawal symptoms. These begin almost immediately after you stop smoking, and are usually at their worst during the first three or four days. Understand that any of the following is possible:

- craving for nicotine
- anxiety, irritability, restlessness, mood changes, nervousness
- disruptions of your sleep
- drowsiness
- trouble concentrating
- increased appetite and weight gain
- headaches, muscular pain, constipation, fatigue.

NicoDerm CQ reduces nicotine withdrawal symptoms such as irritability and nervousness, as well as the craving for nicotine you used to satisfy by having a cigarette.

2. Is NicoDerm CQ just substituting one form of nicotine for another?

NicoDerm CQ does contain nicotine. The purpose of NicoDerm CQ is to provide you with enough nicotine to reduce the physical withdrawal symptoms so you can deal with the mental aspects of quitting.

3. Can I be hurt by using NicoDerm CQ?

For most adults, the amount of nicotine delivered from the patch is less than from smoking. If you believe you may be sensitive to even this amount of nicotine, you should not use this product without advice from your doctor. There are also some important warnings in this User's Guide (See page 4).

4. Will I gain weight?

Many people do tend to gain a few pounds the first 8–10 weeks after they stop smoking. This is a very small price to pay for the enormous gains that you will make in your overall health and attractiveness. If you continue to gain weight after the first two months, try to analyze what you're doing differently. Reduce your fat intake, choose healthy snacks, and increase your physical activity to burn off the extra calories. Drink lots of water. This is good for your body and skin, and also helps to reduce the amount you eat.

5. Is NicoDerm CQ more expensive than smoking?

The total cost of NicoDerm CQ program is similar to what a person who smokes one and a half packs of cigarettes a day would spend on cigarettes for the same period of time. Also, use of NicoDerm CQ is only a short-term cost, while the cost of smoking is a long-term cost, including the health problems smoking causes.

6. What if I slip up?

Discard your cigarettes, forgive yourself and then get back on track. Don't consider yourself a failure or punish yourself.

In fact, people who have already tried to quit are more likely to be successful the next time.

GOOD LUCK!

WALLET CARD

My most important reasons to quit smoking are:

WALLET CARD

Where to call for Help:

| American Lung Association 800-586-4872 | American Cancer Society 800-227-2345 | American Heart Association 800-242-8721 |

For people who smoke more than 10 cigarettes per day:

STEP 1	STEP 2	STEP 3
Use one	Use one	Use one
21 mg	14 mg	7 mg
patch/day	patch/day	patch/day
Weeks 1–6	Weeks 7–8	Weeks 9–10

People who smoke 10 or less cigarettes per day. Do not use STEP 1 (21 mg). Use STEP 2 (14 mg) for six weeks and STEP 3 (7 mg) for two weeks and then stop.

Copyright © 2004 GlaxoSmithKline

For your family's protection, NicoDerm CQ patches are supplied in child resistant pouches. Do not use if individual pouch is open or torn.

Manufactured by ALZA Corporation, Mountain View, CA 94043 for GlaxoSmithKline Consumer Healthcare, L.P. Comments or Questions? Call 1–800–834–5895 Weekdays. (10 a.m.–4:30 p.m. EST).

- **Not for sale to those under 18 years of age.**
- **Proof of age required.**
- **Not for sale in vending machines or from any source where proof of age cannot be verified.**

Available as

NicoDerm CQ Step 1 (21 mg/24 hours)–7 Patches*

NicoDerm CQ Step 1 (21 mg/24 hours)–14 Patches*

NicoDerm CQ Step 2 (14 mg/24 hours)–14 Patches*

NicoDerm CQ Step 3 (7 mg/24 hours)–14 Patches**

NicoDerm CQ Clear Step 1 (21 mg/24 hours)–7 patches*

NicoDerm CQ Clear Step 1 (21 mg/24 hours)–14 patches*

NicoDerm CQ Clear Step 1 (21 mg/24 hours)–21 patches*

NicoDerm CQ Clear Step 2 (14 mg/24 hours)–14 patches*

NicoDerm CQ Clear Step 3 (7 mg/24 hours)–14 patches**

*   User's Guide, CD & Child Resistant Disposal Tray
** User's Guide, & Child Resistant Disposal Tray

NICORETTE®

(GlaxoSmithKline Consumer)
Nicotine Polacrilex Gum/Stop Smoking Aid
Available in Original 2mg and 4mg Strengths,
Mint 2mg and 4mg Strengths and
Orange 2mg and 4mg Strengths

IF YOU SMOKE LESS THAN 25 CIGARETTES A DAY: Use 2 mg

IF YOU SMOKE 25 OR MORE CIGARETTES A DAY: Use 4 mg

Action: Stop Smoking Aid

Drug Facts:

Active Ingredient: **Purpose:**

(In each chewing piece)

Nicotine polacrilex
2 or 4 mg .... stop smoking aid

Use:

- reduces withdrawal symptoms, including nicotine craving, associated with quitting smoking

Warnings:

If you are pregnant or breast-feeding, only use this medicine on the advice of your health care provider. Smoking can seriously harm your child. Try to stop smoking without using any nicotine replacement medicine. This medicine is believed to be safer than smoking. However, the risks to your child from this medicine are not fully known.

Do not use:

- if you continue to smoke, chew tobacco, use snuff, or use a nicotine patch or other nicotine containing products

Ask a doctor before use if you have:

- heart disease, recent heart attack, or irregular heartbeat. Nicotine can increase your heart rate.
- high blood pressure not controlled with medication. Nicotine can increase blood pressure.
- stomach ulcer or diabetes

Ask a doctor or pharmacist before use if you are:

- using a non-nicotine stop smoking drug
- taking prescription medicine for depression or asthma. Your prescription dose may need to be adjusted.

Stop use and ask a doctor if:

- mouth, teeth or jaw problems occur
- irregular heartbeat or palpitations occur
- you get symptoms of nicotine overdose such as nausea, vomiting, dizziness, diarrhea, weakness and rapid heartbeat

Keep out of reach of children and pets. Pieces of nicotine gum may have enough nicotine to make children and pets sick. Wrap used pieces of gum in paper and throw away in the trash. In case of overdose, get medical help or contact a Poison Control Center right away.

Directions:

- **if you are under 18 years of age, ask a doctor before use**
- before using this product, read the enclosed User's Guide for complete directions and other important information
- stop smoking completely when you begin using the gum
- **if you smoke 25 or more cigarettes a day;** use 4 mg nicotine gum
- **if you smoke less than 25 cigarettes a day;** use 2 mg nicotine gum

Use according to the following 12 week schedule:

[See table above]

- nicotine gum is a medicine and must be

Weeks 1 to 6	Weeks 7 to 9	Weeks 10 to 12
1 piece every 1 to 2 hours	1 piece every 2 to 4 hours	1 piece every 4 to 8 hours

used a certain way to get the best results

- chew the gum slowly until it tingles. Then park it between your cheek and gum. When the tingle is gone, begin chewing again, until the tingle returns.
- repeat this process until most of the tingle is gone (about 30 minutes)
- do not eat or drink for 15 minutes before chewing the nicotine gum, or while chewing a piece
- to improve your chances of quitting, use at least 9 pieces per day for the first 6 weeks
- if you experience strong or frequent cravings, you may use a second piece within the hour. However, do not continuously use one piece after another since this may cause you hiccups, heartburn, nausea or other side effects.
- do not use more than 24 pieces a day
- stop using the nicotine gum at the end of 12 weeks. If you still feel the need to use nicotine gum, talk to your doctor.

Other Information:

- store at 20–25°C (68–77°F)
- protect from light

Inactive Ingredients:
Original [2 mg] Inactive Ingredients: Flavors, glycerin, gum base, sodium carbonate, sorbitol, sodium bicarbonate.
Original [4 mg] Inactive Ingredients: Flavors, glycerin, gum base, sodium carbonate, sorbitol, D&C Yellow 10.
Mint [2 mg] Inactive Ingredients: Gum base, magnesium oxide, menthol, peppermint oil, sodium bicarbonate, sodium carbonate, xylitol.
Mint [4 mg] Inactive Ingredients: Gum base, magnesium oxide, menthol, peppermint oil, sodium carbonate, xylitol, D&C yellow #10 Al. lake.
Orange [2 mg] Inactive Ingredients: Flavor, gum base, magnesium oxide, sodium bicarbonate, sodium carbonate, xylitol
Orange [4 mg] Inactive Ingredients: Flavor, gum base, magnesium oxide, sodium carbonate, xylitol, D&C Yellow #10 Al. lake.

TO INCREASE YOUR SUCCESS IN QUITTING:

1. You must be motivated to quit.
2. **Use Enough**—Chew **at least 9 pieces** of Nicorette per day during the first six weeks.
3. **Use Long Enough**—Use Nicorette for the full 12 weeks.
4. **Use with a support program** as directed in the enclosed User's Guide.*

*The American Cancer Society supports the use of a stop smoking aid and counseling as effective tools when quitting smoking but does not endorse any specific product. GlaxoSmithKline pays a fee to the American Cancer Society for the use of its logo.

To remove the gum, tear off single unit.

Peel off backing starting at corner with loose edge.

Push gum through foil.

Blister packaged for your protection. **Do not use if individual seals are open or torn.**

- **not for sale to those under 18 years of age**
- **proof of age required**
- **not for sale in vending machines or from any source where proof of age cannot be verified**

READ THE LABEL

Read the carton and the User's Guide before taking this product. Do not discard carton or User's Guide. They contain important information.

How Supplied: Nicorette Original and Mint are available in:

2 mg or 4 mg Starter kit*—110 pieces
2 mg or 4 mg Refill—48 pieces, 168 pieces or 192 pieces

Nicorette Orange is available in:

2 mg or 4 mg Starter kit*—110 pieces
2 mg or 4 mg Refill—48 pieces

*User's Guide and CD included in kit

Questions or comments? call **1-800-419-4766** weekdays (10:00 a.m.– 4:30 p.m. EST)

Manufactured by Pharmacia AB, Stockholm, Sweden for

Continued on next page

Nicorette—Cont.

GlaxoSmithKline Consumer Healthcare, L.P.
Moon Township, PA 15108

USER'S GUIDE:
HOW TO USE NICORETTE TO HELP YOU QUIT SMOKING
KEYS TO SUCCESS:
1) You must really want to quit smoking for **Nicorette**® to help you.
2) You can greatly increase your chances for success by using at least 9 to 12 pieces every day when you start using **Nicorette**.
3) You should continue to use **Nicorette** as explained in the User's Guide for 12 full weeks.
4) **Nicorette** works best when used together with a support program.
5) If you have trouble using **Nicorette**, ask your doctor or pharmacist or call GlaxoSmithKline at 1-800-419-4766 weekdays (10:00am–4:30pm EST).

SO YOU DECIDED TO QUIT
Congratulations. Your decision to stop smoking is an important one. That's why you've made the right choice in choosing **Nicorette** gum. Your own chances of quitting smoking depend on how much you want to quit, how strongly you are addicted to tobacco, and how closely you follow a quitting program like the one that comes with **Nicorette**.

QUITTING SMOKING IS HARD!
If you've tried to quit before and haven't succeeded, don't be discouraged! Quitting isn't easy. It takes time, and most people try a few times before they are successful. The important thing is to try again until you succeed. This User's Guide will give you support as you become a non-smoker. It will answer common questions about **Nicorette** and give tips to help you stop smoking, and should be referred to often.

WHERE TO GET HELP
You are more likely to stop smoking by using **Nicorette** with a support program that helps you break your smoking habit. There may be support groups in your area for people trying to quit. Call your local chapter of the American Lung Association (1-800-586-4872), American Cancer Society (1-800-227-2345) or American Heart Association (1-800-242-8721) for further information. If you find you cannot stop smoking or if you start smoking again after using **Nicorette**, remember breaking this addiction doesn't happen overnight. You may want to talk to a health care professional who can help you improve your chances of quitting the next time you try **Nicorette** or another method.

LET'S GET ORGANIZED
Your reason for quitting may be a combination of concerns about health, the effect of smoking on your appearance, and pressure from your family and friends to stop smoking. Or maybe you're concerned about the dangerous effect of second-hand smoke on the people you care about. All of these are good reasons. You probably have others. Decide your most important reasons, and write them down on the wallet card inside the back cover of the User's Guide. Carry this card with you. In difficult moments, when you want to smoke, the card will remind you why you are quitting.

WHAT YOU'RE UP AGAINST
Smoking is addictive in two ways. Your need for nicotine has become both physical and mental. You must overcome both addictions to stop smoking. So while **Nicorette** will lessen your body's physical addition to nicotine, you've got to want to quit smoking to overcome the mental dependence on cigarettes. Once you've decided that you're going to quit, it's time to get started. But first, there are some important cautions you should consider.

SOME IMPORTANT WARNINGS. This product is only for those who want to stop smoking.

If you are pregnant or breast-feeding, only use this medicine on the advice of your health care provider. Smoking can seriously harm your child. Try to stop smoking without using any nicotine replacement medicine. This medicine is believed to be safer than smoking. However, the risks to your child from this medicine are not fully known.

Do not use
- if you continue to smoke, chew tobacco, use snuff, or use a nicotine patch or other nicotine containing products.

Ask a doctor before use if you have
- heart disease, recent heart attack, or irregular heartbeat. Nicotine can increase your heart rate.
- high blood pressure not controlled with medication. Nicotine can increase your blood pressure.
- stomach ulcer or diabetes

Ask a doctor or pharmacist before use if you are
- using a non-nicotine stop smoking drug
- taking a prescription medicine for depression or asthma. Your prescription dose may need to be adjusted.

Stop use and ask a doctor if
- mouth, teeth or jaw problems occur
- irregular heartbeat or palpitations occur
- you get symptoms of nicotine overdose such as nausea, vomiting, dizziness, diarrhea, weakness and rapid heartbeat

Keep out of reach of children and pets. Pieces of nicotine gum may have enough nicotine to make children and pets sick. Wrap used pieces of gum in paper and throw away in the trash. In case of overdose, get medical help or contact a Poison Control Center right away.

LET'S GET STARTED
Becoming a non-smoker starts today. First, check that you bought the right starting dose. **If you smoke 25 or more cigarettes a day**, use 4 mg nicotine gum. **If you smoke less than 25 cigarettes a day**, use 2 mg nicotine gum. Next read through the entire User's Guide carefully. Then, set your personalized quitting schedule. Take out a calendar that you can use to track your progress, and identify four dates, using the stickers in the User's Guide.

STEP 1: (Weeks 1–6) Your quit date (and the day you'll start using Nicorette gum). Choose your quit date (it should be soon). This is the day you will quit smoking cigarettes entirely and begin using **Nicorette** to satisfy your cravings for nicotine. For the first six weeks, you'll use a piece of **Nicorette** every hour or two. Be sure to follow the directions starting on pages 9 and 11 of the User's Guide. Place the Step 1 sticker on this date.

STEP 2: (Weeks 7–9) The day you'll start reducing your use of Nicorette. After six weeks, you'll begin gradually reducing your **Nicorette** usage to one piece every two to four hours. Place the Step 2 sticker on this date (the first day of week seven).

STEP 3: (Weeks 10–12) The day you'll further reduce your use of Nicorette. Nine weeks after you begin using **Nicorette**, you will further reduce your nicotine intake by using one piece every four to eight hours. Place the Step 3 sticker on this date (the first day of week ten). For the next three weeks, you'll use a piece of **Nicorette** every four to eight hours. **End of treatment: The day you'll complete Nicorette therapy.**

Nicorette should not be used for longer than twelve weeks. Identify the date thirteen weeks after the date you chose in Step 1 and place the "EX-Smoker" sticker on your calendar.

PLAN AHEAD
Because smoking is an addiction, it is not easy to stop. After you've given up cigarettes, you will still have a strong urge to smoke. Plan ahead NOW for these times, so you're not defeated in a moment of weakness. The following tips may help:
- Keep the phone numbers of supportive friends and family members handy.
- Keep a record of your quitting process. Track the number of **Nicorette** pieces you use each day, and whether you feel a craving for cigarettes. In the event that you slip, immediately stop smoking and resume your quit attempt with **Nicorette**.
- Put together an Emergency Kit that includes items that will help take your mind off occasional urges to smoke. Include cinnamon gum or lemon drops to suck on, a relaxing cassette tape and something for your hands to play with, like a smooth rock, rubber band or small metal balls.
- Set aside some small rewards, like a new magazine or a gift certificate from your favorite store, which you'll 'give' yourself after passing difficult hurdles.
- Think now about the times when you most often want a cigarette, and then plan what else you might do instead of smoking. For instance, you might plan to take your coffee break in a new location, or take a walk right after dinner, so you won't be tempted to smoke.

HOW NICORETTE GUM WORKS
Nicorette's sugar-free chewing pieces provide nicotine to your system—they

work as a temporary aid to help you quit smoking by reducing nicotine withdrawal symptoms. **Nicorette** provides a lower level of nicotine to your blood than cigarettes, and allows you to gradually do away with your body's need for nicotine. Because **Nicorette** does not contain the tar or carbon monoxide of cigarette smoke, it does not have the same health dangers as tobacco. However, it still delivers nicotine, the addictive part of cigarette smoke. Nicotine can cause side effects such as headache, nausea, upset stomach and dizziness.

HOW TO USE NICORETTE GUM

If you are under 18 years of age, ask a doctor before use.

Before you can use **Nicorette** correctly, you have to practice! That sounds silly, but it isn't.

Nicorette isn't like ordinary chewing gum. It's a medicine, and must be chewed a certain way to work right. Chewed like ordinary gum, **Nicorette** won't work well and can cause side effects. An overdose can occur if you chew more than one piece of **Nicorette** at the same time, or if you chew many pieces one after another. Read all the following instructions before using **Nicorette**. Refer to them often to make sure you're using **Nicorette** gum correctly. If you chew too fast, or do not chew correctly, you may get hiccups, heartburn, or other stomach problems. Don't eat or drink for 15 minutes before using **Nicorette**, or while chewing a piece. The effectiveness of **Nicorette** may be reduced by some foods and drinks, such as coffee, juices, wine or soft drinks.

1. Stop smoking completely before you start using **Nicorette**.
2. To reduce craving and other withdrawal symptoms, use **Nicorette** according to the dosage schedule on page 11 of the User's Guide.
3. Chew each **Nicorette** piece <u>very slowly several times.</u>
4. Stop chewing when you notice a peppery taste, or a slight tingling in your mouth. (This usually happens after about 15 chews, but may vary from person to person.)
5. "PARK" the **Nicorette** piece between your cheek and gum and leave it there.
6. When the peppery taste or tingle is almost gone (in about a minute), start to chew a few times slowly again. When the taste or tingle returns, stop again.
7. Park the **Nicorette** piece again (in a different place in your mouth).
8. Repeat steps 3 to 7 (chew, chew, park) until most of the nicotine is gone from the **Nicorette** piece (usually happens in about half an hour; the peppery taste or tingle won't return).
9. Wrap the used **Nicorette** in paper and throw away in the trash.

See the chart in the **"DIRECTIONS"** section above for the recommended usage schedule for **Nicorette**.

[See table above]

To improve your chances of quitting, use at least 9 pieces of **Nicorette** a day. If you experience strong or frequent cravings

The following chart lists the recommended usage schedule for **Nicorette**:

Weeks 1 through 6	Weeks 7 through 9	Weeks 10 through 12
1 piece every 1 to 2 hours	1 piece every 2 to 4 hours	1 piece every 4 to 8 hours

DO NOT USE MORE THAN 24 PIECES PER DAY.

you may use a second piece within the hour. However, do not continuously use one piece after another, since this may cause you hiccups, heartburn, nausea or other side effects.

HOW TO REDUCE YOUR NICORETTE USAGE

The goal of using **Nicorette** is to slowly reduce your dependence on nicotine. The schedule for using **Nicorette** will help you reduce your nicotine craving gradually. Here are some tips to help you cut back during each step:

- After a while, start chewing each **Nicorette** piece for only 10 to 15 minutes, instead of half an hour. Then gradually begin to reduce the number of pieces used.
- Or, try chewing each piece for longer than half an hour, but reduce the number of pieces you use each day.
- Substitute ordinary chewing gum for some of the **Nicorette** pieces you would normally use. Increase the number of pieces of ordinary gum as you cut back on the **Nicorette** pieces.

STOP USING NICORETTE AT THE END OF WEEK 12. If you still feel the need to use **Nicorette** after Week 12, talk with your doctor.

TIPS TO MAKE QUITTING EASIER

Within the first few weeks of giving up smoking, you may be tempted to smoke for pleasure, particularly after completing a difficult task, or at a party or bar. Here are some tips to help get you through the important first stages of becoming a non-smoker.

On your Quit Date:

- Ask your family, friends, and co-workers to support you in your efforts to stop smoking.
- Throw away all your cigarettes, matches, lighters, ashtrays, etc.
- Keep busy on your quit day. Exercise. Go to a movie. Take a walk. Get together with friends.
- Figure out how much money you'll save by not smoking. Most ex-smokers can save more than $1,000 a year.
- Write down what you will do with the money you save.
- Know your high risk situations and plan ahead how you will deal with them.
- Keep **Nicorette** gum near your bed, so you'll be prepared for any nicotine cravings when you wake up in the morning.
- Visit your dentist and have your teeth cleaned to get rid of the tobacco stains.

Right after Quitting:

- During the first few days after you've stopped smoking, spend as much time as possible at places where smoking is not allowed.

- Drink large quantities of water and fruit juices.
- Try to avoid alcohol, coffee and other beverages you associate with smoking.
- Remember that temporary urges to smoke will pass, even if you don't smoke a cigarette.
- Keep your hands busy with something like a pencil or a paper clip.
- Find other activities which help you relax without cigarettes. Swim, jog, take a walk, play basketball.
- Don't worry too much about gaining weight. Watch what you eat, take time for daily exercise, and change your eating habits if you need to.
- Laughter helps. Watch or read something funny.

WHAT TO EXPECT

Your body is now coming back into balance. During the first few days after you stop smoking, you might feel edgy and nervous and have trouble concentrating. You might get headaches, feel dizzy and a little out of sorts, feel sweaty or have stomach upsets. You might even have trouble sleeping at first. These are typical withdrawal symptoms that will go away with time. Your smoker's cough will get worse before it gets better. But don't worry, that's a good sign. Coughing helps clear the tar deposits out of your lungs.

After a Week or Two.

By now you should be feeling more confident that you can handle those smoking urges. Many of your withdrawal symptoms have left by now, and you should be noticing some positive signs: less coughing, better breathing and an improved sense of taste and smell, to name a few.

After a Month.

You probably have the urge to smoke much less often now. But urges may still occur, and when they do, they are likely to be powerful ones that come out of nowhere. Don't let them catch you off guard. Plan ahead for these difficult times. Concentrate on the ways non-smokers are more attractive than smokers. Their skin is less likely to wrinkle. Their teeth are whiter, cleaner. Their breath is fresher. Their hair and clothes smell better. That cough seems to make even a laugh sound more like a rattle is a thing of the past. Their children and others around them are healthier, too.

What To Do About Relapse.

What should you do if you slip and start smoking again? The answer is simple. A lapse of one or two or even a few cigarettes has not spoiled your efforts! Discard your cigarettes, forgive yourself and try again. If you start smoking again, keep your box

Continued on next page

Nicorette—Cont.

of **Nicorette** for your next quit attempt. If you have taken up regular smoking again, don't be discouraged. Research shows that the best thing you can do is to try again. The important thing is to learn from your last attempt.

- Admit that you've slipped, but don't treat yourself as a failure.
- Try to identify the 'trigger' that caused you to slip, and prepare a better plan for dealing with this problem next time.
- Talk positively to yourself—tell yourself that you have learned something from this experience.
- Make sure you used **Nicorette** gum correctly over the full 12 weeks to reduce your craving for nicotine.
- Remember that it takes practice to do anything, and quitting smoking is no exception.

WHEN THE STRUGGLE IS OVER

Once you've stopped smoking, take a second and pat yourself on the back. Now do it again. You deserve it. Remember now why you decided to stop smoking in the first place. Look at your list of reasons. Read them again. And smile. Now think about all the money you are saving and what you'll do with it. All the non-smoking places you can go, and what you might do there. All those years you may have added to your life, and what you'll do with them. Remember that temptation may not be gone forever. However, the hard part is behind you, so look forward with a positive attitude and enjoy your new life as a non-smoker.

QUESTIONS & ANSWERS

1. How will I feel when I stop smoking and start using Nicorette? You'll need to prepare yourself for some nicotine withdrawal symptoms. These begin almost immediately after you stop smoking, and are usually at their worst during the first three to four days. Understand that any of the following is possible:

- craving for cigarettes
- anxiety, irritability, restlessness, mood changes, nervousness
- drowsiness
- trouble concentrating
- increased appetite and weight gain
- headaches, muscular pain, constipation, fatigue.

Nicorette can help provide relief from withdrawal symptoms such as irritability and nervousness, as well as the craving for nicotine you used to satisfy by having a cigarette.

2. Is Nicorette just substuting one form of nicotine for another? Nicorette does contain nicotine. The purpose of **Nicorette** is to provide you with enough nicotine to help control the physical withdrawal symptoms so you can deal with the mental aspects of quitting. During the 12 week program, you will gradually reduce your nicotine intake by switching to fewer pieces each day. Remember, don't use **Nicorette** together with nicotine patches or other nicotine containing products.

3. Can I be hurt by using Nicorette? For most adults, the amount of nicotine in the gum is less than from smoking. Some people will be sensitive to even this amount of nicotine and should not use this product without advice from their doctor (see page 4 of User's Guide). Because **Nicorette** is a gum-based product, chewing it can cause dental fillings to loosen and aggravate other mouth, tooth and jaw problems. **Nicorette** can also cause hiccups, heartburn and other stomach problems especially if chewed too quickly or not chewed correctly.

4. Will I gain weight? Many people do tend to gain a few pounds in the first 8-10 weeks after they stop smoking. This is a very small price to pay for the enormous gains that you will make in your overall health and attractiveness. If you continue to gain weight after the first two months, try to analyze what you're doing differently. Reduce your fat intake, choose healthy snacks, and increase your physical activity to burn off the extra calories.

5. Is Nicorette more expensive than smoking? The total cost of **Nicorette** for the twelve week program is about equal to what a person who smokes one and a half packs of cigarettes a day would spend on cigarettes for the same period of time. Also use of **Nicorette** is only a short-term cost, while the cost of smoking is a long-term cost, because of the health problems smoking causes.

6. What if I slip up? Discard your cigarettes, forgive yourself and then get back on track. Don't consider yourself a failure or punish yourself. In fact, people who have already tried to quit are more likely to be successful the next time.

GOOD LUCK!

[End User's Guide]

Copyright © 2004 **GlaxoSmithKline** Consumer Healthcare, L.P.

Shown in Product Identification Guide, page 506

Central Nervous System:
Weight Management

BIOLEAN® ACCELERATOR™
(Wellness International)
Herbal & Amino Acid Formulation

Description: BioLean® Accelerator™ is a unique blend of herbal extracts and amino acids that, when used in conjunction with BioLean II® or BioLean Free®, prolongs their adaptogenic and thermogenic properties while adding powerful restorative properties. The restorative properties of the amino acids and herbal extracts in BioLean® Accelerator™ are a strong complement to the energetic and thermogenic properties of BioLean II® and BioLean Free®. When used together, these products provide a well-balanced approach to weight loss, increased energy and detoxification.

Uses: BioLean® Accelerator™ may:
• Enhance weight loss and lipolysis
• Increase thermogenesis
• Increase energy production
• Detoxify

Directions: For maximum effectiveness, use in conjunction with BioLean II® or BioLean Free®. As a dietary supplement, take one tablet in the morning with BioLean II® or BioLean Free®. If desired, BioLean® Accelerator™ may also be taken in the afternoon with or without additional BioLean II® or BioLean Free®. Maximum absorption will be attained if taken with low-calorie food.

Warnings: CAUTION PHENYLKETONURICS: Contains 200 mg phenylalanine per serving. Not for use by children. Consult your physician before using this product if you are taking appetite suppressing drugs or antidepressants, or if you are pregnant or lactating. If symptoms of allergy develop, discontinue use.

Ingredients: Proprietary herbal extract 250mg (Cuscuta Seed, Black Sesame Seed, Rehmannia Root, Achyranthes Root, Cornus Fruit, Chinese Yam, Eclipta Herb, Rosehips, Ligustrum Fruit, Mulberry Fruit, Polygonati Rhizome, Fo Ti Poria Cocos, Euryale Seed, Alisma Rhizome, Moutan Bark, Phellodendron Bark, Anemarrhena Rhizome, Schisandra Berry, Royal Jelly), L-Phenylalanine 200mg, L-Tyrosine 200mg, Calcium Carbonate, Calcium Phosphate Dibasic, Hydroxypropyl Cellulose, Croscarmelose Sodium, Magnesium Stearate, and Silicon Dioxide.

How Supplied: One bottle contains 56 tablets.

Additional Information: For additional information on ingredients or uses, please visit www.winltd.com.

These statements have not been evaluated by the Food & Drug Administration. This product is not intended to diagnose, treat, cure or prevent any disease.

BIOLEAN FREE®
(Wellness International)
Herbal & Amino Acid Dietary Supplement

Description: BioLean Free® is a dietary supplement designed to reduce body fat, suppress the appetite and improve metabolism of dietary carbohydrates, fats, and proteins. BioLean Free® utilizes a strategic blend of vitamins, minerals, amino acids and herbal extracts that enhance fat utilization and energy production through several metabolic pathways. Key ingredients such as quebracho, green tea leaf extract, yerba maté and spices such as ginger and tumeric work together to increase lipolysis, curb cravings, stimulate thermogenesis and increase energy without causing insomnia, which is seen in many other supplements of this type.

Uses: BioLean Free® may:
• Reduce adipose tissue by increasing thermogenesis
• Enhance weight loss via increased lipid mobilization
• Increase energy production
• Suppress appetite
• Improve metabolism of carbohydrates, proteins and fats from the diet
• Reduce free-radical formation (antioxidant)

Directions: As a dietary supplement, take four tablets in mid to late morning with low-calorie food. Some persons may require less than four tablets, or may prefer taking three tablets mid-morning and one additional tablet mid-afternoon to achieve optimum results. Do not exceed recommended daily amounts. Needs may vary with each individual.

Warnings: Not for use by children under the age of 18, pregnant or lactating women. Consult your physician before using this product if you are taking appetite suppressing drugs or cardiovascular medication. Consult your physician if you have hypertension, heart disease, arrhythmias, prostatic hypertrophy, glaucoma, liver disease, renal disease or diabetes. Do not use if you have hyperthyroidism, psychosis, Parkinson's Disease, or are taking monoamine oxidase inhibitors (MAOI). Limit the use of caffeine-containing medications, food, or beverages while taking this product because too much caffeine may cause ner-vousness, irritability, sleeplessness, and occasionally, rapid heart beat. If allergic symptoms develop, discontinue use immediately.

Ingredients: Niacin 40mg (as niacinamide), Vitamin B6 16mg (as pyridoxine HCL), Chromium 400mcg (as chromium Chelavite® chloride), Potassium 100mg (as potassium citrate), Standardized botanical caffeine [Guarana seed (22% methylxanthines), Yerba mate leaf extract (10% methylxanthines), Green tea leaf extract (10% methylxanthines)], Korean ginseng root extract (4% ginsenosides), Uva ursi leaf (20% arbutin), Quebracho bark extract (10% quebrachine), Non-irradiated pure herbs and thermogenic spices 1440mg [Gotu kola leaf (Centella asiatica), Ceylon cinnamon bark, Chinese horseradish root, Jamaican ginger root, Turmeric rhizome, Nigerian cayenne pepper (fruit), English mustard seed, Ho shou wu root, Ginkgo biloba leaf (24% ginkgoflavoneslycosides and 6% bilobalides)], L-Tyrosine 500mg, L-Methionine 100mg, Vanadium 400mcg (as BMOV), Dicalcium phosphate, Cellulose, Cellulose gum, Vegetable stearic acid, Silica, Vegetable magnesium stearate and Vegetable resin glaze.

How Supplied: One box contains 28 packets, four tablets per packet.

Additional Information: For additional information on ingredients or uses, please visit www.winltd.com.

These statements have not been evaluated by the Food & Drug Administration. This product is not intended to diagnose, treat, cure or prevent any disease.

BIOLEAN® LIPOTRIM™
(Wellness International)
All-Natural Dietary Supplement

Description: BioLean® LipoTrim™ contains two dynamic and powerful ingredients that synergistically inhibit new fat deposition and prevent sharp increases in blood glucose levels. Garcinia cambogia extract and chromium polynicotinate help to reduce the rate of lipogenesis and prevent hyperglycemia, especially when used in conjunction with either BioLean II® or BioLean Free®. These potent ingredients combine to discourage body fat accumulation as well as produce an appetite suppressant effect that together can contribute to weight loss.

Uses: BioLean® LipoTrim™ may:
• Facilitate weight loss
• Maintain healthy blood glucose levels
• Suppress appetite

BioLean LipoTrim—Cont.

• Enhance endurance and recovery during periods of exercise

Directions: As a dietary supplement, take one capsule three times daily, 30 minutes before each meal. BioLean® LipoTrim™ should be used in conjunction with a healthy diet and exercise program.

Warnings: Not for use by children under the age of 18, pregnant or lactating women. Consult your physician before using this product if your diet consists of less than 1,000 calories per day.

Ingredients: Chromium 100mcg (as Chromium Polynicotinate), Garcinia Cambogia Fruit Extract 500mg, Hydroxypropylmethylcellulose, Calcium Sulfate, Starch, and Silicone Dioxide.

How Supplied: One bottle contains 84 easy-to-swallow capsules.

Additional Information: For additional information on ingredients or uses, please visit www.winltd.com.

These statements have not been evaluated by the Food & Drug Administration. This product is not intended to diagnose, treat, cure or prevent any disease.

Dermatologic Conditions:
Alopecia

MEN'S ROGAINE®
EXTRA STRENGTH
(Pfizer Consumer Healthcare)
(5% Minoxidil Topical Solution)
Hair Regrowth Treatment
Ocean Rush™ Scent

Drug Facts

Active Ingredient: Minoxidil 5% w/v

Use: to regrow hair on the top of the scalp (vertex only)

Warnings:

For external use only. For use by men only.

Flammable Keep away from fire or flame

Do not use if

- you are a woman
- your amount of hair loss is different than that shown on the side of the product carton or your hair loss is on the front of the scalp. 5% minoxidil topical solution is not intended for frontal baldness or receding hairline.
- you have no family history of hair loss
- your hair loss is sudden and/or patchy
- you do not know the reason for your hair loss
- you are under 18 years of age. Do not use on babies and children.
- your scalp is red, inflamed, infected, irritated, or painful
- you use other medicines on the scalp

Ask a doctor before use if you have heart disease

When using this product

- do not apply on other parts of the body
- avoid contact with the eyes. In case of accidental contact, rinse eyes with large amounts of cool tap water.
- some people have experienced changes in hair color and/or texture
- it takes time to regrow hair. Results may occur at 2 months with twice a day usage. For some men, you may need to use this product for at least 4 months before you see results.
- the amount of hair regrowth is different for each person. This product will not work for all men.

Stop use and ask a doctor if

- chest pain, rapid heartbeat, faintness, or dizziness occurs
- sudden, unexplained weight gain occurs
- your hands or feet swell
- scalp irritation or redness occurs
- unwanted facial hair growth occurs
- you do not see hair regrowth in 4 months

May be harmful if used when pregnant or breast-feeding. Keep out of reach of children. If swallowed, get medical help or contact a Poison Control Center right away.

Directions:

- apply one mL with dropper 2 times a day directly onto the scalp in the hair loss area
- using more or more often will not improve results
- continued use is necessary to increase and keep your hair regrowth, or hair loss will begin again.

Other Information: See hair loss pictures on side of product carton. Before use, read all information on product carton and enclosed booklet. Keep the product carton. It contains important information. Hair regrowth has not been shown to last longer than 48 weeks in large clinical trials with continuous treatment with 5% minoxidil topical solution for men. In clinical studies with mostly white men aged 18–49 years with moderate degrees of hair loss, 5% minoxidil topical solution for men provided more hair regrowth than 2% minoxidil topical solution. Store at controlled room temperature 20° to 25°C (68° to 77° F)

Inactive Ingredients: Alcohol, fragrance, propylene glycol, and purified water.

How Supplied: Men's RogaineExtra Strength Ocean Rush™ Scent is available in one 60 mL bottle. Men's Rogaine Extra Strength Original Formula Unscented is available in packs of three or four 60 mL bottles. (One 60 mL bottle is a one month supply.)

MEN'S ROGAINE FOAM
(Pfizer Consumer Healthcare)
(5% Minoxidil Topical Aerosol)
[ro-gān]
Hair Regrowth Treatment

Drug Facts

Active Ingredient: **Purpose:**
Minoxidil 5% w/w
(without propellant) .... Hair regrowth treatment for men

Use: to regrow hair on the top of the scalp (vertex only, see pictures inside label)

Warnings:

For external use only. For use by men only.

Extremely Flammable: Avoid fire, flame, or smoking during and immediately following application.

Do not use if

- you are a woman
- your amount of hair loss is different than that shown on the inside of this label or your hair loss is on the front of

the scalp. 5% minoxidil topical foam is not intended for frontal baldness or receding hairline.

- you have no family history of hair loss
- your hair loss is sudden and/or patchy
- you do not know the reason for your hair loss
- you are under 18 years of age. Do not use on babies and children.
- your scalp is red, inflamed, infected, irritated, or painful
- you use other medicines on the scalp

Ask a doctor before use if you have heart disease

When using this product

- do not apply on other parts of the body
- avoid contact with the eyes. In case of accidental contact, rinse eyes with large amounts of cool tap water.
- some people have experienced changes in hair color and/or texture
- it takes time to regrow hair. Results may occur at 2 months with twice a day usage. For some men, you may need to use this product for at least 4 months before you see results.
- the amount of hair regrowth is different for each person. This product will not work for all men.

Stop use and ask a doctor if

- chest pain, rapid heartheat, faintness, or dizziness occurs
- sudden, unexplained weight gain occurs
- your hands or feet swell
- scalp irritation or redness occurs
- unwanted facial hair growth occurs
- you do not see hair regrowth in 4 months

May be harmful if used when pregnant or breast-feeding.

Keep out of reach of children. If swallowed, get medical help or contact a Poison Control Center right away.

Directions:

- apply half a capful 2 times a day to the scalp in the hair loss area
- massage into scalp with fingers, then wash hands well
- see enclosed booklet for complete directions on how to use
- using more or more often will not improve results
- continued use is necessary to increase and keep your hair regrowth or hair loss will begin again

Using the Product:

- To open container: Match arrow on can ring with arrow on cap. Pull off cap.
- Within the hair thinning area, part the hair into one or more rows to maximize scalp exposure.
- The foam may begin to melt right away on contact with your warm skin. If your

Continued on next page

Men's Rogaine Foam—Cont.

fingers are warm, rinse them in cold water first. (Be sure to dry them thoroughly before handling the foam.)
- Hold the can upside down and press nozzle to dispense the topical foam product onto your fingers. The total amount of foam applied should not exceed half a capful.
- Using your fingers, spread the foam over the hair loss area and gently massage into scalp and then wash your hands well.
- After each use, close the container to make child resistant by snapping the cap back on to the can.

Other Information:
- hair growth has been shown in a clinical study of men (mostly white) aged 18-49 years who used it for 4 months
- see hair loss pictures on right
- before use, read all information on package and enclosed booklet
- keep the package. It contains important information.
- store at controlled room temperature 20° to 25°C (68° to 77°F)
- contents under pressure. Do not puncture or incinerate container. Do not expose to heat or store at temperatures above 120°F (49°C).

Inactive Ingredients:
butane, butylated hydroxytoluene, cetyl alcohol, citric acid, fragrance, glycerin, isobutane, lactic acid, polysorbate 60, propane, purified water, SD alcohol 40-B, stearyl alcohol

Questions?
- call us at **1-800-ROGAINE** (1-800-764-2463)
- visit **www.rogaine.com**

How Supplied:
- One 60 g (2.11 oz) Can of *Men's Rogaine®* Foam (one month supply)

WOMEN'S ROGAINE®
(Pfizer Consumer Healthcare)
(2% Minoxidil Topical Solution)
Hair Regrowth Treatment
Spring Bloom™ Scent

Drug Facts
Active Ingredient: Minoxidil 2% w/v

Use: to regrow hair on the scalp

Warnings:
For external use only
Flammable: Keep away from fire or flame
Do not use if
- your degree of hair loss is more than that shown on the side of the product carton, because this product may not work for you
- you have no family history of hair loss
- your hair loss is sudden and/or patchy
- your hair loss is associated with childbirth
- you do not know the reason for your hair loss
- you are under 18 years of age. Do not use on babies and children.
- your scalp is red, inflamed, infected, irritated, or painful
- you use other medicines on the scalp

Ask a doctor before use if you have heart disease

When using this product
- do not apply on other parts of the body
- avoid contact with the eyes. In case of accidental contact, rinse eyes with large amounts of cool tap water.
- some people have experienced changes in hair color and/or texture
- it takes time to regrow hair. You may need to use this product 2 times a day for at least 4 months before you see results.
- the amount of hair regrowth is different for each person. This product will not work for everyone

Stop use and ask a doctor if
- chest pain, rapid heartbeat, faintness, or dizziness occurs

- sudden, unexplained weight gain occurs
- your hands or feet swell
- scalp irritation or redness occurs
- unwanted facial hair growth occurs
- you do not see hair regrowth in 4 months

May be harmful if used when pregnant or breast-feeding.
Keep out of reach of children. If swallowed, get medical help or contact a Poison Control Center right away.

Directions:
- apply one mL with dropper 2 times a day directly onto the scalp in the hair loss area
- using more or more often will not improve results
- continued use is necessary to increase and keep your hair regrowth, or hair loss will begin again

Other Information: See hair loss pictures on side of product carton. Before use, read all information on product carton and enclosed booklet. Keep the product carton. It contains important information. In clinical studies of mostly white women aged 18–45 years with mild to moderate degrees of hair loss, the following response to 2% minoxidil topical solution was reported: 19% of women reported moderate hair regrowth after using 2% minoxidil topical solution for 8 months (19% had moderate regrowth; 40% had minimal regrowth). This compares with 7% of women reporting moderate hair regrowth after using the placebo, the liquid without minoxidil in it, for 8 months (7% had moderate regrowth; 33% had minimal regrowth). Store at controlled room temperature 20° to 25°C (68° to 77° F)

Inactive Ingredients: Alcohol, fragrance, propylene glycol, and purified water.

How Supplied: Women's ROGAINE Spring Bloom™ Scent is available in one 60 mL bottle. Women's Rogaine Original Unscented is available in packs of three or four 60 mL bottles. (One 60 mL bottle is a one-month supply.)

Dermatologic Conditions:
Athlete's Foot (Tinea pedis)

DESENEX™ CREAM
(Novartis Consumer Health, Inc.)
1% clotrimazole cream, USP, antifungal

Drug Facts

Active Ingredient: **Purpose:**
Clotrimazole USP, 1% .... Antifungal

Uses:
- cures most athlete's foot (tinea pedis), most jock itch (tinea cruris), and ringworm (tinea corporis)
- relieves itching, burning, cracking, and discomfort which accompany these conditions

Warnings:
For external use only
Do not use
- in or near the mouth or the eyes
- for vaginal yeast infections
- on nail or scalp

Stop use and ask a doctor if
- irritation occurs or gets worse
- there is no improvement within 4 weeks for athlete's foot or ringworm or within 2 weeks for jock itch

Keep out of reach of children. If swallowed, get medical help or contact a poison control center right away.

Directions:
- Adults and children 2 years of age and older.
- use tip of cap to break the seal and open the tube
- wash the affected skin with soap and water and dry completely before applying
- for athlete's foot and ringworm, apply a thin layer over affected area morning and evening for 4 weeks or as directed by a doctor
- for athlete's foot, pay special attention to the spaces between the toes. Wear well-fitting, ventilated shoes and change shoes and socks at least once a day.
- for jock itch, apply a thin layer over affected area morning and evening for 2 weeks or as directed by a doctor
- Children under 2 years: ask a doctor

Other Information:
- store between 2°-30°C (36°-86°F)
- do not use if seal on tube is broken or is not visible

Inactive Ingredients: benzyl alcohol (1%), cetostearyl alcohol, cetyl esters wax, 2-octyldodecanol, polysorbate 60, purified water, sorbitan monostearate

Questions? call 1-800-452-0051 24 hours a day, 7 days a week.

How Supplied: ½ oz cartons.
Shown in Product Identification Guide, page 513

DESENEX™ ANTIFUNGALS
(Novartis Consumer Health, Inc.)
All products are Prescription Strength
Shake Powder
Liquid Spray
Spray Powder
Jock Itch Spray Powder

Drug Facts

Active Ingredient: **Purpose:**
Miconazole nitrate 2% .... Antifungal

Uses: *Shake Powder, Liquid Spray, and Spray Powder*
- cures most athlete's foot (tinea pedis) and ringworm (tinea corporis) • relieves itching, scaling, burning, and discomfort that can accompany athlete's foot
Jock Itch Spray Powder
- cures most jock itch (tinea cruris) • relieves itching, scaling, burning and discomfort that can accompany jock itch
For Spray Powder, Spray Liquid, and Jock Itch Spray Powder
Liquid Spray, Spray Powder and Jock Itch Spray Powder

Warnings:
For external use only
Flammability Warning: Contents under pressure. Do not puncture or incinerate. Flammable mixture; do not use near fire or flame, or expose to heat or temperatures above 49°C (120°F). Use only as directed. Intentional misuse by deliberately concentrating and inhaling the contents can be harmful or fatal.
Do not use
- in or near the mouth or the eyes • for nail or scalp infections
When using this product
- do not get into the eyes or mouth
Stop use and ask a doctor if
- irritation occurs or gets worse
- no improvement within 4 weeks for athlete's foot and ringworm, or no improvement within 2 weeks for jock itch.
Keep out of reach of children. If swallowed, get medical help or contact a poison control center right away.

Directions:
- adults and children 2 years and older
- wash the affected area with soap and water and dry completely before applying

Shake Powder
- apply a thin layer over affected area twice a day (morning and night) or as directed by a doctor
- pay special attention to the spaces between the toes. Wear well-fitting, ventilated shoes and change shoes and socks at least once a day.
- use every day for 4 weeks
- supervise children in the use of this product
- children under 2 years of age: ask a doctor
Liquid Spray and Spray Powder
- shake can well, hold 4″ to 6″ from skin
- spray a thin layer over affected area twice a day (morning and night) or as directed by a doctor
- for athlete's foot pay special attention to the spaces between the toes. Wear well-fitting, ventilated shoes and change shoes and socks at least once a day.
- use daily for 4 weeks
- supervise children in the use of this product
- children under 2 years of age: ask a doctor
Jock Itch Spray Powder
- shake can well, hold 4″ to 6″ from skin
- spray a thin layer over affected area twice a day (morning and night) or as directed by a doctor
- use daily for 2 weeks
- supervise children in the use of this product
- children under 2 years of age: ask a doctor

Other Information: • store at controlled room temperature 20-25°C (68-77°F) • see bottom of can for lot number and expiration date
For Spray Powders and Liquid Spray
- if clogging occurs, remove button and clean nozzle with a pin

Inactive Ingredients: *Shake Powder*—corn starch, corn starch/acrylamide/sodium acrylate polymer, fragrance, talc
Liquid Spray—polyethylene glycol 300, polysorbate 20, SD alcohol 40-B (15%w/w) Propellant: dimethyl ether
Spray Powder, Jock Itch Spray Powder—aloe vera gel, aluminum starch octenyl succinate, isopropyl myristate, propylene carbonate, SD alcohol 40-B (10% w/w), sorbitan monooleate, stearalkonium hectorite Propellant: isobutane/propane

How Supplied: *Shake Powder*-1.5 oz, 3 oz, plastic bottles. *Spray Powder*-4 oz cans. *Liquid Spray*-4.6 oz cans. *Jock Itch Spray Powder*-4 oz cans
Shown in Product Identification Guide, page 513

LAMISIL^{AT}® CREAM
(Novartis Consumer Health, Inc.)

Active Ingredient:	**Purpose:**
Terbinafine hydrochloride 1%	Antifungal

Uses:
- cures most athlete's foot (tinea pedis)
- cures most jock itch (tinea cruris) and ringworm (tinea corporis)
- relieves itching, burning, cracking and scaling which accompany these conditions

Warnings:
For external use only
Do not use • on nails or scalp
- in or near the mouth or the eyes
- for vaginal yeast infections
When using this product do not get into the eyes. If eye contact occurs, rinse thoroughly with water.
Stop use and ask a doctor if too much irritation occurs or gets worse.
Keep out of reach of children. If swallowed, get medical help or contact a poison control center right away.

Directions:
- adults and children 12 years and over
  - use the tip of the cap to break the seal and open the tube
  - wash the affected skin with soap and water and dry completely before applying
  - **for athlete's foot** wear well-fitting, ventilated shoes. Change shoes and socks at least once daily.
    - **between the toes only:** apply twice a day (morning and night) for **1 week** or as directed by a doctor.

1 week between the toes

- **on the bottom or sides of the foot:** apply twice a day (morning and night) for **2 weeks** or as directed by a doctor.

2 weeks on the bottom or sides of the foot

  - **for jock itch and ringworm:** apply once a day (morning **or** night) for **1 week** or as directed by a doctor.
  - wash hands after each use
- children under 12 years: ask a doctor
Other Information: • do not use if seal on tube is broken or is not visible
- store at controlled room temperature 20–25°C (68–77°F)

Inactive Ingredients: benzyl alcohol, cetyl alcohol, cetyl palmitate, isopropyl myristate, polysorbate 60, purified water, sodium hydroxide, sorbitan monostearate, stearyl alcohol.

How Supplied: Athlete's Foot — Net wt. 12g (.42 oz.) tube and 24g (.85 oz.) tube and 30g tube, Jock Itch — Net wt. 12g (.42 oz.) tube.
Questions? call **1-800-452-0051** 24 hours a day, 7 days a week.
Shown in Product Identification Guide, page 514

LAMISIL^{AF} DEFENSE™
(Novartis Consumer Health, Inc.)
TOLNAFTATE 1%, ANTIFUNGAL
Shake Powder
Spray Powder

Drug Facts

Active Ingredient:	**Purpose:**
Tolnaftate 1%	Antifungal

Uses:
- Proven clinically effective in the treatment of most athlete's foot (tinea pedis) and ringworm (tinea corporis)
- Helps prevent most athlete's foot with daily use
- For effective relief of itching, burning and cracking

Warnings:
For external use only
Flammability Warning: (for Spray Powder only): Contents under pressure. Do not puncture or incinerate. Flammable mixture; do not use near fire or flame, or expose to heat or temperatures above 49°C (120°F). Use only as directed. Intentional misuse by deliberately concentrating and inhaling contents can be harmful or fatal.

Do not use
- in or near the mouth or eyes
- on nails or scalp

When using this product
- avoid contact with eyes

Stop use and ask a doctor if
- irritation occurs or gets worse
- no improvement within 4 weeks

Keep out of reach of children. If swallowed, get medical help or contact a poison control center right away.

Directions:
Shake Powder:
- adults and children 2 years and older
  - Wash affected area and dry thoroughly
  - Apply a thin layer over affected area twice daily (morning and night) or as directed by a doctor

- For athlete's foot: pay special attention to spaces between the toes; wear well-fitting, ventilated shoes and change shoes and socks at least once daily
- Use daily for 4 weeks; if condition persists longer, ask a doctor.
- To prevent athlete's foot, apply once or twice daily (morning and/or night)
- Supervise children in the use of this product
- Children under 2 years of age: ask a doctor

Spray Powder:
- adults and children 2 years and older
  - Wash affected area and dry thoroughly
  - Shake can well, hold 4″ to 6″ from skin
  - Spray a thin layer over affected area twice a day (morning and night) or as directed by a doctor
  - For athlete's foot: pay special attention to spaces between the toes; wear well-fitting, ventilated shoes and change shoes and socks at least once daily
- Use daily for 4 weeks; if condition persists longer, ask a doctor
- To prevent athlete's foot, apply once or twice daily (morning and/or night)
- Supervise children in the use of this product
- Children under 2 years of age: ask a doctor

Other Information:
Shake Powder:
- store between 15°C to 25°C (59°F to 77°F)
- see container bottom for lot number and expiration date

Spray Powder:
- store between 20°C to 25°C (68°F to 77°F)
- see container bottom for lot number and expiration date
- In case of clogging, remove button and clean nozzle with a pin

Inactive Ingredients:
Shake Powder: corn starch, fragrance, talc

Spray Powder: aluminum starch octenyl succinate, fragrance, isopropyl myristate, propylene carbonate, SD alcohol 40-B (11% w/w), sorbitan oleate, stearalkonium hectorite, talc.
Propellant: isobutane/propane
Questions call **1-800-452-0051** 24 hours a day, 7 days a week.

How Supplied:
Shake Powder available in 4 oz bottles.
Spray Powder available in 4.6 oz cans.
Shown in Product Identification Guide, page 514

Dermatologic Conditions:

Burns

NEOSPORIN® + PAIN RELIEF
(Pfizer Consumer Healthcare)
MAXIMUM STRENGTH Cream
[nē "uh-spō'rŭn]

For full product information see page 643.

NEOSPORIN® + PAIN RELIEF
(Pfizer Consumer Healthcare)
MAXIMUM STRENGTH Ointment
[nē "uh-spō 'rŭn]

For full product information see page 643.

NEOSPORIN® Ointment
(Pfizer Consumer Healthcare)
[nē "uh-spō' rŭn]

For full product information see page 643.

POLYSPORIN® Ointment
(Pfizer Consumer Healthcare)
[pŏl 'ē-spō 'rŭn]

For full product information see page 643.

Dermatologic Conditions:
Dandruff

HEAD & SHOULDERS INTENSIVE SOLUTIONS (Procter & Gamble)
Dandruff Shampoo for Normal Hair

Head & Shoulders Intensive Solutions Dandruff Shampoo offers effective control of persistent dandruff, seborrheic dermatitis of the scalp, and other symptoms associated with dandruff. Double-blind and expert graded testing have proven that Intensive Solutions Dandruff Shampoo reduces persistent dandruff. It is also gentle enough to use everyday for clean, manageable hair. The formula ingredients below are for the Normal Hair version. Head & Shoulders Intensive Solutions is also available in versions for Oily Hair and Dry Damaged Hair. A 2-in-1 for Normal Hair version is available for increased manageability and prevention of hair damage.

Drug Facts

Active Ingredient: 2% Pyrithione zinc suspended in a mild surfactant base. Shampoo also includes mild conditioning agents.

Purpose: Anti-dandruff

Uses: Helps prevent recurrence of flaking and itching associated with persistent dandruff.

Warnings:
For external use only. When using this product
• Avoid contact with eyes. If contact occurs, rinse eyes thoroughly with water
Stop use and ask a doctor if
• Condition worsens or does not improve after regular use of this product as directed
Keep this and all drugs out of reach of children. If swallowed, get medical help or contact a Poison Control Center right away.

Directions:
• For maximum dandruff control, use every time you shampoo
• Wet hair, massage onto scalp, rinse, repeat if desired

• For best results use at least twice a week or as directed by a doctor

Inactive Ingredients: Water, Sodium Laureth Sulfate, Sodium Lauryl Sulfate, Cocamide MEA, Zinc Carbonate, Glycol Distearate, Dimethicone, Fragrance, Cetyl Alcohol, Guar Hydroxypropyltrimonium Chloride, Magnesium Sulfate, Sodium Benzoate, Ammonium Laureth Sulfate, Magnesium Carbonate Hydroxide, Benzyl Alcohol, Sodium Chloride, Methylchloroisothiazolinone, Methylisothiazolinone, Sodium Xylenesulfonate, Red 4, blue 1.

How Supplied: All versions available in an 8.5 fl. oz. (251 mL) unbreakable plastic bottle.

Questions [or comments]?
1-800-723-9569

NIZORAL® A-D
KETOCONAZOLE SHAMPOO 1%
(McNeil Consumer)

Description:
Nizoral® A-D (Ketoconazole Shampoo 1%) Anti-Dandruff Shampoo is a light-blue liquid for topical application, containing the broad spectrum synthetic antifungal agent Ketoconazole in a concentration of 1%.

Uses:
Controls flaking, scaling and itching associated with dandruff.

Directions:

adults and children 12 years and over	• wet hair thoroughly • apply shampoo, generously lather, rinse thoroughly. Repeat. • use every 3–4 days for up to 8 weeks or as directed by a doctor. Then use only as needed to control dandruff.
children under 12 years	• ask a doctor

Warnings:
For external use only
Do Not Use
• on scalp that is broken or inflamed
• if you are allergic to ingredients in this product
When Using This Product
• avoid contact with eyes
• if product gets into eyes, rinse thoroughly with water
Stop use and ask a doctor if
• rash appears
• condition worsens or does not improve in 2–4 weeks
If pregnant or breast-feeding, ask a doctor before use.
Keep out of the reach of children. If swallowed, get medical help or contact a Poison Control Center right away.
Other Information
• store between 35° and 86°F (2° and 30°C)
• protect from light • protect from freezing

PROFESSIONAL INFORMATION:
OVERDOSAGE INFORMATION
Nizoral® A-D (Ketoconazole) 1% Shampoo is intended for external use only. In the event of accidental ingestion, supportive measures should be employed. Induced emesis and gastric lavage should usually be avoided.

Inactive Ingredients: acrylic acid polymer (carbomer 1342), butylated hydroxytoluene, cocamide MEA, FD&C Blue #1, fragrance, glycol distearate, polyquaternium-7, quaternium-15, sodium chloride, sodium cocoyl sarcosinate, sodium hydroxide and/or hydrochloric acid, sodium laureth sulfate, tetrasodium EDTA, water.

How Supplied:
Available in 4 and 7 fl oz bottles
Shown in Product Identification Guide, page 509

Dermatologic Conditions:
Dry Skin

AMLACTIN® Moisturizing Lotion and Cream (Upsher-Smith)
[ăm-lăk-tĭn]
Cosmetic Lotion and Cream

Description: AMLACTIN® Moisturizing Lotion and Cream are special formulations of 12% lactic acid neutralized with ammonium hydroxide to provide a lotion or cream pH of 4.5–5.5. Lactic acid, an alpha-hydroxy acid, is a naturally occurring humectant for the skin. AMLACTIN® moisturizes and softens rough, dry skin.

How Supplied: 225g (8oz) plastic bottle: List No. 0245-0023-22
400g (14oz) plastic bottle: List No. 0245-0023-40
140g (4.9oz) tube: List No. 0245-0024-14

AMLACTIN AP® Anti-Itch Moisturizing Cream (Upsher-Smith)
[ăm-lăk'-tĭn]
1% Pramoxine HCl

Description: AMLACTIN AP® Anti-Itch Moisturizing Cream is a special formulation containing 12% lactic acid neutralized with ammonium hydroxide to provide a cream pH of 4.5–5.5 with pramoxine HCl. Lactic acid, an alpha-hydroxy acid, is a naturally occurring humectant which moisturizes and softens rough, dry skin. Pramoxine HCl, USP, 1% is an effective antipruritic ingredient used to relieve itching associated with dry skin.

How Supplied: 140g (4.9oz) tube: NDC No. 0245-0025-14

AMLACTIN® XL™ (Upsher-Smith) Moisturizing Lotion
ULTRAPLEX™ Formulation
[ăm-lăk'-tĭn]

Description: AmLactin® XL™ Moisturizing Lotion is a clinically proven moisturizer which provides powerful moisturizing for rough, dry skin. AmLactin® XL™ Moisturizing Lotion contains ULTRAPLEX™ formulation, a proprietary blend of alpha-hydroxy moisturizing compounds.

How Supplied: 160g (5.6oz) tube: List No. 0245-0022-16

Dermatologic Conditions:
Jock Itch (Tinea cruris)

DESENEX™ CREAM
(Novartis Consumer Health, Inc.)
1% clotrimazole cream, USP, antifungal

For full product information see page 635.

DESENEX™ ANTIFUNGALS
(Novartis Consumer Health, Inc.)
All products are Prescription
Strength
Shake Powder
Liquid Spray
Spray Powder
Jock Itch Spray Powder

For full product information see page 635.

LAMISIL^AT® CREAM
(Novartis Consumer Health, Inc.)

For full product information see page 636.

Dermatologic Conditions:
Pediculosis (Lice)

PERMETHRIN LOTION 1%
(Actavis, Inc.)
Lice Treatment

Description:
EACH FLUID OUNCE CONTAINS: Active Ingredient: Permethrin 280 mg (1%). Inactive Ingredients: Balsam fir canada, cetyl alcohol, citric acid, FD&C Yellow No. 6, fragrance, hydrolyzed animal protein, hydroxyethylcellulose, polyoxyethylene 10 cetyl ether, propylene glycol, stearalkonium chloride, water, isopropyl alcohol 5.6 g (20%), methylparaben 56 mg (0.2%), and propylparaben 22 mg (0.08%).
Permethrin Lotion 1% kills lice and their unhatched eggs with usually only one application. Permethrin Lotion 1% protects against head lice reinfestation for 14 days. The creme rinse formula leaves hair manageable and easy to comb.

Indications: For the treatment of head lice. For prophylactic use during head lice epidemics.

Warnings: For external use only. Keep out of eyes when rinsing hair. Adults and children: Close eyes and do not open eyes until product is rinsed out. If product gets into the eyes, immediately flush with water. Do not use near the eyes or permit contact with mucous membranes, such as inside the nose, mouth, or vagina, as irritation may occur. Children: Also protect children's eyes with a washcloth, towel or other suitable material or method. This product should not be used on pediatric patients less than 2 months of age. Itching, redness, or swelling of the scalp may occur. If skin irritation persists or infection is present or develops, discontinue use and consult a doctor. Consult a doctor if infestation of eyebrows or eyelashes occurs. This product may cause breathing difficulty or an asthmatic episode in susceptible persons. As with any drug, if you are pregnant or nursing a baby, seek the advice of a health professional before using this product. Keep this and all drugs out of the reach of children. In case of accidental ingestion, seek professional assistance or contact a Poison Control Center immediately.

Dosage and Administration:
Treatment: Permethrin Lotion 1% should be used after hair has been washed with patient's regular shampoo, rinsed with water and towel dried. A sufficient amount should be applied to saturate hair and scalp (especially behind the ears and on the nape of the neck). Leave on hair for 10 minutes but not longer. Rinse with water. A single application is usually sufficient. If live lice are observed seven days or more after the first application of this product, a second treatment should be given. For proper head lice management, remove nits with the nit comb provided. Head lice live on the scalp and lay small white eggs (nits) on the hair shaft close to the scalp. The nits are most easily found on the nape of the neck or behind the ears. All personal headgear, scarfs, coats, and bed linen should be disinfected by machine washing in hot water and drying, using the hot cycle of a dryer for at least 20 minutes. Personal articles of clothing or bedding that cannot be washed may be dry-cleaned, sealed in a plastic bag for a period of about 2 weeks, or sprayed with a product specifically designed for this purpose. Personal combs and brushes may be disinfected by soaking in hot water (above 130°F) for 5 to 10 minutes. Thorough vacuuming of rooms inhabited by infected patients is recommended.
Prophylaxis: Prophylactic use of Permethrin Lotion 1% is only recommended for individuals exposed to head lice epidemics in which at least 20% of the population at an institution are infested and for immediate household members of infested individuals. Casual use is strongly discouraged.
The method of application of Permethrin Lotion 1% for prophylaxis is identical to that described above for treatment of a lice infestation except nit removal is not required.

Directions For Use: One application of Permethrin Lotion 1% has been shown to protect greater than 95% of patients against reinfestation for at least two weeks. In epidemic settings, a second prophylactic application is recommended two weeks after the first because the life cycle of a head louse is approximately four weeks.

How Supplied: Bottles of 2 fl. oz. (59 mL) with nit removal comb and Family Pack of 2 bottles, 2 fl. oz. (59 mL) each, with 2 nit removal combs.
Store at 15° to 25°C (59° to 77°F).
Alpharma USPD Inc.
Baltimore, MD 21244
FORM NO. 5242   Rev. 9/99
                       VC1587

Dermatologic Conditions:
Ringworm (Tinea corporis)

DESENEX™ CREAM
(Novartis Consumer Health, Inc.)
1% clotrimazole cream, USP, antifungal

For full product information see page 635.

DESENEX™ ANTIFUNGALS
(Novartis Consumer Health, Inc.)
All products are Prescription
Strength
Shake Powder
Liquid Spray
Spray Powder
Jock Itch Spray Powder

For full product information see page 635.

LAMISIL^AT® CREAM
(Novartis Consumer Health, Inc.)

For full product information see page 636.

LAMISIL^AF DEFENSE™
(Novartis Consumer Health, Inc.)
TOLNAFTATE 1%, ANTIFUNGAL
Shake Powder
Spray Powder

For full product information see page 636.

Dermatologic Conditions:
Wound Care

NEOSPORIN® + PAIN RELIEF
(Pfizer Consumer Healthcare)
MAXIMUM STRENGTH Cream
[nē "uh-spō'rŭn]

Drug Facts:

Active Ingredient: **Purpose:**
(in each gram)
Neomycin 3.5 mg ..... First aid antibiotic
Polymyxin B
    10,000 units .... First aid antibiotic
Pramoxine HCl
    10 mg .... External analgesic

Uses: first aid to help prevent infection and for temporary relief of pain or discomfort in minor:
• cuts • scrapes • burns

Warnings:

For external use only.
Do not use
• if you are allergic to any of the ingredients
• in the eyes
• over large areas of the body
Ask a doctor before use if you have
• deep or puncture wounds
• animal bites • serious burns
Stop use and ask a doctor if
• you need to use longer than 1 week
• condition persists or gets worse
• symptoms persist for more than 1 week, or clear up and occur again within a few days
• rash or other allergic reaction develops
Keep out of reach of children. If swallowed, get medical help or contact a Poison Control Center right away.

Directions:
• adults and children 2 years of age and older
    • clean the affected area
    • apply a small amount of this product (an amount equal to the surface area of the tip of a finger) on the area 1 to 3 times daily
    • may be covered with a sterile bandage
• children under 2 years of age: ask a doctor

Other Information:
• store at 20° to 25°C (68° to 77° F)

Inactive Ingredients: emulsifying wax, methylparaben, mineral oil, propylene glycol, purified water, and white petrolatum
Questions? call **1-800-223-0182**, weekdays, 9 AM–5 PM EST

How Supplied: ½ oz (14.2 g) tubes

NEOSPORIN® + PAIN RELIEF
(Pfizer Consumer Healthcare)
MAXIMUM STRENGTH Ointment
[nē "uh-spō'rŭn]

Drug Facts:

Active Ingredient: **Purpose:**
(in each gram)
Bacitracin
    500 units .... First aid antibiotic
Neomycin 3.5 mg ..... First aid antibiotic
Polymyxin B
    10,000 units .... First aid antibiotic
Pramoxine HCl
    10 mg .... External analgesic

Uses: first aid to help prevent infection and for temporary relief of pain or discomfort in minor:
• cuts • scrapes • burns

Warnings:

For external use only.
Do not use
• if you are allergic to any of the ingredients
• in the eyes
• over large areas of the body
Ask a doctor before use if you have
• deep or puncture wounds
• animal bites
• serious burns
Stop use and ask a doctor if
• you need to use longer than 1 week
• condition persists or gets worse
• symptoms persist for more than 1 week, or clear up and occur again within a few days
• rash or other allergic reaction develops
Keep out of reach of children. If swallowed, get medical help or contact a Poison Control Center right away.

Directions:
• adults and children 2 years of age and older
    • clean the affected area
    • apply a small amount of this product (an amount equal to the surface area of the tip of a finger) on the area 1 to 3 times daily
    • may be covered with a sterile bandage
• children under 2 years of age: ask a doctor

Other Information:
• store at 20° to 25°C (68° to 77° F)

Inactive Ingredient: white petrolatum
Questions? call **1-800-223-0182**, weekdays, 9 AM - 5 PM EST

How Supplied: ½ oz (14.2 g) and 1 oz (28.3 g) tubes

NEOSPORIN® Ointment (Pfizer
Consumer Healthcare)
[nē "uh-spō'rŭn]

Drug Facts

Active Ingredients   **Purpose:**
(in each gram):
Bacitracin
    400 units .... First aid antibiotic
Neomycin 3.5 mg ..... First aid antibiotic
Polymyxin B
    5,000 units .... First aid antibiotic

Use: first aid to help prevent infection in minor:
• cuts • scrapes • burns
Warnings:
For external use only.
Do not use
• if you are allergic to any of the ingredients
• in the eyes
• over large areas of the body
Ask a doctor before use if you have
• deep or puncture wounds
• animal bites
• serious burns
Stop use and ask a doctor if
• you need to use longer than 1 week
• condition persists or gets worse
• rash or other allergic reaction develops
Keep out of reach of children. If swallowed, get medical help or contact a Poison Control Center right away.

Directions:
• clean the affected area
• apply a small amount of this product (an amount equal to the surface area of the tip of a finger) on the area 1 to 3 times daily
• may be covered with a sterile bandage

Other Information:
• store at 20° to 25°C (68° to 77° F)

Inactive Ingredients: cocoa butter, cottonseed oil, olive oil, sodium pyruvate, vitamin E, and white petrolatum
Questions? call **1-800-223-0182**, weekdays, 9 AM - 5 PM EST

How Supplied: Tubes, ½ oz (14.2 g), 1 oz (28.3 g), ¹/₃₂ oz (0.9 g) foil packets packed 10 per box (Neo To Go®) or 144 per box.

POLYSPORIN® Ointment (Pfizer
Consumer Healthcare)
[pŏl 'ē-spō'rŭn]

Drug Facts

Active Ingredient: **Purpose:**
(in each strip)
Bacitracin
    500 units .... First aid antibiotic

Polysporin Ointment—Cont.

Polymyxin B
  10,000 units .... First aid antibiotic

Use: first aid to help prevent infection in minor:
• cuts • scrapes • burns

Warnings:
For external use only.
Do not use
• if you are allergic to any of the ingredients
• in the eyes
• over large areas of the body
Ask a doctor before use if you have
• deep or puncture wounds
• animal bites
• serious burns
Stop use and ask a doctor if
• you need to use longer than 1 week
• condition persists or gets worse
• rash or other allergic reaction develops
Keep out of reach of children. If swallowed, get medical help or contact a Poison Control Center right away.

Directions:
• clean the affected area
• apply a small amount of this product (an amount equal to the surface area of the tip of a finger) on the area 1 to 3 times daily
• may be covered with a sterile bandage

Other Information:
• store at 20° to 25°C (68° to 77° F)

Inactive Ingredient: white petrolatum base
Questions? call **1-800-223-0182**, weekdays, 9 AM - 5 PM EST

How Supplied: Tubes, $1/2$ oz (14.2 g), 1 oz (28.3 g); $1/32$ oz (0.9 g) foil packets packed in cartons of 144.

Gastrointestinal/Genitourinary System:
Acid Indigestion

GAS-X® REGULAR STRENGTH
(Novartis Consumer Health, Inc.)
Antigas Chewable Tablets
GAS-X® EXTRA STRENGTH
Antigas Softgels and Chewable
Tablets
GAS-X® MAXIMUM STRENGTH
Antigas Softgels
GAS-X® WITH MAALOX®
Antigas/Antacid Softgels and
Chewable Tablets

For full product information see page 656.

GAVISCON® EXTRA STRENGTH
(GlaxoSmithKline Consumer)
Antacid Tablets
[găv 'ĭs-kŏn]

For full product information see page 658.

GAVISCON® EXTRA STRENGTH
Liquid Antacid
(GlaxoSmithKline Consumer)
[găv 'ĭs-kŏn]

For full product information see page 658.

GAVISCON® Regular Strength
(GlaxoSmithKline Consumer)
Liquid Antacid
[găv 'ĭs-kŏn]

For full product information see page 658.

CHEWABLE
MAALOX® Regular Strength
(Novartis Consumer Health, Inc.)
Calcium Carbonate Antacid
Chewable Tablets
Lemon and Wild Berry
flavors Chewable Tablets

For full product information see page 659.

MAALOX MAX® MAXIMUM
STRENGTH ANTACID/ANTI-GAS
LIQUID
(Novartis Consumer Health, Inc.)
Oral Suspension Antacid/Anti-Gas

For full product information see page 659.

MAALOX REGULAR STRENGTH
(Novartis Consumer Health, Inc.)
Liquid Antacid/Anti-Gas

For full product information see page 660.

MAXIMUM STRENGTH
MAALOX TOTAL STOMACH
RELIEF®
(Novartis Consumer Health, Inc.)
Bismuth Subsalicylate/Upset
Stomach Reliever
Peppermint

For full product information see page 660.

MAALOX® TOTAL STOMACH
RELIEF®
(Novartis Consumer Health, Inc.)

For full product information see page 672.

ORIGINAL PEPCID AC®
(J&J — Merck)
TABLETS AND GELCAPS
MAXIMUM STRENGTH PEPCID® AC
Tablets
Acid reducer

For full product information see page 661.

PEPCID® COMPLETE
(J&J — Merck)
Acid Reducer + Antacid
with DUAL ACTION
Reduces and Neutralizes Acid

For full product information see page 662.

CHILDREN'S PEPTO
(Procter & Gamble)
Calcium carbonate/antacid

For full product information see page 662.

PEPTO-BISMOL®
(Procter & Gamble)
ORIGINAL LIQUID,
MAXIMUM STRENGTH LIQUID,
ORIGINAL AND CHERRY FLAVOR
CHEWABLE TABLETS
AND EASY-TO-SWALLOW CAPLETS
For upset stomach, indigestion,
heartburn, nausea and diarrhea.

For full product information see page 672.

TAGAMET HB® 200
(GlaxoSmithKline Consumer)
Cimetidine Tablets 200 mg/
Acid Reducer

For full product information see page 664.

TUMS® Regular Antacid/Calcium
Supplement Tablets
(GlaxoSmithKline Consumer)

TUMS E–X® and TUMS E–X®
Sugar Free Antacid/Calcium
Supplement Tablets

TUMS ULTRA® Antacid/Calcium
Supplement Tablets

For full product information see page 664.

Gastrointestinal/Genitourinary System:
Anal Itching

PREPARATION H®
(Wyeth Consumer)
Hemorrhoidal Ointment and
Maximum Strength Cream
PREPARATION H®
Hemorrhoidal Suppositories
PREPARATION H®
Hemorrhoidal Cooling Gel

For full product information see page 666.

PREPARATION H®
HYDROCORTISONE CREAM
(Wyeth Consumer)
Anti-itch cream

Active Ingredient:
Hydrocortisone 1%

Uses:
* temporary relief of external anal itching
* temporary relief of itching associated with minor skin irritations and rashes
* other uses of this product should be only under the advice and supervision of a doctor

Warnings:
For external use only
Do not use for the treatment of diaper rash. Consult a doctor.
When using this product
* avoid contact with the eyes
* do not exceed the recommended daily dosage unless directed by a doctor
* do not put into the rectum by using fingers or any mechanical device or applicator
Stop use and ask a doctor if
* bleeding occurs
* condition worsens
* symptoms persist for more than 7 days or clear up and occur again within a few days. Do not begin use of any other hydrocortisone product unless you have consulted a doctor.
Keep out of reach of children. If swallowed, get medical help or contact a Poison Control Center right away.

Directions:
* adults: when practical, cleanse the affected area by patting or blotting with an appropriate cleansing wipe. Gently dry by patting or blotting with a tissue or soft cloth before application of this product.

* when first opening the tube, puncture foil seal with top end of cap
* adults and children 12 years of age and older: apply to the affected area not more than 3 to 4 times daily
* children under 12 years of age: do not use, consult a doctor

Tamper-Evident: Do Not Use if tube seal under cap embossed with "H" is broken or missing.

Inactive Ingredients:
BHA, carboxymethylcellulose sodium, cetyl alcohol, citric acid, edetate disodium, glycerin, glyceryl oleate, glyceryl stearate, lanolin, methylparaben, petrolatum, propyl gallate, propylene glycol, propylparaben, simethicone, sodium benzoate, sodium lauryl sulfate, stearyl alcohol, water, xanthan gum.
Storage: Store at 20–25 °C (68–77 °F)

How Supplied:
0.9 oz. tubes

PREPARATION H® MEDICATED
WIPES (Wyeth Consumer)

For full product information see page 667.

Gastrointestinal/Genitourinary System:
Constipation

CITRUCEL®
(GlaxoSmithKline Consumer)
(methylcellulose)
Soluble Fiber Caplet
Bulk-Forming Fiber Laxative

Uses: Helps restore and maintain regularity. Helps relieve constipation. Also useful in treatment of constipation (irregularity) associated with other bowel disorders when recommended by a physician. This product generally produces a bowel movement in 12 to 72 hours.

Active Ingredient: Each caplet contains 500mg Methylcellulose.

Inactive Ingredients: Crospovidone, Dibasic Calcium Phosphate, FD&C Yellow No. 6 Aluminum Lake, Magnesium Stearate, Maltodextrin, Povidone, Sodium Lauryl Sulfate.

Directions: Adult dose: Take two caplets as needed with 8 ounces of liquid, up to six times daily. Children (6–12 years): Take one caplet with 8 ounces of liquid, up to six times per day. The dosage requirement may vary according to the severity of constipation. Children under 6 years: consult a physician. **TAKE THIS PRODUCT (CHILD OR ADULT DOSE) WITH AT LEAST 8 OUNCES (A FULL GLASS) OF WATER OR OTHER FLUID. TAKING THIS PRODUCT WITHOUT ENOUGH LIQUID MAY CAUSE CHOKING. SEE WARNINGS.**

Directions for Use: Take each dose with 8oz. of liquid.

Age	Dose	Daily Maximum
Adults & Children over 12 years	2 Caplets	Up to 6 times daily*
Children (6 to 12 years)	1 Caplet	Up to 6 times daily*
Children under 6 years	Consult a physician	

*Refer to directions below.

Warnings: Consult a physician before using any laxative product if you have noticed a sudden change in bowel habits which persists for two weeks. Unless directed by a physician, do not use laxative products when abdominal pain, nausea, or vomiting are present. Discontinue use and consult a physician if rectal bleeding or failure to produce a bowel movement occurs after use of any laxative product. Unless recommended by a physician, do not exceed recommended maximum daily dose. Laxative products should not be used for a period longer than a week unless directed by a physician. If sensitive to any of the ingredients, do not use. **TAKING THIS PRODUCT WITHOUT ADEQUATE FLUID MAY CAUSE IT TO SWELL AND BLOCK YOUR THROAT OR ESOPHAGUS AND MAY CAUSE CHOKING. DO NOT TAKE THIS PRODUCT IF YOU HAVE DIFFICULTY IN SWALLOWING. IF YOU EXPERIENCE CHEST PAIN, VOMITING, OR DIFFICULTY IN SWALLOWING OR BREATHING AFTER TAKING THIS PRODUCT, SEEK IMMEDIATE MEDICAL ATTENTION. KEEP THIS AND ALL DRUGS OUT OF THE REACH OF CHILDREN.**

Store at room temperature 15–30°C (59–86°F). Protect contents from moisture. Tamper evident feature: Bottle sealed with printed foil under cap. Do not use if foil is torn or broken.

How Supplied: Bottles of 100 and 164 caplets

Questions or comments?
Call toll-free 1-800-897-6081 weekdays. Patents Pending
The various Citrucel Logos and design elements of the packaging are Registered Trademarks of GlaxoSmithKline.
©2004 GlaxoSmithKline
Distributed by:
GlaxoSmithKline Consumer Healthcare
GlaxoSmithKline Consumer Healthcare, L.P.
Moon Township, PA 15108, Made in Canada.

ORANGE FLAVOR
CITRUCEL®
(GlaxoSmithKline Consumer)
[sĭt ′rə-sĕl]
(Methylcellulose)
Bulk-forming Fiber Laxative

Description: Each 19 g adult dose (approximately one heaping measuring tablespoonful) contains Methylcellulose 2 g. Each 9.5 g child's dose (one-half the adult dose) contains Methylcellulose 1 g. Methylcellulose is a nonallergenic fiber. Also contains: Citric Acid, FD&C Yellow No. 6 Lake, Orange Flavors (natural and artificial), Potassium Citrate, Riboflavin, Sucrose, and other ingredients. Each adult dose contains approximately 3 mg of sodium and contributes 60 calories from Sucrose.

Actions: Promotes elimination by providing additional fiber (bulk) to the diet. This product generally produces bowel movement in 12 to 72 hours.

Indications: For relief of constipation (irregularity). May also be used for relief of constipation associated with other bowel disorders such as irritable bowel syndrome, diverticular disease, and hemorrhoids as well as for bowel management during postpartum, postsurgical, and convalescent periods when recommended by a physician.

Contraindications: Intestinal obstruction, fecal impaction, known hypersensitivity to formula ingredients.

Warnings: Patients should be instructed to consult their physician before using any laxative if they have noticed a sudden change in bowel habits which persists for two weeks. Unless directed by a physician, patients should be advised not to use laxative products when abdominal pain, nausea, or vomiting is present. Patients should also be advised to discontinue use and consult a physician if rectal bleeding or failure to have a bowel movement occurs after use of any laxative product. Unless recommended by a physician, patients should not exceed the recommended maximum daily dose. Patients should not use laxative products for a period longer than one week unless directed by a physician.
TAKING THIS PRODUCT WITHOUT ADEQUATE FLUID MAY CAUSE IT TO SWELL AND BLOCK YOUR THROAT OR ESOPHAGUS AND MAY CAUSE CHOKING. DO NOT TAKE THIS PRODUCT IF YOU HAVE DIFFICULTY IN SWALLOWING. IF YOU EXPERIENCE CHEST PAIN, VOMITING, OR DIFFICULTY IN SWALLOWING OR BREATHING AFTER TAKING THIS PRODUCT, SEEK IMMEDIATE MEDICAL ATTENTION. KEEP THIS AND ALL DRUGS OUT OF THE REACH OF CHILDREN.

Dosage and Administration: Adult Dose: dissolve one leveled scoop (one heaping tablespoon – 19g) in 8 ounces of cold water up to three times daily at the first sign of constipation. Children age 6 to 12 years of age: *one-half the adult dose* stirred briskly in 8 ounces of cold water, once daily at the first sign of constipation. The mixture should be administered promptly and drinking another glass of water is highly recommended (see Warnings). Children under 6 years of age: *Use only as directed by a physician.* Continued

Continued on next page

Citrucel—Cont.

use for 12 to 72 hours may be necessary for full benefit.

TAKE THIS PRODUCT (CHILD OR ADULT DOSE) WITH AT LEAST 8 OZ. (A FULL GLASS) OF WATER OR OTHER FLUID. TAKING THIS PRODUCT WITHOUT ENOUGH LIQUID MAY CAUSE CHOKING. SEE WARNINGS.

How Supplied: 16 oz., 30 oz., and 50 oz. containers.
Boxes of 20-single-dose packets.
Store below 86°F (30°C). Protect contents from humidity; keep tightly closed.

Shown in Product Identification Guide, page 504

SUGAR FREE ORANGE FLAVOR CITRUCEL®

(GlaxoSmithKline Consumer)
[sĭt 'rə-sĕl]
(Methylcellulose)
Bulk-forming Fiber Laxative

Description: Each 10.2 g adult dose (approximately one rounded measuring tablespoonful) contains Methylcellulose 2 g. Each 5.1 g child's dose (one-half the adult dose) contains Methylcellulose 1 g. Methylcellulose is a nonallergenic fiber. Also contains: Aspartame, Dibasic Calcium Phosphate, FD&C Yellow No. 6 Lake, Malic Acid, Maltodextrin, Orange Flavors (natural and artificial), Potassium Citrate, and Riboflavin. Each 10.2 g dose contains approximately 3 mg of sodium and contributes 24 calories from Maltodextrin.

Actions: Promotes elimination by providing additional fiber (bulk) to the diet. This product generally produces bowel movement in 12 to 72 hours.

Indications: For relief of constipation (irregularity). May also be used for relief of constipation associated with other bowel disorders such as irritable bowel syndrome, diverticular disease, and hemorrhoids as well as for bowel management during postpartum, postsurgical, and convalescent periods when recommended by a physician.

Contraindications and Warnings: See entry for "Orange Flavor Citrucel".

Phenylketonurics: CONTAINS PHENYLALANINE 52 mg per adult dose. Individuals with phenylketonuria and other individuals who must restrict their intake of phenylalanine should be warned that each 10.2 g adult dose contains aspartame which provides 52 mg of phenylalanine.

Dosage and Administration: Adult Dose: dissolve one leveled scoop (one rounded measuring tablespoon – 10.2 g) in 8 ounces of cold water up to three times daily at the first sign of constipation. Children age 6 to 12 years of age: *one-half the adult dose* stirred briskly into at least

8 ounces of cold water, once daily at the first sign of constipation. The mixture should be administered promptly and drinking another glass of water is highly recommended (see Warnings). Children under 6 years of age: *Use only as directed by a physician.* Continued use for 12 to 72 hours may be necessary for full benefit.

TAKE THIS PRODUCT (CHILD OR ADULT DOSE) WITH AT LEAST 8 OZ. (A FULL GLASS) OF WATER OR OTHER FLUID. TAKING THIS PRODUCT WITHOUT ENOUGH LIQUID MAY CAUSE CHOKING. SEE WARNINGS.

How Supplied:

8.6 oz, 16.9 oz, and 32 oz containers.
Boxes of 20 single-dose packets.
Store below 86°F (30°C). Protect contents from humidity; keep tightly closed.

Shown in Product Identification Guide, page 504

DULCOLAX® (Boehringer Ingelheim Consumer)

[dul' cō-lax]

Drug Facts

Active Ingredient:
(in each liquid gel)   **Purpose:**
Docusate sodium
100 mg .... Stool softener Laxative

Uses:
• temporary relief of occasional constipation
• this product produces bowel movement within 12 to 72 hours

Warnings:

Do not use if abdominal pain, nausea or vomiting are present
Ask a doctor before use if you
• have noticed a sudden change in bowel habits that persists over a period of 2 weeks
• are presently taking mineral oil
Stop use and ask a doctor if
• rectal bleeding or failure to have a bowel movement occur after use, which may indicate a serious condition
• you need to use a laxative for more than 1 week
If pregnant or breast-feeding, ask a health professional before use.
Keep out of reach of children. In case of overdose, get medical help or contact a Poison Control Center immediately.

Directions:

adults and children 12 years and over	take 1 to 3 liquid gels daily
children 6 to under 12 years	take 1 liquid gel daily
children under 6 years	ask a doctor

Other Information:
• **each liquid gel contains:** sodium 5 mg
• store at 15–30°C
• protect from excessive moisture

Inactive Ingredients: FD&C Red #40, FD&C Yellow #6, gelatin, glycerin, hypromellose, polyethylene glycol, propylene glycol, purified water, sorbitol special, titanium dioxide

How Supplied: Bottles of 25, 50, 100 and 180 Liquid Gels

Boehringer Ingelheim Consumer Healthcare Products.
Division of Boehringer Ingelheim Pharmaceuticals, Inc., Ridgefield, CT 06877
©Boehringer Ingelheim Pharmaceuticals, Inc. 2006

Questions about DULCOLAX?
Call toll-free **1-888-285-9159**
Or visit **www.Dulcolax.com**
Se habla Español.
Shown in Product Identification Guide, page 504

DULCOLAX® (Boehringer Ingelheim Consumer)

[dul' cō-lax]
brand of bisacodyl USP
Suppositories of 10 mg Laxative

Drug Facts

Active Ingredient:
(in each suppository)   **Purpose:**
Bisacodyl USP 10 mg .... Laxative

Uses:
• relieves occasional constipation and irregularity
• this product usually causes bowel movement in 15 minutes to 1 hour

Warnings:
For rectal use only
Do not use when abdominal pain, nausea or vomiting are present
Ask a doctor before use if you have
• stomach pain, nausea or vomiting
• a sudden change in bowel habits that lasts more than 2 weeks
When using this product you may have abdominal discomfort, faintness, rectal burning and mild cramps
Stop use and ask a doctor if
• rectal bleeding or failure to have a bowel movement occurs after using laxative. This may indicate a serious condition.
• you need to use a laxative for more than 1 week
If pregnant or breast-feeding, ask a doctor before use. **Keep out of reach of children.** If swallowed, get medical help or contact a Poison Control Center right away.

Directions:

adults and children 12 years and over	1 suppository once daily. Remove foil. Insert suppository well into rectum, pointed end first. Retain about 15 to 20 minutes.

children 6 to under 12 years	½ suppository daily
children under 6 years	ask a doctor

Other Information:
- store at controlled room temperature 20-25°C (68-77°F)

Inactive Ingredients: hydrogenated vegetable oil

How Supplied: Boxes of 4, 8, 16 and 28 comfort shaped suppositories
Boehringer Ingelheim Consumer Healthcare Products.
Division of Boehringer Ingelheim Pharmaceuticals, Inc., Ridgefield, CT 06877
Made in Italy ©Boehringer Ingelheim Pharmaceuticals, Inc. 2006

Questions about DULCOLAX?
Call toll-free **1-888-285-9159**
Or visit **www.Dulcolax.com**
Se habla Español.

Shown in Product Identification Guide, page 504

DULCOLAX® (Boehringer Ingelheim Consumer)
[dul' cō-lax]
brand of bisacodyl USP
Tablets of 5 mg Laxative

Drug Facts
Active Ingredient:
(in each tablet)   **Purpose:**

Bisacodyl USP 5 mg .... Laxative

Uses:
- relieves occasional constipation and irregularity
- this product usually causes bowel movement in 6 to 12 hours

Warnings:
Do not use if you cannot swallow without chewing
Ask a doctor before use if you have
- stomach pain, nausea or vomiting
- a sudden change in bowel habits that lasts more than 2 weeks

When using this product
- do not chew or crush tablet
- do not use within 1 hour after taking an antacid or milk
- you may have stomach discomfort, faintness or cramps

Stop use and ask a doctor if
- rectal bleeding or failure to have a bowel movement occurs after use of a laxative. These could be signs of a serious condition.
- you need to use a laxative for more than 1 week

If pregnant or breast-feeding, ask a doctor before use. **Keep out of reach of children.** In case of overdose, get medical help or contact a Poison Control Center right away.

Directions:

adults and children 12 years and over	take 1 to 3 tablets (usually 2) daily
children 6 to under 12 years	take 1 tablet daily
children under 6 years	ask a doctor

Other Information:
- store at 20-25°C (68-77°F)
- avoid excessive humidity

Inactive Ingredients: acacia, acetylated monoglyceride, carnauba wax, cellulose acetate phthalate, corn starch, dibutyl phthalate, docusate sodium, gelatin, glycerin, iron oxides, kaolin, lactose, magnesium stearate, methylparaben, pharmaceutical glaze, polyethylene glycol, povidone, propylparaben, Red No. 30 lake, sodium benzoate, sorbitan monooleate, sucrose, talc, titanium dioxide, white wax, Yellow No. 10 lake

How Supplied: Boxes of 10, 25, 50 100 and 150 comfort coated tablets
Boehringer Ingelheim Consumer Healthcare Products.
Division of Boehringer Ingelheim Pharmaceuticals, Inc., Ridgefield, CT 06877
Made in Mexico ©Boehringer Ingelheim Pharmaceuticals, Inc. 2006

Questions about DULCOLAX?
Call toll-free **1-888-285-9159**
Or visit **www.Dulcolax.com**
Se habla Español.

EX•LAX® CHOCOLATED STIMULANT LAXATIVE
(Novartis Consumer Health, Inc.)
Sennosides, USP, 15mg

Drug Facts
Active Ingredient   **Purpose:**
(in each piece):
Sennosides, USP,
15 mg .... Stimulant laxative

Uses:
- relieves occasional constipation (irregularity)
- generally produces bowel movement in 6 to 12 hours

Warnings:
Do not use laxative products when abdominal pain, nausea, or vomiting are present unless directed by a doctor

Ask a doctor before use if you have
- noticed a sudden change in bowel habits that persists over a period of 2 weeks

Ask a doctor or pharmacist before use if you
- are taking a prescription drug. Laxatives may affect how other drugs

work. Take this product 2 or more hours before or after other drugs.

When using this product
- do not use for a period longer than 1 week

Stop use and ask a doctor if
- rectal bleeding or failure to have a bowel movement occur after use of a laxative. These may be signs of a serious condition.

If pregnant or breast-feeding, ask a health professional before use.
Keep out of reach of children. In case of overdose, get medical help or contact a Poison Control Center right away.

Directions:

adults and children 12 years of age and older	chew 2 chocolated pieces once or twice daily
children 6 to under 12 years of age	chew 1 chocolated piece once or twice daily
children under 6 years of age	ask a doctor

Other Information:
- each piece contains: potassium 10mg
- sodium free
- store at controlled room temperature 20-25°C (68-77°F)

Inactive Ingredients: cocoa, confectioners sugar, hydrogenated palm kernel oil, lecithin, non-fat dry milk, vanillin

Questions? call 1-800-452-0051
24 hours a day, 7 days a week.

How Supplied: Carton of 18ct. pieces
Shown in Product Identification Guide, page 514

EX•LAX® Laxative Pills
(Novartis Consumer Health, Inc.)
Regular Strength
Maximum Strength
Laxative Pills
Senosides, USP, 15mg
Senosides, USP, 25mg

Active Ingredients: Regular Strength: Sennosides, USP, 15 mg.
Maximum Strength: Sennosides, USP, 25 mg.

Purpose: Stimulant Laxative

Uses:
- relieves occasional constipation (irregularity)
- generally produces bowel movement in 6 to 12 hours

Warnings:
Do not use laxative products when abdominal pain, nausea, or vomiting are present unless directed by a doctor

Ask a doctor before use if you have

Continued on next page

Ex-Lax—Cont.

- noticed a sudden change in bowel habits that persists over a period of 2 weeks

Ask a doctor or pharmacist before use if you

- are taking a prescription drug. Laxatives may affect how other drugs work. Take this product 2 or more hours before or after other drugs.

When using this product

- do not use for a period longer than 1 week

Stop use and ask a doctor if

- rectal bleeding or failure to have a bowel movement occur after use of a laxative. These may be signs of a serious condition.

If pregnant or breast-feeding, ask a health professional before use.

Keep out of reach of children. In case of overdose, get medical help or contact a Poison Control Center right away.

Directions:

- swallow pill(s) with a glass of water
- swallow pill(s) whole, do not crush, break or chew

adults and children 12 years of age and older	2 pills once or twice daily
children 6 to under 12 years of age	1 pill once or twice daily
children under 6 years of age	ask a doctor

Other Information:

- each pill contains: calcium 50mg
- sodium free
- store at controlled room temperature 20-25°C (68-77°F)

Inactive Ingredients:

Regular Strength:

acacia, alginic acid, carnauba wax, colloidal silicon dioxide, dibasic calcium phosphate, iron oxides, magnesium stearate, microcrystalline cellulose, sodium benzoate, sodium lauryl sulfate, starch, stearic acid, sucrose, talc, titanium dioxide

Maximum Strength:

acacia, alginic acid, carnauba wax, colloidal silicon dioxide, dibasic calcium phosphate, FD&C blue no. 1 aluminium lake, magnesium stearate, microcrystalline cellulose, sodium benzoate, sodium lauryl sulfate, starch, slearic acid, sucrose, talc, titanium dioxide

Questions? call 1-800-452-0051 24 hours a day, 7 days a week.

How Supplied: Available in cartons of 24ct. and 30ct. pills.

FIBERCON® Caplets
(Wyeth Consumer)
Calcium Polycarbophil
Bulk-Forming Laxative

Active Ingredient
(in each caplet):

Calcium polycarbophil 625 mg (equivalent to 500 mg polycarbophil)

Uses:

- relieves occasional constipation to help restore and maintain regularity
- this product generally produces bowel movement in 12 to 72 hours

Warnings:

Choking: Taking this product without adequate fluid may cause it to swell and block your throat or esophagus and may cause choking. Do not take this product if you have difficulty in swallowing. If you experience chest pain, vomiting, or difficulty in swallowing or breathing after taking this product, seek immediate medical attention.

Ask a doctor before use if you have

- abdominal pain, nausea, or vomiting
- a sudden change in bowel habits that persists over a period of 2 weeks

Ask a doctor or pharmacist before use if you are taking any other drug. Take this product 2 or more hours before or after other drugs. All laxatives may affect how other drugs work.

When using this product

- do not use for more than 7 days unless directed by a doctor
- do not take more than 8 caplets in a 24 hour period unless directed by a doctor

Stop use and ask a doctor if rectal bleeding occurs or if you fail to have a bowel movement after use of this or any other laxative. These could be signs of a serious condition.

Keep out of reach of children. In case of overdose, get medical help or contact a Poison Control Center right away.

Directions:

- take each dose of this product with at least 8 ounces (a full glass) of water or other fluid. Taking this product without enough liquid may cause choking. See choking warning.
- FiberCon works naturally so continued use for one to three days is normally required to provide full benefit. Dosage may vary according to diet, exercise, previous laxative use or severity of constipation.

[See table below]

Inactive Ingredients: caramel, crospovidone, hypromellose, magnesium stearate, microcrystalline cellulose, polyethylene glycol, silicon dioxide, sodium lauryl sulfate

Each caplet contains: 140 mg calcium and 10 mg magnesium.
Storage: Protect contents from moisture. Store at 20–25°C (68–77°F)

How Supplied: Film-coated scored caplets.
Package of 36 caplets, and Bottles of 60, 90 and 140 caplets.

METAMUCIL® DIETARY FIBER SUPPLEMENT (Procter & Gamble)
[met uh-mū sil]
(psyllium husk)

Description: Metamucil contains psyllium husk (from the plant *Plantago ovata*), a concentrated source of soluble fiber which can be used to increase one's dietary fiber intake. When used as part of a diet low in saturated fat and cholesterol, 7g per day of soluble fiber from psyllium husk (the amount in 3 doses of Metamucil) may reduce the risk of heart disease by lowering cholesterol. Each dose of Metamucil powder and Metamucil Fiber Wafers contains approximately 3.4 grams of psyllium husk (or 2.4 grams of soluble fiber). A listing of ingredients and nutrition information is available in the listing of Metamucil Fiber Laxative in the Nonprescription Drug section. Metamucil Smooth Texture Sugar-Free Unflavored, Metamucil capsules and Metamucil plus Calcium capsules contains no sugar and no artificial sweeteners. Metamucil Plus Calcium Capsules also helps build strong bones. Metamucil Smooth Texture Sugar-Free Orange Flavor contains aspartame (phenylalanine content of 25 mg per dose). Metamucil powdered products are gluten-free.

Fibersure from the makers of Metamucil, is an all natural, clear-mixing powder that is flavor-free, non-thickening and quickly dissolves in water or most other liquids and won't change the flavor or texture. Fibersure is made of 100% Inulin (a natural vegetable fiber), and can easily be included into cooking and baking.

[See table at top of next page]

Uses: Metamucil Dietary Fiber Supplement can be used as a concentrated source of soluble fiber to increase the dietary intake of fiber. Diets low in saturated fat and cholesterol that include 7 grams of soluble fiber per day from psyllium husk, as in Metamucil, may reduce the risk of heart disease by lowering cholesterol. One adult dose of Metamucil has 2.4 grams of this soluble fiber. Consult a doctor if you are considering use of this product as part of a cholesterol-lowering program.

Age	Recommended dose	Daily maximum
adults & children 12 years of age and over	2 caplets once a day	up to 4 times a day
children under 12 years	consult a physician	

Metamucil Dietary Fiber Supplements

Versions/Flavors	Ingredients (alphabetical order)	Sodium mg/ dose	Calcium mg/ dose	Potas- sium mg/ dose	Calories kcal/ dose	Total Carbo- hydrate g/dose	Dietary Fiber/ (Soluble) g/dose	Serving (Weight in gms)	How Supplied
Capsules plus Calcium	Psyllium husk, Calcium carbonate, Geltain, Crosprovidone, Titanium dioxide, Polysorbate 80, Caramel color, Red 40 Lake, Blue 1 Lake, Yellow 6 Lake	0	300	30	10	12	3 (2.4)	5 capsules (2.6)	Bottles: 75 ct, 120 ct, 150 ct.
Fibersure	Inulin	0	0	0	25	6	5 (5)	1 heaping teaspoon (5.8)	Bottles: 34 servings, 57 servings, 100 servings.
Smooth Texture Orange Flavor Metamucil Powder	Citric Acid, FD&C Yellow #6, Natural and Artificial Flavor, Psyllium Husk, Sucrose	5	7	30	45	12	3 (2.4)	1 rounded tablespoon ~12g	Canisters: Doses: 48, 72, 114, 188; Cartons: 30 single-dose packets.
Smooth Texture Sugar-Free Orange Flavor Metamucil Powder	Aspartame, Citric Acid, FD&C Yellow #6, Maltodextrin, Natural and Artificial Flavor, Psyllium Husk	5	7	30	20	5	3 (2.4)	1 rounded teaspoon ~5.8g	Canisters: Doses: 30, 48, 72, 114, 180, 220; Cartons: 30 single-dose packets.
Smooth Texture Sugar-Free Unflavored Metamucil Powder	Citric Acid, Maltodextrin, Psyllium Husk	4	7	30	20	5	3 (2.4)	1 rounded teaspoon ~5.4g	Canisters: Doses: 48, 72 114.
Coarse Milled Unflavored Metamucil Powder	Psyllium Husk, Sucrose	3	6	30	25	7	3 (2.4)	1 rounded teaspoon ~7g	Canisters: Doses: 48, 72 114.
Coarse Milled Orange Flavor Metamucil Powder	Citric Acid, FD&C Yellow #6, Natural and Artificial Flavor, Psyllium Husk, Sucrose	5	6	30	40	11	3 (2.4)	1 rounded tablespoon ~11g	Canisters: Doses: 48,72 114.
Metamucil Capsules	Caramel color, FD&C Blue No. 1 Aluminum Lake, FD&C Red No. 40 Aluminum Lake, FD&C Yellow No. 6 Aluminum Lake, gelatin, polysorbate 80, psyllium husk	0	5	30	10	3	3 (2.4)	6 capsules 3.2g	Bottles: 100 ct, 160 ct, 300 ct
Fiber Laxative Wafers **Apple** Metamucil Wafers	(1)	20	14	60	120	17	6	2 wafers 24 g	Cartons: 12 doses
Cinnamon Metamucil Wafers	(2)	20	14	60	120	17	6	2 wafers 24 g	Cartons: 12 doses

(1) ascorbic acid, brown sugar, cinnamon, corn oil, corn starch, fructose, lecithin, molasses, natural and artificial flavors, oat hull fiber, psyllium husk, sodium bicarbonate, sucrose, water, wheat flour
(2) ascorbic acid, cinnamon, corn oil, corn starch, fructose, lecithin, molasses, natural and artificial flavors, nutmeg, oat hull fiber, oats, psyllium husk, sodium bicarbonate, sucrose, water, wheat flour

Warnings: Read entire Drug Facts section in listing for Metamucil Fiber Laxative in the Nonprescription Drug section.
Directions: Adults 12 yrs. & older: 1 dose in 8 oz of liquid *3 times daily.*
Capsules: 2–6 capsules for increasing daily fiber intake; 6 capsules for cholesterol lowering use. Up to three times daily. Under 12 yrs.: Consult a doctor. See mixing directions in Drug Facts in listing for Metamucil Fiber Laxative in the Nonprescription Drug section.
NOTICE: Mix this product with at least 8 oz (a full glass) of liquid. Taking without enough liquid may cause choking. Do not take if you have difficulty swallowing.

Capsules plus Calcium: 2-5 capsules as an easy way to increase daily fiber and calcium intake. May be taken up to 4

Continued on next page

Metamucil—Cont.

times daily. Under 12 yrs: Consult a doctor.

Fibersure: Stir 1 heaping teaspoon briskly in 8 oz or more water or other beverages. Product dissolves best in room temperature or warmer liquid. Not recommended for carbonated beverages. Add desired amount directly to foods as you prepare them. For best results use in moist foods or recipes.

For listing of ingredients and nutritional information for Metamucil Dietary Fiber Supplement, and for laxative indications and directions for use, see Metamucil Fiber Laxative in the Nonprescription Drug section.

Notice to Health Care Professionals: To minimize the potential for allergic reaction, health care professionals who frequently dispense powdered psyllium products should avoid inhaling airborne dust while dispensing these products. Handling and Dispensing: To minimize generating airborne dust, spoon product from the canister into a glass according to label directions.

How Supplied: Powder: canisters and cartons of single-dose packets. Capsules: 100 and 160 count bottles. For complete ingredients and sizes for each version, see Metamucil Table 1, page 718, Nonprescription Drug section.

Questions? 1-800-983-4237

METAMUCIL® FIBER LAXATIVE
(Procter & Gamble)
[met uh-mü sil]
(psyllium husk)

Description: Metamucil contains psyllium husk (from the plant *Plantago ovata*), a bulk forming, natural therapeutic fiber for restoring and maintaining regularity when recommended by a physician. Metamucil contains no chemical stimulants and does not disrupt normal bowel function. Each dose of Metamucil powder and Metamucil Fiber Wafers contains approximately 3.4 grams of psyllium husk (or 2.4 grams of soluble fiber). Each dose of Metamucil capsules fiber laxative (5 capsules) contains approximately 2.6 grams of psyllium husk (or 2.0 grams of soluble fiber). Inactive ingredients, sodium, calcium, potassium, calories, carbohydrate, dietary fiber, and phenylalanine content are shown in the following table for all versions and flavors. Metamucil Smooth Texture Sugar-Free Unflavored and Metamucil capsules contain no sugar and no artificial sweeteners; Metamucil Smooth Texture Sugar-Free Orange Flavor contains aspartame (phenylalanine content per dose is 25 mg). Metamucil powdered products and Metamucil capsules are gluten-free. Metamucil Fiber Wafers contain gluten:

Apple contains 0.7g/dose, Cinnamon contains 0.5g/dose. Each two-wafer dose contains 5 grams of fat.

Actions: The active ingredient in Metamucil is psyllium husk, a natural fiber which promotes elimination due to its bulking effect in the colon. This bulking effect is due to both the water-holding capacity of undigested fiber and the increased bacterial mass following partial fiber digestion. These actions result in enlargement of the lumen of the colon, and softer stool, thereby decreasing intraluminal pressure and straining, and speeding colonic transit in constipated patients.

Indications: Metamucil is indicated for the treatment of occasional constipation, and when recommended by a physician, for chronic constipation and constipation associated with irritable bowel syndrome, diverticulosis, hemorrhoids, convalescence, senility and pregnancy. Pregnancy: Category B. If considering use of Metamucil as part of a cholesterol-lowering program, see **Metamucil Dietary Fiber Supplement** in Dietary Supplement Section.

Drug Facts

Active Ingredient: **Purpose:**
(in each DOSE)
Psyllium husk
    approximately 3.4 g .... Fiber therapy
                        for regularity

For Metamucil capsules each dose of 5 capsules contains approximately 2.6 gm of psyllium husk.

Uses:
• effective in treating occasional constipation and restoring regularity

Warnings:

Choking: Taking this product without adequate fluid may cause it to swell and block your throat or esophagus and may cause choking. Do not take this product if you have difficulty in swallowing. If you experience chest pain, vomiting, or difficulty in swallowing or breathing after taking this product, seek immediate medical attention.

Allergy alert: This product may cause allergic reaction in people sensitive to inhaled or ingested psyllium.

Ask a doctor before use if you have:
• a sudden change in bowel habits persisting for 2 weeks
• abdominal pain, nausea or vomiting
Stop use and ask a doctor if:
• constipation lasts more than 7 days
• rectal bleeding occurs
These may be signs of a serious condition.
Keep out of reach of children. In case of overdose, get medical help or contact a Poison Control Center right away.

Directions: For Powders: Put one dose into an empty glass. Fill glass with at least 8 oz of water or your favorite beverage. Stir briskly and drink promptly. If mixture thickens, add more liquid and

stir. Mix this product (child or adult dose) with at least 8 ounces (a full glass) of water or other fluid. **For Capsules:** Take product with 8 oz of liquid (swallow 1 capsule at a time) up to 3 times daily. Take this product with at least 8 oz (a full glass) of liquid. **For Wafers:** Take this product (child or adult dose) with at least 8 ounces (a full glass) of liquid. Taking these products without enough liquid may cause choking. See choking warning.

Adults 12 yrs. & older	Powders: 1 dose in 8 oz of liquid. Capsules: 5 capsules with 8 oz of liquid (swallow one capsule at a time). Wafers: 1 dose with 8 oz of liquid. Take at the first sign of irregularity; can be taken up to 3 times daily. Generally produces effect in 12 – 72 hours.
6 – 11 yrs.	Powders: ½ adult dose in 8 oz of liquid. Wafers: 1 wafer with 8 oz of liquid. Can be taken up to 3 times daily. Capsules: consider use of powder or wafer products
Under 6 yrs.	consult a doctor

Laxatives, including bulk fibers, may affect how well other medicines work. If you are taking a prescription medicine by mouth, take this product at least 2 hours before or 2 hours after the prescribed medicine. As your body adjusts to increased fiber intake, you may experience changes in bowel habits or minor bloating. **New Users:** Start with 1 dose per day; gradually increase to 3 doses per day as necessary.

Other Information:
• **Each product contains:** Potassium; sodium (See table for amount/dose)
• **PHENYLKETONURICS:**   **Smooth Texture Sugar Free Orange product contains phenylalanine** 25 mg per dose
• Each product contains a 100% natural, therapeutic fiber

Inactive Ingredients: See table Notice to Health Care Professionals:
To minimize the potential for allergic reaction, health care professionals who frequently dispense powdered psyllium products should avoid inhaling airborne dust while dispensing these products. Handling and Dispensing: To minimize generating airborne dust, spoon product from the canister into a glass according to label directions.

How Supplied: Powder: canisters and cartons of single-dose packets. Capsules: 100, 160 and 300 count bottles. Wafers: cartons of single dose packets. (See table) [See table at top of next page]
Questions? 1-800-983-4237
Shown in Product Indentification Guide, page 516

Metamucil Fiber Laxative/Dietary Fiber Supplement

Versions/Flavors	Ingredients (alphabetical order)	Sodium mg/ dose	Calcium mg/ dose	Potas- sium mg/ dose	Calories kcal/ dose	Total Carbo- hydrate g/dose	Dietary Fiber/ (Soluble) g/dose	Dosage (Weight in gms)	How Supplied
Smooth Texture Orange Flavor Metamucil Powder	Citric Acid, FD&C Yellow #6, Natural and Artificial Flavor, Psyllium Husk, Sucrose	5	7	30	45	12	3 (2.4)	1 rounded tablespoon ~12g	Canisters: Doses: 48, 72, 114, 188; Cartons: 30 single-dose packets.
Smooth Texture Sugar-Free Orange Flavor Metamucil Powder	Aspartame, Citric Acid, FD&C Yellow #6, Maltodextrin, Natural and Artificial Flavor, Psyllium Husk	5	7	30	20	5	3 (2.4)	1 rounded teaspoon ~5.8g	Canisters: Doses: 30, 48, 72, 114, 180, 220; Cartons: 30 single-dose packets.
Smooth Texture Sugar-Free Unflavored Metamucil Powder	Citric Acid, Maltodextrin, Psyllium Husk	4	7	30	20	5	3 (2.4)	1 rounded teaspoon ~5.4g	Canisters: Doses: 48, 72 114.
Coarse Milled Unflavored Metamucil Powder	Psyllium Husk, Sucrose	3	6	30	25	7	3 (2.4)	1 rounded teaspoon ~7g	Canisters: Doses: 48, 72 114.
Coarse Milled Orange Flavor Metamucil Powder	Citric Acid, FD&C Yellow #6, Natural and Artificial Flavor, Psyllium Husk, Sucrose	5	6	30	40	11	3 (2.4)	1 rounded tablespoon ~11g	Canisters: Doses: 48,72 114.
Metamucil Capsules	Caramel color, FD&C Blue No. 1 Aluminum Lake, FD&C Red No. 40 Aluminum Lake, FD&C Yellow No. 6 Aluminum Lake, gelatin, polysorbate 80, psyllium husk	0	5	30	10	3	3 (2.4)	6 capsules 3.2g	Bottles: 100 ct, 160 ct, 300 ct
Fiber Laxative Wafers **Apple** Metamucil Wafers	(1)	20	14	60	120	17	6	2 wafers 24 g	Cartons: 12 doses
Cinnamon Metamucil Wafers	(2)	20	14	60	120	17	6	2 wafers 24 g	Cartons: 12 doses

(1) ascorbic acid, brown sugar, cinnamon, corn oil, corn starch, fructose, lecithin, molasses, natural and artificial flavors, oat hull fiber, psyllium husk, sodium bicarbonate, sucrose, water, wheat flour

(2) ascorbic acid, cinnamon, corn oil, corn starch, fructose, lecithin, molasses, natural and artificial flavors, nutmeg, oat hull fiber, oats, psyllium husk, sodium bicarbonate, sucrose, water, wheat flour

Gastrointestinal/Genitourinary System:
Diarrhea

IMODIUM® A–D LIQUID AND CAPLETS (loperamide hydrochloride)
(McNeil Consumer)

Description:

Each 7.5 mL (1½ teaspoonful) of *IMODIUM® A-D* liquid contains loperamide hydrochloride 1 mg. *IMODIUM® A-D* liquid is stable, and has a mint flavor.

Each caplet of *IMODIUM® A-D* contains 2 mg of loperamide hydrochloride and is scored and colored green.

Actions:

IMODIUM® A-D contains a clinically proven antidiarrheal medication. Loperamide HCl acts by slowing intestinal motility and by affecting water and electrolyte movement through the bowel.

Uses:

controls symptoms of diarrhea, including Travelers' Diarrhea

Directions:

Imodium A-D Caplets

- **drink plenty of clear fluids to help prevent dehydration caused by diarrhea**
- find right dose on chart. If possible, use weight to dose; otherwise, use age.

adults and children 12 years and over	2 caplets after the first loose stool; 1 caplet after each subsequent loose stool; but no more than 4 caplets in 24 hours
children 9–11 years (60–95 lbs)	1 caplet after first loose stool; ½ caplet after each subsequent loose stool; but no more than 3 caplets in 24 hours
children 6–8 years (48–59 lbs)	1 caplet after first loose stool; ½ caplet after each subsequent loose stool; but no more than 2 caplets in 24 hours
children under 6 years (up to 47 lbs)	ask a doctor

Imodium A-D Liquid

- **drink plenty of clear fluids to help prevent dehydration caused by diarrhea**
- find right dose on chart. If possible, use weight to dose; otherwise use age.
- shake well before using
- only use attached measuring cup to dose product

adults and children 12 years and over	30 mL (6 tsp) after the first loose stool; 15 mL (3 tsp) after each subsequent loose stool; but no more than 60 mL (12 tsp) in 24 hours
children 9–11 years (60–95 lbs)	15 mL (3 tsp) after first loose stool; 7.5 mL (1½ tsp) after each subsequent loose stool; but no more than 45 mL (9 tsp) in 24 hours
children 6–8 years (48–59 lbs)	15 mL (3 tsp) after first loose stool; 7.5 mL (1½ tsp) after each subsequent loose stool; but no more than 30 mL (6 tsp) in 24 hours
children under 6 years (up to 47 lbs)	ask a doctor

Imodium A-D Liquid Professional Dosage Schedule for children 2–5 years old (24–47 lbs): 1½ teaspoonful after first loose bowel movement, followed by 1½ teaspoonful after each subsequent loose bowel movement. Do not exceed 4½ teaspoonful a day.

Warnings:

Allergy alert: Do not use if you have ever had a rash or other allergic reaction to loperamide HCl

Do not use if you have bloody or black stool

Ask a doctor before use if you have

- fever • mucus in the stool • a history of liver disease

Ask a doctor or pharmacist before use if you are taking antibiotics

When using this product tiredness, drowsiness or dizziness may occur. Be careful when driving or operating machinery

Stop use and ask a doctor if

- symptoms get worse • diarrhea lasts for more than 2 days
- you get abdominal swelling or bulging. These may be signs of a serious condition

If pregnant or breast feeding, ask a health professional before use. **Keep out of reach of children.** In case of overdose, get medical help or contact a Poison Control Center right away (1-800-222-1222).

Other Information:

Liquid:	• each 30 mL (6 tsp) contains: **sodium 16 mg**
	• store between 20–25°C (68–77°F)
Caplets:	• each caplet contains: **calcium 10 mg**
	• store between 20–25°C (68–77°F)

PROFESSIONAL INFORMATION:
OVERDOSAGE INFORMATION

Overdosage of loperamide HCl in man may result in constipation, CNS depression and nausea. A slurry of activated charcoal administered promptly after ingestion of loperamide hydrochloride can reduce the amount of drug which is absorbed. If vomiting occurs spontaneously upon ingestion, a slurry of 100 grams of activated charcoal should be administered orally as soon as fluids can be retained. If vomiting has not occurred, and CNS depression is evident, gastric lavage should be performed followed by administration of 100 gms of the activated charcoal slurry through the gastric tube. In the event of overdosage, patients should be monitored for signs of CNS depression for at least 24 hours. Children may be more sensitive to central nervous system effects than adults. If CNS depression is observed, naloxone may be administered. If responsive to naloxone, vital signs must be monitored carefully for recurrence of symptoms of drug overdose for at least 24 hours after the last dose of naloxone.

Inactive Ingredients:

Liquid: cellulose, citric acid, D&C yellow #10, FD&C blue #1, glycerin, flavor, propylene glycol, simethicone, sodium benzoate, sucralose, titanium dioxide, xanthan gum

Caplets: colloidal silicon dioxide, D&C yellow no. 10, dibasic calcium phosphate, FD&C blue no. 1, magnesium stearate, microcrystalline cellulose.

How Supplied:

Liquid: Mint flavored liquid 4 fl. oz. and 8 fl. oz. tamper evident bottles with child resistant safety caps and special dosage cups. Mint flavored liquid 4 fl. oz. for children.

Caplets: Green scored caplets in 6s, 12s, 18s, 24s, 48s and 72s blister packaging which is tamper evident and child resistant, 2s in a tamper resistant pouch.

Shown in Product Identification Guide, page 508

IMODIUM® ADVANCED
(loperamide HCl/simethicone)
Caplets & Chewable Tablets
(McNeil Consumer)

Description:
Each easy to swallow caplet and mint-flavored chewable tablet of *Imodium® Advanced* contains loperamide HCl 2 mg/simethicone 125 mg.

Actions:
Imodium® Advanced combines original prescription strength Imodium® to control the symptoms of diarrhea plus simethicone to relieve bloating, pressure and cramps commonly referred to as gas. Loperamide HCl acts by slowing intestinal motility and by affecting water and electrolyte movement through the bowel. Simethicone acts in the stomach and intestines by altering the surface tension of gas bubbles enabling them to coalesce, thereby freeing and eliminating the gas more easily by belching or passing flatus.

Use:
Controls symptoms of diarrhea plus bloating, pressure, and cramps commonly referred to as gas

Directions:
- **drink plenty of clear fluids to help prevent dehydration caused by diarrhea**
- find right dose on chart. If possible, use weight to dose; otherwise use age

adults and children 12 years and over	swallow 2 caplets or chew 2 tablets and take with water (for chewables) after the first loose stool; 1 caplet/tablet and take with water (for chewables) after each subsequent loose stool; but no more than 4 caplets/tablets in 24 hours
children 9–11 years (60–95 lbs)	swallow 1 caplet or chew 1 tablet and take with water (for chewables) after the first loose stool; ½ caplet/tablet and take with water (for chewables) after each subsequent loose stool; but no more than 3 caplets/tablets in 24 hours
children 6–8 years (48–59 lbs)	swallow 1 caplet or chew 1 tablet and take with water (for chewables) after the first loose stool; ½ caplet/tablet and take with water (for chewables) after each subsequent loose stool; but no more than 2 caplets/tablets in 24 hours
children under 6 years (up to 47 lbs)	ask a doctor

Warnings:
Allergy alert: Do not use if you have ever had a rash or other allergic reaction to loperamide HCl
Do not use if you have bloody or black stool
Ask a doctor before use if you have
• fever • mucus in the stool • a history of liver disease
Ask a doctor or pharmacist before use if you are taking antibiotics
When using this product
• tiredness, drowsiness, or dizziness may occur. Be careful when driving or operating machinery.
Stop use and ask a doctor if • symptoms get worse • diarrhea lasts for more than 2 days • you get abdominal swelling or bulging. These may be signs of a serious condition.
If pregnant or breast-feeding, ask a health professional before use.
Keep out of reach of children. In case of overdose, get medical help or contact a Poison Control Center right away. (1-800-222-1222)

Other Information:
Caplets:
• each caplet contains: **calcium 170 mg**
• store between 20–25°C (68–77°F)
• protect from light
Chewable Tablets:
• each tablet contains: **calcium 50 mg**
• store between 20–25°C (68–77°F)

PROFESSIONAL INFORMATION: OVERDOSAGE INFORMATION
Overdosage of loperamide HCl in man may result in constipation, CNS depression and nausea. A slurry of activated charcoal administered promptly after ingestion of loperamide hydrochloride can reduce the amount of drug which is absorbed. If vomiting occurs spontaneously upon ingestion, a slurry of 100 grams of activated charcoal should be administered orally as soon as fluids can be retained. If vomiting has not occurred, and CNS depression is evident, gastric lavage should be performed followed by administration of 100 gms of the activated charcoal slurry through the gastric tube. In the event of overdosage, patients should be monitored for signs of CNS depression for at least 24 hours. Children may be more sensitive to central nervous system effects than adults. If CNS depression is observed, naloxone may be administered. If responsive to naloxone, vital signs must be monitored carefully for recurrence of symptoms of drug overdose for at least 24 hours after the last dose of naloxone. No treatment is necessary for the simethicone ingestion in this circumstance.

Inactive Ingredients:
Caplets: acesulfame K, cellulose, dibasic calcium phosphate, flavor, sodium starch glycolate, stearic acid **Chewable Tablets:** cellulose acetate, corn starch, D&C Yellow No. 10, dextrates, FD&C Blue No. 1, flavors, microcrystalline cellulose, polymethacrylates, saccharin sodium, sorbitol, stearic acid, sucrose, tribasic calcium phosphate

How Supplied:
Mint Chewable Tablets in 18's, and blister packaging which is tamper evident and child resistant. Each Imodium® Advanced tablet is round, light green in color and has "IMODIUM" embossed on one side and "2/125" on the other side. Imodium Advanced Caplets are available in blister packs of 12's and 18's and bottles of 30's and 42's. Each Imodium® Advanced Caplet is oval, white color and has "IMO" embossed on one side and "2/125" on the other side.
Shown in Product Identification Guide, page 508

PEPTO-BISMOL®
(Procter & Gamble)
ORIGINAL LIQUID,
MAXIMUM STRENGTH LIQUID,
ORIGINAL AND CHERRY FLAVOR
CHEWABLE TABLETS
AND EASY-TO-SWALLOW CAPLETS
For upset stomach, indigestion, heartburn, nausea and diarrhea.

For full product information see page 672.

Gastrointestinal/Genitourinary System:
Gas

GAS-X® REGULAR STRENGTH
(Novartis Consumer Health, Inc.)
Antigas Chewable Tablets
GAS-X® EXTRA STRENGTH
Antigas Softgels and Chewable Tablets
GAS-X® MAXIMUM STRENGTH
Antigas Softgels
GAS-X® WITH MAALOX® EXTRA
STRENGTH Antigas/Antacid Softgels
and Chewable Tablets

Active Ingredients: **Purpose:**

Regular Strength
    Simethicone 80 mg .... Antigas
Extra Strength
    Simethicone 125 mg .... Antigas
Maximum Strength
    Simethicone 166 mg .... Antigas
Gas-X with Maalox Fast tabs
    Calcium carbonate 500 mg ..... Antigas
    Simethicone 125 mg .... Antigas
Gas-X with Maalox Softgels
    Calcium carbonate 250 mg ..... Antigas
    Simethicone 62.5 mg .... Antigas

Inactive Ingredients:
Regular Strength
Cherry Creme
calcium carbonate, D&C Red 30
aluminum lake, dextrose, flavors, maltodextrin, propylene glycol, soy protein isolate
Peppermint Creme
calcium carbonate, dextrose, flavors, maltodextrin, starch
Extra Strength
Softgel
D&C Yellow 10, FD&C Blue 1, FD&C Red
40, gelatin, glycerin, peppermint oil,
purified water, sorbitol, titanium dioxide
Cherry Creme
calcium phosphate tribasic, colloidal
silicon dioxide, D&C Red 30 aluminum
lake, dextrose, flavors, maltodextrin,
propylene glycol soy protein isolate
Peppermint Creme
calcium phosphate tribasic, colloidal
silicon dioxide, D&C Red 30 aluminum
lake, D&C Yellow 10 aluminum lake, dextrose, flavors, maltodextrin, starch
Maximum Strength
FD&C Blue 1, FD&C Red 40, gelatin,
glycerin, peppermint oil, purified water,
sorbitol
Gas-X with Maalox Fast tabs
Orange
colloidal silicon dioxide, dextrose, FD&C
Yellow 6 aluminum lake, flavors, maltodextrin, mannitol, pregelatinized starch,
talc, tribasic calcium phosphate
Wild Berry

colloidal silicon dioxide, D&C Red 30, dextrose, flavors, maltodextrin, mannitol,
pregelatinized starch, talc, tribasic
calcium phosphate
Softgels
D&C Red 28, FD&C Blue 1, gelatin,
glycerin, polyethylene glycol, polysorbate
80, silicon dioxide, sorbitol, titanium
dioxide, purified water

Use:
GAS-X
For the relief of
• pressure and bloating commonly referred to as gas
GAS-X with Maalox
For the relief of
• pressure and bloating commonly referred to as gas
• acid indigestion
• heartburn
• sour stomach
• upset stomach associated with these
  symptoms

Warnings:
GAS-X
Keep out of reach of children.
GAS-X with Maalox
Ask a doctor or pharmacist before use if
you are
• now taking a prescription drug.
  Antacids may interact with certain pre-
  scription drugs.
Keep out of reach of children.

Directions:
Regular Strength
• adults: chew 1 or 2 tablets as needed after meals and at bedtime
• do not exceed 6 tablets in 24 hours except under the advice and supervision of
  a physician
Extra Strength
Tablets
• adults: chew 1 or 2 tablets at needed after meals and at bedtime
• do not exceed 4 tablets in 24 hours except under the advice and supervision of
  a physician
Softgels
• adults: swallow with water one or two
  Softgels as needed after meals and at
  bedtime
• do not exceed 4 Softgels in 24 hours except under the advice and supervision of
  a physician
Maximum Strength
• adults: chew 1 or 2 tablets as needed after meals and at bedtime
• do not exceed 6 tablets in 24 hours except under the advice and supervision of
  a physician
Gas-X with Maalox
Fast tabs

• chew 1 to 2 tablets as symptoms occur
  or as directed by a physician
• do not take more than 4 tablets in a 24-
  hour period or use the maximum dosage
  for more than 2 weeks except under the
  advice and supervision of a physician
Softgels
• adults swallow 2 to 4 Softgels with
  water as symptoms occur or as directed
  by a physician
• do not take more than 8 Softgels in a 24-
  hour period or use the maximum dosage
  for more than 2 weeks except under the
  advice and supervision of a physician

Other Information:
Regular Strength
• each tablet contains: calcium 30mg
• store at controlled room temperature
  20-25°C (68-77°F)
• protect from moisture
Extra Strength
Tablets
• each tablet contains: calcium 45mg
• store at controlled room temperature
  20-25°C (68-77°F)
• protect from moisture
Softgels
• store at controlled room temperature
  20-25°C (68-77°F)
• protect from heat and moisture
Maximum Strength
Gas-X with Maalox
Tablets
• each tablet contains: calcium 45mg
• store at controlled room temperature
  20-25°C (68-77°F)
• protect from moisture
Softgels
• each softgel contains: calcium 102mg
• store at controlled room temperature
  20-25°C (68-77°F)
• protect from heat, moisture and light

Questions?
Call 1-800-452-0051 24 hours a day, 7 days
a week.

How Supplied:
Regular Strength Chewable tablets are
available in peppermint creme and cherry
creme flavored, chewable, scored tablets
in boxes of 36 tablets.
Extra Strength Chewable tablets are
available in peppermint creme and cherry
creme flavored, chewable, scored tablets
in boxes of 18 tablets.
Easy-to-swallow, tasteless/Extra Strength
Softgels are available in boxes of 10 softgels, 30 softgels, 50 softgels and 60 softgels.
Easy-to-swallow, tasteless/Maximum Strength
Softgels are available in boxes of 50 softgels.
Gas-X® With Maalox® Tablets are available in orange and wild berry flavored,

chewable tablets in boxes of 8 tablets and 24 tablets

Easy-to-swallow, tasteless/Gax-X® with Maalox® Softgels are available in boxes of 24 softgels and 48 softgels.

Shown in Product Identification Guide, page 514

GAS-X® THIN STRIPS
(Novartis Consumer Health, Inc.)
Extra Strength
Anti-Gas Simethicone

Description:
Extra Strength Gas-X® Thin Strips™ offers fast, effective, and convenient relief of pressure and bloating. They melt on your tongue so you can discreetly take them anywhere. And they provide a great mouth freshening feel too!

Drug Facts

Active Ingredient (per strip):   Purpose:
Simethicone 62.5 mg .... Antigas

Use:
For the relief of
• Pressure, bloating, and fullness commonly referred to as gas

Warnings:
Keep out of reach of children

Directions:
• Adults: allow 2 to 4 strips to dissolve on tongue as needed after meals and at bedtime
• Do not exceed 8 strips in 24 hours except under the advice and supervision of a physician

Other Information:
• Store at a controlled room temperature 20-25°C (68-77°F)
• Protect from moisture

Inactive Ingredients:
Cinnamon flavor:

corn starch modified, ethyl alcohol, FD&C Red #40, flavor, hypromellose, maltodextrin, polyethylene glycol, sorbitol, sucralose, titanium dioxide, water

Peppermint flavor:

corn starch modified, ethyl alcohol, FD&C Blue #1, flavor, hypromellose, maltodextrin, menthol, polyethylene glycol, sorbitol, sucralose, titanium dioxide, water

Questions?
Call **1-800-452-0051** 24 hours a day, 7 days a week.

How Supplied:
Available in Cinnamon and Peppermint flavors, 18ct. Individually packed strips.
Shown in Product Identification Guide, page 514

IMODIUM® ADVANCED
(loperamide HCl/simethicone)
Caplets & Chewable Tablets
(McNeil Consumer)

For full product information see page 655.

MAALOX MAX® MAXIMUM STRENGTH ANTACID/ANTI-GAS LIQUID
(Novartis Consumer Health, Inc.)
Oral Suspension Antacid/Anti-Gas

For full product information see page 659.

MAALOX REGULAR STRENGTH
(Novartis Consumer Health, Inc.)
Liquid Antacid/Anti-Gas

For full product information see page 660.

QUICK DISSOLVE PHAZYME®–125 MG Chewable Tablets
(GlaxoSmithKline Consumer)
[fay-zime]

Description: A great tasting, smooth cool mint chewable tablet containing simethicone, an antiflatulent to alleviate or relieve the symptoms referred to as gas. Uniquely formulated to dissolve quickly and completely in your mouth. It has no known side effects or drug interactions.

Active Ingredient: Each tablet contains simethicone 125 mg.

Inactive Ingredients: Aspartame, citricacid, colloidal silicon dioxide, crospovidone, dextrates, maltodextrin, mannitol, peppermint flavor, pregelatinized starch, sodium bicarbonate, sorbitol, talc, tribasic calcium phosphate.

Actions: Simethicone minimizes gas formation and relieves gas entrapment in both the stomach and the lower G.I. tract. This action combats the distress due to gastrointestinal gas.

Other Information: Each tablet contains sodium 8 mg. Phenylketonurics: contains phenylalanine 0.4 mg per tablet.

Indication: Relieves pressure, bloating or fullness commonly referred to as gas.

Warnings: Keep this and all drugs out of the reach of children. If condition persists, consult your physician.
Store at room temperature 59°–86°F (15°–30°C).

Dosage: Directions: Chew one or two tablets thoroughly, as needed after a meal]. Do not exceed four tablets per day except under the advice and supervision of a physician.

How Supplied: White, bevel-edged tablets imprinted with "Phazyme 125" in 18 count and 48 count bottles.
Shown in Product Identification Guide, page 506

ULTRA STRENGTH PHAZYME®–180 MG Softgels
(GlaxoSmithKline Consumer)
[fay-zime]

Description: An orange, easy to swallow softgel, containing simethicone, an antiflatulent to alleviate or relieve the symptoms referred to as gas. It has no known side effects or drug interactions.

Active Ingredient: Each softgel contains simethicone 180 mg.

Inactive Ingredients: FD& C Yellow No. 6, gelatin, glycerin, and white edible ink.

Actions: Simethicone minimizes gas formation and relieves gas entrapment in both the stomach and the lower G.I. tract. This action combats the distress due to gastrointestinal gas.

Indication: Relieves pressure, bloating or fullness commonly referred to as gas.

Warnings: Keep this and all drugs out of the reach of children. If condition persists, consult your physician.
Store at room temperature 59°–86°F (15°–30°C).

Dosage: Directions: Swallow one or two softgels as needed after a meal. Do not exceed two softgels per day except under the advice and supervision of a physician.

How Supplied: Orange softgel imprinted with "PZ 180" in 12 count and 36 count blister pack, 60 count and 100 count bottles.
Shown in Product Identification Guide, page 506

Gastrointestinal/Genitourinary System:
Heartburn

**GAS-X® REGULAR STRENGTH
(Novartis Consumer Health, Inc.)
Antigas Chewable Tablets
GAS-X® EXTRA STRENGTH
Antigas Softgels and Chewable Tablets
GAS-X® MAXIMUM STRENGTH
Antigas Softgels
GAS-X® WITH MAALOX®
Antigas/Antacid Softgels and
Chewable Tablets**

For full product information see page 656.

**GAVISCON® EXTRA STRENGTH
(GlaxoSmithKline Consumer)
Antacid Tablets**
[gǎv 'ĭs-kŏn]

Composition: Each chewable tablet contains the following active ingredients:
Aluminum hydroxide .... 160 mg
Magnesium carbonate .... 105 mg
and the following inactive ingredients: alginic acid, calcium stearate, flavor, sodium bicarbonate, and sucrose. May contain stearic acid. Contains sorbitol or mannitol. May contain starch.

Actions: Gavison's unique antacid foam barrier neutralizes stomach acid.

Indications: For the relief of heartburn, sour stomach, acid indigestion and upset stomach associated with these conditions.

Directions: Chew 2 to 4 tablets four times a day or as directed by a physician. Tablets should be taken after meals and at bedtime or as needed. For best results follow by a half glass of water or other liquid. DO NOT SWALLOW WHOLE.

Warnings: Do not take more than 16 tablets in a 24-hour period or 16 tablets daily for more than 2 weeks, except under the advice and supervision of a physician. Do not use this product except under the advice and supervision of a physician if you are on a sodium-restricted diet. Each Extra Strength Gaviscon tablet contains approximately 19 mg of sodium.

Drug Interaction Precaution: Antacids may interact with certain prescription drugs. If you are presently taking a prescription drug, do not take this product without checking with your physician or other health professional. Store at a controlled room temperature in a dry place.
Keep this and all drugs out of the reach of children. In case of accidental overdose, seek professional assistance or contact a poison control center immediately.

How Supplied: Bottles of 100 tablets and in foil-wrapped 2s in boxes of 6 and 30 tablets.
Shown in Product Identification Guide, page 505

**GAVISCON® EXTRA STRENGTH
Liquid Antacid (GlaxoSmithKline
Consumer)**
[gǎv 'ĭs-kŏn]

Composition: Each 2 teaspoonfuls (10 mL) contains the following active ingredients:
Aluminum hydroxide .... 508 mg
Magnesium carbonate .... 475 mg
and the following inactive ingredients: Benzyl alcohol, edetate disodium, flavor, glycerin, saccharin sodium, simethicone emulsion, sodium alginate, sorbitol solution, water, and xanthan gum.

Actions: Gaviscon's unique antacid foam barrier neutralizes stomach acid.

Indications: For the relief of heartburn, sour stomach, acid indigestion and upset stomach associated with these conditions.

Directions: SHAKE WELL BEFORE USING. Take 2 to 4 teaspoonfuls four times a day or as directed by a physician. GAVISCON Extra Strength Liquid should be taken after meals and at bedtime. Dispense product only by spoon or other measuring device.

Warnings: Except under the advice and supervision of a physician, do not take more than 16 teaspoonfuls in a 24-hour period or 16 teaspoonfuls daily for more than 2 weeks. May have laxative effect. Do not use this product if you have a kidney disease. Do not use this product if you are on a sodium-restricted diet except under the advice and supervision of a physician. Each teaspoonful contains approximately 0.9 mEq sodium.
Keep this and all drugs out of the reach of children. In case of accidental overdose, seek professional assistance or contact a poison control center immediately.

Drug Interaction Precaution: Antacids may interact with certain prescription drugs. If you are presently taking a prescription drug, do not take this product without checking with your physician or other health professional.
Keep tightly closed. Avoid freezing. Store at a controlled room temperature.

How Supplied: 12 fl oz (355 mL) bottles.
Shown in Product Identification Guide, page 505

**GAVISCON® Regular Strength
(GlaxoSmithKline Consumer)
Liquid Antacid**
[gǎv 'ĭs-kŏn]

Composition: Each tablespoonful (15 ml) contains the following active ingredients:
Aluminum hydroxide .... 95 mg
Magnesium carbonate .... 358 mg
and the following inactive ingredients: Benzyl alcohol, D&C Yellow #10, edetate disodium, FD&C Blue #1, flavor, glycerin, saccharin sodium, sodium alginate, sorbitol solution, water, and xanthan gum.

Actions: Gaviscon's unique antacid foam barrier neutralizes stomach acid.

Indications: For the relief of heartburn, sour stomach, acid indigestion and upset stomach associated with these conditions.

Directions: SHAKE WELL BEFORE USING. Take 1 or 2 tablespoonfuls four times a day or as directed by a physician. GAVISCON Regular Strength Liquid should be taken after meals and at bedtime. Dispense product only by spoon or other measuring device.

Warnings: Except under the advice and supervision of a physician, do not take more than 8 tablespoonfuls in a 24-hour period or 8 tablespoonfuls daily for more than 2 weeks. May have laxative effect. Do not use this product if you have a kidney disease. Do not use this product if you are on a sodium-restricted diet except under the advice and supervision of a physician. Each tablespoonful of GAVISCON Regular Strength Liquid contains approximately 1.7 mEq sodium.
Keep this and all drugs out of the reach of children. In case of accidental overdose, seek professional assistance or contact a poison control center immediately.

Drug Interaction Precaution: Antacids may interact with certain prescription drugs. If you are presently taking a prescription drug, do not take this product without checking with your physician or other health professional.
Keep tightly closed. Avoid freezing. Store at a controlled room temperature.

How Supplied: 12 fluid oz (355 ml) bottles.
Shown in Product Identification Guide, page 505

**GAVISCON® Regular Strength
Antacid Tablets (GlaxoSmithKline
Consumer)**
[gǎv 'ĭs-kŏn]

Composition: Each chewable tablet contains the following active ingredients:

Aluminum hydroxide dried gel . . . 80 mg
Magnesium trisilicate .... 20 mg
and the following inactive ingredients: alginic acid, calcium stearate, flavor, sodium bicarbonate, starch (may contain corn starch), and sucrose.

Actions: Unique formulation produces soothing foam which floats on stomach contents. Foam containing antacid precedes stomach contents into the esophagus when reflux occurs to help protect the sensitive mucosa from further irritation. GAVISCON® acts locally without neutralizing entire stomach contents to help maintain integrity of the digestive process. Endoscopic studies indicate that GAVISCON Antacid Tablets are equally as effective in the erect or supine patient.

Indications: GAVISCON is specifically formulated for the temporary relief of heartburn (acid indigestion) due to acid reflux. GAVISCON is not indicated for the treatment of peptic ulcers.

Directions: Chew 2 to 4 tablets four times a day or as directed by a physician. Tablets should be taken after meals and at bedtime or as needed. For best results follow by a half glass of water or other liquid. DO NOT SWALLOW WHOLE.

Warnings: Do not take more than 16 tablets in a 24-hour period or 16 tablets daily for more than 2 weeks, except under the advice and supervision of a physician. Do not use this product except under the advice and supervision of a physician if you are on a sodium-restricted diet. Each GAVISCON Tablet contains approximately 19 mg of sodium.

Drug Interaction Precaution: Antacids may interact with certain prescription drugs. If you are presently taking a prescription drug, do not take this product without checking with your physician or other health professional.
Store at a controlled room temperature in a dry place.
Keep this and all drugs out of the reach of children. In case of accidental overdose, seek professional assistance or contact a poison control center immediately.

How Supplied: Bottles of 100 tablets and in foil-wrapped 2s in boxes of 30 tablets.
Shown in Product Identification Guide, page 505

CHEWABLE
MAALOX® Regular Strength
(Novartis Consumer Health, Inc.)
Calcium Carbonate Antacid
Chewable Tablets
Lemon and Wild Berry flavors Chewable Tablets

MAALOX® Regular Strength
Drug Facts:

Active Ingredient:	Purpose:
(in each tablet)	
Calcium carbonate	
600 mg .... Antacid	

Uses: For the relief of
• acid indigestion
• heartburn
• sour stomach
• upset stomach associated with these symptoms

Warnings:
Ask a doctor or pharmacist before use if you are: presently taking a prescription drug. Antacids may interact with certain prescription drugs
Stop use and ask a doctor if symptoms last for more than 2 weeks.
Keep out of reach of children.

Directions:
• Chew 1 to 2 tablets as symptoms occur or as directed by a physician
• do not take more than 12 tablets in a 24-hour period or use the maximum dosage for more than 2 weeks except under the advice and supervision of a physician

Other Information:
• each tablet contains: **calcium 240 mg**
• Phenylketonurics: Contains Phenylalanine, .5 mg per tablet
• store at controlled room temperature 20–25°C (68–77°F)
• keep tightly closed and dry
• Acid neutralizing capacity (per 2 tablets) is 21.6 mEq.

Inactive Ingredients: aspartame, colloidal silicon dioxide, croscarmellose sodium, D&C Red #30 aluminum lake, D&C Yellow #10 aluminum lake (for lemon flavor only), dextrose, flavors, magnesium stearate, maltodextrin, mannitol, pregelatinized starch.

How Supplied:
Lemon — Plastic Bottles of 85 ct. Tablets. Wild Berry — Plastic Bottles of 45 ct. and 150 ct. Tablets.
Questions? call 1-800-452-0051 24 hours a day, 7 days a week.
Shown in Product Identification Guide, page 515

MAALOX MAX® MAXIMUM STRENGTH ANTACID/ANTI-GAS LIQUID
(Novartis Consumer Health, Inc.)
Oral Suspension Antacid/Anti-Gas

Liquids
• **Lemon**
• **Cherry**
• **Mint**
• **Vanilla Crème**
• **Wild Berry**

Drug Facts:

Active Ingredients	Maximum Strength Maalox® Max® Antacid/ Anti-Gas Per Tsp. (5 mL)	Purpose
Aluminum Hydroxide	400 mg	antacid
(equivalent to dried gel, USP)		
Magnesium Hydroxide	400 mg	antacid
Simethicone	40 mg	antigas

Uses: For the relief of
• acid indigestion • heartburn • sour stomach
• upset stomach associated with these symptoms
• bloating and pressure commonly referred to as gas

Warnings:
Ask a doctor before use if you have kidney disease or • a magnesium-restricted diet.
Ask a doctor or pharmacist before use if you are taking a prescription drug. Antacids may interact with certain prescription drugs.
Stop use and ask a doctor if symptoms last for more than 2 weeks
Keep out of reach of children.

Directions:
• shake well before using
• Adults/children 12 years and older: take 2 to 4 teaspoonsful four times a day or as directed by a physician
• do not take more than 12 teaspoonsful in 24 hours or use the maximum dosage for more than 2 weeks.
• Children under 12 years: consult a physician
To aid in establishing proper dosage schedules, the following information is provided:

MAALOX® Max® Maximum Strength Antacid/Anti-Gas	
	Per 2 Tsp. (10 mL)
	(Minimum Recommended Dosage)
Acid neutralizing capacity	38.8 mEq

Inactive Ingredients: butylparaben, carboxymethylcellulose sodium, D&C Yellow #10 (Lemon Flavor only), flavor, glycerin, hypromellose, microcrystalline cellulose, potassium citrate, propylene glycol, propylparaben, purified water, saccharin sodium, sorbitol.

PROFESSIONAL LABELING
Indications:
As an antacid for symptomatic relief of hyperacidity associated with the diagnosis of peptic ulcer, gastritis, peptic esophagitis, gastric hyperacidity, or hiatal hernia.

Continued on next page

Maalox Max—Cont.

As an antiflatulent to alleviate the symptoms of gas, including postoperative gas pain.

Warnings:
Prolonged use of aluminum-containing antacids in patients with renal failure may result in or worsen dialysis osteomalacia. Elevated tissue aluminum levels contribute to the development of the dialysis encephalopathy and osteomalacia syndromes. Small amounts of aluminum are absorbed from the gastrointestinal tract and renal excretion of aluminum is impaired in renal failure. Aluminum is not well removed by dialysis because it is bound to albumin and transferrin, which do not cross dialysis membranes. As a result, aluminum is deposited in bone, and dialysis osteomalacia may develop when large amounts of aluminum are ingested orally by patients with impaired renal function.
Aluminum forms insoluble complexes with phosphate in the gastrointestinal tract, thus decreasing phosphate absorption. Prolonged use of aluminum-containing antacids by normophosphatemic patients may result in hypophosphatemia if phosphate intake is not adequate. In its more severe forms, hypophosphatemia can lead to anorexia, malaise, muscle weakness, and osteomalacia.

Advantages: In addition to the fast acting antacid ingredients, Aluminum Hydroxide and Magnesium Hydroxide, MAALOX® Max® Maximum Strength Antacid/Antigas contains the powerful antigas ingredient, simethicone, to provide concurrent fast relief from discomfort associated with gas.

How Supplied:
Manufacturer: Novartis Consumer
Lemon is available in plastic bottles of 12 fl. oz. (355 mL), and 26 fl. oz. (769 mL).
Cherry is available in plastic bottles of 12 fl. oz. (355 mL) and 26 fl. oz. (769 mL).
Mint is available in plastic bottles of 12 fl. oz. (355 mL) and 26 fl. oz. (769 mL).
Vanilla Crème is available in Plastic Bottles of 12 fl. oz. (355 mL).
Wild Berry is available in Plastic Bottles of 12 fl. oz. (355 mL) and 26 fl. oz. (769 ml).

Shown in Product Identification Guide, page 515

MAALOX MAX® MAXIMUM STRENGTH
(Novartis Consumer Health, Inc.)
ANTACID/ANTIGAS CHEWABLE TABLETS

Drug Facts:
MAALOX Max® Maximum Strength

Active Ingredients:
(in each tablet)   **Purpose:**
Calcium carbonate
    1000 mg .... Antacid

Simethicone 60 mg .... Antigas

Uses:
For the relief of
• acid indigestion • heartburn • sour stomach
• upset stomach associated with these symptoms
• bloating and pressure commonly referred to as gas

Warnings:
Ask a doctor before use if you have:
• kidney stones • a calcium-restricted diet
Ask a doctor or pharmacist before use if you are: presently taking a prescription drug. Antacids may interact with certain prescription drugs.
Stop use and ask a doctor if:
symptoms last for more than 2 weeks.
Keep out of reach of children.

Directions:
• Chew 1 to 2 tablets as symptoms occur or as directed by a physician
• do not take more than 8 tablets in a 24-hour period or use the maximum dosage for more than 2 weeks except under the advice and supervision of a physician

Other Information:
• each tablet contains: **calcium 400 mg**
• store at controlled room temperature 20–25°C (68–77°F)
• keep tightly closed and dry
• Acid neutralizing capacity (per 2 tablets) is 34mEq.

Inactive Ingredients:
Acesulfame K, colloidal silicon dioxide, croscarmellose sodium, D&C Red #30 aluminum lake, D&C Yellow #10 aluminum lake (for lemon & assorted fruit flavor only), dextrose, FD&C Red #40 aluminum lake (for wild berry & assorted fruit flavor only), FD&C Yellow #6 aluminum lake (for assorted fruit flavor only), flavors, magnesium stearate, maltodextrin, mannitol, pregelatinized starch.

How Supplied:
Maalox Max® Lemon — Plastic Bottles of 35 and 65 Tablets.
Maalox Max® Wild Berry — Plastic Bottles of 35 and 65 Tablets.
Maalox Max® Assorted — Plastic Bottles of 35, 65 and 90 tablets.

Questions? call 1-800-452-0051 24 hours a day, 7 days a week.
Manufacturer: Novartis Consumer
Shown in Product Identification Guide, page 515

MAALOX REGULAR STRENGTH
(Novartis Consumer Health, Inc.)
Liquid Antacid/Anti-Gas

Description:
With great flavours, a creamy mouth feel and a pleasant aftertaste, if you haven't tried Maalox® liquids recently, it's time to try them again.

Maalox® Regular Strength Antacid Suspension provides fast, effective relief in two ways. An antacid neutralizes excess stomach acid and an anti-gas ingredient reduces gas pain and pressure.

Uses:
Treatment of moderate symptoms of burning sensation in the stomach or chest area with accompanying bloating and/or gas pain. Usually occurs after a meal.

Medicinal Ingredients: Each teaspoonful (5 mL) contains 200 mg magnesium hydroxide, 200 mg aluminum hydroxide dried gel (equivalent to 153 mg aluminum hydroxide) and 20 mg simethicone.

Non-medicinal Ingredients: butylparaben, flavour, hydroxypropyl methylcellulose, microcrystalline cellulose, propylparaben, sodium carboxymethylcellulose, sodium saccharin, sorbitol and water. Na+ content: 2.84 mg per 5 mL.

Warnings:
KEEP OUT OF REACH OF CHILDREN. Do not take more than 16 teaspoonfuls in a 24 hour period. Do not take this product for more than two weeks, or if symptoms recur, unless directed by a physician. Do not take this product within two hours of another medication because the effectiveness of the other medication may be altered. Individuals with intestinal obstruction or kidney disease should not take this product except on the advice of a physician. SHAKE WELL BEFORE USING.

Directions:
Adults: 2 to 4 teaspoonfuls, four times a day or as directed by a physician. Do not take more than 16 teaspoonfuls in a 24 hour period.
Regular   Strength   Quick   Dissolve Chewable Tablets
Extra-Strength Quick Dissolve Extra-Strength
Chewable Tablets
Nighttime Antacid + Acid Reflux Barrier Quick

How Supplied:
Mint350 mL and 770 mL bottles
Cherry350 mL bottle
Shown in Product Identification Guide, page 514

MAXIMUM STRENGTH MAALOX TOTAL STOMACH RELIEF®
(Novartis Consumer Health, Inc.)
Bismuth Subsalicylate/Upset Stomach Reliever
Peppermint

Drug Facts

Active Ingredient: **Purpose:**
(in each 15 mL*)
Bismuth subsalicylate
    525 mg .... Upset stomach reliever

---
*15 mL = 1 tablespoon

Uses: • upset stomach • heartburn • nausea • fullness • indigestion

Warnings:

Reye's syndrome: Children and teenagers who have or are recovering from chicken pox or flu-like symptoms should not use this product. When using this product, if changes in behavior with nausea and vomiting occur, consult a doctor because these symptoms could be an early sign of Reye's syndrome, a rare but serious illness.

Allergy alert: Do not take this product if you are: • allergic to salicylates (including aspirin)

Ask a doctor or pharmacist before use if you are • taking a prescription drug for anticoagulation (blood thinning), diabetes, gout, or arthritis • taking other salicylate-containing products (such as aspirin)

When using this product a temporary, but harmless, darkening of the stool and/or tongue may occur

Stop use and ask a doctor if
• symptoms last more than 2 days
• ringing in the ears or a loss of hearing occurs

If pregnant or breast-feeding, ask a health care professional before use.

Keep out of reach of children. In case of overdose, get medical help or contact a poison control center right away.

Directions: • shake well before using
• adults and children 12 years of age and older: 2 tablespoons (30 mL) every 1/2 hour to 1 hour, as required, not to exceed 8 tablespoons (120 mL) in 24 hours.
• children under 12 years of age: ask a doctor

Other Information:
• **each tablespoon contains:** sodium 3.3 mg
• each tablespoon contains: salicylate 232 mg
• store at controlled room temperature 20–25°C (68–77°F)
• keep tightly closed and avoid freezing

Inactive Ingredients: carboxymethylcellulose sodium, ethyl alcohol, flavor, methylparaben, microcrystalline cellulose, propylene glycol, propylparaben, purified water, salicylic acid, sodium salicylate, sorbitol, sucralose, xanthan gum
Questions? call **1-800-452-0051** 24 hours a day, 7 days a week.
U.S. Patent No. 5,904,973
Made in Canada

Shown in Product Identification Guide, page 515

MAALOX® TOTAL STOMACH RELIEF®

(Novartis Consumer Health, Inc.)

For full product information see page 672.

ORIGINAL PEPCID AC®
(J&J — Merck)
TABLETS AND GELCAPS
MAXIMUM STRENGTH PEPCID® AC Tablets
Acid reducer

Description: (PEPCID AC)
Each Pepcid AC Tablet and Gelcap contain famotidine 10 mg as an active ingredient.
Each Maximum Strength Pepcid AC Tablet contains famotidine 20 mg as an active ingredient.

Inactive Ingredients:

TABLETS: Hydroxypropyl cellulose, hypromellose, magnesium stearate, microcrystalline cellulose, red iron oxide, starch, talc, titanium dioxide.
GELCAPS: benzyl alcohol, black iron oxide, butylparaben, castor oil, edetate calcium disodium, FD&C red #40, gelatin, hypromellose, magnesium stearate, methylparaben, microcrystalline cellulose, pregelatinized corn starch, propylene glycol, propylparaben, sodium lauryl sulfate, sodium propionate, talc, titanium dioxide.

Inactive Ingredients: (Max. Strength Pepcid AC.)

carnauba wax, hydroxypropyl cellulose, hypromellose, magnesium stearate, microcrystalline cellulose, pregelatinized starch, talc, titanium dioxide.

Product Benefits:
• **1 Tablet or Gelcap** relieves heartburn due to acid indigestion and sour stomach.
• PEPCID AC prevents heartburn associated with acid indigestion and sour stomach brought on by eating or drinking certain food and beverages.
• It contains famotidine, a prescription-proven medicine.

The ingredient in PEPCID AC and Maximum Strength Pepcid AC, famotidine, has been prescribed by doctors for years to treat millions of patients safely and effectively. The active ingredient in PEPCID AC and Maximum Strength Pepcid AC has been taken safely with many frequently prescribed medications.

Action: It is normal for the stomach to produce acid, especially after consuming food and beverages. However, acid in the wrong place (the esophagus), or too much acid, can cause burning pain and discomfort that interfere with everyday activities.

•**Heartburn—Caused by acid in the esophagus**

A valve-like muscle called the lower esophageal sphincter (LES) is relaxed in an open position — Burning pain/discomfort — Excess acid moves up into esophagus

---

Uses:
• Relieves heartburn associated with acid indigestion and sour stomach;
• Prevents heartburn associated with acid indigestion and sour stomach brought on by eating or drinking certain food and beverages.

Tips for Managing Heartburn:
• Do not lie flat or bend over soon after eating.
• Do not eat late at night, or just before bedtime.
• Certain foods or drinks are more likely to cause heartburn, such as rich, spicy, fatty, and fried foods, chocolate, caffeine, alcohol, and even some fruits and vegetables.
• Eat slowly and do not eat big meals.
• If you are overweight, lose weight.
• If you smoke, quit smoking.
• Raise the head of your bed.
• Wear loose fitting clothing around your stomach.

Warnings:

Allergy alert Do not use if you are allergic to famotidine or other acid reducers

Do not use:
• if you have trouble or pain swallowing food, vomiting with blood, or bloody or black stools. These may be signs of a serious condition. See your doctor.
• if you have kidney disease, except under the advice and supervision of a doctor (Maximum Strength Pepcid AC).
• with other acid reducers

Ask a doctor before use if you have
• had heartburn over 3 months. This may be a sign of a more serious condition.
• heartburn with **lightheadedness, sweating, or dizziness**
• chest pain or shoulder pain with shortness of breath; sweating; pain spreading to arms, neck or shoulder; or lightheadedness
• frequent **chest pain**
• frequent wheezing, particularly with heartburn
• unexplained weight loss
• nausea or vomiting
• stomach pain

Stop use and ask a doctor if
• your heartburn continues or worsens
• you need to take this product for more than 14 days.

If pregnant or breast-feeding, ask a health professional before use.

Keep out of reach of children. In case of overdose, get medical help or contact a Poison Control Center right away.

Directions:
Pepcid AC:
• Adults and children 12 years and over:
• Tablet & Gelcap: To **relieve** symptoms, swallow 1 tablet or gelcap with a glass of water. Do not chew.
• Tablet & Gelcap: To **prevent** symptoms, swallow 1 tablet or gelcap with a glass

Continued on next page

Pepcid AC—Cont.

of water at any time from **15 to 60 minutes before** eating food or drinking beverages that cause heartburn.
- Do not use more than 2 tablets or gelcaps in 24 hours.
- Children under 12 years: ask a doctor.

Maximum Strength Pepcid AC:
- adults and children 12 years and over:
- to **relieve** symptoms, swallow 1 tablet with a glass of water. Do not chew.
- to **prevent** symptoms, swallow 1 tablet with a glass of water at any time from **10 to 60 minutes before** eating food or drinking beverages that cause heartburn
- do not use more than 2 tablets in 24 hours
- children under 12 years: ask a doctor

Other Information:
- read the directions and warnings before use
- keep the carton and package insert. They contain important information.
- store at 20°–30°C (68°–86°F)
- protect from moisture

How Supplied:

Pepcid AC Tablet is available as a rose-colored tablet identified as 'PEPCID AC'. NDC 16837-872

Pepcid AC Gelcap is available as a rose and white gelatin coated, capsule shaped tablet identified as 'PEPCID AC'. NDC 16837-856

Maximum Strength Pepcid AC Tablet is a white, "D" shaped, film coated tablet identifed as "PAC 20." NDC 16837 855

Shown in Product Identification Guide, page 506

PEPCID® COMPLETE
(J&J — Merck)
**Acid Reducer + Antacid with DUAL ACTION
Reduces and Neutralizes Acid**

Description:

Active Ingredients	Purpose:
(in each chewablet tablet):	
Famotidine 10mg	Acid Reducer
Calcium carbonate 800 mg	Antacid
Magnesium hydroxide 165 mg	Antacid

Inactive Ingredients:

Mint flavor: cellulose acetate, corn starch, dextrates, flavors, hydroxypropyl cellulose, hypromellose, lactose, magnesium stearate, pregelatinized starch, red iron oxide, sodium lauryl sulfate, sugar
Berry flavor: cellulose acetate, corn starch, D&C red #7, dextrates, FD&C blue #1, FD&C red #40, flavors, hydropropyl cellulose, hypromellose, lactose, magnesium stearate, pregelatinized starch, sodium lauryl sulfate, sugar

Product Benefits: Pepcid Complete combines an acid reducer (famotidine) with antacids (calcium carbonate and magnesium hydroxide) to relieve heartburn in two different ways: Acid reducers decrease the production of new stomach acid; antacids neutralize acid that is already in the stomach. The active ingredients in PEPCID COMPLETE have been used for years to treat acid-related problems in millions of people safely and effectively.

Uses:
Relieves heartburn associated with acid indigestion and sour stomach.

Action:

It is normal for the stomach to produce acid, especially after consuming food and beverages. However, acid in the stomach may move up into the wrong place (the esophagus), causing burning pain and discomfort that interfere with everyday activities.

Heartburn—Caused by acid in the esophagus
- Burning pain/discomfort in esophagus
- A valve-like muscle called the lower esophageal sphincter (LES) is relaxed in an open position
- Acid moves up from stomach

Tips For Managing Heartburn
- Do not lie flat or bend over soon after eating.
- Do not eat late at night, or just before bedtime.
- Certain foods or drinks are more likely to cause heartburn, such as rich, spicy, fatty, and fried foods, chocolate, caffeine, alcohol, and even some fruits and vegetables.
- Eat slowly and do not eat big meals.
- If you are overweight, lose weight.
- If you smoke, quit smoking.
- Raise the head of your bed.
- Wear loose fitting clothing around your stomach.

Warnings:
- **Allergy alert:** Do not use if you are allergic to famotidine or other acid reducers

Do not use
- if you have trouble or pain swallowing food, vomiting with blood, or bloody or black stools. These may be signs of a serious condition. See your doctor.
- with other acid reducers

Ask a doctor before use if you have
- had heartburn over 3 months. This may be a sign of a more serious condition.
- heartburn with **lightheadedness, sweating, or dizziness**
- chest pain or shoulder pain with shortness of breath; sweating; pain spreading to arms, neck or shoulders; or lightheadedness
- frequent **chest pain**
- frequent wheezing, particularly with heartburn
- unexplained weight loss

- nausea or vomiting
- stomach pain

Ask a doctor or pharmacist before use if you are presently taking a prescription drug. Antacids may interact with certain prescription drugs.

Stop use and ask a doctor if
- your heartburn continues or worsens
- you need to take this product for more than 14 days
- **If pregnant or breast-feeding,** ask a health professional before use.
- **Keep out of reach of children.** In case of overdose, get medical help or contact a Poison Control Center right away.

Directions:
- Adults and children 12 years and over:
  - **do not swallow tablet whole; chew completely.**
  - to relieve symptoms, **chew** 1 tablet before swallowing
  - do not use more than 2 chewable tablets in 24 hours
- Children under 12 years: ask a doctor.

Other Information:
- each tablet contains: **calcium 321 mg; magnesium 71 mg.**
- read the directions and warnings before use
- keep the carton and package insert. They contain important information. (Berry)
- read the bottle label. It contains important information. (Mint and Berry pull-out Bottle label)
- store at 20°–30°C (68°–86°F).
- protect from moisture

How Supplied:
Pepcid Complete is available as a rose-colored chewable tablet identified by 'P'. NDC 16837-888– Mint flavor; NDC 16837-291– Pepcid Complete Berry flavor
Shown in Product Identification Guide, page 507

CHILDREN'S PEPTO
(Procter & Gamble)
Calcium carbonate/antacid

Drug Facts

Active Ingredient: (in each tablet)	Purpose:
Calcium carbonate 400 mg	Antacid

Uses:
- relieves:
  - heartburn
  - sour stomach
  - acid indigestion
  - upset stomach due to these symptoms or overindulgence in food and drink

Warnings:
Ask a doctor or pharmacist before use if the child is • presently taking a prescription drug.
Antacids may interact with certain prescription drugs.

Stop use and ask a doctor if symptoms last more than two weeks.
Keep this and all drugs out of the reach of children.

Directions:
- find the right dose on chart below based on weight (preferred), otherwise use age
- repeat dose as needed
- do not take more than 3 tablets (ages 2–5) or 6 tablets (ages 6–11) in a 24-hour period, or use the maximum dosage for more than two weeks, except under the advice and supervision of a doctor.

Dosing Chart

Weight (lbs.)	Age	Dose
under 24	under 2 yrs	ask a doctor
24–47	2–5 yrs	1 tablet
48–95	6–11 yrs	2 tablets

Other Information:
- each tablet contains: calcium 161 mg
- very low sodium
- store at room temperature, avoid excessive humidity

Inactive Ingredients: [Editor's note: "flavor" is applicable to both BUBBLE-GUM AND WATERMELON] flavor, magnesium stearate, mannitol, povidone, red 27 aluminum lake, sorbitol, sugar, talc

Questions? 1-800-717-3786

How Supplied: Available in 24ct

PEPTO-BISMOL®
(Procter & Gamble)
ORIGINAL LIQUID,
MAXIMUM STRENGTH LIQUID,
ORIGINAL AND CHERRY FLAVOR
CHEWABLE TABLETS
AND EASY-TO-SWALLOW CAPLETS
For upset stomach, indigestion, heartburn, nausea and diarrhea.

For full product information see page 672.

PRILOSEC OTC® TABLETS
(Procter & Gamble)
[prĭ-lō-sĕk]

Drug Facts

Active Ingredient: **Purpose:**
(in each tablet)
Omeprazole magnesium
   delayed-release tablet
   20.6 mg (equivalent to 20 mg
   omeprazole) .... Acid reducer

Use:
- treats frequent heartburn (occurs 2 or more days a week)
- not intended for immediate relief of heartburn; this drug may take 1 to 4 days for full effect

Warnings:
Allergy alert: Do not use if you are allergic to omeprazole
Do not use if you have
- trouble or pain swallowing food
- vomiting with blood
- bloody or black stools
These may be signs of a serious condition. See your doctor.
Ask a doctor before use if you have
- had heartburn over 3 months. This may be a sign of a more serious condition.
- heartburn with **lightheadedness, sweating or dizziness**
- chest pain or shoulder pain with shortness of breath; sweating; pain spreading to arms, neck or shoulders; or lightheadedness
- frequent **chest pain**
- frequent wheezing, particularly with heartburn
- unexplained weight loss
- nausea or vomiting
- stomach pain
Ask a doctor or pharmacist before use if you are taking
- warfarin (blood-thinning medicine)
- prescription antifungal or anti-yeast medicines
- diazepam (anxiety medicine)
- digoxin (heart medicine)
Stop use and ask a doctor if
- your heartburn continues or worsens
- you need to take this product for more than 14 days
- you need to take more than 1 course of treatment every 4 months
If pregnant or breast-feeding, ask a health professional before use.
Keep out of reach of children. In case of overdose, get medical help or contact a Poison Control Center right away.

Directions:
- adults 18 years of age and older
- this product is to be used once a day (every 24 hours), every day for 14 days
- it may take 1 to 4 days for full effect, although some people get complete relief of symptoms within 24 hours
  14-Day Course of Treatment
  - swallow 1 tablet with a glass of water before eating in the morning
  - take every day for 14 days
  - do not take more than 1 tablet a day
  - do not chew or crush the tablets
  - do not crush tablets in food
  - do not use for more than 14 days unless directed by your doctor
  Repeated 14-Day Courses (if needed)
  - you may repeat a 14-day course every 4 months
  - **do not take for more than 14 days or more often than every 4 months unless directed by a doctor**
- children under 18 years of age: ask a doctor

Other Information:
- read the directions, warnings and package insert before use
- keep the carton and package insert. They contain important information.
- store at 20–25°C (68–77°F)

- keep product out of high heat and humidity
- protect product from moisture
How Prilosec OTC Works For Your Frequent Heartburn
Prilosec OTC works differently from other OTC heartburn products, such as antacids and other acid reducers. Prilosec OTC stops acid production at the source – the **acid pump** that produces stomach acid. Prilosec OTC is to be used once a day (every 24 hours), every day for 14 days.
What to Expect When Using Prilosec OTC
Prilosec OTC is a different type of medicine from antacids and other acid reducers. Prilosec OTC may take 1 to 4 days for full effect, although some people get complete relief of symptoms within 24 hours. Make sure you take the entire 14 days of dosing to treat your frequent heartburn.
Safety Record
For years, doctors have prescribed Prilosec to treat acid-related conditions in millions of people safely.
Who Should Take Prilosec OTC
This product is for adults (18 years and older) with **frequent heartburn**-when you have heartburn 2 or more days a week.
- Prilosec OTC is **not** intended for those who have heartburn infrequently, one episode of heartburn a week or less, or for those who want immediate relief of heartburn.
Tips for Managing Heartburn
- Do not lie flat or bend over soon after eating.
- Do not eat late at night or just before bedtime.
- Certain foods or drinks are more likely to cause heartburn, such as rich, spicy, fatty and fried foods, chocolate, caffeine, alcohol and even some fruits and vegetables.
- Eat slowly and do not eat big meals.
- If you are overweight, lose weight.
- If you smoke, quit smoking.
- Raise the head of your bed.
- Wear loose-fitting clothing around your stomach.

Inactive Ingredients:
glyceryl monostearate, hydroxypropyl cellulose, hypromellose, iron oxide, magnesium stearate, methacrylic acid copolymer, microcrystalline cellulose, paraffin, polyethylene glycol 6000, polysorbate 80, polyvinylpyrrolidone, sodium stearyl fumarate, starch, sucrose, talc, titanium dioxide, triethyl citrate

How Supplied:
Prilosec OTC is available in 14 tablet, 28 tablet and 42 tablet sizes. These sizes contain one, two and three 14-day courses of treatment, respectively. Do not use for more than 14 days in a row unless directed by your doctor. For the 28 count (two 14-day courses) and the 42 count (three 14-day courses), you may repeat a 14-day course every 4 months.

Continued on next page

Prilosec—Cont.

Safety Feature – Do not use if tablet blister unit is open or torn.
Questions? 1-800-289-9181
Shown in Product Identification Guide, page 516

TAGAMET HB® 200
(GlaxoSmithKline Consumer)
Cimetidine Tablets 200 mg/
Acid Reducer

Tagamet HB® 200 relieves and prevents heartburn, acid indigestion and sour stomach when used as directed. It contains the same ingredient found in prescription strength Tagamet. Tagamet HB 200 reduces the production of stomach acid.

Active Ingredient: Cimetidine, 200 mg.

Inactive Ingredients: Cellulose, cornstarch, hypromellose, magnesium stearate, polyethylene glycol, polysorbate 80, povidone, sodium lauryl sulfate, sodium starch glycolate, titanium dioxide.

Uses:
• For relief of heartburn associated with acid indigestion and sour stomach.
• For prevention of heartburn associated with acid indigestion and sour stomach brought on by eating or drinking certain food and beverages.

Directions:
• For **relief** of symptoms, swallow 1 tablet with a glass of water.
• For **prevention** of symptoms, swallow 1 tablet with a glass of water **right before or anytime up to 30 minutes before** eating food or drinking beverages that cause heartburn.
• Tagamet HB 200 can be used up to twice daily (up to 2 tablets in 24 hours).
• This product should not be given to children under 12 years old unless directed by a doctor.

Warnings:

Allergy Warning: Do not use if you are allergic to Tagamet HB 200 (cimetidine) or other acid reducers.

Ask a Doctor Before Use If You are Taking:
• theophylline (oral asthma medicine)
• warfarin (blood thinning medicine)
• phenytoin (seizure medicine)
If you are not sure whether your medication contains one of these drugs or have any other questions about medicines you are taking, call our consumer affairs specialist at 1-800-482-4394.
• Do not take the maximum daily dosage for more than 2 weeks continuously except under the advice and supervision of a doctor.
• If you have trouble swallowing, or persistent abdominal pain, see your doctor promptly. You may have a serious condition that may need a different treatment.

• As with any drug, if you are pregnant or nursing a baby, seek the advice of a health professional before using this product.
• Keep this and all medications out of the reach of children.
• In case of accidental overdose, seek professional assistance or contact a poison control center immediately.

READ THE LABEL
Read the directions and warnings before taking this medication.
Store at 15°–30°C (59°–86°F).
Comments or questions? Call Toll-Free 1-800-482-4394 weekdays.

PHARMACOKINETIC INTERACTIONS
Cimetidine at prescription doses is known to inhibit various P450 metabolizing isoenzymes, which could affect metabolism of other drugs and increase their blood concentration. Investigation of pharmacokinetic interactions at the recommended OTC doses of cimetidine have thus far shown only small effects.
A pharmacokinetic study conducted in 26 normal male subjects (mean age, 38 years) at steady state using the maximum recommended OTC dose level (200 mg twice a day), showed that Tagamet HB 200, on average, increased the 24 hour AUC of theophylline by 14% and increased peak theophylline levels by 15%. This interaction should be borne in mind in advising patients on the use of Tagamet HB 200. At the prescription doses of cimetidine, clinically significant pharmacokinetic interactions between cimetidine and warfarin, phenytoin, and theophylline have been reported. At prescription doses, pharmacokinetic interactions have been reported for a number of other drugs as well, such as with dihydropyridine calcium channel blockers or some short acting benzodiazepines. At the maximum recommended OTC dose level (200 mg twice a day), a pharmacokinetic study conducted in 21 normal male subjects (mean age, 38 years) showed that Tagamet HB 200, on average, increased the total AUC of triazolam by 26–28% and increased peak triazolam levels by 11–23%. Tagamet HB 200 did not alter the apparent terminal elimination half-life of triazolam.

How Supplied: Tagamet HB 200 (Cimetidine Tablets 200 mg) is available in boxes of blister packs in 6, 30, 50, & 70 tablet sizes.
Shown in Product Identification Guide, page 506

TUMS® Regular Antacid/Calcium Supplement Tablets
(GlaxoSmithKline Consumer)
TUMS E-X® and TUMS E-X®
Sugar Free Antacid/Calcium Supplement Tablets
TUMS ULTRA® Antacid/Calcium Supplement Tablets

Professional Labeling: Indicated for the symptomatic relief of hyperacidity

associated with the diagnosis of peptic ulcer, gastritis, peptic esophagitis, gastric hyperacidity, and hiatal hernia.

Indications: For fast relief of acid indigestion, heartburn, sour stomach, and upset stomach associated with these symptoms.

Active Ingredient:
Tums, Calcium Carbonate 500 mg
Tums E-X, Calcium Carbonate 750 mg
Tums ULTRA, Calcium Carbonate 1000 mg

Actions: Tums provides rapid neutralization of stomach acid. Each Tums tablet has an acid-neutralizing capacity (ANC) of 10 mEq. Each Tums E-X tablet has an ANC of 15 mEq and each Tums ULTRA tablet, an ANC of 20 mEq. This high neutralization capacity makes Tums tablets an ideal antacid for management of conditions associated with hyperacidity. It effectively neutralizes free acid yet does not cause systemic alkalosis in the presence of normal renal function. A double-blind placebo-controlled clinical study demonstrated that calcium carbonate taken at a dosage of 16 Tums tablets daily for a two-week period was non-constipating/non-laxative.

Warnings: Tums: Do not take more than 15 tablets in a 24-hour period or use the maximum dosage of this product for more than 2 weeks, except under the advice and supervision of a physician. If symptoms persist for 2 weeks, stop using this product and see a physician. Keep this and all drugs out of the reach of children.

Tums E-X: Do not take more than 10 tablets in a 24-hour period or use the maximum dosage of this product for more than two weeks, except under the advice and supervision of a physician. If symptoms persist for two weeks, stop using this product and see a physician. Keep this and all drugs out of the reach of children. Additionally, for Tums Ex Sugar Free: Phenylketonurics: Contains phenylalanine, less than 1 mg per tablet.

Tums ULTRA: Do not take more than 7 tablets in 24-hour period or use the maximum dosage of this product for more than two weeks, except under the advice and supervision of a physician. If symptoms persist for two weeks, stop using and see a physician. Keep this and all drugs out of the reach of children.

Drug Interaction Precaution: Antacids may interact with certain prescription drugs. If you are presently taking a prescription drug, do not take this product without checking with your physician or other health professional.

Dosage and Administration: Tums: Chew 2–4 tablets as symptoms occur. Repeat hourly if symptoms return, or as directed by physician.

Tums E-X: Chew 2–4 tablets as symptoms occur. Repeat hourly if symptoms return, or as directed by a physician.

Tums ULTRA: Chew 2-3 tablets as symptoms occur. Repeat hourly if symptoms return, or as directed by a physician.

AS A DIETARY SUPPLEMENT:
Calcium Supplement Directions

Tums, Tums E-X, & Tums ULTRA:
USES: As a daily source of extra calcium. Tums is recommended by the National Osteoporosis Foundation.

IMPORTANT INFORMATION ON OSTEOPOROSIS: Research shows that certain ethnic, age and other groups are at higher risk for developing osteoporosis, including Caucasian and Asian teen and young adult women, menopausal women, older persons and those persons with a family history of fragile bones.
A balanced diet with enough calcium and regular exercise throughout life will help you to build and maintain healthy bones and may reduce your risk of developing osteoporosis. Adequate calcium intake is important, but daily intakes above 2,000 mg are not likely to provide any additional benefit.

Directions: Chew 2 tablets twice daily.

[See table above]

Ingredients (all variants except sugar free): Sucrose, Corn Starch, Talc,

Supplement Facts

	Tums 2 Tablets	Tums E-X 2 Tablets	Tums E-X Sugar Free 2 Tablets	Tums Ultra 2 Tablets
Serving Size				
Amount Per Serving	5	10	5	10
Calories				
Sorbitol (g)	—	—	1	—
Sugars (g)	1	2	—	3
Calcium (mg)	400	600	600	800
% Daily Value	40	60	60	80
Sodium (mg)	—	5	—	10
% Daily Value	—	<1%	—	<1%

Mineral Oil, Flavors (natural and/or artificial), Sodium Polyphosphate. May also contain 1% or less of Adipic Acid, Blue 1 Lake, Yellow 6 Lake, Yellow 5 Lake, Red 40 Lake.

Ingredients (Sugar Free): Sorbitol, Acacia, Natural and Artificial Flavors, Calcium Stearate, Adipic Acid, Yellow 6 Lake, Aspartame.

How Supplied:

Tums: **Peppermint flavor** is available in 12-tablet rolls, 3-roll wraps, and bottles of 75, 150, and 180. **Assorted Flavors** (Cherry, Lemon, Orange, and Lime), are available in 12-tablet rolls, 3-roll wraps, and bottles of 75, 150, and 320.

Tums E-X: **Wintergreen** 3-roll wraps and bottles of 48, 96, and 116.

Tums E-X: Assorted Fruit, Assorted Tropical Fruit, and Assorted Berries, Fresh Blend 8 tablet rolls, 3-roll wraps, 6-roll wraps, and bottles of 48, 96, and 116. Assorted Tropical Fruit and Assorted Berries are also available in bottles of 200 tablets.

Tums EX Sugar Free: Orange Cream; bottles of 48 and 80 tablets.

Tums ULTRA: Assorted Berries, and **Spearmint** bottles of 160 tablets. **Assorted Fruit** and **Assorted Mint** bottles of 36, 72, and 86 tablets. Assorted Fruit also available in bottles of 160 tablets. **Tropical Fruit** bottles of 160 tablets.

Shown in Product Identification Guide, page 506

Gastrointestinal/Genitourinary System:
Hemorrhoids

PREPARATION H®
(Wyeth Consumer)
Hemorrhoidal Ointment and
Maximum Strength Cream
PREPARATION H®
Hemorrhoidal Suppositories
PREPARATION H®
Hemorrhoidal Cooling Gel

Active Ingredients: Preparation H is available in ointment, cream, gel, and suppository product forms. The **Ointment** contains Petrolatum 71.9%, Mineral Oil 14%, Shark Liver Oil 3% and Phenylephrine HCl 0.25%.

The **Maximum Strength Cream** contains White Petrolatum 15%, Glycerin 14.4%, Pramoxine HCl 1% and Phenylephrine HCl 0.25%.

The **Suppositories** contain Cocoa Butter 85.5%, Shark Liver Oil 3%, and Phenylephrine HCl 0.25%.

The **Cooling Gel** contains Phenylephrine HCl 0.25% and Witch Hazel 50%.

Uses: Preparation H Ointment and Suppositories
- helps relieve the local itching and discomfort associated with hemorrhoids
- temporarily shrinks hemorrhoidal tissue and relieves burning
- temporarily provides a coating for relief of anorectal discomforts
- temporarily protects the inflamed, irritated anorectal surface to help make bowel movements less painful

Maximum Strength Cream
- for temporary relief of pain, soreness and burning
- helps relieve the local itching and discomfort associated with hemorrhoids
- temporarily shrinks hemorrhoidal tissue
- temporarily provides a coating for relief of anorectal discomforts
- temporarily protects the inflamed, irritated anorectal surface to help make bowel movements less painful

Cooling Gel
- helps relieve the local itching and discomfort associated with hemorrhoids
- temporarily relieves irritation and burning
- temporarily shrinks hemorrhoidal tissue
- aids in protecting irritated anorectal areas

Warnings:
For all product forms:
Ask a doctor before use if you have
- heart disease
- high blood pressure
- thyroid disease
- diabetes

- difficulty in urination due to enlargement of the prostate gland

Ask a doctor or pharmacist before use if you are presently taking a prescription drug for high blood pressure or depression.

When using this product do not exceed the recommended daily dosage unless directed by a doctor.

Stop use and ask a doctor if
- bleeding occurs
- condition worsens or does not improve within 7 days

If pregnant or breast-feeding, ask a health professional before use.

Keep out of reach of children. If swallowed, get medical help or contact a Poison Control Center right away.

Ointment: For external and/or intra-rectal use only. Stop use and ask a doctor if introduction of applicator into the rectum causes additional pain.

Maximum Strength Cream: For external use only. When using this product do not put into the rectum by using fingers or any mechanical device or applicator. **Stop use and ask a doctor if** an allergic reaction develops; or if the symptom being treated does not subside or if redness, irritation, swelling, pain, or other symptoms develop or increase.

Cooling Gel: For external use only. When using this product do not put into the rectum by using fingers or any mechanical device or applicator.

Suppositories: For rectal use only.

Directions:
Ointment—
- adults: when practical, cleanse the affected area by patting or blotting with an appropriate cleansing wipe. Gently dry by patting or blotting with a tissue or a soft cloth before applying ointment.
- when first opening the tube, puncture foil seal with top end of cap
- apply to the affected area up to 4 times daily, especially at night, in the morning or after each bowel movement
- intrarectal use:
  - remove cover from applicator, attach applicator to tube, lubricate applicator well and gently insert applicator into the rectum
  - thoroughly cleanse applicator after each use and replace cover
- also apply ointment to external area
- regular use provides continual therapy for relief of symptoms
- children under 12 years of age: ask a doctor

Tamper-Evident: Do Not Use if tube seal under cap embossed with "H" is broken or missing.

Maximum Strength Cream—
- adults: when practical, cleanse the affected area by patting or blotting with an appropriate cleansing wipe. Gently dry by patting or blotting with a tissue or a soft cloth before applying cream.
- when first opening the tube, puncture foil seal with top end of cap
- apply externally or in the lower portion of the anal canal only
- apply externally to the affected area up to 4 times daily, especially at night, in the morning or after each bowel movement
- for application in the lower anal canal: remove cover from dispensing cap. Attach dispensing cap to tube. Lubricate dispensing cap well, then gently insert dispensing cap partway into the anus.
- thoroughly cleanse dispensing cap after each use and replace cover
- children under 12 years of age: ask a doctor

Tamper-Evident: Do Not Use if tube seal under cap embossed with "H" is broken or missing.

Suppositories—
- adults: when practical, cleanse the affected area by patting or blotting with an appropriate cleansing wipe. Gently dry by patting or blotting with a tissue or a soft cloth before insertion of this product.
- detach one suppository from the strip; remove the foil wrapper before inserting into the rectum as follows:
  - hold suppository with rounded end up
  - carefully separate foil tabs by inserting tip of fingernail at end marked "peel down"
  - slowly and evenly peel apart (do not tear) foil by pulling tabs down both sides, to expose the suppository
  - remove exposed suppository from wrapper
  - insert one suppository into the rectum up to 4 times daily, especially at night, in the morning or after each bowel movement
- children under 12 years of age: ask a doctor

Tamper-Evident: Individually quality sealed for your protection. Do Not Use if foil imprinted "PREPARATION H" is torn or damaged.

Cooling Gel—
- adults: when practical, cleanse the affected area by patting or blotting with an appropriate cleansing wipe. Gently dry by patting or blotting with a tissue or a soft cloth before applying gel.
- when first opening the tube, puncture foil seal with top end of cap
- apply externally to the affected area up to 4 times daily, especially at night, in

the morning or after each bowel movement
- children under 12 years of age: ask a doctor

Tamper-Evident: Do Not Use if tube seal under cap embossed with "H" is broken or missing.

Inactive Ingredients: **Ointment**—benzoic acid, BHA, BHT, corn oil, glycerin, lanolin, lanolin alcohol, methylparaben, paraffin, propylparaben, thyme oil, tocopherol, water, wax

Maximum Strength Cream—aloe barbadensis leaf extract, BHA, carboxymethylcellulose sodium, cetyl alcohol, citric acid, edeteth disodium, glyceryl stearate, laureth-23, methylparaben, mineral oil, panthenol, propyl gallate, propylene glycol, propylparaben, purified water, sodium benzoate, steareth-2, steareth-20, stearyl alcohol, tocopherol, vitamin E, xanthan gum

Suppositories—methylparaben, propylparaben, starch

Cooling Gel—aloe barbadensis gel, benzophenone-4, edetate disodium, hydroxyethylcellulose, methylparaben, polysorbate 80, propylene glycol, propylparaben, sodium citrate, vitamin E, water

Storage: Store at 20–25°C (68–77°F).

How Supplied: Ointment: Net Wt. 1 oz and 2 oz **Cream:** Net Wt. 0.9 oz and 1.8 oz **Suppositories:** 12's, 24's and 48's. **Cooling Gel:** Net Wt. 0.9 oz and 1.8 oz

PREPARATION H® MEDICATED WIPES (Wyeth Consumer)

Active Ingredient: Witch Hazel 50%.

Uses:
- helps relieve the local itching and discomfort associated with hemorrhoids
- temporary relief of irritation and burning
- aids in protecting irritated anorectal areas
- **for vaginal care**—cleanse the area by gently wiping, patting or blotting. Repeat as needed.
- **for use as a moist compress**—if necessary, first cleanse the area as described below. Fold wipe to desired size and place in contact with tissue for a soothing and cooling effect. Leave in place for up to 15 minutes and repeat as needed.

Warnings:
For external use only
When using this product
- do not exceed the recommended daily dosage unless directed by a doctor
- do not put this product into the rectum by using fingers or any mechanical device or applicator
Stop use and ask a doctor if
- bleeding occurs
- condition worsens or does not improve within 7 days
If pregnant or breast-feeding, ask a health professional before use. **Keep out of reach of children.** If swallowed, get

medical help or contact a Poison Control Center right away.
Directions:
Container and Refill:
- remove tab on right side of wipes pouch label and peel back to open
- grab the top wipe at the edge of the center fold and pull out of pouch
- carefully reseal label on pouch after each use to retain moistness
Travel Pack, Container and Refill:
- adults: unfold wipe and cleanse the area by gently wiping, patting or blotting. If necessary, repeat until all matter is removed from the area.
- use up to 6 times daily or after each bowel movement and before applying topical hemorrhoidal treatments, and then discard
- children under 12 years of age: consult a doctor
- for best results, flush only one or two wipes at a time

Tamper-Evident (Container & Refill): Pouch quality sealed for your protection. Do Not Use if tear strip imprinted "Safety Sealed" is torn or missing
Tamper-Evident (Travel Pack): Each wipe is enclosed in a sealed foil pouch. Do Not Use if the pouch is broken or torn.

Inactive Ingredients: aloe barbadensis gel, capryl/capramidopropyl betaine, citric acid, diazolidinyl urea, glycerin, methylparaben, propylene glycol, propylparaben, sodium citrate, water.

Storage: store at 20-25°C (68-77°F)
How Supplied: Containers of 48 wipes. Refills of 48 wipes. 10 count portable pack.

Gastrointestinal/Genitourinary System:
Lactose Intolerance

LACTAID® ORIGINAL STRENGTH CAPLETS (McNeil Consumer)
(lactase enzyme)

LACTAID® FAST ACT CAPLETS AND CHEWABLE TABLETS
(lactase enzyme)

Description:
Each serving size (3 caplets) of *LACTAID® Original Strength Caplets* contains 9000 FCC (Food Chemical Codex) units of lactase enzyme (derived from *Aspergillus oryzae*).
Each serving size (1 caplet) of *LACTAID® Fast Act Caplet* contains 9000 FCC units of lactase enzyme (derived from *Aspergillus oryzae*).
Each serving size (1 tablet) of *LACTAID® Fast Act Chewable Tablet* contains 9000 FCC units of lactase enzyme (derived from *Aspergillus oryzae*).
LACTAID® is the original lactase dietary supplement that makes milk and dairy foods more digestible for individuals with lactose intolerance. *LACTAID®* lactase enzyme hydrolyzes lactose into two digestible simple sugars: glucose and galactose. *LACTAID®* *Caplets/Chewable Tablets* are taken orally for *in vivo* hydrolysis of lactose.

Actions:
LACTAID® *Caplets/Chewable Tablets* work by providing the enzyme that hydrolyzes the milk sugar lactose (disaccharide) into the two monosaccharides, glucose and galactose.

Uses:
LACTAID® Supplements help prevent the gas, bloating, or diarrhea that many people may experience after eating foods containing dairy.*

*This statement has not been evaluated by the Food and Drug Administration. This product is not intended to diagnose, treat, cure, or prevent any disease.

Directions:
Original Strength: Swallow or chew 3 LACTAID® Original Strength Caplets with **your first bite of dairy foods** to help **prevent** symptoms. **LACTAID® Fast Act Caplets:** Swallow 1 caplet with your **FIRST BITE** of dairy foods. If necessary, you may swallow 2 caplets at one time. If you continue to eat foods containing dairy after 30–45 minutes, we recommend taking another caplet. **LACTAID® Fast Act Chewable Tablets:** Chew 1 tablet with your **FIRST BITE** of dairy foods. If necessary, you may take 2 chewable tablets at one time. If you continue to eat foods containing dairy after 30–45 minutes, we recommend taking another chewable tablet.

Warnings:
Consult your doctor if your symptoms continue after using the product or if your symptoms are unusual and seem unrelated to eating dairy. Keep out of reach of children. **Do not use if carton is open or if printed plastic neckwrap is broken or if single serve packet is open.**

Ingredients: *LACTAID® Original Strength Caplets:* Lactase Enzyme (9000 FCC Lactase units/3 caplets), Mannitol, Cellulose, Sodium Citrate, Magnesium Stearate.
LACTAID® Fast Act Chewable Tablets: Lactase Enzyme (9000 FCC Lactase units/tablet), Mannitol, Microcrystalline Cellulose, Croscarmellose Sodium, Crospovidone, Magnesium Stearate, Natural and Artificial Flavor, Citric Acid, Sucralose.
LACTAID® Fast Act Caplets: Lactase Enzyme (9000 FCC Lactase units/caplet), Microcrystalline Cellulose, Croscarmellose Sodium, Crospovidone, Magnesium Stearate, Colloidal Silicon Dioxide.

How Supplied:
LACTAID® Original Strength Caplets are available in bottles of 120 count. Store at or below room temperature (below 77°F) but do not refrigerate. Keep away from heat. *LACTAID® Fast Act Caplets and Chewables* are available in single serve packets of 12, 32, and 60 count packages. Store at below 77°F.
Also available: 100% lactose-free LACTAID® Milk.

Shown in Product Identification Guide, page 508

Gastrointestinal/Genitourinary System:
Nausea

**MAXIMUM STRENGTH
MAALOX TOTAL STOMACH
RELIEF®**
(Novartis Consumer Health, Inc.)
**Bismuth Subsalicylate/Upset
Stomach Reliever
Peppermint**

For full product information see page 660.

**MAALOX® TOTAL STOMACH
RELIEF®**
(Novartis Consumer Health, Inc.)

For full product information see page 672.

PEPTO-BISMOL®
(Procter & Gamble)
**ORIGINAL LIQUID,
MAXIMUM STRENGTH LIQUID,
ORIGINAL AND CHERRY FLAVOR
CHEWABLE TABLETS
AND EASY-TO-SWALLOW CAPLETS**
**For upset stomach, indigestion,
heartburn, nausea and diarrhea.**

For full product information see page 672.

Gastrointestinal/Genitourinary System:
Pinworm Infection

REESE'S PINWORM TREATMENTS (Reese)
[rēsĭs]

Directions for Use: For the treatment of pinworms. Read package insert carefully before taking this medication. Take according to directions. Do not exceed recommended dosage unless directed by a doctor. Medication should be taken only one time as a single dose: do not repeat treatment unless directed by a doctor. When one individual in a household has pinworms, the entire household should be treated unless otherwise advised. These products can be taken any time of day, with or without food. If you are pregnant, nursing a baby, or have liver disease, do not take this product unless directed by a doctor.

DOSAGE GUIDE		
under 25 lbs or 2 yrs of age, consult a doctor		
WEIGHT LBS.	DOSAGE Teaspoons	Caplets
25–37	1/2	2
38–62	1	4
63–87	1-1/2	6
88–112	2	8
113–137	2-1/2	10
138–162	3	12
163–187	3-1/2	14
188 & over	4	16

Warnings: Keep this and all drugs out of the reach of children. In case of accidental overdose, seek professional assistance or contact a poison control center immediately.

How Supplied:
Oral Suspension Liquid
NDC: 10956-618-01
Each 1 mL contains: pyrantel pamoate 144mg
(equivalent of 50 mg pyrantel base)
Pre-Measured Caplet
NDC: 10956-658-24
Packaged in boxes of 24 caplets.
Each caplet contains: pyrantel pamoate 180mg
(equivalent of 62.5 mg pyrantel base)
Shown in Product Identification Guide, page 517

Gastrointestinal/Genitourinary System:
Sour Stomach

GAS-X® REGULAR STRENGTH
(Novartis Consumer Health, Inc.)
Antigas Chewable Tablets
GAS-X® EXTRA STRENGTH
Antigas Softgels and Chewable
Tablets
GAS-X® MAXIMUM STRENGTH
Antigas Softgels
GAS-X® WITH MAALOX®
Antigas/Antacid Softgels and
Chewable Tablets

For full product information see page 656.

GAVISCON® EXTRA STRENGTH
(GlaxoSmithKline Consumer)
Antacid Tablets
[găv 'ĭs-kŏn]

For full product information see page 658.

GAVISCON® EXTRA STRENGTH
Liquid Antacid (GlaxoSmithKline
Consumer)
[găv 'ĭs-kŏn]

For full product information see page 658.

CHEWABLE
MAALOX® Regular Strength
(Novartis Consumer Health, Inc.)
Calcium Carbonate Antacid
Chewable Tablets
Lemon and Wild Berry
flavors Chewable Tablets

For full product information see page 659.

MAALOX MAX® MAXIMUM
STRENGTH ANTACID/ANTI-GAS
LIQUID
(Novartis Consumer Health, Inc.)
Oral Suspension Antacid/Anti-Gas

For full product information see page 659.

MAALOX REGULAR STRENGTH
(Novartis Consumer Health, Inc.)
Liquid Antacid/Anti-Gas

For full product information see page 660.

ORIGINAL PEPCID AC®
(J&J — Merck)
TABLETS AND GELCAPS
MAXIMUM STRENGTH PEPCID® AC
Tablets
Acid reducer

For full product information see page 661.

PEPCID® COMPLETE
(J&J — Merck)
Acid Reducer + Antacid
with DUAL ACTION
Reduces and Neutralizes Acid

For full product information see page 662.

CHILDREN'S PEPTO
(Procter & Gamble)
Calcium carbonate/antacid

For full product information see page 662.

TAGAMET HB® 200
(GlaxoSmithKline Consumer)
Cimetidine Tablets 200 mg/
Acid Reducer

For full product information see page 664.

TUMS® Regular Antacid/Calcium
Supplement Tablets
(GlaxoSmithKline Consumer)
TUMS E–X® and TUMS E–X®
Sugar Free Antacid/Calcium
Supplement Tablets
TUMS ULTRA® Antacid/Calcium
Supplement Tablets

For full product information see page 664.

Gastrointestinal/Genitourinary System:
Upset Stomach

GAVISCON® EXTRA STRENGTH
(GlaxoSmithKline Consumer)
Antacid Tablets
[găv 'ĭs-kŏn]

For full product information see page 658.

GAVISCON® EXTRA STRENGTH
Liquid Antacid (GlaxoSmithKline Consumer)
[găv 'ĭs-kŏn]

For full product information see page 658.

GAVISCON® Regular Strength
(GlaxoSmithKline Consumer)
Liquid Antacid
[găv 'ĭs-kŏn]

For full product information see page 658.

CHEWABLE
MAALOX® Regular Strength
(Novartis Consumer Health, Inc.)
Calcium Carbonate Antacid
Chewable Tablets
Lemon and Wild Berry
flavors Chewable Tablets

For full product information see page 659.

MAALOX MAX® MAXIMUM
STRENGTH ANTACID/ANTI-GAS
LIQUID
(Novartis Consumer Health, Inc.)
Oral Suspension Antacid/Anti-Gas

For full product information see page 659.

MAALOX REGULAR STRENGTH
(Novartis Consumer Health, Inc.)
Liquid Antacid/Anti-Gas

For full product information see page 660.

MAXIMUM STRENGTH
MAALOX TOTAL STOMACH
RELIEF®
(Novartis Consumer Health, Inc.)
Bismuth Subsalicylate/Upset
Stomach Reliever
Peppermint

For full product information see page 660.

MAALOX® TOTAL STOMACH
RELIEF®
(Novartis Consumer Health, Inc.)
Drug Facts
Active Ingredient:

(in each 15 mL*)	Purpose:
Bismuth subsalicylate 525 mg	Upset stomach reliever/Antidiarrheal

*15 mL = 1 tablespoon

Uses:
- upset stomach
- indigestion
- nausea
- diarrhea
- gas
- heartburn

Warnings:
Do not use
- if you have bloody or black stool
- an ulcer
- a bleeding problem

Reye's syndrome: Children and teenagers who have or are recovering from chicken pox or flu-like symptoms should not use this product. When using this product, if changes in behavior with nausea and vomiting occur, consult a doctor because these symptoms could be an early sign of Reye's syndrome, a rare but serious illness.

Allergy alert: Do not take this product if you are
- allergic to salicylates (including aspirin)
- taking other salicylate-containing products (such as aspirin)

Ask a doctor or pharmacist before use if you
- are taking a prescription drug for anticoagulation (blood thinning), diabetes, gout, or arthritis
- have fever
- have mucus in the stool

When using this product a temporary, but harmless, darkening of the stool and/or tongue may occur

Stop use and ask a doctor if
- symptoms get worse
- ringing in the ears or a loss of hearing occurs
- diarrhea or symptoms last more than 2 days

If pregnant or breast-feeding, ask a health care professional before use.
Keep out of reach of children. In case of overdose, get medical help or contact a poison control center right away.
Directions:
- shake well before using
- adults and children 12 years of age and older: 2 tablespoons (30 mL) every 1/2 hour to 1 hour, as required, not to exceed 8 tablespoons (120 mL) in 24 hours

- use until diarrhea stops but not more than 2 days
- children under 12 years of age: ask a doctor
- drink plenty of clear liquids to prevent dehydration caused by diarrhea

Other Information:
- **each tablespoon contains:** sodium 6 mg
- each tablespoon contains: salicylate 232 mg
- store at controlled room temperature 20-25°C (68-77°F)
- keep tightly closed and avoid freezing

Inactive Ingredients:
carboxymethylcellulose sodium, ethyl alcohol, flavor, methylparaben, microcrystalline cellulose, propylene glycol, propylparaben, purified water, salicylic acid, sodium salicylate, sorbitol, sucralose, xanthan gum

Stawberry flavor:
Other Information:
- **each tablespoon contains:** sodium 6 mg
- each tablespoon contains: salicylate 232 mg
- store at controlled room temperature 20-25°C (68-77°F)
- keep tightly closed and avoid freezing

Inactive Ingredients:
carboxymethylcellulose sodium, flavor, methylparaben, microcrystalline cellulose, propylene glycol, propylparaben, purified water, salicylic acid, sodium salicylate, sorbitol, sucralose, xanthan gum

Questions?
call **1-800-452-0051** 24 hours a day, 7 days a week.
Novartis Consumer Health, Inc.
Parsippany, NJ 07054-0622
© 2005
Made in Canada
www.maaloxus.com
Shown in Product Identification Guide, page 515

CHILDREN'S PEPTO
(Procter & Gamble)
Calcium carbonate/antacid

For full product information see page 662.

PEPTO-BISMOL®
(Procter & Gamble)
ORIGINAL LIQUID,
MAXIMUM STRENGTH LIQUID,
ORIGINAL AND CHERRY FLAVOR
CHEWABLE TABLETS
AND EASY-TO-SWALLOW CAPLETS
For upset stomach, indigestion, heartburn, nausea and diarrhea.

Multi-symptom Pepto-Bismol® contains bismuth subsalicylate and is the only

leading OTC stomach remedy clinically proven effective for both upper and lower GI symptoms. It has been clinically proven in double-blind placebo-controlled trials for relief of upset stomach symptoms and diarrhea.

Active Ingredient:

(per tablespoon/per tablet/per caplet) Original Liquid/Tablets/Caplets
Bismuth subsalicylate 262 mg
Maximum Strength Liquid
Bismuth subsalicylate 525 mg

Inactive Ingredients:

[**Original Liquid**] benzoic acid, flavor, magnesium aluminum silicate, methylcellulose, red 22, red 28, saccharin sodium, salicylic acid, sodium salicylate, sorbic acid, water

[**Maximum Strength Liquid**] benzoic acid, flavor, magnesium aluminum silicate, methylcellulose, red 22, red 28, saccharin sodium, salicylic acid, sodium salicylate, sorbic acid, water

[**Original Tablets**] calcium carbonate, flavor, magnesium stearate, mannitol, povidone, red 27 aluminum lake, saccharin sodium, talc

[**Cherry Tablets**] adipic acid, calcium carbonate, flavor, magnesium stearate, mannitol, povidone, red 27 aluminum lake, red 40 aluminum lake, saccharin sodium, talc

[**Caplets**] calcium carbonate, magnesium stearate, mannitol, microcrystalline cellulose, polysorbate 80, povidone, red 27 aluminum lake, silicon dioxide, sodium starch glycolate.

Other Information:

Sodium Content
Original Liquid—each Tbsp contains: sodium 6 mg • low sodium
Maximum Strength Liquid—each Tbsp contains: sodium 6 mg • low sodium
Chewable Tablets—each Original or Cherry Flavor Tablet contains: calcium 140 mg, sodium less than 1 mg • very low sodium
Caplets—each Caplet contains: calcium 27 mg, sodium 3 mg • low sodium
Salicylate Content
Original Liquid—each Tbsp contains: salicylate 130 mg
Maximum Strength Liquid—each Tbsp contains: salicylate 236 mg
Chewable Tablets—each tablet contains:
[original] salicylate 102 mg
[cherry] salicylate 99 mg
Caplets—each caplet contains: salicylate 99 mg
All Forms are sugar free.

Indications:

- relieves upset stomach symptoms (i.e., indigestion, heartburn, nausea and fullness caused by over-indulgence in food and drink) without constipating; and,
- controls diarrhea.

Actions: For upset stomach symptoms, the active ingredient is believed to work via a topical effect on the stomach mucosa. For diarrhea, it is believed to work by several mechanisms in the gastrointestinal tract, including: 1) normalizing fluid movement via an antisecretory merchanism, 2) binding bacterial toxins and 3) antimicrobial activity.

Warnings:

Reye's syndrome: Children and teenagers who have or are recovering from chicken pox or flu-like symptoms should not use this product. When using this product, if changes in behavior with nausea and vomiting occur, consult a doctor because these symptoms could be an early sign of Reye's syndrome, a rare but serious illness.

Allergy alert: Contains salicylate. Do not take if you are

- allergic to salicylates (including aspirin)
- taking other salicylate products

Do not use if you have

- an ulcer
- a bleeding problem
- bloody or black stool

Ask a doctor before use if you have

- fever
- mucus in the stool

Ask a doctor or pharmacist before use if you are taking any drug for

- anticoagulation (thinning the blood)
- diabetes
- gout
- arthritis

When using this product a temporary, but harmless, darkening of the stool and/or tongue may occur

Stop use and ask a doctor if

- symptoms get worse
- ringing in the ears or loss of hearing occurs
- diarrhea lasts more than 2 days

If pregnant or breast feeding, ask a health professional before use.

Keep out of reach of children. In case of overdose, get medical help or contact a Poison Control Center right away.

Notes: May cause a temporary and harmless darkening of the tongue or stool. Stool darkening should not be confused with melena.

While no lead is intentionally added to Pepto-Bismol, this product contains certain ingredients that are mined from the ground and thus contain small amounts of naturally occurring lead. For example, bismuth, contained in the active ingredient of Pepto-Bismol, is mined and therefore contains some naturally occurring lead. The small amounts of naturally occurring lead in Pepto-Bismol are low in comparison to average daily lead exposure; this is for the information of healthcare professionals. Pepto-Bismol is indicated for treatment of acute upset stomach symptoms and diarrhea. It is not intended for chronic use.

Overdosage: In case of overdose, patients are advised to contact a physician or Poison Control Center. Emesis induced by ipecac syrup is indicated in large ingestions provided ipecac can be administered within one hour of ingestion. Activated charcoal should be administered after gastric emptying. Patients should be evaluated for signs and symptoms of salicylate toxicity.

Directions:
Pepto-Bismol® Original Liquid, Original & Cherry Flavor Chewable Tablets, and Caplets
[Original Liquid]
- shake well before using
- for accurate dosing, use dose cup
[Original Tablet, Cherry Tablets]
- chew or dissolve in mouth
[Caplets]
- swallow with water, do not chew
- adults and children 12 years and over: 1 dose (2 Tbsp or 30 ml; 2 tablets or 2 caplets) every 1/2 to 1 hour as needed
- do not exceed 8 doses (16 Tbsp or 240 ml); 16 tablets or capsules in 24 hours
- use until diarrhea stops but not more than 2 days
- children under 12 years: ask a doctor
- drink plenty of clear fluids to help prevent dehydration caused by diarrhea

Pepto-Bismol® Maximum Strength Liquid
- shake well before use
- for accurate dosing, use dose cup
- adults and children 12 years and over: 1 dose (2 Tbsp 30 ml) every 1 hour as needed
- do not exceed 4 doses (8 Tbsp or 120 ml) in 24 hours
- use until diarrhea stops but not more than 2 days
- children under 12 years: ask a doctor
- drink plenty of clear fluids to help prevent dehydration caused by diarrhea

How Supplied: Pepto-Bismol® Original and Maximum Strength Liquids are pink. Pepto-Bismol® Original Liquid is available in: 4, 8, 12 and 16 fl oz bottles. Pepto-Bismol®   Maximum   Strength Liquid is available in: 4, 8 and 12 fl oz bottles. Pepto-Bismol® Original and Cherry Flavor Tablets are pink, round, chewable tablets imprinted with a debossed triangle and "Pepto-Bismol" on one side. Tablets are available in: boxes of 30 and 48. Pepto-Bismol® Caplets are pink and imprinted with "Pepto-Bismol" on one side. Caplets are available in bottles of 24 and 40.

- avoid excessive heat (over 104°F or 40°C)
- protect liquids from freezing
Questions: 1-800-717-3786
www.pepto-bismol.com
Shown in Product Identification Guide, page 516

TUMS® Regular Antacid/Calcium Supplement Tablets (GlaxoSmithKline Consumer)

TUMS E–X® and TUMS E–X® Sugar Free Antacid/Calcium Supplement Tablets

TUMS ULTRA® Antacid/Calcium Supplement Tablets

For full product information see page 664.

Musculoskeletal System:
Aches and Pains

ADVIL® (Wyeth Consumer)
Ibuprofen Tablets, USP
Ibuprofen Caplets (Oval-Shaped Tablets)
Ibuprofen Gel Caplets (Oval-Shaped Gelatin Coated Tablets)
Ibuprofen Liqui-Gel Capsules
Pain reliever/Fever Reducer (NSAID)

Active Ingredient: Each tablet, caplet, or gel caplet, contains Ibuprofen 200 mg (NSAID)*
*nonsteroidal anti-inflammatory drug
Each Liqui-gel capsule contains solubilized Ibuprofen equal to 200 mg ibuprofen (NSAID)* (present as the free acid and potassium salt)
*nonsteroidal anti-inflammatory drug

Uses:
temporarily relieves minor aches and pains due to the common cold, headache, toothache, muscular aches, backache, minor pain of arthritis, menstrual cramps; and temporarily reduces fever.

Warnings:
Allergy alert: Ibuprofen may cause a severe allergic reaction, especially in people allergic to aspirin. Symptoms may include:
• hives
• facial swelling
• asthma (wheezing)
• shock
• skin reddening
• rash
• blisters
If an allergic reaction occurs, stop use and seek medical help right away.
Stomach bleeding warning: This product contains a nonsteroidal anti-inflammatory drug (NSAID), which may cause stomach bleeding. The chance is higher if you:
• are age 60 or older
• have had stomach ulcers or bleeding problems
• take a blood thinning (anticoagutant) or steroid drug
• take other drugs containing an NSAID [aspirin, ibuprofen, naproxen, or others]
• have 3 or more alcoholic drinks every day while using this product
• take more or for a longer time than directed
Do not use
• if you have ever had an allergic reaction to any other pain reliever/fever reducer
• right before or after heart surgery
Ask a doctor before use if you have
• problems or serious side effects from taking pain relievers or fever reducers
• stomach problems that last or come

back, such as heartburn, upset stomach, or stomach pain
• ulcers
• bleeding problems
• high blood pressure
• heart or kidney disease
• taken a diuretic
• reached age 60 or older
Ask a doctor or pharmacist before use if you are
• taking any other drug containing an NSAID (prescription or nonprescription)
• taking a blood thinning (anticoagulant) or steroid drug
• under a doctor's care for any serious condition
• taking aspirin to prevent heart attack or stroke, because ibuprofen may decrease this benefit of aspirin
• taking any other drug
When using this product
• take with food or milk if stomach upset occurs
• long term continuous use may increase the risk of heart attack or stroke
Stop use and ask a doctor if
• you feel faint, vomit blood, or have bloody or black stools. These are signs of stomach bleeding.
• pain gets worse or lasts more than 10 days
• fever gets worse or lasts more than 3 days
• stomach pain or upset gets worse or lasts
• redness or swelling is present in the painful area
• any new symptoms appear
If pregnant or breast-feeding, ask a health professional before use. It is especially important not to use ibuprofen during the last 3 months of pregnancy unless definitely directed to do so by a doctor because it may cause problems in the unborn child or complications during delivery.
Keep out of reach of children. In case of overdose, get medical help or contact a Poison Control Center right away.

Directions:
• **do not take more than directed**
• **the smallest effective dose should be used**
• do not take longer than 10 days, unless directed by a doctor (see Warnings)
Adults and children 12 years and over:
• take 1 tablet, caplet, gelcap or liquigel capsule every 4 to 6 hours while symptoms persist
• if pain or fever does not respond to 1 tablet, caplet, gelcap, or liquigel capsule, 2 tablets, caplets, gelcaps or liquigel capsules may be used • do not exceed 6 tablets, caplets, gelcaps or liquigel

capsules in 24 hours, unless directed by a doctor
Children under 12 years: ask a doctor

Inactive Ingredients:
Tablets and Caplets: acetylated monoglyceride, beeswax and/or carnauba wax, croscarmellose sodium, iron oxides, lecithin, methylparaben, microcrystalline cellulose, pharmaceutical glaze, povidone, propylparaben, silicon dioxide, simethicone, sodium benzoate, sodium lauryl sulfate, starch, stearic acid, sucrose, titanium dioxide.
Gel Caplets: colloidal silicon dioxide, croscarmellose sodium, FD&C red no. 40, FD&C yellow no. 6, fractionated coconut oil, gelatin, glycerin, hypromellose, iron oxide, pharmaceutical ink, pregelatinized starch, propyl gallate, sodium lauryl sulfate, starch, stearic acid, titanium dioxide, triacetin
Liqui-Gels: FD& C green no. 3, gelatin, light mineral oil, pharmaceutical ink, polyethylene glycol, potassium hydroxide, purified water, sorbitan, sorbitol.

Other Information:
• **each Liqui-gel capsule contains:** potassium 20 mg
• read all warnings and directions before use. Keep carton.
• store at 20–25°C (68–77°F)
• avoid excessive heat 40°C (above 104°F)

How Supplied:
Coated tablets in a 10 ct. vial and bottles of 24, 50, 100, 165 (non-child resistant), and 225. Coated caplets in bottles of 24, 50, 100, 165 (non-child resistant), and 225.
Gel caplets in bottles of 24, 50, 100, 165 (non-child resistant) and 225.
Liqui-Gels in bottles of 20, 40, 80, 135 (non-child resistant) and 180.

ADVIL® ALLERGY SINUS CAPLETS (Wyeth Consumer)
ADVIL® MULTI-SYMPTOM COLD CAPLETS
Pain Reliever/Fever Reducer (NSAID)
Nasal Decongestant
Antihistamine

For full product information see page 770.

ADVIL® COLD & SINUS
Caplets, and Liqui-Gels
Pain Reliever/Fever Reducer/(NSAID)
Nasal Decongestant

For full product information see page 723.

ADVIL PM CAPLETS
(Wyeth Consumer)
Pain reliever (NSAID)/Nighttime sleep-aid

For full product information see page 615.

CHILDREN'S ADVIL CHEWABLE TABLETS (Wyeth Consumer)
Fever Reducer/Pain Reliever (NSAID)

For full product information see page 603.

CHILDREN'S ADVIL SUSPENSION (Wyeth Consumer)
Fever Reducer/Pain Reliever (NSAID)

For full product information see page 603.

INFANTS' ADVIL CONCENTRATED DROPS
(Wyeth Consumer)
INFANT'S ADVIL WHITE GRAPE CONCENTRATED DROPS
(DYE-FREE)
Fever Reducer/Pain Reliever (NSAID)

For full product information see page 604.

JUNIOR STRENGTH ADVIL® SWALLOW TABLETS
(Wyeth Consumer)
Fever Reducer/Pain Reliever (NSAID)

For full product information see page 605.

ALEVE CAPLETS (Bayer Healthcare)
(NSAID Labeling)
[a-lēv]

Drug Facts

Active Ingredient
(in each caplet):   **Purposes:**

Naproxen sodium 220 mg
(naproxen 200 mg)
(NSAID)* .... Pain reliever/
fever reducer

---

* nonsteroidal anti-inflammatory drug

Uses:
• temporarily relieves minor aches and pains due to:
  • minor pain of arthritis
  • muscular aches
  • backache
  • menstrual cramps
  • headache
  • toothache
  • the common cold
• temporarily reduces fever

Warnings:

Allergy alert: Naproxen sodium may cause a severe allergic reaction, especially in people allergic to aspirin. Symptoms may include:
• hives
• facial swelling
• asthma (wheezing)
• shock
• skin reddening
• rash
• blisters
If an allergic reaction occurs, stop use and seek medical help right away.

Stomach bleeding warning: This product contains a nonsteroidal anti-inflammatory drug (NSAID), which may cause stomach bleeding. The chance is higher if you:
• are age 60 or older
• have had stomach ulcers or bleeding problems
• take a blood thinning (anticoagulant) or steroid drug
• take other drugs containing an NSAID (aspirin, ibuprofen, naproxen, or others)
• have 3 or more alcoholic drinks every day while using this product
• take more or for a longer time than directed

Do not use
• if you have ever had an allergic reaction to any other pain reliever/fever reducer
• right before or after heart surgery

Ask a doctor before use if you have
• problems or serious side effects from taking pain relievers or fever reducers
• stomach problems that last or come back, such as heartburn, upset stomach, or stomach pain
• ulcers
• bleeding problems
• high blood pressure
• heart or kidney disease
• taken a diuretic
• reached age 60 or older

Ask a doctor or pharmacist before use if you are
• taking any other drug containing an NSAID (prescription or nonprescription)
• taking a blood thinning (anticoagulant) or steroid drug
• under a doctor's care for any serious condition
• taking any other drug

When using this product
• take with food or milk if stomach upset occurs
• long term continuous use may increase the risk of heart attack or stroke

Stop use and ask a doctor if
• you feel faint, vomit blood, or have bloody or black stools. These are signs of stomach bleeding.
• pain gets worse or lasts more than 10 days
• fever gets worse or lasts more than 3 days
• you have difficulty swallowing
• it feels like the pill is stuck in your throat
• you develop heartburn
• stomach pain or upset gets worse or lasts
• redness or swelling is present in the painful area
• any new symptoms appear

If pregnant or breast-feeding, ask a health professional before use. It is especially important not to use naproxen sodium during the last 3 months of pregnancy unless definitely directed to do so by a doctor because it may cause problems in the unborn child or complications during delivery.

Keep out of reach of children. In case of overdose, get medical help or contact a Poison Control Center right away.

Directions:
• do not take more than directed
• the smallest effective dose should be used
• do not take longer than 10 days, unless directed by a doctor (see Warnings)
• drink a full glass of water with each dose

Adults and children 12 years and older	• take 1 caplet every 8 to 12 hours while symptoms last • for the first dose you may take 2 caplets within the first hour • do not exceed 2 caplets in any 8- to 12-hour period • do not exceed 3 caplets in a 24-hour period
Children under 12 years	• ask a doctor

Other Information:
• **each caplet contains:** sodium 20 mg
• store at 20–25°C (68–77°F). Avoid high humidity and excessive heat above 40°C (104°F).

Inactive Ingredients: FD&C blue #2 lake, hypromellose, magnesium stearate, microcrystalline cellulose, polyethylene glycol, povidone, talc, titanium dioxide

Questions or comments?
1-800-395-0689 (Mon – Fri 9AM – 5PM EST) or www.aleve.com

How Supplied: Available in 8, 24, 50, 100, 150 and 200 ct. and in a 100 ct. Easy Open Arthritis Cap Bottle.

Shown in Product Identification Guide, page 503

ALEVE COLD & SINUS CAPLETS
(Bayer Healthcare)
(NSAID Labeling)
[a-lēv]

For full product information see page 724.

ALEVE GELCAPS
(Bayer Healthcare)
(NSAID Labeling)
[a-lēv]

Drug Facts
Active Ingredient
(in each gelcap):   **Purposes:**
Naproxen sodium 220 mg (naproxen 200 mg)
(NSAID)* ..... Pain reliever/fever reducer

---

* nonsteroidal anti-inflammatory drug

Continued on next page

Aleve Gelcaps—Cont.

Uses:

- temporarily relieves minor aches and pains due to:
  - minor pain of arthritis
  - muscular aches
  - backache
  - menstrual cramps
  - headache
  - toothache
  - the common cold
- temporarily reduces fever

Warnings:

Allergy alert: Naproxen sodium may cause a severe allergic reaction, especially in people allergic to aspirin. Symptoms may include:

- hives
- facial swelling
- asthma (wheezing)
- shock
- skin reddening
- rash
- blisters

If an allergic reaction occurs, stop use and seek medical help right away.

Stomach bleeding warning: This product contains a nonsteroidal anti-inflammatory drug (NSAID), which may cause stomach bleeding. The chance is higher if you:

- are age 60 or older
- have had stomach ulcers or bleeding problems
- take a blood thinning (anticoagulant) or steroid drug
- take other drugs containing an NSAID (aspirin, ibuprofen, naproxen, or others)
- have 3 or more alcoholic drinks every day while using this product
- take more or for a longer time than directed

Do not use

- if you have ever had an allergic reaction to any other pain reliever/fever reducer
- right before or after heart surgery

Ask a doctor before use if you have

- problems or serious side effects from taking pain relievers or fever reducers
- stomach problems that last or come back, such as heartburn, upset stomach, or stomach pain
- ulcers
- bleeding problems
- high blood pressure
- heart or kidney disease
- taken a diuretic
- reached age 60 or older

Ask a doctor or pharmacist before use if you are

- taking any other drug containing an NSAID (prescription or nonprescription)
- taking a blood thinning (anticoagulant) or steroid drug
- under a doctor's care for any serious condition
- taking any other drug

When using this product

- take with food or milk if stomach upset occurs
- long term continuous use may increase the risk of heart attack or stroke

Stop use and ask a doctor if

- you feel faint, vomit blood, or have bloody or black stools. These are signs of stomach bleeding.
- pain gets worse or lasts more than 10 days
- fever gets worse or lasts more than 3 days
- you have difficulty swallowing
- it feels like the pill is stuck in your throat
- you develop heartburn
- stomach pain or upset gets worse or lasts
- redness or swelling is present in the painful area
- any new symptoms appear

If pregnant or breast-feeding, ask a health professional before use. It is especially important not to use naproxen sodium during the last 3 months of pregnancy unless definitely directed to do so by a doctor because it may cause problems in the unborn child or complications during delivery.

Keep out of reach of children. In case of overdose, get medical help or contact a Poison Control Center right away.

Directions:

- **do not take more than directed**
- **the smallest effective dose should be used**
- do not take longer than 10 days, unless directed by a doctor (see Warnings)
- drink a full glass of water with each dose

Adults and children 12 years and older	• take 1 caplet every 8 to 12 hours while symptoms last • for the first dose you may take 2 Gelcaps within the first hour • do not exceed 2 Gelcaps in any 8- to 12-hour period • do not exceed 3 Gelcaps in a 24-hour period
Children under 12 years	• ask a doctor

Other Information:

- **each caplet contains:** sodium 20 mg
- store at 20–25°C (68–77°F). Avoid high humidity and excessive heat above 40°C (104°F).

Inactive Ingredients: D&C yellow #10 aluminum lake, edetate disodium, edible ink, FD&C blue #1, FD&C yellow #6 aluminum lake, gelatin, glycerin, hypromellose, magnesium stearate, microcrystalline cellulose, polyethylene glycol, povidone, stearic acid, talc, titanium dioxide

Questions or comments?

1-800-395-0689 (Mon – Fri 9AM – 5PM EST) or www.aleve.com

How Supplied: Available in 20, 40, 80 ct. and in a 40 ct. Easy Open Arthritis Cap Bottle.

Shown in Product Identification Guide, page 503

ALEVE TABLETS (Bayer Healthcare) (NSAID Labeling)

[*a-lēv*]

Drug Facts

Active Ingredient (in each tablet):   Purposes:

Naproxen sodium 220 mg (naproxen 200 mg) (NSAID)* ..... Pain reliever/fever reducer

---

* nonsteroidal anti-inflammatory drug

Uses:

- temporarily relieves minor aches and pains due to:
  - minor pain of arthritis
  - muscular aches
  - backache
  - menstrual cramps
  - headache
  - toothache
  - the common cold
- temporarily reduces fever

Warnings:

Allergy alert: Naproxen sodium may cause a severe allergic reaction, especially in people allergic to aspirin. Symptoms may include:

- hives
- facial swelling
- asthma (wheezing)
- shock
- skin reddening
- rash
- blisters

If an allergic reaction occurs, stop use and seek medical help right away.

Stomach bleeding warning: This product contains a nonsteroidal anti-inflammatory drug (NSAID), which may cause stomach bleeding. The chance is higher if you:

- are age 60 or older
- have had stomach ulcers or bleeding problems
- take a blood thinning (anticoagulant) or steroid drug
- take other drugs containing an NSAID (aspirin, ibuprofen, naproxen, or others)
- have 3 or more alcoholic drinks every day while using this product
- take more or for a longer time than directed

Do not use

- if you have ever had an allergic reaction to any other pain reliever/fever reducer
- right before or after heart surgery

Ask a doctor before use if you have

- problems or serious side effects from taking pain relievers or fever reducers

- stomach problems that last or come back, such as heartburn, upset stomach, or stomach pain
- ulcers
- bleeding problems
- high blood pressure
- heart or kidney disease
- taken a diuretic
- reached age 60 or older

Ask a doctor or pharmacist before use if you are

- taking any other drug containing an NSAID (prescription or nonprescription)
- taking a blood thinning (anticoagulant) or steroid drug
- under a doctor's care for any serious condition
- taking any other drug

When using this product

- take with food or milk if stomach upset occurs
- long term continuous use may increase the risk of heart attack or stroke

Stop use and ask a doctor if

- you feel faint, vomit blood, or have bloody or black stools. These are signs of stomach bleeding.
- pain gets worse or lasts more than 10 days
- fever gets worse or lasts more than 3 days
- you have difficulty swallowing
- it feels like the pill is stuck in your throat
- you develop heartburn
- stomach pain or upset gets worse or lasts
- redness or swelling is present in the painful area
- any new symptoms appear

If pregnant or breast-feeding, ask a health professional before use. It is especially important not to use naproxen sodium during the last 3 months of pregnancy unless definitely directed to do so by a doctor because it may cause problems in the unborn child or complications during delivery.

Keep out of reach of children. In case of overdose, get medical help or contact a Poison Control Center right away.

Directions:

- **do not take more than directed**
- **the smallest effective dose should be used**
- do not take longer than 10 days, unless directed by a doctor (see Warnings)
- drink a full glass of water with each dose

Adults and children 12 years and older	• take 1 tablet every 8 to 12 hours while symptoms last • for the first dose you may take 2 tablets within the first hour • do not exceed 2 tablets in any 8- to 12-hour period • do not exceed 3 tablets in a 24-hour period
Children under 12 years	• ask a doctor

Other Information:

- **each caplet contains:** sodium 20 mg
- store at 20–25°C (68–77°F). Avoid high humidity and excessive heat above 40°C (104°F).

Inactive Ingredients: FD&C blue #2 lake, hypromellose, magnesium stearate, microcrystalline cellulose, polyethylene glycol, povidone, talc, titanium dioxide

Questions or comments?
1-800-395-0689 (Mon – Fri 9AM – 5PM EST) or www.aleve.com

How Supplied: Available in 8, 24, 50, 100, 150, 200 ct. and in a 200 ct. Easy Open Arthritis Cap Bottle.

Shown in Product Identification Guide, page 503

BC® POWDER
(GlaxoSmithKline Consumer)
ARTHRITIS STRENGTH BC®
POWDER
BC® COLD POWDER LINE

Description: BC® POWDER: **Active Ingredients:** Each powder contains Aspirin 650 mg, Salicylamide 195 mg and Caffeine 33.3 mg. **Inactive Ingredients:** Docusate Sodium, Fumaric Acid, Lactose Monohydrate and Potassium Chloride. ARTHRITIS STRENGTH BC® POWDER: **Active Ingredients:** Each powder contains Aspirin 742 mg, Salicylamide 222 mg and Caffeine 38 mg. **Inactive Ingredients:** Docusate Sodium, Fumaric Acid, Lactose Monohydrate and Potassium Chloride.
BC® ALLERGY SINUS COLD POWDER

Active Ingredients: Aspirin 650 mg, Pseudoephedrine Hydrochloride 60 mg and Chlorpheniramine Maleate 4 mg per powder. **Inactive Ingredients:** Fumaric Acid, Glycine, Lactose, Potassium Chloride, Silica, Sodium Lauryl Sulfate. BC® SINUS COLD POWDER. **Active Ingredients:** Aspirin 650 mg and Pseudoephedrine Hydrochloride 60 mg. per powder. **Inactive Ingredients:** Colloidal Silicon Dioxide, Microcrystalline Cellulose, Povidone, Pregelatinized Starch, Stearic Acid.

Indications: BC Powder is for relief of simple headache; for temporary relief of minor arthritic pain, for relief of muscular aches, discomfort and fever of colds; and for relief of normal menstrual pain and pain of tooth extraction.
Arthritis Strength BC Powder is specially formulated to fight occasional minor pain and inflammation of arthritis. Like Original Formula BC, Arthritis Strength BC provides fast temporary relief of minor arthritis pain and inflammation, relief of muscular aches, discomfort and fever of colds; and pain of tooth extraction.

BC Allergy Sinus Cold Powder is for relief of multiple symptoms such as body aches, fever, nasal congestion, sneezing, running nose, and watery itchy eyes associated with allergy and sinus attacks and the onset of colds. BC Sinus Cold Powder is for relief of such symptoms as body aches, fever, and nasal congestion.
BC Powder®, Arthritis Strength BC® Powder and BC Cold Powder Line:

Warnings: Children and teenagers should not use this medicine for chicken pox or flu symptoms before a doctor is consulted about Reye's Syndrome, a rare but serious illness reported to be associated with aspirin. Keep this and all medicines out of children's reach. In case of accidental overdose, contact a physician or poison control center immediately.
As with any drug, if you are pregnant or nursing a baby seek the advice of a health professional before using this product.
IT IS ESPECIALLY IMPORTANT NOT TO USE ASPIRIN DURING THE LAST 3 MONTHS OF PREGNANCY UNLESS SPECIFICALLY DIRECTED TO DO SO BY A DOCTOR BECAUSE IT MAY CAUSE PROBLEMS IN THE UNBORN CHILD OR COMPLICATIONS DURING DELIVERY.

Alcohol Warning: If you consume 3 or more alcoholic drinks every day, ask your doctor whether you should take aspirin or other pain relievers/fever reducers. Aspirin may cause stomach bleeding.

Allergy Alert: Aspirin may cause a severe allergic reaction which may include hives, facial swelling, shock or asthma (wheezing). **Ask a doctor before use if you have** asthma, ulcers, a bleeding problem, stomach problems that last or come back such as heartburn, upset stomach or pain. **Ask a doctor or pharmacist before use** if you are taking a prescription drug for gout, diabetes, arthritis or anticoagulation (blood thinning). **Stop use and ask a doctor if** an allergic reaction occurs, ringing in ears or loss of hearing occurs, pain gets worse or persists for more than 10 days, fever lasts more than 3 days, redness or swelling is present, or new symptoms occur.

For BC Powder and Arthritis Strength BC Powder:
When using these products limit the use of caffeine containing drugs, foods, or drinks, because too much caffeine may cause nervousness, irritability, sleeplessness, and occasionally, rapid heartbeat.

For BC Cold Powder Line:
Do not exceed recommended dosage. If nervousness, dizziness, or sleeplessness occur, discontinue use and consult a doctor. If symptoms do not improve within 7 days, or are accompanied by fever that lasts more than 3 days, or if new symptoms occur, consult a physician before continuing use. Do not take BC if

Continued on next page

BC Powders—Cont.

you are sensitive to aspirin, or have heart disease, high blood pressure, thyroid disease, diabetes, asthma, glaucoma, emphysema, chronic pulmonary disease, shortness of breath, difficulty in breathing or difficulty in urination due to enlargement of the prostate gland, or if you are presently taking a prescription antihypertensive or antidepressant drug unless directed by a doctor. "*Drug interaction precaution.* Do not use this product if you are now taking a prescription monoamine oxidase inhibitor (MAOI) (certain drugs for depression, psychiatric or emotional conditions, or Parkinson's disease), or for 2 weeks after stopping the MAOI drug. If you are uncertain whether your prescription drug contains an MAOI, consult a health professional before taking this product." BC Allergy Sinus Cold Powder with antihistamine may cause drowsiness. Avoid alcoholic beverages when taking this product because it may increase drowsiness. Use caution when driving a motor vehicle or operating machinery. May cause excitability, especially in children.

Overdosage: In case of accidental overdosage, contact a physician or poison control center immediately.

Dosage and Administration: BC® Powder, Arthritis Strength BC® Powder, BC® Cold Powder Line:
Place one powder on tongue and follow with liquid. If you prefer, stir powder into glass of water or other liquid.
For BC Powder and Arthritis Strength BC Powder:
Adults and children 12 years and over: Take one powder every 3–4 hours not to exceed 4 powders in 24 hours.
For BC Cold Powder Line:
Adults and children 12 years and over: Take one powder every 6 hours not to exceed 4 powders in 24 hours. For children under 12, consult a physician.

How Supplied: BC Powder: Available in tamper evident overwrapped envelopes of 2 or 6 powders, as well as tamper evident boxes of 24 and 50 powders.
Arthritis Strength BC Powder: Available in tamper evident over wrapped envelopes of 6 powders, and tamper evident overwrapped boxes of 24 and 50 powders.
BC Cold Powder Line:
Available in tamper-evident overwrapped envelopes of 6 powders, as well as tamper-evident boxes of 12 powders (For BC Allergy Sinus Cold Powder only).

BIOFREEZE® PAIN RELIEVING PRODUCTS (Performance Health)

Active Ingredients (US Market Label): "Roll on/Gel" Menthol 3.5%, "Cryospray™" Menthol 10%

Inactive Ingredients:

Roll on/Gel (US Market Label): Carbomer FD&C Blue #1, FD&C Yellow #5, glycerine, herbal extract (Ilex Paraguariensis), isopropyl alcohol USP, methylparaben, natural camphor USP (for scent), propylene glycol, silicon dioxide, triethanolamine, water.

Cryospray™ (US Market Label): Arnica Extract, Eucalyptus Oil, Ilex Herbal Extract, Lavender Oil, Lime Oil, Natural Camphor USP, Nutmeg Oil, Orange Oil, Peppermint Oil, Pine Oil, Polysorbate 20, SD Alcohol 39-C, Thyme Oil, Water, White Tea Extract.

Indications (US Market Label): Temporary relief from minor aches and pains of muscles and joints associated with arthritis, backache, strains and sprains.

Warnings (US Market Label): Ask a doctor before use if you have sensitive skin. Keep away from excessive heat or open flame. Avoid contact with the eyes or mucous membranes. Do not apply to wounds or damaged skin. Do not use with other ointments, creams, sprays or liniments. Do not apply to irritated skin or if excessive irritation develops. Do not bandage. Wash hands after use. If pregnant or breast-feeding, ask a health professional before use. Do not use with heating pad or device. Keep out of reach of children. If accidentally ingested, get medical help or contact a Poison Control Center.

Directions:

Roll on/Gel (US Market Label): Adults and children 2 years of age and older apply to the affected areas not more than 4 times daily; massage not necessary. Children under 2 years of age, consult physician.

Cryospray™ (US Market Label): Adults and children 12 years of age and older apply to affected areas not more than 4 times daily; massage not necessary. Children under 12 years of age, consult a physician.

How Supplied (US Market Label): 4 oz Gel Tube, 4 oz Cryospray™, 3 oz. Roll-on and 5 gram packets for home use. 16 oz, 32 oz and Gallon Gel bottles, and 16 oz Cryospray™ for professional use.

BUFFERIN®
(Novartis Consumer Health, Inc.)
Regular/Extra Strength
Pain Reliever/Fever Reducer

Drug Facts
Regular Strength
Active Ingredients: **Purpose:**
(in each tablet)
Buffered aspirin equal to
325 mg aspirin .... Pain reliever/
fever reducer
(buffered with calcium carbonate, magnesium oxide and magnesium carbonate)

Extra Strength
Active Ingredients: **Purpose:**
(in each tablet)
Buffered aspirin equal to
500 mg aspirin .... Pain reliever/
fever reducer
(buffered with calcium carbonate, magnesium oxide and magnesium carbonate)

Uses:
• for the temporary relief of minor aches and pains associated with:
  • headache   • cold
  • muscular aches   • arthritis
  • toothache   • premenstrual & menstrual cramps
• temporarily reduces fever

Warnings:

Reye's syndrome: Children and teenagers who have or are recovering from chicken pox or flu-like symptoms should not use this product. When using this product, if changes in behavior with nausea and vomiting occur, consult a doctor because these symptoms could be an early sign of Reye's syndrome, a rare but serious illness.

Allergy alert: Aspirin may cause a severe allergic reaction, which may include:
• facial swelling • asthma (wheezing)
• shock   • hives

Alcohol warning: If you consume 3 or more alcoholic drinks every day, ask your doctor whether you should take aspirin or other pain relievers/fever reducers. Aspirin may cause stomach bleeding.

Do not use if you have ever had an allergic reaction to any other pain reliever/fever reducer.

Ask a doctor before use if you have
• kidney disease
• a magnesium-restricted diet
• asthma • bleeding problems • ulcers
• stomach problems that last or come back, such as heartburn, upset stomach, or pain

Ask a doctor or pharmacist before use if you are
taking a prescription drug for:
• anticoagulation (thinning the blood)
• diabetes • gout • arthritis

Stop use and ask a doctor if
• allergic reaction occurs. Seek medical help right away.
• pain gets worse or lasts for more than 10 days
• new symptoms occur
• fever gets worse or lasts for more than 3 days
• painful area is red or swollen
• ringing in the ears or loss of hearing occurs

If pregnant or breast-feeding, ask a health professional before use.

It is especially important not to use aspirin during the last 3 months of pregnancy unless definitely directed to do so by a doctor because it may cause problems in the unborn child or complications during delivery.

Keep out of reach of children. In case of overdose, get medical help or contact a Poison Control Center right away.

Directions:
Regular Strength
Drink a full glass of water with each dose.
- adults and children 12 years and over: take 2 tablets every 4 hours; not more than 12 tablets in 24 hours
- children under 12 years: ask a doctor

Extra Strength
Drink a full glass of water with each dose.
- adults and children 12 years and over: take 2 tablets every 6 hours; not more than 8 tablets in 24 hours
- children under 12 years: ask a doctor

Other Information:
Regular Strength
- **each tablet contains:** calcium 65 mg and magnesium 50 mg
- store at room temperature
- read all product information before using.

Extra Strength
- **each tablet contains:** calcium 90 mg and magnesium 70 mg
- store at room temperature
- read all product information before using.

Inactive Ingredients:
benzoic acid, carnauba wax, citric acid, corn starch, FD&C blue #1, hypromellose, magnesium stearate, mineral oil, polysorbate 20, povidone, propylene glycol, simethicone emulsion, sodium phosphate, sorbitan monolaurate, titanium dioxide, zinc stearate

Questions or comments?
1-800-468-7746

How Supplied:
Regular Strength and Extra Strength are available in 39 ct., 65 ct., and 130 ct. cartons.
Shown in Product Identification Guide, page 513

COMTREX®
(Novartis Consumer Health, Inc.)
MAXIMUM STRENGTH
Pain Reliever/Fever Reducer, Cough Suppressant, Nasal Decongestant
Acetaminophon, Dextromethorphan HBr, Phenylephrine HCI
Non-Drowsy Cold & Cough

For full product information see page 725.

COMTREX®
(Novartis Consumer Health, Inc.)
MAXIMUM STRENGTH
Day/Night Severe Cold & Sinus
Pain Reliever/Fever Reducer – Nasal Decongestant – Antihistamine*
Acetaminophen, Phenylephrine HCI, Chlorpheniramine Maleate*

For full product information see page 725.

COMTREX® Cold & Cough Day/Night
(Novartis Consumer Health, Inc.)
Pain Reliever/Fever Reducer

For full product information see page 726.

CONCENTRATED TYLENOL®
acetaminophen Infants' Drops
(McNeil Consumer)

CHILDREN'S TYLENOL®
acetaminophen Suspension Liquid and Meltaways

JR. TYLENOL®
acetaminophen Meltaways

CHILDREN'S TYLENOL®
Suspension with Flavor Creator

Product information for all dosages of Children's TYLENOL have been combined under this heading

Description:
Concentrated TYLENOL® Infants' Drops are stable, alcohol-free, grape-flavored and purple in color, cherry-flavored and red in color or dye-free cherry flavored. Each 1.6 mL contains 160 mg acetaminophen. *Concentrated TYLENOL® Infants' Drops* features the SAFE-TY-LOCK™ Bottle. The SAFE-TY-LOCK® Bottle has a unique safety barrier inside the bottle which helps make administration easier. The integrated dropper promotes proper administration. The innovative design eliminates excess product on dropper. The star-shaped barrier inside the bottle minimizes spills and discourages pouring into a spoon. *Children's TYLENOL® Suspension Liquid* is stable, alcohol-free, cherry blast-flavored and red in color, bubblegum yum-flavored and pink in color, grape splash-flavored and purple in color, or very berry strawberry-flavored and red in color. Each 5 mL (one teaspoonful) contains 160 mg acetaminophen. Each *Children's TYLENOL® Meltaways* contains 80 mg acetaminophen in a grape punch, bubblegum burst or wacky watermelon flavor. Each *Jr. TYLENOL® Meltaways* contains 160 mg acetaminophen in grape punch or bubblegum burst flavor.

Actions:
Acetaminophen is a clinically proven analgesic/antipyretic. Acetaminophen produces analgesia by elevation of the pain threshold and antipyresis through action on the hypothalamic heat-regulating center. Acetaminophen is equal to aspirin in analgesic and antipyretic effectiveness and it is unlikely to produce many of the side effects associated with aspirin and aspirin-containing products.

Uses:
Concentrated TYLENOL® Infants' Drops: temporarily:

- reduces fever
- relieves minor aches and pains due to:
  - the common cold • flu • headache
  - sore throat • toothache

Children's TYLENOL® Suspension Liquid and Children's TYLENOL® Meltaways: temporarily relieves minor aches and pains due to: • the common cold • flu • headache • sore throat • toothache • temporarily reduces fever

Jr. TYLENOL® Meltaways: temporarily relieves minor aches and pains due to:
- the common cold • flu • headache
- temporarily reduces fever

Children's TYLENOL® Suspension with Flavor Creator:
- temporarily relieves minor aches and pains due to:
  - the common cold • flu • headache
  - sore throat • toothache
- temporarily reduces fever

Directions:
See Table 1: Children's Tylenol Dosing Chart on pgs. 757–758.

Warnings:
Sore throat warning: if sore throat is severe, persists for more than 2 days, is accompanied or followed by fever, headache, rash, nausea, or vomiting, consult a doctor promptly (excluding *Jr. TYLENOL® Meltaways*).

Do not use
- with any other product containing acetaminophen

When using this product
- **do not exceed recommended dose (see overdose warning)** *(Children's TYLENOL® Cherry Blast Liquid, Dye-Free Liquid, Children's TYLENOL® Suspension with Flavor Creator and Infants' Cherry Dye-Free Liquid)*

Stop use and ask a doctor if
- new symptoms occur
- redness or swelling is present
- pain gets worse or lasts for more than 5 days
- fever gets worse or lasts for more than 3 days

These could be signs of a serious condition *(Children's TYLENOL® Cherry Blast Liquid, Dye-Free Liquid and Children's TYLENOL® Suspension with Flavor Creator)*

Keep out of reach of children.
Overdose warning: Taking more than the recommended dose (overdose) may cause liver damage. In case of overdose, get medical help or contact a Poison Control Center (1-800-222-1222) right away. Quick medical attention is critical even if you do not notice any signs or symptoms.

Other Information:
Concentrated TYLENOL® Infants' Drops:
- store between 20–25°C (68–77°F)

Children's TYLENOL® Suspension Liquid:
- each teaspoon contains: **sodium 2mg** (excludes Dye-Free Cherry)

Continued on next page

Tylenol Infants—Cont.

- store between 20–25°C (68–77°F)

Children's TYLENOL® Meltaways:
- store between 20–25°C (68–77°F). Avoid high humidity. (Grape Punch: Protect from light).

Jr. TYLENOL® Meltaways:
- store between 20–25°C (68–77°F). Avoid high humidity. (Grape Punch: Protect from light).

Children's TYLENOL® with Flavor Creator:
- each teaspoon contains: **sodium 2mg**
- store between 20–25°C (68–77°F)

PROFESSIONAL INFORMATION: OVERDOSAGE INFORMATION for all Infants', Children's & Jr. Tylenol® Products

Acetaminophen: Acetaminophen in massive overdosage may cause hepatic toxicity in some patients. In adults and adolescents (≥ 12 years of age), hepatic toxicity may occur following ingestion of greater than 7.5 to 10 grams over a period of 8 hours or less. Fatalities are infrequent (less than 3–4% of untreated cases) and have rarely been reported with overdoses of less than 15 grams. In children (<12 years of age), an acute overdosage of less than 150 mg/kg has not been associated with hepatic toxicity. Early symptoms following a potentially hepatotoxic overdose may include: nausea, vomiting, diaphoresis and general malaise. Clinical and laboratory evidence of hepatic toxicity may not be apparent until 48 to 72 hours post-ingestion. In adults and adolescents, any individual presenting with an unknown amount of acetaminophen ingested or with a questionable or unreliable history about the time of ingestion should have a plasma acetaminophen level drawn and be treated with *N*-acetylcysteine. For full prescribing information, refer to the *N*-acetylcysteine package insert. Do not await results of assays for plasma acetaminophen levels before initiating treatment with *N*-acetylcysteine. The following additional procedures are recommended: Promptly initiate gastric decontamination of the stomach. A plasma acetaminophen assay should be obtained as early as possible, but no sooner than four hours following ingestion. If an acetaminophen *extended release* product is involved, it may be appropriate to obtain an additional plasma acetaminophen level 4–6 hours following the initial acetaminophen level. If either acetaminophen level plots above the treatment line on the acetaminophen overdose nomogram, *N*-acetylcysteine treatment should be continued for a full course of therapy. Liver function studies should be obtained initially and repeated at 24-hour intervals. Serious toxicity or fatalities have been extremely infrequent following an acute acetaminophen overdose in young children, possibly because of differences in the way they metabolize acetaminophen. In children, the maximum potential amount ingested can be more easily estimated. If more than 150 mg/kg or an unknown amount was ingested, obtain a plasma acetaminophen level as soon as possible, but no sooner than 4 hours following ingestion. If an acetaminophen *extended release* product is involved, it may be appropriate to obtain an additional plasma acetaminophen level 4–6 hours following the initial acetaminophen level. If either acetaminophen level plots above the treatment line on the acetaminophen overdose nomogram, *N*-acetylcysteine treatment should be initiated and continued for a full course of therapy. If an assay cannot be obtained and the estimated acetaminophen ingestion exceeds 150 mg/kg, dosing with *N*-acetylcysteine should be initiated and continued for a full course of therapy. For additional emergency information, call your regional poison center or call the Rocky Mountain Poison Center toll-free, (1-800-525-6115).

Our pediatric Tylenol® combination products contain active ingredients in addition to acetaminophen. The following is basic overdose information regarding those ingredients.

Chlorpheniramine: Chlorpheniramine toxicity should be treated as you would an anthihistamine/anticholinergic overdose and is likely to be present within a few hours after acute ingestion.

Dextromethorphan: Acute dextromethorphan overdose usually does not result in serious signs and symptoms unless massive amounts have been ingested. Signs and symptoms of a substantial overdose may include nausea and vomiting, visual disturbances, CNS disturbances and urinary retention.

Diphenhydramine: Diphenhydramine toxicity should be treated as you would an antihistamine/anticholinergic overdose and is likely to be present within a few hours after acute ingestion.

Phenylephrine: Symptoms from phenylephrine overdose most often consist of hypertension, anxiety, nervousness, restlessness, tachycardia, bradycardia, headache, dizziness and/or palpitations. Symptoms usually are transient and typically require no treatment.

For additional emergency information, please contact your local poison control center.

Inactive Ingredients:

Concentrated TYLENOL® Infants' Drops: **Cherry-Flavored:** cellulose, citric acid, corn syrup, FD&C Red #40, flavors, glycerin, purified water, sodium benzoate, sorbitol, xanthan gum. **Grape-Flavored:** cellulose, citric acid, corn syrup, D&C Red #33, FD&C Blue #1, flavors, glycerin, purified water, sodium benzoate, sorbitol, xanthan gum.

Dye-Free Cherry Flavored: butylparaben, carboxymethylcellulose sodium, cellulose, citric acid, flavors, glycerin, propylene glycol, propylparaben, purified water, sorbitol, sucralose, xanthan gum.

Children's TYLENOL® Suspension Liquid: butylparaben, carboxymethylcellulose sodium, cellulose, citric acid, corn syrup, flavors, glycerin, propylene glycol, purified water, sodium benzoate, sorbitol, sucralose, xanthan gum. In addition to the above ingredients cherry blast-flavored suspension contains FD&C red #40, bubblegum-yum-flavored suspension contains D&C red #33 and FD&C red #40, grape splash-flavored suspension contains D&C red #33 and FD&C blue #1 and very berry strawberry-flavored suspension contains FD&C red #40.

Dye-Free Cherry Flavored: butylparaben, carboxymethylcellulose sodium, cellulose, citric acid, flavors, glycerin, propylene glycol, propylparaben, purified water, sorbitol, sucralose, sucrose, xanthan gum.

Children's TYLENOL® Meltaways: Wacky Watermelon-Flavored: cellulose acetate, citric acid, crospovidone, D&C red #30, dextrose, flavors, magnesium stearate, povidone, sucralose. **Grape-Punch-Flavored:** cellulose acetate, citric acid, crospovidone, dextrose, D&C red #7, D&C red #30, FD&C blue #1, flavors, magnesium stearate, povidone, sucralose. **Bubblegum Burst-Flavored:** cellulose acetate, citric acid, crospovidone, D&C red #7, dextrose, flavors, magnesium stearate, povidone, sucralose.

Jr. TYLENOL® Meltaways Bubblegum Burst Flavored: cellulose acetate, citric acid, crospovidone, D&C red #7, dextrose, flavors, magnesium stearate, povidone, sucralose. **Grape Punch Flavored:** cellulose acetate, citric acid, crospovidone, D&C red #7, D&C red #30, dextrose, FD&C blue #1, flavors, magnesium stearate, povidone, sucralose.

Children's TYLENOL® Suspension with Flavor Creator: apple flavor*, bubblegum flavor*, butylparaben, carboxymethylcellulose sodium, cellulose, chocolate powder*, citric acid, corn syrup, FD&C blue #1, FD&C red #3*, FD&C red #40, flavors, glycerin, gum arabic*, malic acid*, powered cellulose*, propylene glycol, purified water, sodium alginate*, sodium benzoate, sorbitol, strawberry flavor*, sucralose, tumeric extract*, xanthan gum.
* each dose contains one or more of these ingredients.

How Supplied:

Concentrated TYLENOL® Infants' Drops: (purple-colored grape): bottles of ½ oz (15 mL) and 1 oz (30 mL); (red-colored cherry): bottles of ½ oz and 1 oz, and dye-free cherry each with calibrated plastic dropper.
Children's TYLENOL® Suspension Liquid: (red-colored cherry blast): bottles of 2 and 4 fl oz. (pink-colored bubblegum yum, purple-colored grape splash, red-colored very berry strawberry and dye-free cherry): bottles of 4 fl. oz.

Children's TYLENOL® with Flavor Creator: contains (1) 4 fl. oz. Cherry Blast Liquid (red-colored) plus 20 sugar free flavor packets in 4 flavors (apple, strawberry, chocolate and bubblegum).
Children's TYLENOL® Meltaways: (red-colored wacky watermelon, purple-colored grape punch, pink-colored bubble-gum burst, scored, imprinted "TY80"). Bottles of 30 and also blister packaged 48's and 64's.
Jr. TYLENOL® Meltaways: (purple-colored grape punch or pink-colored bubblegum burst, imprinted "TY 160"). Blister packaged 24's and 48's. All packages listed above are safety sealed and use child-resistant safety caps or blisters.

Shown in Product Identification Guide, page 509 & 510

CONTAC® COLD AND FLU DAY AND NIGHT
(GlaxoSmithKline Consumer)

For full product information see page 727.

CONTAC COLD AND FLU NON-DROWSY MAXIMUM STRENGTH
(GlaxoSmithKline Consumer)

For full product information see page 728.

CONTAC® COLD AND FLU MAXIMUM STRENGTH
(GlaxoSmithKline Consumer)

For full product information see page 728.

ECOTRIN
(GlaxoSmithKline Consumer)
Enteric-Coated Aspirin
Antiarthritic, Antiplatelet
COMPREHENSIVE PRESCRIBING INFORMATION

Description: Ecotrin enteric coated aspirin (acetylsalicylic acid) tablets available in 81mg, 325mg and 500 mg tablets for oral administration. The 325 mg and 500 mg tablets contain the following inactive ingredients: Carnuba Wax, Colloidal Silicon Dioxide, FD&C Yellow No. 6, Hypromellose, Methacrylic Acid Copolymer, Microcrystalline Cellulose, Pregelatinized Starch, Propylene Glycol, Simethicone, Sodium Starch Glycolate, Stearic Acid, Talc, Titanium Dioxide, and Triethyl Citrate. The 81 mg tablets contain Carnuba Wax, Corn Starch, D&C Yellow No. 10, FD&C Yellow No. 6, Hypromellose, Methacrylic Acid Copolymer, Microcrystalline Cellulose, Propylene Glycol, Simethicone, Stearic Acid, Talc and Triethyl Citrate.
Aspirin is an odorless white, needle-like crystalline or powdery substance. When exposed to moisture, aspirin hydrolyzes into salicylic and acetic acids, and gives off a vinegary-odor. It is highly lipid soluble and slightly soluble in water.

Clinical Pharmacology: Mechanism of Action: Aspirin is a more potent inhibitor of both prostaglandin synthesis and platelet aggregation than other salicylic acid derivatives. The differences in activity between aspirin and salicylic acid are thought to be due to the acetyl group on the aspirin molecule. This acetyl group is responsible for the inactivation of cyclooxygenase via acetylation.

PHARMACOKINETICS
Absorption: In general, immediate release aspirin is well and completely absorbed from the gastrointestinal (GI) tract. Following absorption, aspirin is hydrolyzed to salicylic acid with peak plasma levels of salicylic acid occurring within 1–2 hours of dosing (see Pharmacokinetics—Metabolism). The rate of absorption from the GI tract is dependent upon the dosage form, the presence or absence of food, gastric pH (the presence or absence of GI antacids or buffering agents), and other physiologic factors. Enteric coated aspirin products are erratically absorbed from the GI tract.
Distribution: Salicylic acid is widely distributed to all tissues and fluids in the body including the central nervous system (CNS), breast milk, and fetal tissues. The highest concentrations are found in the plasma, liver, renal cortex, heart, and lungs. The protein binding of salicylate is concentration-dependent, i.e., non-linear. At low concentrations (<100 mcg/mL) approximately 90 percent of plasma salicylate is bound to albumin while at higher concentrations (>400 mcg/mL), only about 75 percent is bound. The early signs of salicylic overdose (salicylism), including tinnitus (ringing in the ears), occur at plasma concentrations approximating 200 mcg/mL. Severe toxic effects are associated with levels > 400 mcg/mL (See section Adverse Reactions and Overdosage.)
Metabolism: Aspirin is rapidly hydrolyzed in the plasma to salicylic acid such that plasma levels of aspirin are essentially undetectable 1–2 hours after dosing. Salicylic acid is primarily conjugated in the liver to form salicyluric acid, a phenolic glucuronide, an acyl glucuronide, and a number of minor metabolites. Salicylic acid has a plasma half-life of approximately 6 hours. Salicylate metabolism is saturable and total body clearance decreases at higher serum concentrations due to the limited ability of the liver to form both salicyluric acid and phenolic glucuronide. Following toxic doses (10–20 grams (g)), the plasma half-life may be increased to over 20 hours.
Elimination: The elimination of salicylic acid follows zero order pharmacokinetics; (i.e., the rate of drug elimination is constant in relation to plasma concentration). Renal excretion of unchanged drug depends upon urine pH. As urinary pH rises above 6.5, the renal clearance of free salicylate increases from < 5 percent to > 80 percent. Alkalinization of the urine is a key concept in the management of salicylate overdose. (See Overdosage.) Following therapeutic doses, approximately 10 percent is found excreted in the urine as salicylic acid, 75 percent as salicyluric acid, and 10 percent phenolic and 5 percent acyl glucuronides of salicylic acid.
Pharmacodynamics: Aspirin affects platelet aggregation by irreversibly inhibiting prostaglandin cyclo-oxygenase. This effect lasts for the life of the platelet and prevents the formation of the platelet aggregating factor thromboxane A2. Nonacetylated salicylates do not inhibit this enzyme and have no effect on platelet aggregation. At somewhat higher doses, aspirin reversibly inhibits the formation of prostaglandin 1_2 (prostacyclin), which is an arterial vasodilator and inhibits platelet aggregation.
At higher doses aspirin is an effective anti-inflammatory agent, partially due to inhibition of inflammatory mediators via cyclooxygenase inhibition in peripheral tissues. In vitro studies suggest that other mediators of inflammation may also be suppressed by aspirin administration, although the precise mechanism of action has not been elucidated. It is this non-specific suppression of cyclooxygenase activity in peripheral tissues following large doses that leads to its primary side effect of gastric irritation. (See Adverse Reactions.)

Clinical Studies: Ischemic Stroke and Transient Ischemic Attack (TIA): In clinical trials of subjects with TIA's due to fibrin platelet emboli or ischemic stroke, aspirin has been shown to significantly reduce the risk of the combined endpoint of stroke or death and the combined endpoint of TIA, stroke, or death by about 13–18 percent.
Suspect Acute Myocardial Infarction (MI): In a large, multi-center study of aspirin, streptokinase, and the combination of aspirin and streptokinase in 17,187 patients with suspected acute MI, aspirin treatment produced a 23-percent reduction in the risk of vascular mortality. Aspirin was also shown to have an additional benefit in patients given a thrombolytic agent.
Prevention of Recurrent MI and Unstable Angina Pectoris: These indications are supported by the results of six large, randomized, multi-center, placebo-controlled trials of predominantly male post-MI subjects and one randomized placebo-controlled study of men with unstable angina pectoris. Aspirin therapy in MI subjects was associated with a significant reduction (about 20 percent) in the risk of the combination endpoint of subsequent death and/or nonfatal reinfarction in these patients. In aspirin-treated unstable angina patients the event rate was reduced to 5 percent from the 10 percent rate in the placebo group.
Chronic Stable Angina Pectoris: In a randomized, multi-center, double-blind

Continued on next page

Ecotrin—Cont.

trial designed to assess the role of aspirin for prevention of MI in patients with chronic stable angina pectoris, aspirin significantly reduced the primary combined endpoint of nonfatal MI, fatal MI, and sudden death by 34 percent. The secondary endpoint for vascular events (first occurrence of MI, stroke, or vascular death) was also significantly reduced (32 percent).

Revascularization Procedures: Most patients who undergo coronary artery revascularization procedures have already had symptomatic coronary artery disease for which aspirin is indicated. Similarly, patients with lesions of the carotid bifurcation sufficient to require carotid endarterectomy are likely to have had a precedent event. Aspirin is recommended for patients who undergo revascularization procedures if there is a preexisting condition for which aspirin is already indicated.

Rheumatologic Diseases: In clinical studies in patients with rheumatoid arthritis, juvenile rheumatoid arthritis, ankylosing spondylitis and osteoarthritis, aspirin has been shown to be effective in controlling various indices of clinical disease activity.

Animal Toxicology: The acute oral 50 percent lethal dose in rats is about 1.5 g/kg and in mice 1.1 g/kg. Renal papillary necrosis and decreased urinary concentrating ability occur in rodents chronically administered high doses. Dose-dependent gastric mucosal injury occurs in rats and humans. Mammals may develop aspirin toxicosis associated with GI symptoms, circulatory effects, and central nervous system depression. (See Overdosage.)

Indications and Usage: Vascular Indications (Ischemic Stroke, TIA, Acute MI, Prevention of Recurrent MI, Unstable Angina Pectoris, and Chronic Stable Angina Pectoris): Aspirin is indicated to: (1) Reduce the combined risk of death and nonfatal stroke in patients who have had ischemic stroke or transient ischemia of the brain due to fibrin platelet emboli, (2) reduce the risk of vascular mortality in patients with a suspected acute MI, (3) reduce the combined risk of death and non-fatal MI in patients with a previous MI or unstable angina pectoris, and (4) reduce the combined risk of MI and sudden death in patients with chronic stable angina pectoris.

Revascularization Procedures (Coronary Artery Bypass Graft (CABG), Percutaneous Transluminal Coronary Angioplasty (PTCA), and Carotid Endarterectomy): Aspirin is indicated in patients who have undergone revascularization procedures (i.e., CABG, PTCA, or carotid endarterectomy) when there is a preexisting condition for which aspirin is already indicated.

Rheumatologic Disease Indications (Rheumatoid Arthritis, Juvenile Rheumatoid Arthritis, Spondyloarthropathies, Osteoarthritis, and the Arthritis and Pleurisy of Systemic Lupus Erythematosus (SLE)): Aspirin is indicated for the relief of the signs and symptoms of rheumatoid arthritis, juvenile rheumatoid arthritis, osteoarthritis, spondyloarthropathies, and arthritis and pleurisy associated with SLE.

Contraindications: Allergy: Aspirin is contraindicated in patients with known allergy to nonsteroidal anti-inflammatory drug products and in patients with the syndrome of asthma, rhinitis, and nasal polyps. Aspirin may cause severe urticaria, angioedema, or bronchospasm (asthma).

Reye's Syndrome: Aspirin should not be used in children or teenagers for viral infections, with or without fever, because of the risk of Reye's syndrome with concomitant use of aspirin in certain viral illnesses.

Warnings: Alcohol Warning: Patients who consume three or more alcoholic drinks every day should be counseled about the bleeding risks involved with chronic, heavy alcohol use while taking aspirin.

Coagulation Abnormalities: Even low doses of aspirin can inhibit platelet function leading to an increase in bleeding time. This can adversely affect patients with inherited (hemophilia) or acquired (liver disease or vitamin K deficiency) bleeding disorders.

GI Side Effects: GI side effects include stomach pain, heartburn, nausea, vomiting, and gross GI bleeding. Although minor upper GI symptoms, such as dyspepsia, are common and can occur anytime during therapy, physicians should remain alert for signs of ulceration and bleeding, even in the absence of previous GI symptoms. Physicians should inform patients about the signs and symptoms of GI side effects and what steps to take if they occur.

Peptic Ulcer Disease: Patients with a history of active peptic ulcer disease should avoid using aspirin, which can cause gastric mucosal irritation and bleeding.

Precautions
General
Renal Failure: Avoid aspirin in patients with severe renal failure (glomerular filtration rate less than 10 mL/minute).

Hepatic Insufficiency: Avoid aspirin in patients with severe hepatic insufficiency. Sodium Restricted Diets: Patients with sodium-retaining states, such as congestive heart failure or renal failure, should avoid sodium-containing buffered aspirin preparations because of their high sodium content.

Laboratory Tests: Aspirin has been associated with elevated hepatic enzymes, blood urea nitrogen and serum creatinine, hyperkalemia, proteinuria, and prolonged bleeding time.

Drug Interactions
Angiotensin Converting Enzyme (ACE) Inhibitors: The hyponatremic and hypotensive effects of ACE inhibitors may be diminished by the concomitant administration of aspirin due to its direct effect on the renin-angiotensin conversion pathway.

Acetazolamide: Concurrent use of aspirin and acetazolamide can lead to high serum concentrations of acetazolamide (and toxicity) due to competition at the renal tubule for secretion.

Anticoagulant Therapy (Heparin and Warfarin): Patients on anticoagulation therapy are at increased risk for bleeding because of drug-drug interactions and the effect on platelets. Aspirin can displace warfarin from protein binding sites, leading to prolongation of both the prothrombin time and the bleeding time. Aspirin can increase the anticoagulant activity of heparin, increasing bleeding risk.

Anticonvulsants: Salicylate can displace protein-bound phenytoin and valproic acid, leading to a decrease in the total concentration of phenytoin and an increase in serum valproic acid levels.

Beta Blockers: The hypotensive effects of beta blockers may be diminished by the concomitant administration of aspirin due to inhibition of renal prostaglandins, leading to decreased renal blood flow, and salt and fluid retention.

Diuretics: The effectiveness of diuretics in patients with underlying renal or cardiovascular disease may be diminished by the concomitant administration of aspirin due to inhibition of renal prostaglandins, leading to decreased renal blood flow and salt and fluid retention.

Methotrexate: Salicylate can inhibit renal clearance of methotrexate, leading to bone marrow toxicity, especially in the elderly or renal impaired.

Nonsteroidal Anti-inflammatory Drugs (NSAID's): The concurrent use of aspirin with other NSAID's should be avoided because this may increase bleeding or lead to decreased renal function.

Oral Hypoglycemics: Moderate doses of aspirin may increase the effectiveness of oral hypoglycemic drugs, leading to hypoglycemia.

Uricosuric Agents (Probenecid and Sulfinpyrazone): Salicylates antagonize the uricosuric action of uricosuric agents.

oCarcinogenesis, Mutagenesis, Impairment of Fertility: Administration of aspirin for 68 weeks at 0.5 percent in the feed of rats was not carcinogenic. In the Ames Salmonella assay, aspirin was not mutagenic; however, aspirin did induce chromosome aberrations in cultured human fibroblasts. Aspirin inhibits ovulation in rats. (See Pregnancy.)

Pregnancy: Pregnant women should only take aspirin if clearly needed. Because of known effects of NSAID's on the fetal cardiovascular system (closure of the ductus arteriosus), use during the third trimester of pregnancy should be avoided. Salicylate products have also been associated with alterations in maternal and neonatal hemostasis mechanisms, decreased birth weight, and with perinatal mortality.

Labor and Delivery: Aspirin should be avoided 1 week prior to and during labor and delivery because it can result in excessive blood loss at delivery. Prolonged gestation and prolonged labor due to prostaglandin inhibition have been reported.
Nursing Mothers: Nursing mothers should avoid using aspirin because salicylate is excreted in breast milk. Use of high doses may lead to rashes, platelet abnormalities, and bleeding in nursing infants.
Pediatric Use: Pediatric dosing recommendations for juvenile rheumatoid arthritis are based on well-controlled clinical studies. An initial dose of 90–130 mg/kg/day in divided doses, with an increase as needed for anti-inflammatory efficacy (target plasma salicylate levels of 150–300 mcg/mL) are effective. At high doses (i.e., plasma levels of greater than 200 mg/mL), the incidence of toxicity increases.

Adverse Reactions: Many adverse reactions due to aspirin ingestion are dose-related. The following is a list of adverse reactions that have been reported in the literature. (See Warnings.)
Body as a Whole: Fever, hypothermia, thirst.
Cardiovascular: Dysrhythmias, hypotension, tachycardia.
Central Nervous System: Agitation, cerebral edema, coma, confusion, dizziness, headache, subdural or intracranial hemorrhage, lethargy, seizures.
Fluid and Electrolyte: Dehydration, hyperkalemia, metabolic acidosis, respiratory alkalosis.
Gastrointestinal: Dyspepsia, GI bleeding, ulceration and perforation, nausea, vomiting, transient elevations of hepatic enzymes, hepatitis, Reye's Syndrome, pancreatitis.
Hematologic: Prolongation of the prothrombin time, disseminated intravascular coagulation, coagulopathy, thrombocytopenia.
Hypersensitivity: Acute anaphylaxis, angioedema, asthma, bronchospasm, laryngeal edema, urticaria.
Musculoskeletal: Rhabdomyolysis.
Metabolism: Hypoglycemia (in children), hyperglycemia.
Reproductive: Prolonged pregnancy and labor, stillbirths, lower birth weight infants, antepartum and postpartum bleeding.
Respiratory: Hyperpnea, pulmonary edema, tachypnea.
Special Senses: Hearing loss, tinnitus. Patients with high frequency hearing loss may have difficulty perceiving tinnitus. In these patients, tinnitus cannot be used as a clinical indicator of salicylism.
Urogenital: Interstitial nephritis, papillary necrosis, proteinuria, renal insufficiency and failure.

Drug Abuse and Dependence: Aspirin is non-narcotic. There is no known potential for addiction associated with the use of aspirin.

Overdosage: Salicylate toxicity may result from acute ingestion (overdose) or chronic intoxication. The early signs of salicylic overdose (salicylism), including tinnitus (ringing in the ears), occur at plasma concentrations approaching 200 mcg/mL. Plasma concentrations of aspirin above 300 mcg/mL are clearly toxic. Severe toxic effects are associated with levels above 400 mcg/mL. (See Clinical Pharmacology.) A single lethal dose of aspirin in adults is not known with certainty but death may be expected at 30 g. For real or suspected overdose, a Poison Control Center should be contacted immediately. Careful medical management is essential.
Signs and Symptoms: In acute overdose, severe acid-base and electrolyte disturbances may occur and are complicated by hyperthermia and dehydration. Respiratory alkalosis occurs early while hyperventilation is present, but is quickly followed by metabolic acidosis.
Treatment: Treatment consists primarily of supporting vital functions, increasing salicylate elimination, and correcting the acid-base disturbance. Gastric emptying and/or lavage is recommended as soon as possible after ingestion, even if the patient has vomited spontaneously. After lavage and/or emesis, administration of activated charcoal, as a slurry, is beneficial, if less than 3 hours have passed since ingestion. Charcoal adsorption should not be employed prior to emesis and lavage.
Severity of aspirin intoxication is determined by measuring the blood salicylate level. Acid-base status should be closely followed with serial blood gas and serum pH measurements. Fluid and electrolyte balance should be maintained.
In severe cases, hyperthermia and hypovolemia are the major immediate threats to life. Children should be sponged with tepid water. Replacement fluid should be administered intravenously and augmented with correction of acidosis. Plasma electrolytes and pH should be monitored to promote alkaline diuresis of salicylate if renal function is normal. Infusion of glucose may be required to control hypoglycemia.
Hemodialysis and peritoneal dialysis can be performed to reduce the body drug content. In patients with renal insufficiency or in cases of life-threatening intoxication, dialysis is usually required. Exchange transfusion may be indicated in infants and young children.

Dosage and Administration: Each dose of aspirin should be taken with a full glass of water unless patient is fluid restricted. Anti-inflammatory and analgesic dosages should be individualized. When aspirin is used in high doses, the development of tinnitus may be used as a clinical sign of elevated plasma salicylate levels except in patients with high frequency hearing loss.
Ischemic Stroke and TIA: 50–325 mg once a day. Continue therapy indefinitely.

Suspected Acute MI: The initial dose of 160–162.5 mg is administered as soon as an MI is suspected. The maintenance dose of 160–162.5 mg a day is continued for 30 days post infarction. After 30 days, consider further therapy based on dosage and administration for prevention of recurrent MI.
Prevention of Recurrent MI: 75–325 mg once a day. Continue therapy indefinitely.
Unstable Angina Pectoris: 75–325 mg once a day. Continue therapy indefinitely.
Chronic Stable Angina Pectoris: 75–325 mg once a day. Continue therapy indefinitely.
CABG: 325 mg daily starting 6 hours post-procedure. Continue therapy for 1 year post-procedure.
PTCA: The initial dose of 325 mg should be given 2 hours pre-surgery. Maintenance dose is 160–325 mg daily. Continue therapy indefinitely.
Carotid Endarterectomy: Doses of 80 mg once daily to 650 mg twice daily, started presurgery, are recommended. Continue therapy indefinitely.
Rheumatoid Arthritis: The initial dose is 3 g a day in divided doses. Increase as needed for anti-inflammatory efficacy with target plasma salicylate levels of 150–300 mcg/mL. At high doses (i.e., plasma levels of greater than 200 mg/mL), the incidence of toxicity increases.
Juvenile Rheumatoid Arthritis: Initial dose is 90–130 mg/kg/day in divided doses. Increase as needed for anti-inflammatory efficacy with target plasma salicylate levels of 150–300 mcg/mL. At high doses (i.e., plasma levels of greater than 200 mg/mL), the incidence of toxicity increases.
Spondyloarthropathies: Up to 4 g per day in divided doses.
Osteoarthritis: Up to 3 g per day in divided doses.
Arthritis and Pleurisy of SLE: The initial dose is 3 g a day in divided doses. Increase as needed for anti-inflammatory efficacy with target plasma salicylate levels of 150–300 mcg/mL. At high doses (i.e., plasma levels of greater than 200 mg/mL), the incidence of toxicity increases.

How Supplied: 81 mg convex orange film coated tablet with ECOTRIN LOW printed in black ink on one side of the tablet. Available as follows
NDC 0108-0117-82 Bottle of 36 tablets
NDC 0108-0117-83 Bottle of 120 tablets
325 mg convex orange film coated tablet with ECOTRIN REG printed in black ink on one side of the tablet. Available as follows:
NDC 0108-0014-26 Bottle of 100 tablets
NDC 0108-0014-29 Bottle of 250 tablets
500 mg convex orange film coated tablet with ECOTRIN MAX printed in black ink on one side of the tablet. Available as follows:
NDC 0108-0016-23 Bottle of 60 tablets
NDC 0108-0016-27 Bottle of 150 tablets

Continued on next page

Ecotrin—Cont.

Store in a tight container at 25°C (77° F); excursions permitted to 15–30° C (59–86°F).

Shown in Product Identification Guide, page 505

EXCEDRIN PM®
(Novartis Consumer Health, Inc.)
PAIN RELIEVER/NIGHTTIME SLEEP AID

For full product information see page 610.

EXCEDRIN® SINUS HEADACHE
(Novartis Consumer Health, Inc.)
Acetaminophen and Phenylephrine HCl

For full product information see page 610.

EXCEDRIN® TENSION HEADACHE
(Novartis Consumer Health, Inc.)
PAIN RELIEVER

For full product information see page 611.

EXCEDRIN® EXTRA STRENGTH
(Novartis Consumer Health, Inc.)
PAIN RELIEVER

Drug Facts

Active Ingredients: **Purpose:**
(in each caplet/tablet/geltab)
Acetaminophen 250 mg ..... Pain reliever
Aspirin 250 mg .... Pain reliever
Caffeine 65 mg .... Pain reliever aid

Uses:
- temporarily relieves minor aches and pains due to:
  - headache
  - a cold • arthritis • muscular aches
  - sinusitis   • toothache
  - premenstrual & menstrual cramps

Warnings:

Reye's syndrome: Children and teenagers who have or are recovering from chicken pox or flu-like symptoms should not use this product. When using this product, if changes in behavior with nausea and vomiting occur, consult a doctor because these symptoms could be an early sign of Reye's syndrome, a rare but serious illness.

Allergy alert: Aspirin may cause a severe allergic reaction, which may include:
- hives • facial swelling
- asthma (wheezing) • shock

Alcohol warning: If you consume 3 or more alcoholic drinks every day, ask your doctor whether you should take acetaminophen and aspirin or other pain relievers/fever reducers. Acetaminophen and aspirin may cause liver damage and stomach bleeding.

Caffeine warning: The recommended dose of this product contains about as much caffeine as a cup of coffee. Limit the use of caffeine-containing medications, foods, or beverages while taking this product because too much caffeine may cause nervousness, irritability, sleeplessness, and, occasionally, rapid heart beat.

Do not use
- if you have ever had an allergic reaction to any other pain reliever/fever reducer
- with any other products containing acetaminophen. Taking more than directed may cause liver damage.

Ask a doctor before use if you have
- asthma
- ulcers
- bleeding problems
- stomach problems such as heartburn, upset stomach, or stomach pain that do not go away or return

Ask a doctor or pharmacist before use if you are taking a prescription drug for:
- anticoagulation (thinning of the blood)
- diabetes • gout • arthritis

Stop use and ask a doctor if
- an allergic reaction occurs. Seek medical help right away.
- new symptoms occur
- symptoms do not get better or worsen
- ringing in the ears or loss of hearing occurs
- painful area is red or swollen
- pain gets worse or lasts for more than 10 days
- fever gets worse or lasts for more than 3 days

If pregnant or breast-feeding, ask a health professional before use. It is especially important not to use aspirin during the last 3 months of pregnancy unless definitely directed to do so by a doctor because it may cause problems in the unborn child or complications during delivery.

Keep out of reach of children.

Overdose warning: Taking more than the recommended dose can cause serious health problems. In case of overdose, get medical help or contact a Poison Control Center right away. Quick medical attention is critical for adults as well as for children even if you do not notice any signs or symptoms.

Directions:
- do not use more than directed (see overdose warning)
- drink a full glass of water with each dose
- adults and children 12 years and over: take 2 caplets, tablets, or geltabs every 6 hours; not more than 8 caplets, tablets, or geltabs in 24 hours
- children under 12 years: ask a doctor

Other Information:
- store at room temperature
- read all product information before using.

Inactive Ingredients:
Tablets/Caplets
benzoic acid, carnauba wax, FD&C blue #1*, hydroxypropyl cellulose, hypromel-

lose, microcrystalline cellulose, mineral oil, polysorbate 20, povidone, propylene glycol, simethicone emulsion, sorbitan monolaurate, stearic acid, titanium dioxide*

* may also contain these ingredients.

Inactive Ingredients:
Geltabs
benzoic acid, D&C yellow #10 lake, disodium EDTA, FD&C blue #1 lake, FD&C red #40 lake, ferric oxide, gelatin, glycerin, hydroxypropyl cellulose, hypromellose, maltitol solution, microcrystalline cellulose, mineral oil, pepsin, polysorbate 20, povidone, propylene glycol, propyl gallate, simethicone emulsion, sorbitan monolaurate, stearic acid, titanium dioxide

Questions or comments?
1-800-468-7746

How Supplied: Caplets available in 24 ct., 50 ct., 100 ct., and 250 ct. cartons. Tablets available in 2 ct., 10 ct., 24 ct., 50 ct., 100 ct. and 250 ct. cartons. Geltabs available in 24 ct., 50 ct. and 100 ct. cartons.

Shown in Product Identification Guide, page 513

GOODY'S
(GlaxoSmithKline Consumer)
Body Pain Formula Powder

Indications: For temporary relief of minor body aches & pains due to muscular aches, arthritis & headaches.

Directions: Adults: Place one powder on tongue and follow with liquid, or stir powder into a glass of water or other liquid. May be repeated in 4 to 6 hours. Do not take more than 4 powders in any 24-hour period. Children under 12 years of age: Consult a doctor.

Warnings: Children and teenagers should not use this medicine for chicken pox or flu symptoms before a doctor is consulted about Reye's Syndrome, a rare but serious illness reported to be associated with aspirin. Do not use with any other product containing acetaminophen. **Ask a doctor before use if you have** asthma, ulcers, a bleeding problem, stomach problems that last or come back such as heartburn, upset stomach or pain. **Ask a doctor or pharmacist before use** if you are taking a prescription drug for gout, diabetes, arthritis or anticoagulation (blood thinning). **Stop use and ask a doctor if** an allergic reaction occurs, ringing in ears or loss of hearing occurs, pain gets worse or persists for more than 10 days, fever lasts more than 3 days, redness or swelling is present, or new symptoms occur. As with any drug, if you are pregnant, or nursing a baby, seek the advice of a health professional before using this product. **IT IS ESPECIALLY IMPORTANT NOT TO USE ASPIRIN DURING THE LAST 3 MONTHS OF PREGNANCY UNLESS SPECIFICALLY DIRECTED TO DO SO BY**

A DOCTOR BECAUSE IT MAY CAUSE PROBLEMS IN THE UNBORN CHILD OR COMPLICATIONS DURING DELIVERY.

Alcohol Warning: If you consume 3 or more alcoholic drinks every day, ask your doctor whether you should take acetaminophen and aspirin or other pain relievers/fever reducers. Acetaminophen and aspirin may cause liver damage and stomach bleeding.

Keep this and all medicines out of the reach of children. Overdose warning: Taking more than the recommended dose can cause serious health problems. In case of overdose, contact a doctor or poison control center immediately.

Active Ingredients: Each powder contains: 500 mg. aspirin and 325 mg. acetaminophen.

Inactive Ingredients: Each powder contains: Lactose Monohydrate and Potassium Chloride.

GOODY'S®
(GlaxoSmithKline Consumer)
Extra Strength Headache Powder

For full product information see page 611.

GOODY'S®
(GlaxoSmithKline Consumer)
Extra Strength Pain Relief Tablets

Indications: Goody's EXTRA STRENGTH tablets are a specially developed pain reliever that provide fast & effective temporary relief from minor aches & pain due to headaches, arthritis, colds or "flu," muscle strain, backache & menstrual discomfort. It is recommended for temporary relief of toothaches and to reduce fever.

Dosage: Adults: Two tablets with water or other liquid. May be repeated in 4 to 6 hours. Do not take more than 8 tablets in any 24-hour period. Children under 12 years of age: Consult a doctor.

Warnings: Children and teenagers should not use this medicine for chicken pox or flu symptoms before a doctor is consulted about Reye's Syndrome, a rare but serious illness reported to be associated with aspirin. Do not use with any other product containing acetaminophen. **Ask a doctor before use if you have** asthma, ulcers, a bleeding problem, stomach problems that last or come back such as heartburn, upset stomach or pain. **Ask a doctor or pharmacist before use** if you are taking a prescription drug for gout, diabetes, arthritis or anticoagulation (blood thinning) **When using this product** limit the use of caffeine containing drugs, foods, or drinks, because too much caffeine may cause nervousness, irritability, sleeplessness, and occasionally, rapid heartbeat. **Stop use and ask a doctor if** an allergic reaction

occurs, ringing in ears or loss of hearing occurs, pain gets worse or persists for more than 10 days, fever lasts more than 3 days, redness or swelling is present, or new symptoms occur.

As with any drug, if you are pregnant, or nursing a baby, seek the advice of a health professional before using this product. IT IS ESPECIALLY IMPORTANT NOT TO USE ASPIRIN DURING THE LAST 3 MONTHS OF PREGNANCY UNLESS SPECIFICALLY DIRECTED TO DO SO BY A DOCTOR BECAUSE IT MAY CAUSE PROBLEMS IN THE UNBORN CHILD OR COMPLICATIONS DURING DELIVERY. **Alcohol Warning:** If you consume 3 or more alcoholic drinks every day, ask your doctor whether you should take acetaminophen and aspirin or other pain relievers/fever reducers. Acetaminophen and aspirin may cause liver damage and stomach bleeding. **Keep this and all medicines out of the reach of children. Overdose warning:** Taking more than the recommended dose can cause serious health problems. In case of overdose, contact a doctor or poison control center immediately.

Active Ingredients: Each tablet contains 260 mg. aspirin in combination with 130 mg. acetaminophen and 16.25 mg. caffeine. **Inactive Ingredients:** Corn Starch, Crospovidone, Povidone, Pregelatinized Starch and Stearic Acid.

GOODY'S PM® POWDER
(GlaxoSmithKline Consumer)
For Pain with Sleeplessness

For full product information see page 612.

HYLAND'S COMPLETE FLU CARE 4 KIDS (Standard Homeopathic)

For full product information see page 732.

MINERAL ICE®
(Novartis Consumer Health, Inc.)
Pain Reliever

Drug Facts

Active Ingredient: **Purpose:**
Menthol 2% .... Topical analgesic

Uses:
- temporarily relieves minor aches and pains of muscles and joints associated with:
  - arthritis • simple backache • strains
  - bruises • sport injuries • sprains
- provides cooling penetrating relief

Warnings:
For external use only
Do not use
- with other topical pain relievers
- with heating pads or heating devices
When using this product
- do not use in or near the eyes

- do not apply to wounds or damaged skin
- do not bandage tightly
Stop use and ask a doctor if
- condition worsens
- symptoms last more that 7 days or clear up and occur again within a few days
- redness or irritation develops
If pregnant or breast-feeding, ask a health professional before use.
Keep out of reach of children. If swallowed, get medical help or contact a Poison Control Center right away.

Directions:
- clean affected area before applying product
- adults and children 2 years of age and older: apply to affected area not more than 3 to 4 times daily
- children under 2 years of age: ask a doctor

Other Information:
- store in a cool place
- keep lid tightly closed
- do not use, pour, spill or store near heat or open flame

Inactive Ingredients:
ammonium hydroxide, carbomer, cupric sulfate, FD&C blue no. 1, isopropyl alcohol, magnesium sulfate, sodium hydroxide, thymol, water

Questions or comments?
1-800-468-7746

How Supplied:
Available in 3.5 oz, 8.0 oz &, 16.0 oz jar.
Shown in Product Identification Guide, page 515

CHILDREN'S MOTRIN® Cold
(McNeil Consumer)
ibuprofen/pseudoephedrine HCl
Oral Suspension

For full product information see page 733.

INFANTS' MOTRIN® ibuprofen
Concentrated Drops
(McNeil Consumer)

CHILDREN'S MOTRIN® ibuprofen
Oral Suspension

JUNIOR STRENGTH MOTRIN®
ibuprofen Caplets and Chewable Tablets
Product information for all dosages of Children's MOTRIN have been combined under this heading

Description:
Infants' MOTRIN® Concentrated Drops are available in an alcohol-free, berry-flavored suspension and a non-staining, dye-free, berry-flavored suspension. Each 1.25 mL contains ibuprofen 50 mg. *Children's MOTRIN® Oral Suspension is*

Continued on next page

Motrin Infants'—Cont.

available as an alcohol-free, berry, dye-free berry, bubblegum, grape or tropical punch flavored suspension. Each 5 mL (teaspoon) of *Children's MOTRIN® Oral Suspension* contains ibuprofen 100 mg. *Junior Strength MOTRIN® Chewable Tablets* and *Junior Strength MOTRIN® Caplets* contain ibuprofen 100 mg. *Junior Strength MOTRIN® Chewable Tablets* are available in orange or grape flavors. *Junior Strength MOTRIN® Caplets* are available as easy-to-swallow caplets (capsule-shaped tablet).

Uses:

temporarily:
- reduces fever
- relieves minor aches and pains due to the common cold, flu, sore throat, headaches and toothaches

Directions:

See Table 2: Children's Motrin Dosing Chart on pgs. 757–758.

Warnings:

Allergy alert: Ibuprofen may cause a severe allergic reaction, especially in people allergic to aspirin. Symptoms may include:
- hives • facial swelling • asthma (wheezing) • shock • skin reddening • rash • blisters

If an allergic reaction occurs, stop use and seek medical help right away.

Stomach bleeding warning: This product contains a nonsteroidal anti-inflammatory drug (NSAID), which may cause stomach bleeding. The chance is higher if the child:
- has had stomach ulcers or bleeding problems
- takes a blood thinning (anticoagulant) or steroid drug
- takes other drugs containing an NSAID (aspirin, ibuprofen, naproxen, or others)
- takes more or for a longer time than directed

Sore throat warning:

Severe or persistent sore throat or sore throat accompanied by high fever, headache, nausea, and vomiting may be serious. Consult doctor promptly. Do not use more than 2 days or administer to children under 3 years of age unless directed by doctor.

Do not use

- if the child has ever had an allergic reaction to any other pain reliever/fever reducer
- right before or after heart surgery

Ask a doctor before use if the child has:

- problems or serious side effects from taking pain relievers or fever reducers
- stomach problems that last or come back, such as heartburn, upset stomach, or stomach pain
- ulcers
- bleeding problems
- not been drinking fluids

- lost a lot of fluid due to vomiting or diarrhea
- high blood pressure
- heart or kidney disease
- taken a diuretic

Ask a doctor or pharmacist before use if the child is

- taking any other drug containing an NSAID (prescription or nonprescription)
- taking a blood thinning (anticoagulant) or steroid drug
- under a doctor's care for any serious condition
- taking any other drug

When using this product

- mouth or throat burning may occur; give with food or water (*Junior Strength MOTRIN® Chewable Tablets* only)
- take with food or milk if stomach upset occurs
- long term continuous use may increase the risk of heart attack or stroke

Stop use and ask a doctor if

- the child feels faint, vomits blood, or has bloody or black stools. These are signs of stomach bleeding.
- stomach pain or upset gets worse or lasts
- the child does not get any relief within first day (24 hours) of treatment
- fever or pain gets worse or lasts more than 3 days
- redness or swelling is present in the painful area
- any new symptoms appear

Keep out of reach of children. In case of overdose, get medical help or contact a Poison Control Center (1-800-222-1222) right away.

Other Information: *Infants', Children's and Junior Strength MOTRIN® products:*
- store between 20–25°C (68–77°F)

Children's MOTRIN® Suspension Liquid:
- each teaspoon contains: **sodium 2 mg**

Junior Strength MOTRIN® Chewable Tablets:
- phenylketonurics: contains phenylalanine 2.8 mg per tablet

PROFESSIONAL INFORMATION: OVERDOSAGE INFORMATION FOR ALL INFANTS', CHILDREN'S & JUNIOR STRENGTH MOTRIN® PRODUCTS

IBUPROFEN: The *toxicity of ibuprofen* overdose is dependent upon the amount of drug ingested and the time elapsed since ingestion, though individual response may vary, which makes it necessary to evaluate each case individually. Although uncommon, serious toxicity and death have been reported in the medical literature with ibuprofen overdosage. The most frequently reported symptoms of ibuprofen overdose include abdominal pain, nausea, vomiting, lethargy and drowsiness. Other central nervous system symptoms include headache, tinnitus, CNS depression and seizures. Metabolic acidosis, coma, acute renal failure and apnea (primarily in very young children) may rarely occur. Cardiovascular toxicity, including hypotension, bradycardia,

tachycardia and atrial fibrillation, also have been reported.

The *treatment of acute ibuprofen overdose* is primarily supportive. Management of hypotension, acidosis and gastrointestinal bleeding may be necessary. In cases of acute overdose, the stomach should be emptied through ipecac-induced emesis or lavage. Emesis is most effective if initiated within 30 minutes of ingestion. Orally administered activated charcoal may help in reducing the absorption and reabsorption of ibuprofen. In children, the estimated amount of ibuprofen ingested per body weight may be helpful to predict the potential for development of toxicity although each case must be evaluated. Ingestion of less than 100 mg/kg is unlikely to produce toxicity. Children ingesting 100 to 200 mg/kg may be managed with induced emesis and a minimal observation time of four hours. Children ingesting 200 to 400 mg/kg of ibuprofen should have immediate gastric emptying and at least four hours observation in a health care facility. Children ingesting greater than 400 mg/kg require immediate medical referral, careful observation and appropriate supportive therapy. Ipecac-induced emesis is not recommended in overdoses greater than 400 mg/kg because of the risk of convulsions and the potential for aspiration of gastric contents.

In adult patients the history of the dose reportedly ingested does not appear to be predictive of toxicity. The need for referral and follow-up must be judged by the circumstances at the time of the overdose ingestion. Symptomatic adults should be admitted to a health care facility for observation.

Our Children's MOTRIN® Cold product contains pseudoephedrine in addition to ibuprofen. The following is basic overdose information regarding pseudoephedrine.

PSEUDOEPHEDRINE: Symptoms from pseudoephedrine overdose consist most often of mild anxiety, tachycardia and/or mild hypertension. Symptoms usually appear in 4 to 8 hours of ingestion and are transient, usually requiring no treatment.

For additional emergency information, please contact your local poison control center.

Inactive Ingredients:

Infants' MOTRIN® Concentrated Drops: **Berry-Flavored:** citric acid, corn starch, FD&C Red #40, flavors, glycerin, polysorbate 80, purified water, sodium benzoate, sorbitol, sucrose, xanthan gum. **Dye-Free Berry-Flavored:** artificial flavors, citric acid, corn starch, glycerin, polysorbate 80, purified water, sodium benzoate, sorbitol, sucrose, xanthan gum. *Children's MOTRIN® Oral Suspension:* **Berry-Flavored:** acesulfame potassium, citric acid, corn starch, D&C Yellow #10, FD&C Red #40, flavors, glycerin, polysorbate 80, purified water, sodium benzoate, sucrose, xanthan gum. **Dye-Free Berry-Flavored:** acesulfame potassium, citric acid, corn starch, glycerin,

natural and artificial flavors, polysorbate 80, purified water, sodium benzoate, sucrose, xanthan gum. **Bubble Gum-Flavored:** acesulfame potassium, citric acid, corn starch, FD&C Red #40, flavors, glycerin, polysorbate 80, purified water, sodium benzoate, sucrose, xanthan gum. **Grape-Flavored:** acesulfame potassium, citric acid, corn starch, D&C Red #33, FD&C Blue #1, FD&C Red #40, flavors, glycerin, polysorbate 80, purified water, sodium benzoate, sucrose, xanthan gum. **Tropical Punch Flavored:** acesulfame potassium, citric acid, corn starch, FD&C Red #40, flavors, glycerin, polysorbate 80, purified water, sodium benzoate, sucralose, sucrose, xanthan gum.

Junior Strength MOTRIN® Chewable Tablets: **Orange-Flavored:** acesulfame potassium, aspartame, cellulose, citric acid, FD&C yellow #6, flavor, fumaric acid, hydroxyethyl cellulose, hypromellose, magnesium stearate, mannitol, povidone, sodium lauryl sulfate, sodium starch glycolate. **Grape-Flavored:** acesulfame potassium, aspartame, cellulose, citric acid, D&C red #7, D&C red #30, FD&C blue #1, flavor, fumaric acid, hydroxyethyl cellulose, hypromellose, magnesium stearate, mannitol, povidone, sodium lauryl sulfate, sodium starch glycolate. **Easy-To-Swallow Caplets:** carnauba wax, cellulose, corn starch, D&C yellow #10, FD&C yellow #6, hypromellose, polydextrose, polyethylene glycol, propylene glycol, silicon dioxide, sodium starch glycolate, titanium dioxide, triacetin.

How Supplied:

Infants' MOTRIN® Concentrated Drops: Berry-flavored, pink-colored liquid and Berry-Flavored, Dye-Free, white-colored liquid in ½ fl. oz. bottles w/calibrated plastic syringe. Dye-Free Berry also available in 1 oz. size

Children's MOTRIN® Oral Suspension: Berry-flavored, pink-colored; (2 and 4 fl. oz) Berry-Flavored, Dye-Free white-colored, Bubble Gum-flavored, pink-colored, Grape-flavored, purple-colored, and Tropical Punch flavored liquid in tamper evident bottles (4 fl. oz.)

Junior Strength MOTRIN® Chewable Tablets: Orange-flavored, orange-colored chewable tablets or Grape-flavored, purple-colored chewable tablets in 24 count bottles.

Junior Strength MOTRIN® Caplets: Easy-to-swallow caplets (capsule shaped tablets) in 24 count bottles.

Shown in Product Identification Guide, page 508

MOTRIN® IB (Ibuprofen)
Pain Reliever/Fever Reducer
Tablets and Caplets
(McNeil Consumer)

Description:

Each *MOTRIN® IB Tablet and Caplet* contains ibuprofen 200 mg.

Uses:
- temporarily relieves minor aches and pains due to:
  - headache • muscular aches • minor pain of arthritis • toothache
  - backache • the common cold
  - menstrual cramps
- temporarily reduces fever

Directions:
- **do not take more than directed**
- **the smallest effective dose should be used**
- do not take longer than 10 days, unless directed by a doctor (see Warnings)

adults and children 12 years and older	• take 1 tablet or caplet every 4 to 6 hours while symptoms persist • if pain or fever does not respond to 1 tablet or caplet, 2 tablets or caplets may be used • do not exceed 6 tablets or caplets in 24 hours, unless directed by a doctor
children under 12 years	• ask a doctor

Warnings:

Allergy alert: Ibuprofen may cause a severe allergic reaction, especially in people allergic to aspirin. Symptoms may include:
- hives • facial swelling • asthma (wheezing) • shock • skin reddening • rash • blisters
If an allergic reaction occurs, stop use and seek medical help right away.

Stomach bleeding warning:　　　This product contains a nonsteroidal anti-inflammatory drug (NSAID), which may cause stomach bleeding. The chance is higher if you:
- are age 60 or older
- have had stomach ulcers or bleeding problems
- take a blood thinning (anticoagulant) or steroid drug
- take other drugs containing an NSAID (aspirin, ibuprofen, naproxen, or others)
- have 3 or more alcoholic drinks every day while using this product
- take more or for a longer time than directed

Do not use
- if you have ever had an allergic reaction to any other pain reliever/fever reducer
- right before or after heart surgery

Ask a doctor before use if you have
- problems or serious side effects from taking pain relievers or fever reducers
- stomach problems that last or come back, such as heartburn, upset stomach, or stomach pain
- ulcers

- bleeding problems
- high blood pressure
- heart or kidney disease
- taken a diuretic
- reached age 60 or older

Ask a doctor or pharmacist before use if you are
- taking any other drug containing an NSAID (prescription or nonprescription)
- taking a blood thinning (anticoagulant) or steroid drug
- under a doctor's care for any serious condition
- taking any other drug

When using this product
- take with food or milk if stomach upset occurs
- long term continuous use may increase the risk of heart attack or stroke

Stop use and ask a doctor if
- you feel faint, vomit blood, or have bloody or black stools. These are signs of stomach bleeding.
- pain gets worse or lasts more than 10 days
- fever gets worse or lasts more than 3 days
- stomach pain or upset gets worse or lasts
- redness or swelling is present in the painful area
- any new symptoms appear.

If pregnant or breast-feeding, ask a health professional before use. It is especially important not to use ibuprofen during the last 3 months of pregnancy unless definitely directed to do so by a doctor because it may cause problems in the unborn child or complications during delivery.

Keep out of reach of children. In case of overdose, get medical help or contact a Poison Control Center right away (1-800-222-1222).

Other Information:
- store between 20–25°C (68–77°F)

PROFESSIONAL INFORMATION: OVERDOSAGE INFORMATION FOR ADULT MOTRIN®

IBUPROFEN

The *toxicity of ibuprofen* overdose is dependent upon the amount of drug ingested and the time elapsed since ingestion, though individual response may vary, which makes it necessary to evaluate each case individually. Although uncommon, serious toxicity and death have been reported in the medical literature with ibuprofen overdosage. The most frequently reported symptoms of ibuprofen overdose include abdominal pain, nausea, vomiting, lethargy and drowsiness. Other central nervous system symptoms include headache, tinnitus, CNS depression and seizures. Metabolic acidosis, coma, acute renal failure and apnea (primarily in very young children) may rarely occur. Cardiovascular toxicity, including hypotension, bradycardia, tachycardia and atrial fibrillation, also have been reported. The *treat-*

Continued on next page

Motrin IB—Cont.

ment of acute ibuprofen overdose is primarily supportive. Management of hypotension, acidosis and gastrointestinal bleeding may be necessary. In cases of acute overdose, the stomach should be emptied through ipecac-induced emesis or lavage. Emesis is most effective if initiated within 30 minutes of ingestion. Orally administered activated charcoal may help in reducing the absorption and reabsorption of ibuprofen. In children, the estimated amount of ibuprofen ingested per body weight may be helpful to predict the potential for development of toxicity although each case must be evaluated. Ingestion of less than 100 mg/kg is unlikely to produce toxicity. Children ingesting 100 to 200 mg/kg may be managed with induced emesis and a minimal observation time of four hours. Children ingesting 200 to 400 mg/kg of ibuprofen should have immediate gastric emptying and at least four hours observation in a health care facility. Children ingesting greater than 400 mg/kg require immediate medical referral, careful observation and appropriate supportive therapy. Ipecac-induced emesis is not recommended in overdoses greater than 400 mg/kg because of the risk of convulsions and the potential for aspiration of gastric contents. In adult patients the history of the dose reportedly ingested does not appear to be predictive of toxicity. The need for referral and follow-up must be judged by the circumstances at the time of the overdose ingestion. Symptomatic adults should be admitted to a health care facility for observation.

Inactive Ingredients:

Tablets and Caplets: carnauba wax, corn starch, FD&C Yellow #6, hypromellose, iron oxide, polydextrose, polyethylene glycol, silicon dioxide, stearic acid, titanium dioxide.

How Supplied:

Tablets: (orange, printed "MOTRIN IB" in black) in tamper evident packaging of 24, 50, 100, and 165.
Caplets: (orange, printed "MOTRIN IB" in black) in tamper evident packaging of 24, 50, 100, 165, 225, and 300.

Shown in Product Identification Guide, page 509

ST. JOSEPH 81 mg Aspirin
ST. JOSEPH 81 mg Adult Low Strength Aspirin Chewable & Enteric Coated Tablets (McNeil Consumer)

Description:
Each St. Joseph Adult Low Strength Aspirin tablet contains 81 mg of aspirin.

Uses:
• temporarily relieves minor aches and pains

Directions:
• drink a full glass of water with each dose

adults and children 12 years and over	• take 4 to 8 tablets every 4 hours while symptoms last • do not exceed 48 tablets in 24 hours or as directed by a doctor
children under 12	do not use unless directed by a doctor

Warnings:

Reye's syndrome: Children and teenagers who have or are recovering from chicken pox or flu-like symptoms should not use this product. When using this product, if changes in behavior with nausea and vomiting occur, consult a doctor because these symptoms could be an early sign of Reye's syndrome, a rare but serious illness.

Allergy alert: Aspirin may cause a severe allergic reaction which may include:
• hives
• facial swelling
• asthma (wheezing)
• shock

Alcohol warning: If you consume 3 or more alcoholic drinks every day, ask your doctor whether you should take aspirin or other pain relievers or fever reducers. Aspirin may cause stomach bleeding.

Do not use
• if you have ever had an allergic reaction to any pain reliever or fever reducer
• for at least 7 days after tonsillectomy or oral surgery unless directed by a doctor *(chewable tablet formulation only)*

Ask a doctor before use if you have
• asthma
• ulcers
• bleeding problems
• stomach problems that last or come back such as heartburn, upset stomach or pain

Ask a doctor or pharmacist before use if you are taking a prescription drug for:
• anticoagulation (blood thinning)
• gout
• diabetes
• arthritis

Stop use and ask a doctor if
• allergic reaction occurs. Seek medical help right away.
• ringing in the ears or loss of hearing occurs
• pain gets worse or lasts more than 10 days
• new symptoms occur
• redness or swelling is present
These could be signs of a serious condition.

If pregnant or breast-feeding, ask a health professional before use. It is especially important not to use aspirin during the last three months of pregnancy unless definitely directed to do so by a doctor because it may cause problems in the un-

born child or complications during delivery.

Keep out of reach of children. In case of overdose, get medical help or contact a Poison Control Center right away (1-800-222-1222).

Other Information:
• store between 20–25°C (68–77°F). Avoid high humidity.

Inactive Ingredients: *St. Joseph 81 mg Adult Low Strength Aspirin Chewable Tablets:* corn starch, FD&C Yellow #6 aluminum lake, flavor, mannitol, saccharin, silicon dioxide, stearic acid. *Enteric Coated Tablets:* cellulose, corn starch, FD&C Red #40, FD&C Yellow #6, glyceryl monostearate, iron oxide, methacrylic acid, silicon dioxide, simethicone, stearic acid, triethyl citrate.

How Supplied:
St. Joseph 81 mg Adult Low Strength Chewable Aspirin Tablets: tamper evident bottles of 36 and 108 (Tri-Pack). *Enteric Coated Tablets:* tamper evident bottles of 36, 100, 180, 300 and 395.

COMPREHENSIVE PRESCRIBING INFORMATION

Description:
St. Joseph Adult Low Strength Aspirin Chewable & Enteric Coated Tablets (acetylsalicylic acid) are available in 81 mg for oral administration. *St. Joseph 81 mg Adult Low Strength Aspirin Chewable Tablets* contain the following inactive ingredients: corn starch, FD&C yellow #6 aluminum lake, flavor, mannitol, saccharin, silicon dioxide, stearic acid. *St. Joseph 81 mg Adult Low Strength Aspirin Enteric Coated Tablets* contain the following inactive ingredients: cellulose, corn starch, FD&C Red #40, FD&C Yellow #6, glyceryl monostearate, iron oxide, methacrylic acid, silicon dioxide, simethicone, stearic acid, triethyl citrate. Aspirin is an odorless white, needle-like crystalline or powdery substance. When exposed to moisture, aspirin hydrolyzes into salicylic and acetic acids, and gives off a vinegary-odor. It is highly lipid soluble and slightly soluble in water.

Clinical Pharmacology:

Mechanism of Action: Aspirin is a more potent inhibitor of both prostaglandin synthesis and platelet aggregation than other salicylic acid derivatives. The differences in activity between aspirin and salicylic acid are thought to be due to the acetyl group on the aspirin molecule. This acetyl group is responsible for the inactivation of cyclo-oxygenase via acetylation.

Pharmacokinetics: Absorption: In general, immediate release aspirin is well and completely absorbed from the gastrointestinal (GI) tract. Following absorption, aspirin is hydrolyzed to salicylic acid with peak plasma levels of salicylic acid occurring within 1–2 hours of dosing (see Pharmacokinetics—Metabolism). The rate of absorption from the GI tract is dependent upon the dosage form, the pres-

ence or absence of food, gastric pH (the presence or absence of GI antacids or buffering agents), and other physiologic factors. Enteric coated aspirin products are erratically absorbed from the GI tract. Distribution: Salicylic acid is widely distributed to all tissues and fluids in the body including the central nervous system (CNS), breast milk, and fetal tissues. The highest concentrations are found in the plasma, liver, renal cortex, heart, and lungs. The protein binding of salicylate is concentration-dependent, i.e., nonlinear. At low concentrations (<100 micrograms/milliliter μg/mL), approximately 90 percent of plasma salicylate is bound to albumin while at higher concentrations (400 μg/mL), only about 75 percent is bound. The early signs of salicylic overdose (salicylism), including tinnitus (ringing in the ears), occur at plasma concentrations approximating 200 μg/mL. Severe toxic effects are associated with levels 400 μg/mL. (See Adverse Reactions and Overdosage.)

Metabolism: Aspirin is rapidly hydrolyzed in the plasma to salicylic acid such that plasma levels of aspirin are essentially undetectable 1–2 hours after dosing. Salicylic acid is primarily conjugated in the liver to form salicyluric acid, a phenolic glucuronide, an acyl glucuronide, and a number of minor metabolites. Salicylic acid has a plasma half-life of approximately 6 hours. Salicylate metabolism is saturable and total body clearance decreases at higher serum concentrations due to the limited ability of the liver to form both salicyluric acid and phenolic glucuronide. Following toxic doses (10–20 grams (g)), the plasma half-life may be increased to over 20 hours.

Elimination: The elimination of salicylic acid follows zero order pharmacokinetics; (i.e., the rate of drug elimination is constant in relation to plasma concentration). Renal excretion of unchanged drug depends upon urine pH. As urinary pH rises above 6.5, the renal clearance of free salicylate increases from <5 percent to 80 percent. Alkalinization of the urine is a key concept in the management of salicylate overdose. (See Overdosage.) Following therapeutic doses, approximately 10 percent is found excreted in the urine as salicylic acid, 75 percent as salicyluric acid, and 10 percent phenolic and 5 percent acyl glucuronides of salicylic acid.

Pharmacodynamics: Aspirin affects platelet aggregation by irreversibly inhibiting prostaglandin cyclo-oxygenase. The effect lasts for the life of the platelet and prevents the formation of the platelet aggregating factor thromboxane A2. Nonacetylated salicylates do not inhibit this enzyme and have no effect on platelet aggregation. At somewhat higher doses, aspirin reversibly inhibits the formation of prostaglandin I2 (prostacyclin), which is an arterial vasodilator and inhibits platelet aggregation.

At higher doses, aspirin is an effective anti-inflammatory agent, partially due to inhibition of inflammatory mediators via cyclo-oxygenase inhibition in peripheral tissues. In vitro studies suggest that other mediators of inflammation may also be suppressed by aspirin administration, although the precise mechanism of action has not been elucidated. It is this nonspecific suppression of cyclo-oxygenase activity in peripheral tissues following large doses that leads to its primary side effect of gastric irritation. (See Adverse Reactions.)

Clinical Studies:

Ischemic Stroke and Transient Ischemic Attack (TIA): In clinical trials of subjects with TIA's due to fibrin platelet emboli or ischemic stroke, aspirin has been shown to significantly reduce the risk of the combined endpoint of stroke or death and the combined endpoint of TIA, stroke, or death by about 13–18 percent.

Suspected Acute Myocardial Infarction (MI): In a large, multi-center study of aspirin, streptokinase, and the combination of aspirin and streptokinase in 17,187 patients with suspected acute MI, aspirin treatment produced a 23-percent reduction in the risk of vascular mortality. Aspirin was also shown to have an additional benefit in patients given a thrombolytic agent.

Prevention of Recurrent MI and Unstable Angina Pectoris: These indications are supported by the results of six large, randomized, multi-center, placebo-controlled trials of predominantly male post-MI subjects and one randomized placebo-controlled study of men with unstable angina pectoris. Aspirin therapy in MI subjects was associated with a significant reduction (about 20 percent) in the risk of the combined endpoint of subsequent death and/or nonfatal reinfarction in these patients. In aspirin-treated unstable angina patients, the event rate was reduced to 5 percent from the 10 percent rate in the placebo group.

Chronic Stable Angina Pectoris: In a randomized, multi-center, double-blind trial designed to assess the role of aspirin for prevention of MI in patients with chronic stable angina pectoris, aspirin significantly reduced the primary combined endpoint of nonfatal MI, fatal MI, and sudden death by 34 percent. The secondary endpoint for vascular events (first occurrence of MI, stroke, or vascular death) was also significantly reduced (32 percent).

Revascularization Procedures: Most patients who undergo coronary artery revascularization procedures have already had symptomatic coronary artery disease for which aspirin is indicated. Similarly, patients with lesions of the carotid bifurcation sufficient to require carotid endarterectomy are likely to have had a precedent event. Aspirin is recommended for patients who undergo revascularization procedures if there is a preexisting condition for which aspirin is already indicated.

Rheumatologic Diseases: In clinical studies in patients with rheumatoid arthritis, juvenile rheumatoid arthritis, ankylosing spondylitis and osteoarthritis, aspirin has been shown to be effective in controlling various indices of clinical disease activity.

ANIMAL TOXICOLOGY

The acute oral 50 percent lethal dose in rats is about 1.5 g/kilogram (kg) and in mice 1.1 g/kg. Renal papillary necrosis and decreased urinary concentrating ability occur in rodents chronically administered high doses. Dose-dependent gastric mucosal injury occurs in rats and humans. Mammals may develop aspirin toxicosis associated with GI symptoms, circulatory effects, and central nervous system depression. (See Overdosage.)

Indications and Usage:

Vascular Indications (Ischemic Stroke, TIA, Acute MI, Prevention of Recurrent MI, Unstable Angina Pectoris, and Chronic Stable Angina Pectoris): Aspirin is indicated to: (1) Reduce the combined risk of death and nonfatal stroke in patients who have had ischemic stroke or transient ischemia of the brain due to fibrin platelet emboli, (2) reduce the risk of vascular mortality in patients with a suspected acute MI, (3) reduce the combined risk of death and nonfatal MI in patients with a previous MI or unstable angina pectoris, and (4) reduce the combined risk of MI and sudden death in patients with chronic stable angina pectoris.

Revascularization Procedures (Coronary Artery Bypass Graft (CABG), Percutaneous Transminase Coronary Angioplasty (PTCA), and Carotid Endarterectomy): Aspirin is indicated in patients who have undergone revascularization procedures (i.e., CABG, PTCA, or carotid endarterectomy) when there is a preexisting condition for which aspirin is already indicated.

Rheumatologic Disease Indications (Rheumatoid Arthritis, Juvenile Rheumatoid Arthritis, Spondyloarthropathies, Osteoarthritis, and the Arthritis and Pleurisy of Systemic Lupus Erythematosus (SLE)): Aspirin is indicated for the relief of the signs and symptoms of rheumatoid arthritis, juvenile rheumatoid arthritis, osteoarthritis, spondyloarthropathies, and arthritis and pleurisy associated with SLE.

Contraindications:

Allergy: Aspirin is contraindicated in patients with known allergy to nonsteroidal anti-inflammatory drug products and in patients with the syndrome of asthma, rhinitis, and nasal polyps. Aspirin may cause severe urticaria, angioedema, or bronchospasm (asthma).

Reye's Syndrome: Aspirin should not be used in children or teenagers for viral infections, with or without fever, because of the risk of Reye's syndrome with concom-

Continued on next page

St. Joseph Aspirin—Cont.

itant use of aspirin in certain viral illnesses.

Warnings:

Alcohol Warning: Patients who consume three or more alcoholic drinks every day should be counseled about the bleeding risks involved with chronic, heavy alcohol use while taking aspirin.

Coagulation Abnormalities: Even low doses of aspirin can inhibit platelet function leading to an increase in bleeding time. This can adversely affect patients with inherited (hemophilia) or acquired (liver disease or vitamin K deficiency) bleeding disorders.

GI Side Effects: GI side effects include stomach pain, heartburn, nausea, vomiting, and gross GI bleeding. Although minor upper GI symptoms, such as dyspepsia, are common and can occur anytime during therapy, physicians should remain alert for signs of ulceration and bleeding, even in the absence of previous GI symptoms. Physicians should inform patients about the signs and symptoms of GI side effects and what steps to take if they occur.

Peptic Ulcer Disease: Patients with a history of active peptic ulcer disease should avoid using aspirin, which can cause gastric mucosal irritation and bleeding.

Precautions:

General: Renal Failure: Avoid aspirin in patients with severe renal failure (glomerular filtration rate less than 10 mL/minute)
Hepatic Insufficiency: Avoid aspirin in patients with severe hepatic insufficiency. Sodium Restricted Diets: Patients with sodium-retaining states, such as congestive heart failure or renal failure, should avoid sodium-containing buffered aspirin preparations because of their high sodium content.

Laboratory Tests: Aspirin has been associated with elevated hepatic enzymes, blood urea nitrogen and serum creatinine, hyperkalemia, proteinuria, and prolonged bleeding time.

Drug Interactions: Angiotensin Converting Enzyme (ACE) Inhibitors: The hyponatremic and hypotensive effects of ACE inhibitors may be diminished by the concomitant administration of aspirin due to its indirect effect on the renin-angiotensin conversion pathway.
Acetazolamide: Concurrent use of aspirin and acetazolamide can lead to high serum concentrations of acetazolamide (and toxicity) due to competition at the renal tubule for secretion. Anticoagulant Therapy (Heparin and Warfarin): Patients on anticoagulation therapy are at increased risk for bleeding because of drug-drug interactions and the effect on platelets. Aspirin can displace warfarin from protein binding sites, leading to prolongation of both the prothrom-

bin time and the bleeding time. Aspirin can increase the anticoagulant activity of heparin, increasing bleeding risk.
Anticonvulsants: Salicylate can displace protein-bound phenytoin and valproic acid, leading to a decrease in the total concentration of phenytoin and an increase in serum valproic acid levels.
Beta Blockers: The hypotensive effects of beta blockers may be diminished by the concomitant administration of aspirin due to inhibition of renal prostaglandins, leading to decreased renal blood flow, and salt and fluid retention.
Diuretics: The effectiveness of diuretics in patients with underlying renal or cardiovascular disease may be diminished by the concomitant administration of aspirin due to inhibition of renal prostaglandins, leading to decreased renal blood flow and salt and fluid retention.
Methotrexate: Salicylate can inhibit renal clearance of methotrexate, leading to bone marrow toxicity, especially in the elderly or renal impaired.
Nonsteroidal Anti-Inflammatory Drugs (NSAID's): The concurrent use of aspirin with other NSAID's should be avoided because this may increase bleeding or lead to decreased renal function.
Oral Hypoglycemics: Moderate doses of aspirin may increase the effectiveness of oral hypoglycemic drugs, leading to hypoglycemia.
Uricosuric Agents (Probenecid and Sulfinpyrazone): Salicylates antagonize the uricosuric action of uricosuric agents.

Carcinogenesis, Mutagenesis, Impairment of Fertility: Administration of aspirin for 68 weeks at 0.5 percent in the feed of rats was not carcinogenic. In the Ames Salmonella assay, aspirin was not mutagenic; however, aspirin did induce chromosome aberrations in cultured human fibroblasts. Aspirin inhibits ovulation in rats. (See Pregnancy.)

Pregnancy: Pregnant women should only take aspirin if clearly needed. Because of the known effects of NSAID's on the fetal cardiovascular system (closure of the ductus arteriosus), use during the third trimester of pregnancy should be avoided. Salicylate products have also been associated with alterations in maternal and neonatal hemostasis mechanisms, decreased birth weight, and with perinatal mortality.

Labor and Delivery: Aspirin should be avoided 1 week prior to and during labor and delivery because it can result in excessive blood loss at delivery. Prolonged gestation and prolonged labor due to prostaglandin inhibition have been reported.

Nursing Mothers: Nursing mothers should avoid using aspirin because salicylate is excreted in breast milk. Use of high doses may lead to rashes, platelet abnormalities, and bleeding in nursing infants.

Pediatric Use: Pediatric dosing recommendations for juvenile rheumatoid arthritis are based on well-controlled clinical studies. An initial dose of 90–

130 mg/kg/day in divided doses, with an increase as needed for anti-inflammatory efficacy (target plasma salicylate levels of 150–300 µg/mL) are effective. At high doses (i.e., plasma levels of greater than 200 µg/mL), the incidence of toxicity increases.

Adverse Reactions:

Many adverse reactions due to aspirin ingestion are dose-related. The following is a list of adverse reactions that have been reported in the literature. (See Warnings.)
Body as a Whole: Fever, hypothermia, thirst.
Cardiovascular: Dysrhythmias, hypotension, tachycardia.
Central Nervous System: Agitation, cerebral edema, coma, confusion, dizziness, headache, subdural or intracranial hemorrhage, lethargy, seizures.
Fluid and Electrolyte: Dehydration, hyperkalemia, metabolic acidosis, respiratory alkalosis.
Gastrointestinal: Dyspepsia, GI bleeding, ulceration and perforation, nausea, vomiting, transient elevations of hepatic enzymes, hepatitis, Reye's Syndrome, pancreatitis.
Hematologic: Prolongation of the prothrombin time, disseminated intravascular coagulation, coagulopathy, thrombocytopenia.
Hypersensitivity: Acute anaphylaxis, angioedema, asthma, bronchospasm, laryngeal edema, urticaria.
Musculoskeletal: Rhabdomyolysis.
Metabolism: Hypoglycemia (in children), hyperglycemia.
Reproductive: Prolonged pregnancy and labor, stillbirths, lower birth weight infants, antepartum and postpartum bleeding.
Special Senses: Hearing loss, tinnitus. Patients with high frequency hearing loss may have difficulty perceiving tinnitus. In these patients, tinnitus cannot be used as a clinical indicator of salicylism.
Urogenital: Interstitial nephritis, papillary necrosis, proteinuria, renal insufficiency and failure.

Drug Abuse and Dependence:

Aspirin is nonnarcotic. There is no known potential for addiction associated with the use of aspirin.

Overdosage:

Salicylate toxicity may result from acute ingestion (overdose) or chronic intoxication. The early signs of salicylic overdose (salicylism), including tinnitus (ringing in the ears), occur at plasma concentrations approaching 200 µg/mL. Plasma concentrations of aspirin above 300 µg/mL are clearly toxic. Severe toxic effects are associated with levels above 400 µg/mL (See Clinical Pharmacology.) A single lethal dose of aspirin in adults is not known with certainty but death may be expected at 30 g. For real or suspected overdose, a Poison Control Center should be contacted immediately. Careful medical management is essential.
Signs and Symptoms: In acute overdose, severe acid-base and electrolyte distur-

bances may occur and are complicated by hyperthermia and dehydration. Respiratory alkalosis occurs early while hyperventilation is present, but is quickly followed by metabolic acidosis.

Treatment: Treatment consists primarily of supporting vital functions, increasing salicylate elimination, and correcting the acid-base disturbance. Gastric emptying and/or lavage is recommended as soon as possible after ingestion, even if the patient has vomited spontaneously. After lavage and/or emesis, administration of activated charcoal, as a slurry, is beneficial, if less than 3 hours have passed since ingestion. Charcoal adsorption should not be employed prior to emesis and lavage. Severity of aspirin intoxication is determined by measuring the blood salicylate level. Acid-base status should be closely followed with serial blood gas and serum pH measurements. Fluid and electrolyte balance should also be maintained. In severe cases, hyperthermia and hypovolemia are the major immediate threats to life. Children should be sponged with tepid water. Replacement fluids should be administered intravenously and augmented with correction of acidosis. Plasma electrolytes and pH should be monitored to promote alkaline diuresis of salicylate if renal function is normal. Infusion of glucose may be required to control hypoglycemia. Hemodialysis and peritoneal dialysis can be performed to reduce the body drug content. In patients with renal insufficiency or in cases of life-threatening intoxication, dialysis is usually required. Exchange transfusion may be indicated in infants and young children.

Dosage and Administration:

Each dose of aspirin should be taken with a full glass of water unless the patient is fluid restricted. Anti-inflammatory and analgesic dosages should be individualized. When aspirin is used in high doses, the development of tinnitus may be used as a clinical sign of elevated plasma salicylate levels except in patients with high frequency hearing loss.

Ischemic Stroke and TIA: 50–325 mg once a day. Continue therapy indefinitely

Suspected Acute MI: The initial dose of 160–162.5 mg is administered as soon as an MI is suspected. The maintenance dose of 160–162.5 mg a day is continued for 30 days post-infarction. After 30 days, consider further therapy based on dosage and administration for prevention of recurrent MI.

Prevention of Recurrent MI: 75–325 mg once a day. Continue therapy indefinitely.

Unstable Angina Pectoris: 75–325 mg once a day. Continue therapy indefinitely.

Chronic Stable Angina Pectoris: 75–325 mg once a day. Continue therapy indefinitely.

CABG: 325 mg daily starting 6 hours post-procedure. Continue therapy for 1 year post-procedure.

PTCA: The initial dose of 325 mg daily should be given 2 hours pre-surgery.

Maintenance dose is 160–325 mg daily. Continue therapy indefinitely.

Carotid Endarterectomy: Doses of 80 mg once a day to 650 mg twice daily, started presurgery, are recommended. Continue therapy indefinitely.

Rheumatoid Arthritis: The initial dose is 3 g a day in divided doses. Increase as needed for anti-inflammatory efficacy with target plasma salicylate levels of 150–300 µg/mL. At high doses (i.e., plasma levels of greater than 200 µg/mL), the incidence of toxicity increases.

Juvenile Rheumatoid Arthritis: Initial dose is 90–130 mg/kg/day in divided doses. Increase as needed for anti-inflammatory efficacy with target plasma salicylate levels of 150–300 µg/mL. At high doses (i.e., plasma levels of greater than 200 µg/mL), the incidence of toxicity increases.

Spondyloarthropathies: Up to 4 g per day in divided doses.

Osteoarthritis: Up to 3 g per day in divided doses.

Arthritis and Pleurisy of SLE: The initial dose is 3 g a day in divided doses. Increase as needed for anti-inflammatory efficacy with target plasma salicylate levels of 150–300 µg/mL. At high doses (i.e., plasma levels of greater than 200 µg/mL), the incidence of toxicity increases.

How Supplied:

St. Joseph Adult Low Strength Aspirin Chewable Tablets are round, concave, orange-flavored, orange-colored tablets that are debossed with the "SJ" logo. Available as follows:
NDC 50580-173-36 Bottle of 36 tablets
NDC 50580-173-08 Tri-Pack
St Joseph Adult Low Strength Enteric Coated Tablets are round, concave, pink-coated tablets that are printed with the "St J" logo. Available as follows:
NDC 50580-126-36 Bottle of 36 tablets
NDC 50580-126-10 Bottle of 100 tablets
NDC 50580-126-18 Bottle of 180 tablets
NDC 50580-126-03 Bottle of 300 tablets
NDC 50580-126-39 Bottle of 395 tablets
Store in tight container at 25 deg.C (77 deg.F); excursions permitted to 15–30 deg.C (59–86 deg.F).

Shown in Product Identification Guide, page 509

THERAFLU® Nighttime Severe Cold
(Novartis Consumer Health, Inc.)
Pain Reliever-Fever Reducer (Acetaminophen)
Antihistamine (Pheniramine maleate)
Nasal Decongestant (Phenylephrine HCl)

For full product information see page 740.

THERAFLU® Cold & Cough
(Novartis Consumer Health, Inc.)
Cough Suppressant (Dextromethorphan HBr)
Antihistamine (Pheniramine maleate)
Nasal Decongestant (Phenylephrine HCl)

For full product information see page 740.

THERAFLU® Cold & Sore Throat
(Novartis Consumer Health, Inc.)
Pain Reliever-Fever Reducer (Acetaminophen)
Antihistamine (Pheniramine maleate)
Nasal Decongestant (Phenylephrine HCl)

For full product information see page 741.

THERAFLU® Flu & Chest Congestion
(Novartis Consumer Health, Inc.)
Pain Reliever-Fever Reducer (Acetaminophen)
Expectorant (Guaifenesin)

For full product information see page 741.

THERAFLU® Flu & Sore Throat
(Novartis Consumer Health, Inc.)
Pain Reliever-Fever Reducer (Acetaminophen)
Antihistamine (Pheniramine maleate)
Nasal Decongestant (Phenylephrine HCl)

For full product information see page 742.

THERAFLU® Daytime Severe Cold
(Novartis Consumer Health, Inc.)
Pain Reliever-Fever Reducer (Acetaminophen)
Nasal Decongestant (Phenylephrine HCl)

For full product information see page 742.

THERAFLU® DAYTIME WARMING RELIEF
(Novartis Consumer Health, Inc.)
Pain Reliever/Fever Reducer/Cough Suppressant/Nasal Decongestant

For full product information see page 743.

THERAFLU® NIGHTTIME WARMING RELIEF
(Novartis Consumer Health, Inc.)
Cough Suppressant/Antihistamine/Pain Reliever/Fever Reducer/Nasal Decongestant

For full product information see page 743.

THERA-GESIC® Maximum Strength Analgesic Pain Relieving Creme
(Mission Pharmacal)
pain relieving crème

Drug Facts

Active Ingredients:	Purpose:
Menthol 1%	Analgesic

Continued on next page

Thera-Gesic—Cont.

Methyl Salicylate 15% .. Counterirritant

Use:

temporary relief of minor aches and pains of muscles and joints associated with:
- arthritis • simple backaches • strains
- bruises • sprains

Warnings:

For external use only. Use only as directed. Avoid contact with eyes or mucous membranes.

Do not bandage tightly, wrap or cover until after washing the areas where THERA-GESIC® has been applied.

Do not use
- immediately after shower or bath
- if skin is sensitive to oil of wintergreen (methyl salicylate)
- on wounds or damaged skin

Ask a doctor before use
- for children under 2 and to 12 years of age
- if prone or sensitive to allergic reactions from aspirin or salicylate

When using this product
- discontinue use if skin irritation develops, or redness is present
- do not swallow
- do not use a heating pad after application of THERA-GESIC®

Stop use and ask a doctor if condition worsens, or if symptoms persist for more than 7 days or clear up and occur again within a few days.

If pregnant or breast-feeding, ask a health professional before use.

Keep out of reach of children to avoid accidental poisoning. If swallowed, get medical help or contact a Poison Control Center right away.

Directions:

Adults and children 12 or more years of age: Apply thin layers of creme into and around the sore or painful area, not more than 3 to 4 times daily. The number of thin layers controls the intensity of the action of THERA-GESIC®. One thin layer provides a mild effect, two thin layers provide a strong effect and three thin layers provide a very strong effect. SEE WARNINGS. Wash hands thoroughly after application.

Other Information:

Once THERA-GESIC® has penetrated the skin, the area may be washed, leaving it dry, clean and fragrance-free without decreasing the effectiveness of the product. Avoid contact with clothing or other surfaces. Store at 20–25°C (68–77°F).

Inactive Ingredients:

Carbomer 934, Dimethicone, Glycerine, Methylparaben, Propylparaben, Sodium Lauryl Sulfate, Trolamine, Water.

Questions?

(210) 696–8400 (M-F 8:30–5:00 CST)

How Supplied: Net wt. 3 oz., NDC 0178-0320-03; Net wt. 5 oz., NDC 0178-0320-05.

THERMA-CARE HEAT ACTIVATED WRAPS (Procter & Gamble)

Therapeutic heat wraps

Back/Hip

PLEASE READ ALL INSTRUCTIONS AND WARNINGS BEFORE USE. ADDITIONAL WARNINGS ARE INCLUDED IN THE PACKAGE INSERT. TO REDUCE THE RISK OF BURNS, FIRE, AND PERSONAL INJURY, THIS PRODUCT MUST BE USED IN ACCORDANCE WITH THE USE INSTRUCTIONS AND WARNINGS. CHOOSE THE RIGHT SIZE THERMACARE® BACK/HIP WRAP FOR YOU

	Women's Pant Size	Men's Pant Size
S/M	Up to size 8	Up to 34-inch waist
L/XL	Size 9 up to size 20	35 inches to 47 inches

Uses: Provides temporary relief of minor muscular and joint aches and pains associated with overexertion, strains, sprains, and arthritis.

Directions: Tear open pouch when ready to use. It may take up to 30 minutes for ThermaCare® to reach its therapeutic temperature. Place on pain area on lower back or hip with darker discs toward skin. Over-tightening may cause discomfort. Adjust as needed. For maximum effectiveness, we recommend you wear ThermaCare® for 8 hours. Do not wear for more than 8 hours in any 24-hour period.

WARNING: THIS PRODUCT CAN CAUSE BURNS. CHECK SKIN FREQUENTLY DURING USE. IF YOU FIND IRRITATION OR A BURN, REMOVE PRODUCT IMMEDIATELY.

55 OR OLDER: YOUR RISK OF BURNING INCREASES AS YOU AGE. IF YOU ARE 55 YEARS OF AGE OR OLDER, WEAR THERMACARE® OVER A LAYER OF CLOTHING, NOT DIRECTLY AGAINST YOUR SKIN, AND DO NOT WEAR WHILE SLEEPING.

ASK A DOCTOR BEFORE USE if you have
- DIABETES
- poor circulation or heart disease
- rheumatoid arthritis
- or are pregnant

ADDITIONAL WARNINGS: Each heat disc contains iron (~2 grams), which can be harmful if ingested. If ingested, rinse mouth with water and call a Poison Control Center immediately. If heat disc contents come in contact with your skin or eyes, rinse right away with water. Never heat product in a microwave or attempt to reheat as wrap could catch fire. Keep out of reach of children and pets.

WHEN USING THIS PRODUCT check skin frequently for signs of burns or blisters – if found stop use

- if product feels too hot – stop use or wear over clothing
- do not place extra pressure, a tight waistband or belt over the product
- do not use for more than 8 hours in a 24-hour period

DO NOT USE with pain rubs, medicated lotions, creams or ointments
- on unhealthy, damaged or broken skin
- on areas of bruising or swelling that have occurred within 48 hours
- on people unable to follow all use instructions
- on areas of the body where you can't feel heat
- with other forms of heat
- on people unable to remove the product, including children, infants, and some elderly

STOP USE AND ASK A DOCTOR if you experience any discomfort, burning, swelling, rash or other changes in your skin that persist where the wrap is worn
- if after 7 days your pain gets worse or remains unchanged as this may be a sign of a more serious condition

Menstrual

PLEASE READ ALL INSTRUCTIONS AND WARNINGS BEFORE USE. ADDITIONAL WARNINGS ARE INCLUDED IN THE PACKAGE INSERT. TO REDUCE THE RISK OF BURNS, FIRE, AND PERSONAL INJURY, THIS PRODUCT MUST BE USED IN ACCORDANCE WITH THE USE INSTRUCTIONS AND WARNINGS.

Uses: Provides temporary relief of minor menstrual cramp pain and associated back aches.

Directions: Tear open pouch when ready to use. It may take up to 30 minutes for ThermaCare® to reach its therapeutic temperature. Peel away paper to reveal adhesive side. Place on pain area with adhesive side against underwear and not against the skin. Attach firmly. For maximum effectiveness, we recommend you wear ThermaCare® for 8 hours. Do not wear for more than 8 hours in any 24-hour period.

WARNING: THIS PRODUCT CAN CAUSE BURNS. CHECK SKIN FREQUENTLY DURING USE. IF YOU FIND IRRITATION OR A BURN, REMOVE PRODUCT IMMEDIATELY.

55 OR OLDER: YOUR RISK OF BURNING INCREASES AS YOU AGE. IF YOU ARE 55 YEARS OF AGE OR OLDER DO NOT USE DURING SLEEP.

ASK A DOCTOR BEFORE USE if you have
- DIABETES
- poor circulation or heart disease
- rheumatoid arthritis
- or are pregnant

ADDITIONAL WARNINGS: Each heat disc contains iron (~2 grams), which can be harmful if ingested. If ingested, rinse mouth with water and call a Poison Control Center immediately. If heat disc contents come in contact with your skin or eyes, rinse right away with water.

Never heat product in a microwave or attempt to reheat as wrap could catch fire. Keep out of reach of children and pets.

WHEN USING THIS PRODUCT check skin frequently for signs of burns or blisters – if found stop use

- if product feels too hot – stop use or wear over clothing
- do not place extra pressure, a tight waistband or belt over the product
- do not use for more than 8 hours in a 24-hour period

DO NOT USE with pain rubs, medicated lotions, creams or ointments

- on unhealthy, damaged or broken skin
- on areas of bruising or swelling that have occurred within 48 hours
- on people unable to follow all use instructions
- on areas of the body where you can't feel heat
- with other forms of heat
- on people unable to remove the product, including children, infants, and some elderly

STOP USE AND ASK A DOCTOR if you experience any discomfort, burning, swelling, rash or other changes in your skin that persist where the wrap is worn

- if after 4 days your pain gets worse or remains unchanged as this may be a sign of a more serious condition.

Neck, Shoulder & Wrist

PLEASE READ ALL INSTRUCTIONS AND WARNINGS BEFORE USE. ADDITIONAL WARNINGS ARE INCLUDED IN THE PACKAGE INSERT. TO REDUCE THE RISK OF BURNS, FIRE, AND PERSONAL INJURY, THIS PRODUCT MUST BE USED IN ACCORDANCE WITH THE USE INSTRUCTIONS AND WARNINGS.

Uses: Provides temporary relief of minor muscular and joint aches and pains associated with overexertion, strains, sprains, and arthritis.

Directions: Tear open pouch when ready to use. It may take up to 30 minutes for ThermaCare® to reach its therapeutic temperature. Peel away paper to reveal adhesive side. Place on pain area with adhesive against the skin. Attach firmly. Be careful when applying to the wrist – do not overlap the heat cells. For maximum effectiveness, we recommend you wear ThermaCare® for 8 hours. Do not wear for more than 8 hours in any 24-hour period.

WARNING: **THIS PRODUCT CAN CAUSE BURNS. CHECK SKIN FREQUENTLY DURING USE. IF YOU FIND IRRITATION OR A BURN, REMOVE PRODUCT IMMEDIATELY.**

55 OR OLDER: YOUR RISK OF BURNING INCREASES AS YOU AGE. IF YOU ARE 55 YEARS OF AGE OR OLDER DO NOT USE DURING SLEEP.

ASK A DOCTOR BEFORE USE if you have

- DIABETES
- poor circulation or heart disease
- rheumatoid arthritis,
- or are pregnant

ADDITIONAL WARNINGS: Each heat disc contains iron (~2 grams), which can be harmful if ingested. If ingested, rinse mouth with water and call a Poison Control Center immediately. If heat disc contents come in contact with your skin or eyes, rinse right away with water. Never heat product in a microwave or attempt to reheat as wrap could catch fire. Keep out of reach of children and pets.

WHEN USING THIS PRODUCT check skin frequently for signs of burns or blisters – if found stop use

- if product feels too hot – stop use or wear over clothing
- do not place extra pressure over the product
- do not use for more than 8 hours in a 24-hour period

DO NOT USE with pain rubs, medicated lotions, creams or ointments

- on unhealthy, damaged or broken skin
- on areas of bruising or swelling that have occurred within 48 hours
- on people unable to follow all use instructions
- on areas of the body where you can't feel heat
- with other forms of heat
- on people unable to remove the product, including children, infants, and some elderly

STOP USE AND ASK A DOCTOR if you experience any discomfort, burning, swelling, rash or other changes in your skin that persist where the wrap is worn

- if after 7 days your pain gets worse or remains unchanged as this may be a sign of a more serious condition.

Knee/Elbow

PLEASE READ ALL INSTRUCTIONS AND WARNINGS BEFORE USE. ADDITIONAL WARNINGS ARE INCLUDED IN THE PACKAGE INSERT. TO REDUCE THE RISK OF BURNS, FIRE, AND PERSONAL INJURY, THIS PRODUCT MUST BE USED IN ACCORDANCE WITH THE USE INSTRUCTIONS AND WARNINGS.

Uses: Provides temporary relief of minor muscular and joint aches and pains associated with overexertion, strains, sprains, and arthritis.

Directions: Tear open pouch when ready to use. It may take up to 30 minutes for ThermaCare® to reach its therapeutic temperature. Peel away paper to reveal adhesive tabs. Using adhesive is optional if you have sensitive skin or have body hair around the knee or elbow area.

Knee: Do not place heat cells on the back of the knee. Bend knee slightly and place opening over kneecap. Secure tabs to skin (optional). Wrap straps around knee and fasten. Over-tightening may cause discomfort. Adjust as needed.

Elbow: Do not place heat cells on the inside of the bend of the arm. Bend elbow slightly and place opening over elbow. Secure tabs to skin (optional). Wrap straps around elbow and fasten. Over-tightening may cause discomfort. Adjust as needed. For maximum effectiveness, we recommend you wear ThermaCare® for 8 hours.

Do not wear for more than 8 hours in any 24-hour period.

WARNING: **THIS PRODUCT CAN CAUSE BURNS. CHECK SKIN FREQUENTLY DURING USE. IF YOU FIND IRRITATION OR A BURN, REMOVE PRODUCT IMMEDIATELY.**

55 OR OLDER: YOUR RISK OF BURNING INCREASES AS YOU AGE. IF YOU ARE 55 YEARS OF AGE OR OLDER, WEAR THERMACARE® OVER A TOWEL OR CLOTH SUCH AS A WASHCLOTH, NOT DIRECTLY AGAINST YOUR SKIN, AND DO NOT WEAR WHILE SLEEPING.

ASK A DOCTOR BEFORE USE if you have

- DIABETES
- poor circulation or heart disease
- rheumatoid arthritis
- or are pregnant

ADDITIONAL WARNINGS: Each heat disc contains iron (~2 grams), which can be harmful if ingested. If ingested, rinse mouth with water and call a Poison Control Center immediately. If heat disc contents come in contact with your skin or eyes, rinse right away with water. Never heat product in a microwave or attempt to reheat as wrap could catch fire. Keep out of reach of children and pets.

WHEN USING THIS PRODUCT check skin frequently for signs of burns or blisters – if found stop use

- if product feels too hot – stop use or wear over clothing
- do not place extra pressure or tight clothing over the product
- do not use for more than 8 hours in a 24-hour period

DO NOT USE with pain rubs, medicated lotions, creams or ointments

- on unhealthy, damaged or broken skin
- on areas of bruising or swelling that have occurred within 48 hours
- on people unable to follow all use instructions
- on areas of the body where you can't feel heat
- with other forms of heat
- on people unable to remove the product, including children, infants, and some elderly

STOP USE AND ASK A DOCTOR if you experience any discomfort, burning, swelling, rash or other changes in your skin that persist where the wrap is worn

- if after 7 days your pain gets worse or remains unchanged as this may be a sign of a more serious condition.

QUESTIONS

1-800-323-3383 or visit www.thermacare.com ThermaCare®/Universal SKUs/Current Business March 28, 2006 New Universal SKU Format/Updated Safety/Caution Warnings

How Supplied:

Available in boxes of 3 or in single use pouches.

Shown in Product Identification Guide, page 516

TRIAMINIC® COUGH & SORE THROAT

(Novartis Consumer Health, Inc.)
Pain Reliever/Fever Reducer/Cough Suppressant

For full product information see page 747.

CHILDREN'S TYLENOL® Plus Cold & Allergy (McNeil Consumer)

For full product information see page 716.

CHILDREN'S TYLENOL® Plus Flu (McNeil Consumer)

For full product information see page 749.

CONCENTRATED TYLENOL®
acetaminophen Infants' Drops
(McNeil Consumer)

CHILDREN'S TYLENOL®
acetaminophen Suspension Liquid and Meltaways

JR. TYLENOL®
acetaminophen Meltaways

CHILDREN'S TYLENOL®
Suspension with Flavor Creator

Product information for all dosages of Children's TYLENOL have been combined under this heading

For full product information see page 754.

EXTRA STRENGTH TYLENOL® PM
Pain Reliever/Sleep Aid Caplets, Vanilla Caplets, Geltabs, Gelcaps, and Liquid (McNeil Consumer)

Description:
Each *Extra Strength TYLENOL® PM Caplet, Vanilla Caplet, Geltab or Gelcap* contains acetaminophen 500 mg and diphenhydramine HCl 25 mg. Each 30 mL = 2 Tablespoonfuls of TYLENOL® PM Liquid contains acetaminophen 1000 mg and diphenhydramine HCl 50 mg.

Actions:
Extra Strength TYLENOL® PM Caplets, Vanilla Caplets, Geltabs, Gelcaps, and *Liquid* contain a clinically proven analgesic-antipyretic and an antihistamine. Maximum allowable nonprescription levels of acetaminophen and diphenhydramine provide temporary relief of occasional headaches and minor aches and pains with accompanying sleeplessness. Acetaminophen is equal to aspirin in analgesic and antipyretic effectiveness and it is unlikely to produce many of the side effects associated with aspirin-containing products. Acetamino-

phen produces analgesia by elevation of the pain threshold. Diphenhydramine HCl is an antihistamine with sedative properties.

Uses:
temporary relief of occasional headaches and minor aches and pains with accompanying sleeplessness

Directions:
• do not take more than directed (see overdose warning)
• use only enclosed measuring cup designed for use with this product. Do not use any other dosing device. (Liquid only).

Extra Strength TYLENOL® PM Caplets, Vanilla Caplets, Geltabs and Gelcaps:

adults and children 12 years and over	• take 2 caplets, geltabs or gelcaps at bedtime • do not take more than 8 caplets, geltabs or gelcaps in 24 hours
children under 12 years	• do not use this adult product in children under 12 years of age; this will provide more than the recommended dose (overdose) and may cause liver damage

Extra Strength TYLENOL® PM Liquid

adults and children 12 years and over	• take 2 tablespoons (tbsp.) or 1 oz in dosing cup provided at bedtime • do not take more than 8 tablespoons in 24 hours
children under 12 years	• do not use this adult product in children under 12 years of age; this will provide more than the recommended dose (overdose) and may cause liver damage

Warnings:
Alcohol Warning: If you consume 3 or more alcoholic drinks every day, ask your doctor whether you should take acetaminophen or other pain relievers or fever reducers. Acetaminophen may cause liver damage.
Do not use
• with any other product containing acetaminophen
• with any other product containing diphenhydramine, even one used on skin
• in children under 12 years of age
Ask a doctor before use if you have
• a breathing problem such as emphysema or chronic bronchitis
• trouble urinating due to an enlarged prostate gland

• glaucoma
Ask a doctor or pharmacist before use if you are taking sedatives or tranquilizers
When using this product
• drowsiness will occur
• avoid alcoholic drinks
• do not drive a motor vehicle or operate machinery
Stop use and ask a doctor if
• sleeplessness persists continuously for more than 2 weeks. Insomnia may be a symptom of serious underlying medical illness.
• pain gets worse or lasts for more than 10 days
• fever gets worse or lasts for more than 3 days
• new symptoms occur
• redness or swelling is present
These could be signs of a serious condition.
If pregnant or breast-feeding, ask a health professional before use.
Keep out of reach of children.

Overdose warning: Taking more than the recommended dose (overdose) may cause liver damage. In case of overdose, get medical help or contact a Poison Control Center right away (1-800-222-1222). Quick medical attention is critical for adults as well as for children even if you do not notice any signs or symptoms.

Other Information:
• each tablespoon contains: **sodium 11 mg** (applies to TYLENOL® PM Liquid)
• store between 20–25°C (68–77°F).
• Avoid high humidity. (Applies only to Tylenol® PM Geltabs/Gelcaps)

PROFESSIONAL INFORMATION:
OVERDOSAGE INFORMATION

For overdosage information, please refer to pgs. 696–697.

Inactive Ingredients:
Caplets: carnauba wax, cellulose, corn starch, FD&C Blue #1, FD&C Blue #2, hypromellose, magnesium stearate, polyethylene glycol, polysorbate 80, sodium citrate, sodium starch glycolate, titanium dioxide.
Vanilla Caplets: carnauba wax, cellulose, corn starch, FD&C blue #1, FD&C blue #2, flavor, hypromellose, magnesium stearate, polyethylene glycol, polysorbate 80, sodium citrate, sodium starch glycolate, sucralose, titanium dioxide, yellow iron oxide.
Geltabs/Gelcaps: benzyl alcohol, butylparaben, castor oil, cellulose, corn starch, D&C Red #28, edetate calcium disodium, FD&C Blue #1, gelatin, hypromellose, iron oxide, magnesium stearate, methylparaben, propylparaben, sodium citrate, sodium lauryl sulfate, sodium propionate, sodium starch glycolate, titanium dioxide.
Liquid: caramel color, carboxymethylcellulose sodium, citric acid, FD&C red #40, flavors, polyethylene glycol, propylene glycol, purified water, sodium benzoate, sorbitol, sucralose, sucrose.

How Supplied:

Caplets (colored light blue imprinted "Tylenol PM") tamper evident bottles of 24, 50, 100, and 150 and 225.

Vanilla Caplets (colored off white and blue imprinted "TYLENOL PM") tamper evident bottles of 6, 24, 100 and 225.

Gelcaps (colored blue and white imprinted "TYLENOL PM") tamper-evident bottles of 24 and 50.

Geltabs (colored blue and white imprinted "TYLENOL PM") tamper-evident bottles of 24, 50, 100 and 150.

Liquid (brown colored vanilla liquid) Bottles of 1 oz and 8 fl. oz.

Shown in Product Identification Guide, page 512

REGULAR STRENGTH TYLENOL®
acetaminophen Tablets
(McNeil Consumer)

EXTRA STRENGTH TYLENOL®
acetaminophen Geltabs, Caplets, Cool Caplets, and EZ Tabs

EXTRA STRENGTH TYLENOL®
acetaminophen Rapid Release Gels

EXTRA STRENGTH TYLENOL®
acetaminophen Adult Liquid Pain Reliever

TYLENOL® Arthritis Pain
Acetaminophen Extended Release Geltabs/Caplets

TYLENOL® 8 Hour Acetaminophen
Extended Release Caplets

Product information for all dosage forms of Adult TYLENOL acetaminophen have been combined under this heading.

Description:

Each Regular Strength TYLENOL® Tablet contains acetaminophen 325 mg. *Each Extra Strength TYLENOL® Geltab, Caplet, Cool Caplet, EZ Tab or Rapid Release Gel* contains acetaminophen 500 mg. *Extra Strength TYLENOL® Adult Liquid* is alcohol-free and each 15 mL (1 tablespoonful) contains 500 mg acetaminophen. *Each TYLENOL® Arthritis Pain Extended Relief Geltab/Caplet* and each *TYLENOL® 8 Hour Extended Release Caplet* contains acetaminophen 650 mg.

Actions:

Acetaminophen is a clinically proven analgesic/antipyretic. Acetaminophen produces analgesia by elevation of the pain threshold and antipyresis through action on the hypothalamic heat-regulating center. Acetaminophen is equal to aspirin in analgesic and antipyretic effectiveness and it is unlikely to produce many of the side effects associated with aspirin and aspirin-containing products. *Tylenol Arthritis*

Pain Extended Release and *TYLENOL 8 Hour Extended Release* use a unique, patented, bilayer geltab/caplet. The first layer dissolves quickly to provide prompt relief while the second layer is time released to provide up to 8 hours of relief.

Uses:

Regular Strength TYLENOL® Tablets: temporarily relieves minor aches and pains due to:
• headache • muscular aches • backache
• arthritis • the common cold
• toothache • premenstrual and menstrual cramps
• temporarily reduces fever

Extra Strength TYLENOL® Geltabs, Caplets, EZ Tabs, or Rapid Release Gels:
• temporarily relieves minor aches and pains due to:
  • headache • muscular aches
  • backache • minor pain of arthritis
  • the common cold • toothache
  • premenstrual and menstrual cramps
• temporarily reduces fever

Extra Strength TYLENOL® Cool Caplets:
• temporarily relieves minor aches and pains due to:
  • the common cold • headache
  • backache • toothache • muscular aches • premenstrual and menstrual cramps • minor pain of arthritis
• temporarily reduces fever

Extra Strength TYLENOL® Adult Liquid:
• temporarily relieves minor aches and pains due to:
  • headache • muscular aches
  • backache • minor pain of arthritis
  • the common cold • toothache
  • premenstrual and menstrual cramps
• temporarily reduces fever

TYLENOL® Arthritis Pain Extended Release Caplets: temporarily relieves minor aches and pains due to:
• arthritis • the common cold • headache
• toothache • muscular aches • backache
• menstrual cramps

TYLENOL® Arthritis Pain Extended Geltabs: temporarily relieves minor aches and pains due to:
• minor pain of arthritis • muscular aches
• backache • premenstrual and menstrual cramps • the common cold
• headache • toothache

TYLENOL® 8 Hour Extended Release Caplets:
• temporarily relieves minor aches and pains due to:
  • muscular aches • backache
  • headache • toothache
  • the common cold • menstrual cramps
  • minor pain of arthritis
• temporarily reduces fever

Directions:

Regular Strength TYLENOL® Tablets:
• **do not take more than directed (see overdose warning)**

adults and children 12 years and over	• take 2 tablets every 4 to 6 hours as needed • do not take more than 12 tablets in 24 hours
children 6–11 years	• take 1 tablet every 4 to 6 hours as needed • do not take more than 5 tablets in 24 hours
children under 6 years	do not use this adult Regular Strength product in children under 6 years of age; this will provide more than the recommended dose (overdose) of TYLENOL® and may cause liver damage

Extra Strength TYLENOL® Geltabs, Caplets, or Rapid Release Gels:
• **do not take more than directed (see overdose warning)**

adults and children 12 years and over	• take 2 gelcaps, geltabs or caplets every 4 to 6 hours while symptoms last • do not take more than 8 gelcaps, geltabs or caplets in 24 hours • do not use for more than 10 days unless directed by a doctor
children under 12 years	do not use this adult product in children under 12 years of age; this will provide more than the recommended dose (overdose) and may cause liver damage

Extra Strength TYLENOL® Adult Liquid:
• **do not take more than directed (see overdose warning)**
• use only enclosed measuring cup designed for use with this product. Do not use any other dosing device.

adults and children 12 years and over	• take 2 tablespoons (tbsp.) or 1 oz in dose cup provided every 4 to 6 hours while symptoms last • do not take more than 8 tablespoons (tbsp) or 4 oz in 24 hours • do not take for more than 10 days unless directed by a doctor
children under 12 years	do not use this adult product in children under 12 years of age; this will provide more than the recommended dose (overdose) and may cause liver damage

Extra Strength TYLENOL® EZ Tabs:
• **do not take more than directed (see overdose warning)**

Continued on next page

Tylenol Reg. Strength—Cont.

adults and children 12 years and over	• take 2 tablets every 4 to 6 hours while symptoms last • do not take more than 8 tablets in 24 hours • do not use for more than 10 days unless directed by a doctor
children under 12 years	do not use this adult product in children under 12 years of age; this will provide more than the recommended dose (overdose) and may cause liver damage

Extra Strength TYLENOL® Cool Caplets:
• **do not take more than directed (see overdose warning)**

adults and children 12 years and over	• take 2 caplets every 4 to 6 hours while symptoms last • swallow whole - do not crush, chew, or dissolve • do not take more than 8 caplets in 24 hours • do not take for more than 10 days unless directed by a doctor
children under 12 years	do not use this adult product in children under 12 years of age; this will provide more than the recommended dose (overdose) and may cause liver damage

TYLENOL® 8 Hour Extended Release Caplets
• **do not take more than directed (see overdose warning)**

adults and children 12 years and over	• take 2 caplets every 8 hours with water • swallow whole – do not crush, chew or dissolve • do not take more than 6 caplets in 24 hours • do not use for more than 10 days unless directed by a doctor
children under 12 years	• do not use

TYLENOL® Arthritis Pain Extended Release Geltabs/Caplets
• **do not take more than directed (see overdose warning)**

adults	• take 2 geltabs or caplets every 8 hours with water

	• swallow whole – do not crush, chew or dissolve • do not take more than 6 geltabs or caplets in 24 hours • do not use for more than 10 days unless directed by a doctor
under 18 years of age	• ask a doctor

Warnings:

Regular Strength TYLENOL® Tablets, Extra Strength TYLENOL® Geltabs, Caplets, Cool Caplets, Rapid Release Gels, and Extra Strength TYLENOL® Liquid

Alcohol warning: If you consume 3 or more alcoholic drinks every day, ask your doctor whether you should take acetaminophen or other pain relievers or fever reducers. Acetaminophen may cause liver damage.

Do not use:
• with any other product containing acetaminophen

Stop use and ask a doctor if:
• pain gets worse or lasts for more than 10 days
• fever gets worse or lasts for more than 3 days
• new symptoms occur
• redness or swelling is present
These could be signs of a serious condition.
If pregnant or breast-feeding, ask a health professional before use.
Keep out of reach of children.

Overdose warning: Taking more than the recommended dose (overdose) may cause liver damage. In case of overdose, get medical help or contact a Poison Control Center (1-800-222-1222) right away. Quick medical attention is critical for adults as well as for children even if you do not notice any signs or symptoms.

TYLENOL® Arthritis Pain Extended Release Geltabs/Caplets and Extra Strength TYLENOL® EZ Tabs:

Alcohol warning: If you consume 3 or more alcoholic drinks every day, ask your doctor whether you should take acetaminophen or other pain relievers or fever reducers. Acetaminophen may cause liver damage.

Do not use
• with any other product containing acetaminophen

Stop use and ask a doctor if
• pain gets worse or lasts for more than 10 days
• fever gets worse or lasts for more than 3 days
• new symptoms occur
• redness or swelling is present
These could be signs of a serious condition.
If pregnant or breast-feeding, ask a health professional before use.

Keep out of reach of children.

Overdose warning: Taking more than the recommended dose (overdose) may cause liver damage. In case of overdose, get medical help or contact a Poison Control Center right away (1-800-222-1222). Quick medical attention is critical for adults as well as for children even if you do not notice any signs or symptoms.

TYLENOL® 8 Hour Extended Release Caplets:

Alcohol warning: If you consume 3 or more alcoholic drinks every day, ask your doctor whether you should take acetaminophen or other pain relievers or fever reducers. Acetaminophen may cause liver damage.

Do not use
• with any other product containing acetaminophen

Stop use and ask a doctor if
• pain gets worse or lasts for more than 10 days
• fever gets worse or lasts for more than 3 days
• new symptoms occur
• redness or swelling is present
These could be signs of a serious condition.
If pregnant or breast-feeding, ask a health professional before use.
Keep out of reach of children.

Overdose warning: Taking more than the recommended dose (overdose) may cause liver damage. In case of overdose, get medical help or contact a Poison Control Center right away (1-800-2222-1222). Quick medical attention is critical for adults as well as for children even if you do not notice any signs or symptoms.

Other Information:
Regular Strength TYLENOL® Tablets
• store between 20–25°C (68–77°F)
Extra Strength TYLENOL® Gelcaps, Geltabs, Caplets, Cool Caplets, EZ Tabs, or Rapid Release Gels:
• store between 20–25°C (68–77°F) (*Caplet, Cool Caplets and EZ Tabs*)
• store between 20–25°C (68–77°F). Avoid high humidity. (*Geltab and Rapid Release Gel*)
Extra Strength TYLENOL® Adult Liquid
• each tablespoon contains: **sodium 9 mg**
• store between 20–25°C (68–77°F)

TYLENOL® Arthritis Pain Extended Release Geltabs/Caplets and *TYLENOL® 8 Hour Extended Release Caplets*
• store at 20–25°C (68–77°F)
• avoid excessive heat 40°C (104°F)

PROFESSIONAL INFORMATION: OVERDOSAGE INFORMATION FOR ALL ADULT TYLENOL PRODUCTS

Acetaminophen: Acetaminophen in massive overdosage may cause hepatic toxicity in some patients. In adults and adolescents ($\geq$ 12 years of age), hepatic toxicity may occur following ingestion of greater than 7.5 to 10 grams over a period of 8 hours or less. Fatalities are infre-

quent (less than 3–4% of untreated cases) and have rarely been reported with overdoses of less than 15 grams. In children (<12 years of age), an acute overdosage of less than 150 mg/kg has not been associated with hepatic toxicity. Early symptoms following a potentially hepatotoxic overdose may include: nausea, vomiting, diaphoresis and general malaise. Clinical and laboratory evidence of hepatic toxicity may not be apparent until 48 to 72 hours postingestion. In adults and adolescents, any individual presenting with an unknown amount of acetaminophen ingested or with a questionable or unreliable history about the time of ingestion should have a plasma acetaminophen level drawn and be treated with N-acetylcysteine. For full prescribing information, refer to the N-acetylcysteine package insert. Do not await results of assays for plasma acetaminophen levels before initiating treatment with N-acetylcysteine. The following additional procedures are recommended: Promptly initiate gastric decontamination of the stomach. A plasma acetaminophen assay should be obtained as early as possible, but no sooner than four hours following ingestion. If an acetaminophen *extended release* product is involved, it may be appropriate to obtain an additional plasma acetaminophen level 4–6 hours following the initial acetaminophen level. If either acetaminophen level plots above the treatment line on the acetaminophen overdose nomogram, N-acetylcysteine treatment should be continued for a full course of therapy. Liver function studies should be obtained initially and repeated at 24-hour intervals. Serious toxicity or fatalities have been extremely infrequent following an acute acetaminophen overdose in young children, possibly because of differences in the way they metabolize acetaminophen. In children, the maximum potential amount ingested can be more easily estimated. If more than 150 mg/kg or an unknown amount was ingested, obtain a plasma acetaminophen level as soon as possible, but no sooner than 4 hours following ingestion. If an acetaminophen *extended release* product is involved, it may be appropriate to obtain an additional plasma acetaminophen level 4–6 hours following the initial acetaminophen level. If either acetaminophen level plots above the treatment line on the acetaminophen overdose nomogram, N-acetylcysteine treatment should be initiated and continued for a full course of therapy. If an assay cannot be obtained and the estimated acetaminophen ingestion exceeds 150 mg/kg, dosing with N-acetylcysteine should be initiated and continued for a full course of therapy. For additional emergency information, call your regional poison center or call the Rocky Mountain Poison Center toll-free, (1-800-525-6115).

Our adult Tylenol® combination products contain active ingredients in addition to acetaminophen. The following is basic overdose information regarding those ingredients.

Chlorpheniramine: Chlorpheniramine toxicity should be treated as you would an antihistamine/anticholinergic overdose and is likely to be present within a few hours after acute ingestion.

Dextromethorphan: Acute dextromethorphan overdose usually does not result in serious signs and symptoms unless massive amounts have been ingested. Signs and symptoms of a substantial overdose may include nausea and vomiting, visual disturbances, CNS disturbances and urinary retention.

Diphenhydramine: Diphenhydramine toxicity should be treated as you would an antihistamine/anticholinergic overdose and is likely to be present within a few hours after acute ingestion.

Doxylamine: Doxylamine toxicity should be treated as you would an antihistamine/anticholinergic overdose and is likely to be present within a few hours after acute ingestion.

Guaifenesin: Guaifenesin should be treated as a nontoxic ingestion.

Pamabrom: Acute overexposure of diuretics is primarily associated with fluid and electrolyte loss. Fluid loss should be treated with the appropriate intravenous and/or oral fluids.

Phenylephrine: Symptoms from phenylephrine overdose most often consist of hypertension, anxiety, nervousness, restlessness, tachycardia, bradycardia, headache, dizziness, and/or palpitations. Symptoms usually are transient and typically require no treatment.

Pseudoephedrine: Symptoms from pseudoephedrine overdose consist most often of mild anxiety, tachycardia and/or mild hypertension. Symptoms usually appear within 4 to 8 hours of ingestion and are transient, usually requiring no treatment. **For additional emergency information, please contact your local poison control center.**

Alcohol Information: Chronic heavy alcohol abusers may be at increased risk of liver toxicity from excessive acetaminophen use, although reports of this event are rare. Reports usually involve cases of severe chronic alcoholics and the dosages of acetaminophen most often exceed recommended doses and often involve substantial overdose. Healthcare professionals should alert their patients who regularly consume large amounts of alcohol not to exceed recommended doses of acetaminophen.

Inactive Ingredients:
Regular Strength TYLENOL® Tablets: cellulose, corn starch, magnesium stearate, sodium starch glycolate.
Extra Strength TYLENOL® Caplets: carnauba wax*, castor oil*, cellulose, corn starch, FD&C red #40, hypromellose, magnesium stearate, polyethylene glycol*, sodium starch glycolate, titanium dioxide. *contains one or more of these ingredients. **Cool Caplets:** castor oil, cellulose, corn starch, FD&C red #40, flavors, hypromellose, magnesium stearate, sodium starch glycolate, sucralose, titanium dioxide. **EZ Tabs:** carnauba wax, cellulose, corn starch, D&C yellow #10, FD&C red #40, FD&C yellow #6, iron oxide, magnesium stearate, polyethylene glycol, polyvinyl alcohol, sodium starch glycolate, sucralose, talc, titanium dioxide. **Geltabs:** benzyl alcohol, butylparaben, castor oil, cellulose, corn starch, D&C Yellow #10, edetate calcium disodium, FD&C Blue #1, FD&C Blue #2, FD&C Red #40, gelatin, hypromellose, magnesium stearate, methylparaben, propylparaben, sodium lauryl sulfate, sodium propionate, sodium starch glycolate, titanium dioxide. **Rapid Release Gels:** benzyl alcohol, black iron oxide, butylparaben, cellulose, corn starch, D&C yellow #10, edetate calcium disodium, FD&C blue #2, FD&C red #40, gelatin, hypromellose, magnesium stearate, methylparaben, polyethylene glycol, polysorbate 80, propylparaben, red iron oxide, sodium lauryl sulfate, sodium propionate, sodium starch glycolate, titanium dioxide, yellow iron oxide.
Extra Strength TYLENOL® Adult Liquid: citric acid, corn syrup, D&C Red #33, FD&C Red #40, flavor, polyethylene glycol, propylene glycol, purified water, saccharin sodium, sodium benzoate, sorbitol
TYLENOL® Arthritis Pain Extended Release **Caplets:** carnauba wax, corn starch, hydroxyethyl cellulose, hypromellose, magnesium stearate, microcrystalline cellulose, povidone, powdered cellulose, pregelatinized starch, sodium starch glycolate, titanium dioxide, triacetin. **Geltabs:** benzyl alcohol, butylparaben, castor oil, cellulose, corn starch, edetate calcium disodium, FD&C Blue #1, FD&C Blue #2, gelatin, hydroxyethyl cellulose, hypromellose, magnesium stearate, methylparaben, povidone, propylparaben, sodium lauryl sulfate, sodium propionate, sodium starch glycolate, titanium dioxide.
Tylenol 8 Hour Extended Release **Caplets:** corn starch, D&C yellow #10, FD&C red #40, FD&C yellow #6, hydroxyethyl cellulose, magnesium stearate, microcrystalline cellulose, polyethylene glycol, polyvinyl alcohol, povidone, powdered cellulose, pregelantinized starch, sodium starch glycolate, sucralose, talc, titanium dioxide.

How Supplied:
Regular Strength TYLENOL® Tablets: (colored white, scored, imprinted "TYLENOL" and "325")—tamper-evident bottles of 100.
Extra Strength TYLENOL® Caplets: (colored white, imprinted "TYLENOL 500 mg")—vials of 10, and tamper-evident bottles of 24, 50, 100, 150, 225, and 325. *Cool Caplets* 8, 24, 50, 100, 150.

Continued on next page

Tylenol Reg. Strength—Cont.

Geltabs (colored yellow and red, imprinted "Tylenol 500") tamper-evident bottles of 50 and 100. *Rapid Release Gels* (colored red and light blue with an exposed grey band; gelcaps are imprinted with "TY 500") tamper-evident bottles of 8, 24, 50, 100, 150, 225, and 290. *EZ Tabs* (colored red, imprinted "TYLENOL EZ Tabs") tamper-evident bottles of 24, 50, 100, 150, and 225.
Extra Strength TYLENOL® Adult Liquid: Cherry-flavored liquid (colored red) 8 fl. oz. tamper-evident bottle with child resistant safety cap and special dosage cup.
TYLENOL® Arthritis Pain Extended Release Caplets: (colored white, engraved "TYLENOL ER") tamper-evident bottles of 24, 50, 100, 150, 225 and 290
Geltabs: available in bottles of 20, 40 and 80
TYLENOL® 8 Hour Extended Release Caplets: (colored red, imprinted "8 hour") available in 24's, 50's, 100's, and 150's.

Shown in Product Identification Guide, page 510 & 511

TYLENOL® Severe Allergy Caplets (McNeil Consumer)

TYLENOL® Allergy Multi-Symptom Caplets with Cool Burst™ and Gelcaps

TYLENOL® Allergy Multi-Symptom Nighttime Caplets with Cool Burst™

For full product information see page 717.

TYLENOL® Chest Congestion Caplets with Cool Burst™ (McNeil Consumer)

TYLENOL® Chest Congestion Liquid with Cool Burst™

For full product information see page 722.

TYLENOL® Cold Head Congestion Daytime Caplets with Cool Burst™ and Gelcaps (McNeil Consumer)

TYLENOL® Cold Head Congestion Nighttime Caplets with Cool Burst™

TYLENOL® Cold Head Congestion Severe Caplets with Cool Burst™

For full product information see page 750.

TYLENOL® COLD Severe Congestion Non-Drowsy Caplets with Cool Burst™ (McNeil Consumer)

For full product information see page 751.

TYLENOL® Cold Multi-Symptom Daytime Caplets with Cool Burst™ and Gelcaps (McNeil Consumer)

TYLENOL® Cold Multi-Symptom Nighttime Caplets with Cool Burst™

TYLENOL® Cold Multi-Symptom Severe Caplets with Cool Burst™

TYLENOL® Cold Multi-Symptom Daytime Liquid

TYLENOL® Cold Multi-Symptom Nighttime Liquid with Cool Burst™

TYLENOL® Cold Multi-Symptom Severe Daytime Liquid

For full product information see page 752.

TYLENOL® Sinus Congestion & Pain Daytime Caplets with Cool Burst™ and Gelcaps (McNeil Consumer)

TYLENOL® Sinus Congestion & Pain Nighttime Caplets with Cool Burst™

TYLENOL® Sinus Congestion & Pain Severe Caplets with Cool Burst™

TYLENOL® Sinus Severe Congestion Caplets with Cool Burst™
Product information for all dosage forms of TYLENOL Sinus have been combined under this heading.
For full product information see page 778.

TYLENOL® Sore Throat Daytime Liquid with Cool Burst™ (McNeil Consumer)

TYLENOL® Sore Throat Nighttime Liquid with Cool Burst™

TYLENOL® Cough & Sore Throat Daytime Liquid with Cool Burst™

TYLENOL® Cough & Sore Throat Nighttime Liquid with Cool Burst™

For full product information see page 790.

CONCENTRATED TYLENOL® Infants' Drops Plus Cold Nasal Decongestant, Fever Reducer & Pain Reliever (McNeil Consumer)

CONCENTRATED TYLENOL® Infants' Drops Plus Cold & Cough Nasal Decongestant, Fever Reducer & Pain Reliever, Cough Suppressant

CHILDREN'S TYLENOL® Plus Cough & Sore Throat Suspension Liquid

CHILDREN'S TYLENOL® Plus Cough & Runny Nose Suspension Liquid

CHILDREN'S TYLENOL® Plus Multi-Symptom Cold Suspension Liquid

CHILDREN'S TYLENOL® Plus Cold Suspension Liquid

For full product information see page 754.

VICKS® DAYQUIL® LIQUID (Procter & Gamble)

VICKS® DAYQUIL® LIQUICAPS® Multi-Symptom Cold/Flu Relief Nasal Decongestant/Pain Reliever/ Cough Suppressant/Fever Reducer Non-drowsy

For full product information see page 761.

VICKS® NYQUIL® LIQUICAPS®/ LIQUID MULTI-SYMPTOM COLD/ FLU RELIEF (Proctor & Gamble)

For full product information see page 763.

VICKS® VAPORUB® (Procter & Gamble)

VICKS® VAPORUB® CREAM (greaseless)
[*vā 'pō-rub*]
Cough Suppressant/Topical Analgesic
For full product information see page 765.

ZICAM® Flu Daytime (Matrixx)

ZICAM® Nighttime

For full product information see page 768.

Musculoskeletal System:
Arthritis

ADVIL® (Wyeth Consumer)
Ibuprofen Tablets, USP
Ibuprofen Caplets (Oval-Shaped Tablets)
Ibuprofen Gel Caplets (Oval-Shaped Gelatin Coated Tablets)
Ibuprofen Liqui-Gel Capsules
Pain reliever/Fever Reducer (NSAID)

For full product information see page 674.

ALEVE CAPLETS (Bayer Healthcare)
(NSAID Labeling)
[a-lēv]

For full product information see page 675.

ALEVE GELCAPS
(Bayer Healthcare)
(NSAID Labeling)
[a-lēv]

For full product information see page 675.

ALEVE TABLETS (Bayer Healthcare)
(NSAID Labeling)
[a-lēv]

For full product information see page 676.

BAYER® ASPIRIN
(Bayer Healthcare)
Comprehensive Prescribing Information

For full product information see page 796.

BC® POWDER
(GlaxoSmithKline Consumer)
ARTHRITIS STRENGTH BC® POWDER
BC® COLD POWDER LINE

For full product information see page 677.

BIOFREEZE® PAIN RELIEVING PRODUCTS (Performance Health)

For full product information see page 678.

BUFFERIN®
(Novartis Consumer Health, Inc.)
Regular/Extra Strength
Pain Reliever/Fever Reducer

For full product information see page 678.

EXCEDRIN® EXTRA STRENGTH
(Novartis Consumer Health, Inc.)
PAIN RELIEVER

For full product information see page 684.

GOODY'S®
(GlaxoSmithKline Consumer)
Extra Strength Pain Relief Tablets

For full product information see page 685.

MINERAL ICE®
(Novartis Consumer Health, Inc.)
Pain Reliever

For full product information see page 685.

MOTRIN® IB (Ibuprofen)
Pain Reliever/Fever Reducer
Tablets and Caplets
(McNeil Consumer)

For full product information see page 687.

THERA-GESIC® Maximum Strength Analgesic Pain Relieving Creme (Mission Pharmacal)
pain relieving crème

For full product information see page 691.

THERMA-CARE HEAT ACTIVATED WRAPS (Procter & Gamble)
Therapeutic heat wraps

For full product information see page 692.

REGULAR STRENGTH TYLENOL®
acetaminophen Tablets
(McNeil Consumer)

EXTRA STRENGTH TYLENOL®
acetaminophen Geltabs, Caplets, Cool Caplets, and EZ Tabs

EXTRA STRENGTH TYLENOL®
acetaminophen Rapid Release Gels

EXTRA STRENGTH TYLENOL®
acetaminophen Adult Liquid Pain Reliever

TYLENOL® Arthritis Pain Acetaminophen Extended Release Geltabs/Caplets

TYLENOL® 8 Hour Acetaminophen Extended Release Caplets

Product information for all dosage forms of Adult TYLENOL acetaminophen have been combined under this heading.

For full product information see page 695.

Musculoskeletal System:
Backache

ADVIL® (Wyeth Consumer)
Ibuprofen Tablets, USP
Ibuprofen Caplets (Oval-Shaped Tablets)
Ibuprofen Gel Caplets (Oval-Shaped Gelatin Coated Tablets)
Ibuprofen Liqui-Gel Capsules
Pain reliever/Fever Reducer (NSAID)

For full product information see page 674.

ALEVE CAPLETS (Bayer Healthcare)
(NSAID Labeling)
[a-lēv]

For full product information see page 675.

ALEVE GELCAPS
(Bayer Healthcare)
(NSAID Labeling)
[a-lēv]

For full product information see page 675.

ALEVE TABLETS (Bayer Healthcare)
(NSAID Labeling)
[a-lēv]

For full product information see page 676.

BIOFREEZE® PAIN RELIEVING PRODUCTS (Performance Health)

For full product information see page 678.

GOODY'S®
(GlaxoSmithKline Consumer)
Extra Strength Pain Relief Tablets

For full product information see page 685.

MINERAL ICE®
(Novartis Consumer Health, Inc.)
Pain Reliever

For full product information see page 685.

MOTRIN® IB (Ibuprofen)
Pain Reliever/Fever Reducer
Tablets and Caplets
(McNeil Consumer)

For full product information see page 687.

THERA-GESIC® Maximum Strength
Analgesic Pain Relieving Creme
(Mission Pharmacal)
pain relieving crème

For full product information see page 691.

THERMA-CARE HEAT ACTIVATED WRAPS (Procter & Gamble)
Therapeutic heat wraps

For full product information see page 692.

REGULAR STRENGTH TYLENOL®
acetaminophen Tablets
(McNeil Consumer)

EXTRA STRENGTH TYLENOL®
acetaminophen Geltabs, Caplets, Cool Caplets, and EZ Tabs

EXTRA STRENGTH TYLENOL®
acetaminophen Rapid Release Gels

EXTRA STRENGTH TYLENOL®
acetaminophen Adult Liquid Pain Reliever

TYLENOL® Arthritis Pain
Acetaminophen Extended Release Geltabs/Caplets

TYLENOL® 8 Hour Acetaminophen Extended Release Caplets

Product information for all dosage forms of Adult TYLENOL acetaminophen have been combined under this heading.

For full product information see page 695.

Musculoskeletal System:
Joint Aches

BIOFREEZE® PAIN RELIEVING PRODUCTS (Performance Health)

For full product information see page 678.

**MINERAL ICE®
(Novartis Consumer Health, Inc.)**
Pain Reliever

For full product information see page 685.

THERA-GESIC® Maximum Strength Analgesic Pain Relieving Creme (Mission Pharmacal)
pain relieving crème

For full product information see page 691.

THERMA-CARE HEAT ACTIVATED WRAPS (Procter & Gamble)
Therapeutic heat wraps

For full product information see page 692.

**VICKS® VAPORUB®
(Procter & Gamble)
VICKS® VAPORUB® CREAM
(greaseless)**
[vā 'pŏ-rub]
Cough
Suppressant/Topical Analgesic

For full product information see page 765.

Musculoskeletal System:
Muscular Aches

ADVIL® (Wyeth Consumer)
Ibuprofen Tablets, USP
Ibuprofen Caplets (Oval-Shaped Tablets)
Ibuprofen Gel Caplets (Oval-Shaped Gelatin Coated Tablets)
Ibuprofen Liqui-Gel Capsules
Pain reliever/Fever Reducer (NSAID)

For full product information see page 674.

ALEVE CAPLETS (Bayer Healthcare)
(NSAID Labeling)
[a-lēv]

For full product information see page 675.

ALEVE GELCAPS
(Bayer Healthcare)
(NSAID Labeling)
[a-lēv]

For full product information see page 675.

ALEVE TABLETS (Bayer Healthcare)
(NSAID Labeling)
[a-lēv]

For full product information see page 676.

BC® POWDER
(GlaxoSmithKline Consumer)
ARTHRITIS STRENGTH BC®
POWDER
BC® COLD POWDER LINE

For full product information see page 677.

BUFFERIN®
(Novartis Consumer Health, Inc.)
Regular/Extra Strength
Pain Reliever/Fever Reducer

For full product information see page 678.

EXCEDRIN® TENSION HEADACHE
(Novartis Consumer Health, Inc.)
PAIN RELIEVER

For full product information see page 611.

EXCEDRIN® EXTRA STRENGTH
(Novartis Consumer Health, Inc.)
PAIN RELIEVER

For full product information see page 684.

MINERAL ICE®
(Novartis Consumer Health, Inc.)
Pain Reliever

For full product information see page 685.

MOTRIN® IB (Ibuprofen)
Pain Reliever/Fever Reducer
Tablets and Caplets (McNeil Consumer)

For full product information see page 687.

THERA-GESIC® Maximum Strength
Analgesic Pain Relieving Creme
(Mission Pharmacal)
pain relieving crème

For full product information see page 691.

THERMA-CARE HEAT ACTIVATED
WRAPS (Procter & Gamble)
Therapeutic heat wraps

For full product information see page 692.

REGULAR STRENGTH TYLENOL®
acetaminophen Tablets (McNeil Consumer)

EXTRA STRENGTH TYLENOL®
acetaminophen Geltabs, Caplets, Cool Caplets, and EZ Tabs

EXTRA STRENGTH TYLENOL®
acetaminophen Rapid Release Gels

EXTRA STRENGTH TYLENOL®
acetaminophen Adult Liquid Pain Reliever

TYLENOL® Arthritis Pain
Acetaminophen Extended Release Geltabs/Caplets

TYLENOL® 8 Hour Acetaminophen
Extended Release Caplets

Product information for all dosage forms of Adult TYLENOL acetaminophen have been combined under this heading.

For full product information see page 695.

TYLENOL® Sore Throat Daytime
Liquid with Cool Burst™ (McNeil Consumer)

TYLENOL® Sore Throat Nighttime
Liquid with Cool Burst™

TYLENOL® Cough & Sore Throat
Daytime Liquid with Cool Burst™

TYLENOL® Cough & Sore Throat
Nighttime Liquid with Cool Burst™

For full product information see page 790.

VICKS® VAPORUB®
(Procter & Gamble)
VICKS® VAPORUB® CREAM
(greaseless)
[vă 'pō-rub]
Cough
Suppressant/Topical Analgesic

For full product information see page 765.

Musculoskeletal System:
Osteoporosis

CITRACAL® CAPLETS
ULTRADENSE® Calcium Citrate
with Vitamin D Dietary
Supplement
(Mission Pharmacal)

Description: Citracal® helps ensure women will have the strong bones necessary to take on a life filled with activity and ambitions. Calcium, together with a healthy diet and regular exercise, can help reduce the risk of osteoporosis. It is important to get adequate calcium; however, intakes above 2,000 mg per day are not likely to provide additional benefits. Make every moment count. Live with determination. Stand strong.

Serving Size: 2 caplets

	Amount Per Serving	%Daily Value
Vitamin D$_3$ (as cholecalciferol)	400 IU	100%
Calcium (as Ultradense® calcium citrate)	630 mg	63%

Ingredients: Calcium citrate, polyethylene glycol, croscarmellose sodium, polyvinyl alcohol-part hydrolyzed, color added, magnesium silicate, magnesium stearate, vitamin D$_3$.

Directions for Use: Take 1 to 2 caplets two times daily or as recommended by your physician, pharmacist, or health professional.

Other Information: STORE AT ROOM TEMPERATURE. KEEP OUT OF THE REACH OF CHILDREN. SAFETY SEALED PACKAGE FOR YOUR PROTECTION. Do not use if inner seal is broken.

How Supplied: 60 coated caplets, UPC 0178-0815-60; 120 coated caplets, UPC 0178-0815-12.

Musculoskeletal System:
Sprains

BIOFREEZE® PAIN RELIEVING PRODUCTS (Performance Health)

For full product information see page 678.

**MINERAL ICE®
(Novartis Consumer Health, Inc.)**
Pain Reliever

For full product information see page 685.

THERA-GESIC® Maximum Strength Analgesic Pain Relieving Creme (Mission Pharmacal)
pain relieving crème

For full product information see page 691.

THERMA-CARE HEAT ACTIVATED WRAPS (Procter & Gamble)
Therapeutic heat wraps

For full product information see page 692.

Musculoskeletal System:
Osteoporosis

CITRACAL® CAPLETS
ULTRADENSE® Calcium Citrate
with Vitamin D Dietary
Supplement
(Mission Pharmacal)

Description: Citracal® helps ensure women will have the strong bones necessary to take on a life filled with activity and ambitions. Calcium, together with a healthy diet and regular exercise, can help reduce the risk of osteoporosis. It is important to get adequate calcium; however, intakes above 2,000 mg per day are not likely to provide additional benefits. Make every moment count. Live with determination. Stand strong.

Serving Size: 2 caplets

	Amount Per Serving	%Daily Value
Vitamin D_3 (as cholecalciferol)	400 IU	100%
Calcium (as Ultradense® calcium citrate)	630 mg	63%

Ingredients: Calcium citrate, polyethylene glycol, croscarmellose sodium, polyvinyl alcohol-part hydrolyzed, color added, magnesium silicate, magnesium stearate, vitamin D_3.

Directions for Use: Take 1 to 2 caplets two times daily or as recommended by your physician, pharmacist, or health professional.

Other Information: STORE AT ROOM TEMPERATURE. KEEP OUT OF THE REACH OF CHILDREN. SAFETY SEALED PACKAGE FOR YOUR PROTECTION. Do not use if inner seal is broken.

How Supplied: 60 coated caplets, UPC 0178-0815-60; 120 coated caplets, UPC 0178-0815-12.

Musculoskeletal System:
Sprains

**BIOFREEZE® PAIN RELIEVING
PRODUCTS (Performance Health)**

For full product information see page 678.

**MINERAL ICE®
(Novartis Consumer Health, Inc.)**
Pain Reliever

For full product information see page 685.

**THERA-GESIC® Maximum Strength
Analgesic Pain Relieving Creme
(Mission Pharmacal)**
pain relieving crème

For full product information see page 691.

**THERMA-CARE HEAT ACTIVATED
WRAPS (Procter & Gamble)**
Therapeutic heat wraps

For full product information see page 692.

Musculoskeletal System:
Strains

**BIOFREEZE® PAIN RELIEVING
PRODUCTS (Performance Health)**

For full product information see page 678.

**MINERAL ICE®
(Novartis Consumer Health, Inc.)**
Pain Reliever

For full product information see page 685.

**THERA-GESIC® Maximum Strength
Analgesic Pain Relieving Creme
(Mission Pharmacal)**
pain relieving crème

For full product information see page 691.

**THERMA-CARE HEAT ACTIVATED
WRAPS (Procter & Gamble)**
Therapeutic heat wraps

For full product information see page 692.

Ophthalmologic System:
Eye Health

BAUSCH & LOMB OCUVITE®
Adult Formula
Eye Vitamin and Mineral Supplement
(Bausch & Lomb)

The #1 recommended supplement brand among eye-care professionals is now available in a new Adult Formula!
New easy to swallow soft gels.
- Essential Eye Nutrition
- Contains 2 mg of Lutein and 100 mg of Omega-3

Description: see supplement facts (table A)
[See first table below]

Other Ingredients: Soybean Oil, Gelatin, Glycerin, Fish Oil (anchovy, sardine), Yellow Beeswax, Silicon Dioxide, Soy Lecithin (Contains peanut oil), Titanium Dioxide, Blue #2, Yellow #6, Green #3

- Ocuvite® Adult formula is an antioxidant supplement with 2 mg of Lutein and 100 mg of Omega-3
- Lutein is clinically proven to help you maintain optimal retinal health.*
- Omega-3 essential fatty acids are structural components of retinal tissues. The retina is particularly rich in long-chain polyunsaturated fatty acids (PUFA) like Omega-3.[1] DHA is a major component of Omega-3. The brain and retina show the highest content of DHA in any tissues. DHA is used continuously for the biogenesis and maintenance of photoreceptor membranes.[2]

> *This statement has not been evaluated by the Food and Drug Administration. This product is not intended to diagnose, treat, cure or prevent any disease.*

References:
1. Uauy R, Lipids, 2001; Vertuani S, Current Pharmac Des, 2004.
2. San Giovanni JP, Progr Ret Eye Res, 2005.

Directions for use: Take 1 Soft Gel daily, in the morning taken with food. Do not exceed the dose indicated without seeking medical advice.
DO NOT USE IF SEAL UNDER CLOSURE IS BROKEN
Keep out of reach of children
STORE AT ROOM TEMPERATURE

How Supplied: NDC 24208-466-30. Available in bottles of 50 count soft gels
FOR MORE INFORMATION, CALL 1–800–553–5340

Bausch & Lomb – Committed to research and leadership in ocular nutritionals
Bausch & Lomb and Ocuvite are registered trademarks of Bausch & Lomb Incorporated.
©Bausch & Lomb Incorporated.
All Rights Reserved
Marketed by:
Bausch & Lomb Incorporated, Rochester, NY 14609
Shown in Product Identification Guide, page 503

BAUSCH & LOMB OCUVITE®
Adult 50+ Formula
Eye Vitamin and Mineral Supplement
(Bausch & Lomb)

The #1 recommended supplement brand among eye-care professionals now in an Adult 50+ Formula!
New easy to swallow soft gels.
- Advanced Eye Nutrition
- Contains 6 mg Lutein and 150 mg of Omega-3

Description: see supplement facts (table A)
[See second table at left]

Other Ingredients: Gelatin, Fish Oil (anchovy, sardine), Glycerin, Yellow Beeswax, Silicon Dioxide, Soy Lecithin (Contains peanut oil), Titanium Dioxide, Blue #1, Blue #2, Yellow #6, Red #40

- Ocuvite® Adult 50+ formula is an antioxidant supplement with 6 mg of Lutein and 150 mg of Omega-3
- As we age, free radicals pose a greater threat to eye health. Our bodies don't neutralize them as effectively as before. The right amount of natural antioxidants, such as 6 mg of Lutein found in Ocuvite Adult 50+ can help maintain eye health as you age.*
- Omega-3 essential fatty acids are structural components of retinal tissues. The retina is particularly rich in long-chain polyunsaturated fatty acids (PUFA) like Omega-3.[1] DHA is a major component of Omega-3. The brain and retina show the highest content of DHA in any tissues. DHA is used continuously for the biogenesis and maintenance of photoreceptor membranes.[2]

> *This statement has not been evaluated by the Food and Drug Administration. This product is not intended to diagnose, treat, cure or prevent any disease.*

References:
1. Uauy R, Lipids, 2001; Vertuani S, Current Pharmac Des, 2004.

Table A

Supplement Facts

Serving Size: 1 Soft Gel
Servings per container: 50

Amount per Serving	1 Soft Gel	% of Daily Value
Vitamin C (ascorbic acid)	100 mg	166.5%
Vitamin E (d-alpha tocopherol)	15 IU	50%
Zinc (as zinc oxide)	9 mg	60%
Copper (as cupric oxide)	1 mg	50%
Lutein	2 mg	+
Omega-3	100mg	+

+ Daily Value not established

Table A

Supplement Facts

Serving Size: 1 Soft Gel
Servings per container: 50

Amount per Serving	1 Soft Gel	% of Daily Value
Vitamin C (ascorbic acid)	150 mg	250%
Vitamin E (d-alpha tocopherol)	30 IU	100%
Zinc (as zinc oxide)	9 mg	60%
Copper (as cupric oxide)	1 mg	50%
Lutein	6 mg	+
Omega-3	150mg	+

+ Daily Value not established

2. San Giovanni JP, Progr Ret Eye Res, 2005.

Directions for use: Take 1 Soft Gel daily, in the morning taken with food. Do not exceed the dose indicated without seeking medical advice.

How Supplied: NDC 24208-465-30. Available in bottles of 50 count soft gels **DO NOT USE IF SEAL UNDER CLOSURE IS BROKEN**
Keep out of reach of children
STORE AT ROOM TEMPERATURE
FOR MORE INFORMATION, CALL
1–800–553–5340
Bausch & Lomb – Committed to research and leadership in ocular nutritionals
Bausch & Lomb and Ocuvite are registered trademarks of Bausch & Lomb Incorporated.
©Bausch & Lomb Incorporated.
All Rights Reserved
Marketed by:
Bausch & Lomb Incorporated, Rochester, NY 14609
Shown in Product Identification Guide, page 503

BAUSCH & LOMB OCUVITE® LUTEIN

[lu 'teen]
Vitamin and Mineral Supplement (Bausch & Lomb)

Description: see supplement facts (table A)
[See table above]

Inactive Ingredients: Lactose monohydrate, Crospovidone, Magnesium Stearate, Silicon dioxide. Contains lactose and casein (milk).

Table A

Supplement Facts
Serving Size: 1 capsule

	Amount	% Daily Value
Vitamin C (ascorbic acid)	60 mg	100%
Vitamin E (dl-alpha tocopheryl acetate)	30 IU	100%
Zinc (zinc oxide)	15 mg	100%
Copper (cupric oxide)	2 mg	100%
Lutein	6 mg	†

†Daily value not established

- Lutein is a carotenoid. Carotenoids are the yellow pigments found in fruits and vegetables, particularly dark, leafy green vegetables such as spinach. Carotenoids are concentrated in the macula, the part of the eye responsible for central vision. Clinical studies suggest that Lutein plays an essential role in maintaining healthy central vision by protecting against free radical damage and filtering blue light.*
- Lutein levels in your eye are related to the amount in your diet. Ocuvite Lutein contains 6 mg of Lutein per capsule. The leading multi-vitamin contains only a fraction of the amount of lutein used in clinical studies.
- Ocuvite Lutein helps supplement your diet with 100% of the US Daily Values for the antioxidant vitamins C, E, and essential minerals, zinc and copper that can play an important role in your ocular health.*
- Ocuvite Lutein is an advanced antioxidant supplement formulated to provide nutritional support for the eye.* The Ocuvite Lutein formulation contains essential antioxidant vitamins, minerals and 6 mg of Lutein.

Recommended Intake: Adults: One capsule, one or two times daily or as directed by their physician.

*These statements have not been evaluated by the Food and Drug Administration. This product is not intended to diagnose, treat, cure or prevent any disease.

How Supplied: Yellow capsule with Ocuvite Lutein printed in black.
NDC 24208-403-19—Bottle of 36
DO NOT USE IF SEAL UNDER CLOSURE IS BROKEN.
Keep this product out of the reach of children.
STORE AT ROOM TEMPERATURE
Made in U.S.A.
Marketed by
Bausch & Lomb
Rochester, NY 14609
© Bausch & Lomb Incorporated. All rights reserved.
Bausch & Lomb, Ocuvite are registered trademarks of Bausch & Lomb Incorporated or its affiliates.
Shown in Product Identification Guide, page 503

Ophthalmologic System:
Itchy, Watery Eyes

ADVIL® ALLERGY SINUS CAPLETS (Wyeth Consumer)
ADVIL® MULTI-SYMPTOM COLD CAPLETS
Pain Reliever/Fever Reducer (NSAID)
Nasal Decongestant
Antihistamine

For full product information see page 770.

ALAVERT (Wyeth Consumer)
Loratadine orally disintegrating tablets
Loratadine swallow tablets
Antihistamine

For full product information see page 771.

ALAVERT ALLERGY & SINUS D-12 HOUR TABLETS (Wyeth Consumer)
Loratadine/Pseudoephedrine Sulfate Extended Release Tablets
Antihistamine/Nasal Decongestant

For full product information see page 771.

BC® POWDER (GlaxoSmithKline Consumer)
ARTHRITIS STRENGTH BC® POWDER
BC® COLD POWDER LINE

For full product information see page 677.

CHILDREN'S CLARITIN ALLERGY (Schering-Plough Healthcare)
loratadine oral solution, grape flavor
5mg/5mL-antihistamine

For full product information see page 771.

CLARITIN 24 HOUR NON-DROWSY REDITABS (Schering-Plough Healthcare)
loratadine 10 mg/antihistamine
CLARITIN 24 HOUR NON-DROWSY TABLETS
Loratadine 10 mg/antihistamine

For full product information see page 772.

CLARITIN-D 12 HOUR NON-DROWSY (Schering-Plough Healthcare)
pseudoephedrine sulfate 120 mg/nasal decongestant
Loratadine 5 mg/antihistamine

CLARITIN-D NON-DROWSY 24 HOUR
pseudoephedrine sulfate 240 mg/nasal decongestant
Loratadine 10 mg/antihistamine

For full product information see page 772.

CHILDREN'S DIMETAPP® COLD & ALLERGY CHEWABLE TABLETS (Wyeth Consumer)
Antihistamine/Nasal decongestant

For full product information see page 730.

CHILDREN'S DIMETAPP® Cold & Allergy Elixir (Wyeth Consumer)
Antihistamine, Nasal Decongestant

For full product information see page 730.

CHILDREN'S DIMETAPP® DM COLD & COUGH Elixir (Wyeth Consumer)
Antihistamine, Cough Suppressant, Nasal Decongestant

For full product information see page 731.

ROBITUSSIN® Cough & Cold Nighttime (Wyeth Consumer)
ROBITUSSIN® Pediatric Cough & Cold Nighttime
ROBITUSSIN® Cough & Allergy
Nasal Decongestant, Cough Suppressant, Antihistamine

For full product information see page 736.

THERAFLU® NIGHTTIME WARMING RELIEF (Novartis Consumer Health, Inc.)
Cough Suppressant/Antihistamine/Pain Reliever/Fever Reducer/Nasal Decongestant

For full product information see page 743.

THERAFLU® THIN STRIPS®-MULTISYMPTOM (Novartis Consumer Health, Inc.)
Antihistamine/Cough Suppressant
(Diphenhydramine HCl)

For full product information see page 744.

TRIAMINIC® COLD & ALLERGY (Novartis Consumer Health, Inc.)
Antihistamine, Nasal Decongestant
Orange Flavor

For full product information see page 746.

TRIAMINIC® NIGHT TIME Cold & Cough (Novartis Consumer Health, Inc.)
Antihistamine/Cough Suppressant, Nasal Decongestant
Grape Flavor

For full product information see page 746.

TRIAMINIC® Softchews® (Novartis Consumer Health, Inc.)
Cough & Runny Nose
Antihistamine, Cough Suppressant
Cherry Flavor

For full product information see page 748.

TRIAMINIC THIN STRIPS® COUGH & RUNNY NOSE (Novartis Consumer Health, Inc.)

For full product information see page 748.

CHILDREN'S TYLENOL® Plus Cold & Allergy (McNeil Consumer)

For full product information see page 716.

TYLENOL® Severe Allergy Caplets (McNeil Consumer)
TYLENOL® Allergy Multi-Symptom Caplets with Cool Burst™ and Gelcaps
TYLENOL® Allergy Multi-Symptom Nighttime Caplets with Cool Burst™

For full product information see page 717.

ZICAM® Allergy Relief (Matrixx)
[zĭ'kăm]

For full product information see page 774.

ZICAM® Flu Daytime (Matrixx)
ZICAM® Nighttime

For full product information see page 768.

Oral Cavity:
Canker Sore

**MAXIMUM STRENGTH
ANBESOL® Gel and Liquid
(Wyeth Consumer)**
Oral Anesthetic

ANBESOL JUNIOR® Gel
Oral Anesthetic

BABY ANBESOL® Gel
Grape Flavor
Oral Anesthetic

For full product information see page 713.

**GLY–OXIDE® Liquid
(GlaxoSmithKline Consumer)**

Description/Active Ingredient:
GLY-OXIDE® Liquid contains carbamide peroxide 10%.

Actions: Gly-Oxide is specially formulated to release peroxide and oxygen bubbles in your mouth. The peroxide and oxygen-rich microfoam help:
• gently remove unhealthy tissue, then cleanse and soothe canker sores and minor wounds and inflammations so natural healing can better occur.
• kill odor-forming germs.
• foam and flush out food particles ordinary brushing can miss.
• clean stains from orthodontics/dentures/bridgework/etc. better than brushing alone.

Indications For Temporary Use: Gly-Oxide liquid is for temporary use in cleansing canker sores and minor wound

or gum inflammation resulting from minor dental procedures, dentures, orthodontic appliances, accidental injury, or other irritations of the mouth and gums. Gly-Oxide can also be used to guard against the risk of infections in the mouth and gums.

Everyday Uses: Gly-Oxide may be used routinely to improve oral hygiene as an aid to regular brushing or when regular brushing is inadequate or impossible such as total care geriatrics, etc. Gly-Oxide kills germs to reduce mouth odors and/or odors on dental appliances. Gly-Oxide penetrates between teeth and other areas of the mouth to flush out food particles ordinary brushing can miss. This can be especially useful when brushing is made more difficult by the presence of orthodontics or other dental appliances. Plus, Gly-Oxide helps remove stains on dental appliances to improve appearance.

Directions For Temporary Use: Do not dilute. Replace tip on bottle when not in use. **Adults and children 2 years of age and older:** Apply several drops directly from bottle onto affected area; spit out after 2 to 3 minutes. Use up to four times daily after meals and at bedtime or as directed by dentist or doctor. OR place 10 drops on tongue, mix with saliva, swish for several minutes, and then spit out. Use by children under 12 years of age should be supervised. **Children under 2 years of age:** Consult a dentist or doctor.
Directions For Everyday Use: The product may be used following the temporary use directions above. OR apply Gly-Oxide to the toothbrush (it will sink

into the brush), cover with toothpaste, brush normally, and spit out.

Warnings: Severe or persistent oral inflammation, denture irritation, or gingivitis may be serious. If sore mouth symptoms do not improve in 7 days, or if irritation, pain, or redness persists or worsens, or if swelling, rash, or fever develops, discontinue use of product and see your dentist or doctor promptly. Avoid contact with eyes. **KEEP THIS AND ALL DRUGS OUT OF THE REACH OF CHILDREN.** In case of accidental overdose, seek professional assistance or contact a poison control center immediately.

Inactive Ingredients: Citric Acid, Flavor, Glycerin, Propylene Glycol, Sodium Stannate, Water, and Other Ingredients. Protect from excessive heat and direct sunlight.

How Supplied: GLY-OXIDE® Liquid is available in $^1/_2$-fl-oz and 2-fl-oz plastic squeeze bottles with applicator spouts. Comments or Questions? Call Toll-free 1-800-245-1040 Weekdays GlaxoSmithKline Consumer Healthcare, L.P.
Moon Township, PA 15108
Made in U.S.A.
Shown in Product Identification Guide, page 505

**HURRICAINE® Topical Anesthetic
20% Benzocaine Oral Anesthetic
(Beutlich LP)**
For full product information see page 712.

Oral Cavity:

Cold Sores/Fever Blisters

ABREVA®
(GlaxoSmithKline Consumer)
Cold Sore/Fever Blister Treatment
Cream
Docosanol 10% Cream

Uses:
- Treats cold sore/fever blisters on the face or lips
- Shortens healing time and duration of symptoms: tingling, pain, burning, and/or itching

Active Ingredient: **Purpose:**

Docosanol 10% .... Cold sore/fever blister treatment

Inactive Ingredients: Benzyl alcohol, light mineral oil, propylene glycol, purified water, sucrose distearate, sucrose stearate.

Directions:
- **adults and children 12 years or over:**
  - wash hands before and after applying cream
  - apply to affected area on face or lips at the first sign of cold sore/fever blister (tingle). **Early treatment ensures the best results.**
  - rub in gently but completely
  - use 5 times a day until healed
- **children under 12 years:** ask a doctor

Warnings:
For external use only.
Do not use
- if you are allergic to any ingredient in this product

When using this product
- apply only to affected areas
- do not use in or near the eyes
- avoid applying directly inside your mouth
- do not share this product with anyone. This may spread infection.

Stop use and ask a doctor if
- your cold sore gets worse or the cold sore is not healed within 10 days
- **Keep out of reach of children.** If swallowed, get medical help or contact a poison control center right away.

Other Information:
- store at 20°–25°C (68°–77°F)
- do not freeze

How Supplied: Abreva Cream is supplied in 2.0 g [.07 oz] tubes.

Question? Call 1-877-709-3539 weekdays

Shown in Product Identification Guide, page 504

ANBESOL COLD SORE THERAPY
(Wyeth Consumer)
Fever blister/Cold sore treatment

Active Ingredients:

Allantoin 1%,
Benzocaine 20%,
Camphor 3%,
White petrolatum 64.9%

Uses:
- temporarily relieves pain associated with fever blisters and cold sores
- relieves dryness and softens fever blisters and cold sores

Warnings: For external use only
Allergy alert: Do not use this product if you have a history of allergy to local anesthetics such as procaine, butacaine, benzocaine, or other "caine" anesthetics.
Do not use over deep or puncture wounds, infections, or lacerations. Consult a doctor.

When using this product
- avoid contact with the eyes
- do not exceed recommended dosage

Stop use and ask a doctor if
- condition worsens
- symptoms persist for more than 7 days
- symptoms clear up and occur again within a few days

Keep out of reach of children. If swallowed, get medical help or contact a Poison Control Center right away.

Directions:
- to open tube, cut tip of the tube on score mark with scissors
- adults and children 2 years of age and older: apply to the affected area not more than 3 to 4 times daily
- children under 12 years of age: adult supervision should be given in the use of this product
- children under 2 years of age: consult a doctor

Tamper-Evident: Safety Sealed Tube. Do Not Use if tube tip is cut prior to opening.

Inactive Ingredients: aloe extract, benzyl alcohol, butylparaben, glyceryl stearate, isocetyl stearate, menthol, methylparaben, propylparaben, sodium lauryl sulfate, vitamin E, white wax

Other Information:
- store at 20–25°C (68–77°F)

How Supplied: 0.33 oz Tube

Oral Cavity:
Dental Care

**SENSODYNE® FRESH MINT
(GlaxoSmithKline Consumer)
SENSODYNE® FRESH IMPACT
SENSODYNE® COOL GEL
SENSODYNE® WITH BAKING
SODA
SENSODYNE® TARTAR CONTROL
SENSODYNE® TARTAR CONTROL
PLUS WHITENING
SENSODYNE® ORIGINAL FLAVOR
SENSODYNE® EXTRA
WHITENING
Anticavity toothpaste for sensitive
teeth**

Active Ingredients: "Fresh Impact" Potassium Nitrate 5% Sodium Fluoride 0.15% w/v fluoride ion 5% Potassium Nitrate and 0.15% w/v Sodium Monofluorophosphate (Extra Whitening) or Sodium Fluoride (Fresh Mint, 0.15% w/v; Baking Soda, 0.15% w/v; Cool Gel, 0.13% w/v; Tartar Control, 0.13% w/v; Tartar Control Plus Whitening 0.145% w/v; Original Flavor, 0.13% w/v), or Sodium Fluoride 0.15% w/v fluoride ion (Fresh Impact). Sensodyne Fresh Mint, Sensodyne Fresh Impact, Sensodyne Cool Gel, Sensodyne with Baking Soda, Sensodyne Tartar Control, Sensodyne Tartar Control Plus Whitening, Sensodyne Original Flavor and Sensodyne Extra Whitening contain fluoride for cavity prevention and Potassium Nitrate clinically proven to reduce pain sensitivity for relief of dentinal hypersensitivity resulting from the exposure of tooth dentin due to periodontal surgery, cervical (gum line) erosion, abrasion or recession which causes pain on contact with hot, cold, or tactile stimuli.

Inactive Ingredients: *Baking Soda:* Flavor, Glycerin, Hydrated Silica, Hydroxyethylcellulose, Methylparaben, Propylparaben, Silica, Sodium Bicarbonate, Sodium Lauryl Sulfate, Sodium Saccharin, Titanium Dioxide, Water.
Extra Whitening: Calcium Peroxide, Flavor, Glycerin, Hydrated Silica, PEG-12, PEG-75, Silica, Sodium Carbonate, Sodium Lauryl Sulfate, Sodium Saccharin, Titanium Dioxide, Water.
Tartar Control: Cellulose Gum, Cocamidopropyl Betaine, Flavor, Glycerin, Hydrated Silica, Silica, Sodium Bicarbonate, Sodium Saccharin, Tetrapotassium Pyrophosphate, Titanium Dioxide, Water.
Tartar Control Plus Whitening: Cellulose Gum, Flavor, Glycerin, Polyethylene Glycol, Silica, Sodium Lauryl Sulfate, Sodium Saccharin, Tetrapotassium Pyrophosphate, Titanium Dioxide, Water.
Cool Gel: Cellulose Gum, FD & C Blue #1, Flavor, Glycerin, Hydrated Silica, Silica, Sodium Methyl Cocoyl Taurate, Sodium Saccharin, Sorbitol, Trisodium Phosphate, Water. *Fresh Impact:* D&C yellow #10 lake, FD & C blue #1 lake, flavor, glycerin, hydrated silica, sodium benzoate, sodium hydroxide, sodium lauryl sulfate, sodium saccharin, sorbitol, titanium dioxide, water, xanthan gum
Fresh Mint: Inactive Ingredients: Carbomer, cellulose gum, D&C yellow #10, FD & C blue #1, flavor, glycerin, hydrated silica, octadecene/MA copolymer, poloxamer 407, potassium hydroxide, sodium lauroyl sarcosinate, sodium saccharin, sorbitol, titanium dioxide, water, xanthan gum.
Original Flavor: Cellulose Gum, D&C Red No. 28, Glycerin, Hydrated Silica, Peppermint Oil, Silica, Sodium Methyl Cocoyl Taurate, Sodium Saccharin, Sorbitol, Titanium Dioxide, Trisodium Phosphate, Water.

Actions: All Sensodyne Formulas significantly reduce tooth hypersensitivity, with response to therapy evident after two weeks of use. Controlled double-blind clinical studies provide substantial evidence of the safety and effectiveness of Potassium Nitrate. The current theory on mechanism of action is that potassium nitrate has an effect on neural transmission, interrupting the signal which would result in the sensation of pain. Fluorides are anticariogenic, forming fluoroapatite in the outer surface of the dental enamel which is resistant to acids and caries.

Warnings: Sensitive teeth may indicate a serious problem that may need prompt care by a dentist. See your dentist if the problem persists or worsens. Do not use this product longer than 4 weeks unless recommended by a dentist or physician. Keep this and all drugs out of the reach of children. If you accidentally swallow more than used for brushing, seek professional assistance or contact a Poison Control Center immediately.

Dosage and Administration: Adults and children 12 years of age and older: Apply a 1-inch strip of the product onto a soft bristle toothbrush. Brush teeth thoroughly for at least 1 minute twice a day (morning and evening) or as recommended by a dentist or physician. Make sure to brush all sensitive areas of the teeth. Children under 12 years of age: consult a dentist or physician.

How Supplied: All Sensodyne formulas are supplied in 2.1 oz. (60g), 4.0 oz. (113g) and 6.0 oz. (170g) tubes. Sensodyne Cool Gel is supplied in 4.0 oz. and 6.0 oz. tubes. Sensodyne Baking Soda is supplied in 4.0 oz and 6.0 oz. only.

Oral Cavity:

Dental Procedure Pain/Sore Gums

HURRICAINE® Topical Anesthetic
20% Benzocaine Oral Anesthetic
(Beutlich LP)

Formats available: Gel, Liquid, Snap-n-Go™ Swabs and Spray

Uses: for the temporary relief of occasional minor irritation and pain, associated with

- Canker sores
- Sore mouth and throat
- Minor dental procedures
- Minor injury of the mouth and gums
- Minor irritation of the mouth and gums dentures or orthodontic appliances

Works fast – within 20 seconds
Safe – available OTC
Tastes good – great flavors
No artificial colors

Packaging Available
GEL

1 oz. jar Wild Cherry - NDC #0283-0871-31
1 oz. jar Pina Colada - NDC #0283-0886-31
1 oz. jar Watermelon - NDC #0283-0293-31
1 oz. jar Fresh Mint - NDC #0283-0998-31
5.25 g. tube - Wild Cherry - NDC #0283-0871-75

LIQUID

1 fl. oz. jar Wild Cherry - NDC #0283-0569-31
1 fl. oz. jar Pina Colada - NDC #0283-1886-31
Snap-n-Go Swabs - 72 each per box NDC #0283-0569-72
Snap-n-Go Swabs - 8 each per travel pack - NDC #0283-0569-08

SPRAY

2 oz. Aerosol Wild Cherry with 1 extension tube NDC #0283-0679-02

SPRAY KIT

2 oz. Aerosol Wild Cherry with 200 extension tubes NDC #0283-0679-60

MAXIMUM STRENGTH
ANBESOL® Gel and Liquid
(Wyeth Consumer)
Oral Anesthetic

ANBESOL JUNIOR® Gel
Oral Anesthetic

BABY ANBESOL® Gel
Grape Flavor
Oral Anesthetic

For full product information see page 713.

Oral Cavity:
Toothache

ADVIL® (Wyeth Consumer)
Ibuprofen Tablets, USP
Ibuprofen Caplets (Oval-Shaped Tablets)
Ibuprofen Gel Caplets (Oval-Shaped Gelatin Coated Tablets)
Ibuprofen Liqui-Gel Capsules
Pain reliever/Fever Reducer (NSAID)

For full product information see page 674.

CHILDREN'S ADVIL CHEWABLE TABLETS (Wyeth Consumer)
Fever Reducer/Pain Reliever (NSAID)

For full product information see page 603.

CHILDREN'S ADVIL SUSPENSION (Wyeth Consumer)
Fever Reducer/Pain Reliever (NSAID)

For full product information see page 603.

INFANTS' ADVIL CONCENTRATED DROPS (Wyeth Consumer)
INFANT'S ADVIL WHITE GRAPE CONCENTRATED DROPS (DYE-FREE)
Fever Reducer/Pain Reliever (NSAID)

For full product information see page 604.

JUNIOR STRENGTH ADVIL® SWALLOW TABLETS (Wyeth Consumer)
Fever Reducer/Pain Reliever (NSAID)

For full product information see page 605.

ALEVE CAPLETS (Bayer Healthcare) (NSAID Labeling)
[a-lēv]

For full product information see page 675.

ALEVE GELCAPS (Bayer Healthcare) (NSAID Labeling)
[a-lēv]

For full product information see page 675.

ALEVE TABLETS (Bayer Healthcare) (NSAID Labeling)
[a-lēv]

For full product information see page 676.

MAXIMUM STRENGTH ANBESOL® Gel and Liquid (Wyeth Consumer)
Oral Anesthetic

ANBESOL JUNIOR® Gel
Oral Anesthetic

BABY ANBESOL® Gel
Grape Flavor
Oral Anesthetic

Active Ingredients: Anbesol is an oral anesthetic which is available in a Maximum Strength gel and liquid. Anbesol Junior, available in a gel, is an oral anesthetic. Baby Anbesol, available in a grape-flavored gel, is an oral anesthetic and is alcohol-free.
Maximum Strength Anbesol Gel and Liquid contain Benzocaine 20%.
Anbesol Junior Gel contains Benzocaine 10%.
Baby Anbesol Gel contains Benzocaine 7.5%.

Uses: **Maximum Strength Anbesol** temporarily relieves pain associated with toothache, canker sores, minor dental procedures, sore gums, braces, and dentures. **Anbesol Junior** temporarily relieves pain associated with braces, sore gums, canker sores, toothaches, and minor dental procedures. **Baby Anbesol Gel** temporarily relieves sore gums due to teething in infants and children 4 months of age and older.

Warnings: **Allergy alert:** Do not use these products if you have a history of allergy to local anesthetics such as procaine, butacaine, benzocaine, or other "caine" anesthetics.
Baby Anbesol: **Do not use** to treat fever and nasal congestion. These are not symptoms of teething and may indicate the presence of infection. If these symptoms persist, consult your doctor.
Maximum Strength Anbesol, Anbesol Junior and Baby Anbesol:
When using this product
• avoid contact with the eyes
• do not exceed recommended dosage
• do not use for more than 7 days unless directed by a doctor/dentist
Stop use and ask a doctor if
• sore mouth symptoms do not improve in 7 days
• irritation, pain, or redness persists or worsens
• swelling, rash, or fever develops
Keep out of reach of children. If more than used for pain is accidentally swallowed, get medical help or contact a Poison Control Center right away.

Directions: **Maximum Strength Anbesol: Gel—**
• adults and children 2 years of age and older: apply to the affected area up to 4 times daily or as directed by a doctor/dentist
• children under 12 years of age: adult supervision should be given in the use of this product
• children under 2 years of age: consult a doctor/dentist
• for denture irritation:
  • apply thin layer to the affected area
  • do not reinsert dental work until irritation/pain is relieved
  • rinse mouth well before reinserting
Do not refrigerate.
Tamper-Evident: Do Not Use if blister is open or the words "SAFETY SEALED" under blister are missing or torn.
Liquid—
• adults and children 2 years of age and older:
  • wipe liquid on with cotton, or cotton swab, or fingertip
  • apply to the affected area up to 4 times daily or as directed by a doctor/dentist
• children under 12 years of age: adult supervision should be given in the use of this product
• children under 2 years of age: consult a doctor/dentist
Tamper-Evident: Do Not Use if plastic blister or backing material is broken or if backing material is separated from the plastic.
Anbesol Junior Gel:
• to open tube, cut tip of the tube on score mark with scissors
• adults and children 2 years of age and older: apply to the affected area up to 4 times daily or as directed by a doctor/dentist
• children under 12 years of age: adult supervision should be given in the use of this product
• children under 2 years of age: consult a doctor/dentist
Tamper-Evident: Safety Sealed Tube. Do Not Use if tube tip is cut prior to opening.
Grape Baby Anbesol Gel:
• to open tube, cut tip of the tube on score mark with scissors
• children 4 months of age and older: apply to the affected area not more than 4 times daily or as directed by a doctor/dentist
• infants under 4 months of age: no recommended dosage or treatment except under the advice and supervision of a doctor/dentist
Tamper-Evident: Safety Sealed Tube. Do Not Use if tube tip is cut prior to opening.

Continued on next page

Anbesol—Cont.

Inactive Ingredients:
Maximum Strength Gel: benzyl alcohol, carbomer 934P, D&C yellow no. 10, FD&C blue no. 1, FD&C red no. 40, flavor, glycerin, methylparaben, polyethylene glycol, propylene glycol, saccharin.
Maximum Strength Liquid: benzyl alcohol, D&C yellow no. 10, FD&C blue no. 1, FD&C red no. 40, flavor, methylparaben, polyethylene glycol, propylene glycol, saccharin.
Junior Gel: artificial flavor, benzyl alcohol, carbomer 934P, D&C red no. 33, glycerin, methylparaben, polyethylene glycol, potassium acesulfame
Grape Baby Gel: benzoic acid, carbomer 934P, D&C red no. 33, edetate disodium, FD&C blue no. 1, flavor, glycerin, methylparaben, polyethylene glycol, propylparaben, saccharin, water

Storage: Store at 20–25°C (68–77°F)

How Supplied: Gels in 0.33 oz (9 g) tubes, Maximum Strength Liquid in 0.41 fl oz (12 mL) bottle.

BUFFERIN®
(Novartis Consumer Health, Inc.)
Regular/Extra Strength
Pain Reliever/Fever Reducer

For full product information see page 678.

EXCEDRIN® EXTRA STRENGTH
(Novartis Consumer Health, Inc.)
PAIN RELIEVER

For full product information see page 684.

GOODY'S®
(GlaxoSmithKline Consumer)
Extra Strength Pain Relief Tablets

For full product information see page 685.

INFANTS' MOTRIN® ibuprofen
Concentrated Drops
(McNeil Consumer)

CHILDREN'S MOTRIN® ibuprofen
Oral Suspension

JUNIOR STRENGTH MOTRIN®
ibuprofen Caplets and Chewable
Tablets
Product information for all dosages of Children's MOTRIN have been combined under this heading

For full product information see page 685.

MOTRIN® IB (Ibuprofen)
Pain Reliever/Fever Reducer
Tablets and Caplets
(McNeil Consumer)

For full product information see page 687.

CONCENTRATED TYLENOL®
acetaminophen Infants' Drops
(McNeil Consumer)

CHILDREN'S TYLENOL®
acetaminophen Suspension Liquid and Meltaways

JR. TYLENOL®
acetaminophen Meltaways

CHILDREN'S TYLENOL®
Suspension with Flavor Creator

Product information for all dosages of Children's TYLENOL have been combined under this heading

For full product information see page 754.

REGULAR STRENGTH TYLENOL®
acetaminophen Tablets
(McNeil Consumer)

EXTRA STRENGTH TYLENOL®
acetaminophen Geltabs, Caplets, Cool Caplets, and EZ Tabs

EXTRA STRENGTH TYLENOL®
acetaminophen Rapid Release Gels

EXTRA STRENGTH TYLENOL®
acetaminophen Adult Liquid Pain Reliever

TYLENOL® Arthritis Pain
Acetaminophen Extended Release Geltabs/Caplets

TYLENOL® 8 Hour Acetaminophen Extended Release Caplets

Product information for all dosage forms of Adult TYLENOL acetaminophen have been combined under this heading.

For full product information see page 695.

Otic Conditions:
Earwax Removal

DEBROX® Drops
(GlaxoSmithKline Consumer)
Ear Wax Removal Aid

Active Ingredient: **Purpose:**
Carbamide peroxide
  6.5% non USP* .... Earwax removal aid

Actions: DEBROX®, used as directed, cleanses the ear with sustained microfoam. DEBROX Drops foam on contact with earwax due to the release of oxygen (there may be an associated crackling sound). DEBROX Drops provide a safe, nonirritating method of softening and removing ear wax.

Uses: For occasional use as an aid to soften, loosen, and remove excessive earwax.

Directions: Adults and children over 12 years of age: tilt head sideways and place 5 to 10 drops into ear. Tip of applicator should not enter ear canal. Keep drops in ear for several minutes by keeping head tilted or placing cotton in the ear. Use twice daily for up to four days if needed, or as directed by a doctor. Any wax remaining after treatment may be removed by gently flushing the ear with warm water, using a soft rubber bulb ear syringe. Children under 12 years of age: consult a doctor.

Warnings: FOR USE IN THE EAR ONLY. Do not use if you have ear drainage or discharge, ear pain, irritation or rash in the ear, or are dizzy; consult a doctor. Do not use if you have an injury or perforation (hole) of the eardrum or after ear surgery unless directed by a doctor. Do not use for more than four days. If excessive earwax remains after use of this product, consult a doctor. Avoid contact with the eyes. In case of accidental ingestion, seek professional assistance or contact a poison control center immediately.

Other Information: Avoid exposing bottle to excessive heat and direct sunlight. Keep tip on bottle when not in use. Product foams on contact with earwax due to release of oxygen. There may be an associated "crackling" sound. Keep this and all drugs out of the reach of children.

Inactive Ingredients: citric acid, flavor, glycerin, propylene glycol, sodium lauroyl sarcosinate, sodium stannate, water

How Supplied: DEBROX Drops are available in ½-fl-oz or 1-fl-oz (15 or 30 ml) plastic squeeze bottles with applicator spouts.

Questions or comments? 1-800-245-1040 weekdays.

Shown in Product Identification Guide, page 505

Respiratory System:
Allergies, Upper Respiratory

4-WAY® MENTHOL (Novartis Consumer Health, Inc.)
Nasal Decongestant

For full product information see page 775.

4-WAY® Fast Acting Nasal Spray (Novartis Consumer Health, Inc.)
Phenylephrine hydrochloride 1%, nasal decongestant

For full product information see page 775.

4-WAY® SALINE (Novartis Consumer Health, Inc.)
Moisturizing Mist

For full product information see page 775.

ADVIL® ALLERGY SINUS CAPLETS (Wyeth Consumer)
ADVIL® MULTI-SYMPTOM COLD CAPLETS
Pain Reliever/Fever Reducer (NSAID)
Nasal Decongestant
Antihistamine

For full product information see page 770.

ALAVERT (Wyeth Consumer)
Loratadine orally disintegrating tablets
Loratadine swallow tablets
Antihistamine

For full product information see page 771.

ALAVERT ALLERGY & SINUS D-12 HOUR TABLETS (Wyeth Consumer)
Loratadine/Pseudoephedrine Sulfate
Extended Release Tablets
Antihistamine/Nasal Decongestant

For full product information see page 771.

CHILDREN'S CLARITIN ALLERGY (Schering-Plough Healthcare)
loratadine oral solution, grape flavor
5mg/5mL-antihistamine

For full product information see page 771.

CLARITIN 24 HOUR NON-DROWSY REDITABS (Schering-Plough Healthcare)
loratadine 10 mg/antihistamine

CLARITIN 24 HOUR NON-DROWSY TABLETS
Loratadine 10 mg/antihistamine

For full product information see page 772.

CLARITIN-D 12 HOUR NON-DROWSY (Schering-Plough Healthcare)
pseudoephedrine sulfate 120 mg/nasal decongestant
Loratadine 5 mg/antihistamine

CLARITIN-D NON-DROWSY 24 HOUR
pseudoephedrine sulfate 240 mg/nasal decongestant
Loratadine 10 mg/antihistamine

For full product information see page 772.

CHILDREN'S DIMETAPP® COLD & ALLERGY CHEWABLE TABLETS (Wyeth Consumer)
Antihistamine/Nasal decongestant

For full product information see page 731.

CHILDREN'S DIMETAPP® COLD & ALLERGY ELIXIR (Wyeth Consumer)
Antihistamine, Nasal Decongestant

For full product information see page 730.

CHILDREN'S DIMETAPP® DM COLD & COUGH Elixir
Antihistamine, Cough Suppressant, Nasal Decongestant

For full product information see page 730.

TODDLER'S DIMETAPP COLD AND COUGH DROPS (Wyeth Consumer)
Cough suppressant/Nasal decongestant

For full product information see page 732.

MUCINEX® D (Adams Respiratory Therapeutics)
600 mg Guaifenesin and 60 mg Pseudoephedrine HCl Extended-Release Bi-Layer Tablets
Expectorant and Nasal Decongestant

For full product information see page 776.

ROBITUSSIN® Cough & Cold Nighttime (Wyeth Consumer)
ROBITUSSIN® Pediatric Cough & Cold Nighttime
ROBITUSSIN® Cough & Allergy
Nasal Decongestant, Cough Suppressant, Antihistamine

For full product information see page 736.

TRIAMINIC® COLD & ALLERGY (Novartis Consumer Health, Inc.)
Antihistamine, Nasal Decongestant
Orange Flavor

For full product information see page 746.

CHILDREN'S TYLENOL® Plus Cold & Allergy (McNeil Consumer)

Description:
Children's TYLENOL® Plus Cold & Allergy is Bubble Gum flavored and contains no alcohol or aspirin. Each teaspoon (5 mL) contains acetaminophen 160 mg, diphenhydramine HCl 12.5 mg and phenylephrine HCl 2.5 mg.

Actions:
Children's TYLENOL® Plus Cold & Allergy combines the analgesic-antipyretic acetaminophen with the antihistamine diphenhydramine hydrochloride and the decongestant phenylephrine hydrochloride to provide fast, effective, temporary relief of all your child's symptoms associated with hay fever and other respiratory allergies including sneezing, sore throat, itchy throat, itchy/watery eyes, runny nose, stuffy nose and nasal congestion. Acetaminophen is equal to aspirin in analgesic and antipyretic effectiveness and it is unlikely to produce the side effects often associated with aspirin or aspirin-containing products.

Uses:
- for the temporary relief of the following cold or other upper respiratory allergy symptoms:
  - minor aches and pains
  - headache
  - sore throat
  - itchy, watery eyes
  - sneezing
  - runny nose
  - stuffy nose
- temporarily reduces fever

Directions:
See Table 1: Children's Tylenol Dosing Chart on pgs. 757–758.

Warnings:
Sore throat warning: If sore throat is severe, persists for more than 2 days, is accompanied or followed by fever, headache, rash, nausea, or vomiting, consult a doctor promptly.
Do not use
- with any other product containing acetaminophen

- with any other product containing diphenhydramine, even one used on skin
- in a child who is taking a prescription monoamine oxidase inhibitor (MAOI) (certain drugs for depression, psychiatric or emotional conditions, or Parkinson's disease) or for 2 weeks after stopping the MAOI drug. If you do not know if your child's prescription drug contains an MAOI, ask a doctor or pharmacist before giving this product.

Ask a doctor before use if the child has
- heart disease • high blood pressure
- thyroid disease • diabetes
- a breathing problem such as chronic bronchitis • glaucoma

Ask a doctor or pharmacist before use if the child is taking sedatives or tranquilizers

When using this product
- **do not exceed recommended dosage (see overdose warning)**
- excitability may occur, especially in children
- marked drowsiness may occur
- sedatives and tranquilizers may increase the drowsiness effect

Stop use and ask a doctor if
- nervousness, dizziness or sleeplessness occur
- pain or nasal congestion gets worse or lasts for more than 5 days
- fever gets worse or lasts for more than 3 days
- new symptoms occur
- redness or swelling is present

These could be signs of a serious condition.
Keep out of reach of children.

Overdose warning:
Taking more than the recommended dose (overdose) may cause liver damage. In case of overdose, get medical help or contact a Poison Control Center right away (1-800-222-1222). Quick medical attention is critical for adults as well as for children even if you do not notice any signs or symptoms.

Other Information:
- store between 20–25° C (68–77° F)

PROFESSIONAL INFORMATION: OVERDOSAGE INFORMATION

For overdosage information, please refer to pg. 680.

Inactive Ingredients:

carboxymethylcellulose sodium, cellulose, citric acid, D&C red #33, FD&C red #40, flavors, glycerin, purified water, sodium benzoate, sorbitol, sucralose, sucrose, xanthan gum

How Supplied:

Pink-colored, Bubble Gum flavored liquid in child resistant tamper-evident bottles of 4 fl. oz.

Shown in Product Identification Guide, page 510

TYLENOL® Severe Allergy Caplets (McNeil Consumer)

TYLENOL® Allergy Multi-Symptom Caplets with Cool Burst™ and Gelcaps

TYLENOL® Allergy Multi-Symptom Nighttime Caplets with Cool Burst™

Product information for all dosage forms of TYLENOL® Allergy have been combined under this heading.

Description:
Each *TYLENOL® Severe Allergy Caplet* contains acetaminophen 500 mg and diphenhydramine HCl 12.5 mg. Each *TYLENOL® Allergy Multi-Symptom Caplet with Cool Burst™ and Gelcap* contains acetaminophen 325 mg, chlorpheniramine maleate 2 mg, and phenylephrine HCl 5 mg. Each *TYLENOL® Allergy Multi-Symptom Nighttime Caplet with Cool Burst™* contains acetaminophen 325 mg, diphenhydramine HCl 25 mg and phenylephrine HCl 5 mg.

Actions:
TYLENOL® Severe Allergy Caplets contain a clinically proven analgesic/antipyretic and antihistamine. Acetaminophen produces analgesia by elevation of the pain threshold and antipyresis through action on the hypothalamic heat regulating center. Acetaminophen is equal to aspirin in analgesic and antipyretic effectiveness, and it is unlikely to produce many of the side effects associated with aspirin and aspirin-containing products. Diphenhydramine HCl is an antihistamine which helps provide temporary relief of itchy, watery eyes, runny nose, sneezing, itching of the nose or throat due to hay fever or other respiratory allergies. *TYLENOL® Allergy Multi-Symptom Caplets with Cool Burst™ and Gelcaps* contain, in addition to acetaminophen, a decongestant, phenylephrine HCl and an antihistamine, chlorpheniramine maleate. Phenylephrine HCl is a sympathomimetic amine which provides temporary relief of nasal and sinus congestion. Chlorpheniramine is an antihistamine which helps provide temporary relief of runny nose, sneezing and watery and itchy eyes. *TYLENOL® Allergy Multi-Symptom Nighttime Caplets with Cool Burst™* contain acetaminophen, phenylephrine HCl and the antihistamine, diphenhydramine HCl.

Uses:
TYLENOL® Severe Allergy:
- temporarily relieves:
  - minor aches and pains • headache • runny nose • sneezing • itching of the nose or throat and itchy, watery eyes due to hay fever

TYLENOL® Allergy Multi-Symptom Caplets with Cool Burst™:

- temporarily relieves these symptoms of hay fever and the common cold:
  - headache • sinus congestion and pressure • nasal congestion • runny nose and sneezing • minor aches and pains
- temporarily relieves these additional symptoms of hay fever:
  - itching of the nose or throat
  - itchy, watery eyes
- helps clear nasal passages

TYLENOL® Allergy Multi-Symptom Gelcaps:
- temporarily relieves these symptoms of hay fever or other upper respiratory allergies:
  - minor aches and pains • headache
  - nasal congestion • runny nose and sneezing • sinus congestion and pressure • itching of the nose or throat
  - itchy, watery eyes
- helps clear nasal passages

TYLENOL® Allergy Multi-Symptom Nighttime Caplets with Cool Burst™:
- temporarily relieves these symptoms of hay fever and other respiratory allergies:
  - headache • sinus congestion and pressure • nasal congestion • runny nose and sneezing • minor aches and pains
- temporarily relieves these additional symptoms of hay fever:
  - itching of the nose or throat
  - itchy, watery eyes
- helps clear nasal passages

Directions:
TYLENOL® Severe Allergy:
- **do not take more than directed (see overdose warning)**

adults and children 12 years and over	• take 2 caplets every 4 to 6 hours • do not take more than 8 caplets in 24 hours
children under 12 years	• do not use this adult product in children under 12 years of age; this will provide more than the recommended dose (overdose) and may cause liver damage

TYLENOL® Allergy Multi-Symptom Caplets with Cool Burst™ and Gelcaps:
- **do not take more than directed (see overdose warning)**

adults and children 12 years and over	• take 2 caplets or gelcaps every 4 hours • swallow whole – do not crush, chew or dissolve (caplets only) • do not take more than 12 caplets or gelcaps in 24 hours

TYLENOL® Allergy Multi-Symptom Caplets with Cool Burst™:

Continued on next page

Tylenol—Cont.

children under 12 years	• do not use this adult product in children under 12 years of age; this will provide more than the recommended dose (overdose) and may cause liver damage.

TYLENOL® Allergy Multi-Symptom Nighttime Caplets with Cool Burst™:

• **do not take more than directed (see overdose warning)**

adults and children 12 years and over	• take 2 caplets every 4 hours • swallow whole – do not crush, chew or dissolve • do not take more than 12 caplets in 24 hours
children under 12 years	• do not use this adult product in children under 12 years of age; this will provide more than the recommended dose (overdose) and may cause liver damage.

Warnings:

Alcohol warning: If you consume 3 or more alcoholic drinks every day, ask your doctor whether your should take acetaminophen or other pain relievers or fever reducers. Acetaminophen may cause liver damage.

Do not use

• if you are now taking a prescription monoamine oxidase inhibitor (MAOI) (certain drugs for depression, psychiatric or emotional conditions, or Parkinson's disease) or for 2 weeks after stopping the MAOI drug. If you do not know if your prescription drug contains an MAOI, ask a doctor or pharmacist before taking this product (does not apply to *TYLENOL® Severe Allergy*)

• with any other product containing acetaminophen

• with any other product containing diphenhydramine, even one used on skin. (does not apply to *TYLENOL® Allergy Multi-Symptom Caplets with Cool Burst™ or Gelcaps*)

TYLENOL® Severe Allergy

Ask a doctor before use if you have

• glaucoma

• trouble urinating due to an enlarged prostate gland

• a breathing problem such as emphysema or chronic bronchitis

TYLENOL® Allergy Multi-Symptom Caplets with Cool Burst™ and Gelcaps and TYLENOL® Allergy Multi-Symptom Nighttime Caplets with Cool Burst™

Ask a doctor before use if you have

• heart disease • high blood pressure

• thyroid disease • diabetes • trouble urinating due to an enlarged prostate gland

• a breathing problem such as emphysema or chronic bronchitis • glaucoma

Ask a doctor or pharmacist before use if you are taking sedatives or tranquilizers

When using this product

• **do not exceed recommended dosage** (*does not apply to TYLENOL® Severe Allergy Caplets*)

• excitability may occur, especially in children

• marked drowsiness may occur (applies to *TYLENOL® Severe Allergy and TYLENOL® Allergy Multi-Symptom Nighttime Caplets with Cool Burst™* only)

• drowsiness may occur (*TYLENOL® Allergy Multi-Symptom Caplets with Cool Burst™ and Gelcaps* only)

• avoid alcoholic drinks

• alcohol, sedatives and tranquilizers may increase the drowsiness effect

• be careful when driving a motor vehicle or operating machinery

Stop use and ask a doctor if

TYLENOL® Severe Allergy Caplets

• pain gets worse or last for more than 10 days

• fever gets worse or last for more than 3 days

• redness or swelling is present

• new symptoms occur

These could be signs of a serious condition.

TYLENOL® Allergy Multi-Symptom Caplets with Cool Burst™ and Gelcaps and TYLENOL® Allergy Multi-Symptom Nighttime Caplets with Cool Burst™

• nervousness, dizziness, or sleeplessness occur

• pain or nasal congestion gets worse or lasts for more than 7 days

• fever gets worse or lasts for more than 3 days

• redness or swelling is present

• new symptoms occur

These could be signs of a serious condition.

If pregnant or breast feeding, ask a health professional before use.

Keep out of reach of children.

Overdose warning: Taking more than the recommended dose (overdose) may cause liver damage. In case of overdose, get medical help or contact a Poison Control Center right away. (1-800-222-1222) Quick medical attention is critical for adults as well as for children even if you do not notice any signs or symptoms.

Other Information:

TYLENOL® Severe Allergy Caplets, TYLENOL® Allergy Multi-Symptom Caplets with Cool Burst™ and TYLENOL® Allergy Multi-Symptom Nighttime Caplets with Cool Burst™:

• store between 20-25°C (68-77°F)

TYLENOL® Allergy Multi-Symptom Gelcaps:

• store between 20-25°C (68-77°F). Avoid high humidity.

PROFESSIONAL INFORMATION: OVERDOSAGE INFORMATION

For overdosage information, please refer to pgs. 696–697.

Inactive Ingredients:

TYLENOL® Severe Allergy:

Caplets: carnauba wax, cellulose, corn starch, D&C yellow #10, FD&C yellow #6, hydroxypropyl cellulose, hypromellose, iron oxide, magnesium stearate, polyethylene glycol, sodium citrate, sodium starch glycolate, titanium dioxide

TYLENOL® Allergy Multi-Symptom:

Caplets with Cool Burst™: black iron oxide, carnauba wax, cellulose, corn starch, flavors, hypromellose, polyethylene glycol, polysorbate 80, silicon dioxide, sodium starch glycolate, stearic acid, sucralose, titanium dioxide, yellow iron oxide. **Gelcaps:** benzyl alcohol, butylparaben, castor oil, cellulose, corn starch, D&C yellow #10, edentate calcium disodium, FD&C blue #1, gelatin, hypromellose, iron oxide, methylparaben, propylparaben, silicon dioxide, sodium lauryl sulfate, sodium propionate, sodium starch glycolate, stearic acid, titanium dioxide

TYLENOL® Allergy Multi-Symptom Nighttime Caplets with Cool Burst™: carnauba wax, cellulose, corn starch, D&C yellow #10, FD&C yellow #6, flavors, hypromellose, iron oxide, magnesium stearate, sodium citrate, sodium starch glycolate, sucralose, titanium dioxide, triacetin

How Supplied:

TYLENOL® Severe Allergy:

Caplets: Yellow film-coated, imprinted with "TYLENOL Severe Allergy" on one side—blister packs of 24.

TYLENOL® Allergy Multi-Symptom:

Caplets *with Cool Burst™:* Off-white, imprinted with "TY C1076" – blister packs of 24 and 48.
Gelcaps: yellow/green, imprinted with "TY C1077" – blister packs of 24.

TYLENOL® Allergy Multi-Symptom Nighttime Caplets with Cool Burst™: light yellow, imprinted with "TY C1082" – blister packs of 24

Shown in Product Identification Guide, page 511

VICKS® SINEX® NASAL SPRAY
(Procter & Gamble)
Ultra Fine Mist for Sinus Relief
[sĭ'nĕx]
Phenylephrine HCl Nasal Decongestant

For full product information see page 781.

ZICAM® Allergy Relief (Matrixx)
[zĭ'kăm]

For full product information see page 774.

Respiratory System:
Asthma

PRIMATENE® Mist
(Wyeth Consumer)
Epinephrine Inhalation Aerosol
Bronchodilator

Active Ingredient: (in each inhalation)
Epinephrine 0.22 mg

Uses:
- for temporary relief of occasional symptoms of mild asthma:
  - wheezing
  - tightness of chest
  - shortness of breath

Warnings:

Asthma alert: Because asthma can be life threatening, see a doctor if you
- are not better in 20 minutes
- get worse
- need 12 inhalations in any day
- use more than 9 inhalations a day for more than 3 days a week
- have more than 2 asthma attacks in a week

For inhalation only

Do not use
- unless a doctor said you have asthma
- if you are now taking a prescription monoamine oxidase inhibitor (MAOI) (certain drugs taken for depression, psychiatric or emotional conditions, or Parkinson's disease), or for 2 weeks after stopping the MAOI drug. If you do not know if your prescription drug contains an MAOI, ask a doctor or pharmacist before taking this product.

Ask a doctor before use if you have
- ever been hospitalized for asthma
- heart disease
- high blood pressure
- diabetes
- thyroid disease
- seizures
- narrow angle glaucoma
- a psychiatric or emotional condition
- trouble urinating due to an enlarged prostate gland

Ask a doctor or pharmacist before use if you are
- taking prescription drugs for asthma, obesity, weight control, depression, or psychiatric or emotional conditions
- taking any drug that contains phenylephrine, pseudoephedrine, ephedrine, or caffeine (such as for allergy, cough-cold, or pain)

When using this product
- **increased blood pressure or heart rate can occur, which could lead to more serious problems such as heart attack and stroke. Your risk may increase if you take more frequently or more than the recommended dose.**
- nervousness, sleeplessness, rapid heart beat, tremor, and seizure may occur. If these symptoms persist or get worse, consult a doctor right away.
- avoid caffeine-containing foods or beverages.
- avoid dietary supplements containing ingredients reported or claimed to have a stimulant effect.
- do not puncture or throw into incinerator. Contents under pressure.
- do not use or store near open flame or heat above 120°F (49°C). May cause bursting.

Contains CFC 12, 114, substances which harm public health and environment by destroying ozone in the upper atmosphere.

If pregnant or breast-feeding, ask a health professional before use.

Keep out of reach of children. In case of overdose, get medical help or contact a Poison Control Center right away.

Directions:
- **do not exceed dosage**
- supervise children using this product
- adults and children 4 years and over: start with one inhalation, then wait at least 1 minute. If not relieved, use once more. Do not use again for at least 3 hours.
- children under 4 years of age: ask a doctor

Directions For Use of Mouthpiece:
The Primatene Mist mouthpiece, which is enclosed in the Primatene Mist 15 mL size (not the refill size), should be used for inhalation only with Primatene Mist.
1. Take plastic cap off mouthpiece. (For refills, use mouthpiece from previous purchase.)
2. Take plastic mouthpiece off bottle.
3. Place short end of mouthpiece on bottle.
4. Turn bottle upside down. Place thumb on bottom of mouthpiece over circular button and forefinger on top of vial. Empty the lungs as completely as possible by exhaling.
5. Place mouthpiece in mouth with lips closed around opening. Inhale deeply while squeezing mouthpiece and bottle together. Release immediately and remove unit from mouth, then complete taking the deep breath, drawing medication into your lungs, holding breath as long as comfortable.
6. Exhale slowly keeping lips nearly closed. This helps distribute the medication in the lungs.
7. For storage, place long end of mouthpiece back on bottle and cover with plastic cap.

Care of the Mouthpiece:

The Primatene Mist mouthpiece should be washed after each use with hot, soapy water, rinsed thoroughly and dried with a clean, lint-free cloth.

Other Information:
- store at room temperature, between 20–25°C (68–77°F) • contains no sulfites

Inactive Ingredients: ascorbic acid, dehydrated alcohol (34%), dichlorodifluoromethane (CFC 12), dichlorotetrafluoroethane (CFC 114), hydrochloric acid, nitric acid, purified water

How Supplied:
½ Fl oz (15 mL) With Mouthpiece.
½ Fl oz (15 mL) Refill
¾ Fl oz (22.5 mL) Refill

Respiratory System:
Chest Congestion (Loosen Phlegm)

HUMIBID® (Adams Respiratory Therapeutics)
1200 mg Guaifenesin Extended-Release Bi-Layer Tablets
Expectorant

Drug Facts

Active Ingredient: **Purpose:**
(in each extended-release bi-layer tablet)
Guaifenesin 1200 mg .... Expectorant

Uses: helps loosen phlegm (mucus) and thin bronchial secretions to rid the bronchial passageways of bothersome mucus and make coughs more productive

Warnings:
Do not use
• for children under 12 years of age
Ask a doctor before use if you have
• persistent or chronic cough such as occurs with smoking, asthma, chronic bronchitis, or emphysema
• cough accompanied by too much phlegm (mucus)
Stop use and ask a doctor if
• cough lasts more than 7 days, comes back, or occurs with fever, rash, or persistent headache. These could be signs of a serious illness.
If pregnant or breast-feeding, ask a health professional before use.
Keep out of reach of children. In case of overdose, get medical help or contact a Poison Control Center right away.

Directions:
• do not crush, chew, or break tablet
• take with a full glass of water
• this product can be administered without regard for the timing of meals
• adults and children 12 years of age and over: 1 tablet every 12 hours. Do not exceed 2 tablets in 24 hours.
• children under 12 years of age: do not use

Other Information:
• tamper evident: do not use if seal on bottle printed "SEALED for YOUR PROTECTION" is broken or missing
• store between 20-25°C (68-77°F)

Inactive Ingredients: carbomer 934P, NF; green lake blend; hypromellose, USP; magnesium stearate, NF; microcrystalline cellulose, NF; sodium starch glycolate, NF

How Supplied: Bottles of 100 tablets (NDC 63824-025-10). A modified oval bi-layer tablet debossed with "Adams" on the green layer and "1200" on the white layer.
US Patent Nos. 6,372,252 B1 and 6,955,821 B2
Shown in Product Identification Guide, page 503

MUCINEX® (Adams Respiratory Therapeutics)
600 mg Guaifenesin Extended-Release Bi-Layer Tablets
Expectorant

Drug Facts

Active Ingredient: **Purpose:**
(in each extended-release bi-layer tablet)
Guaifenesin 600 mg .... Expectorant

Uses: helps loosen phlegm (mucus) and thin bronchial secretions to rid the bronchial passageways of bothersome mucus and make coughs more productive

Warnings:
Do not use
• for children under 12 years of age
Ask a doctor before use if you have
• persistent or chronic cough such as occurs with smoking, asthma, chronic bronchitis, or emphysema
• cough accompanied by too much phlegm (mucus)
Stop use and ask a doctor if
• cough lasts more than 7 days, comes back, or occurs with fever, rash, or persistent headache. These could be signs of a serious illness.
If pregnant or breast-feeding, ask a health professional before use.
Keep out of reach of children. In case of overdose, get medical help or contact a Poison Control Center right away.

Directions:
• do not crush, chew, or break tablet
• take with a full glass of water
• this product can be administered without regard for the timing of meals
• adults and children 12 years of age and over: one or two tablets every 12 hours. Do not exceed 4 tablets in 24 hours.
• children under 12 years of age: do not use

Other Information:
• tamper evident: do not use if seal on bottle printed "SEALED for YOUR PROTECTION" is broken or missing
• store between 20–25°C (68–77°F)

Inactive Ingredients: carbomer 934P, NF; FD&C blue #1 aluminum lake; hypromellose, USP; magnesium stearate, NF; microcrystalline cellulose, NF; sodium starch glycolate, NF

How Supplied:
Bottles of 20 tablets (NDC 63824-008-20), 40 tablets (NDC 63824-008-40), 60 tablets (NDC 63824-008-60), 100 tablets (NDC 63824-008-10) and 500 tablets (NDC 63824-008-50). A round bi-layer tablet debossed with "A" on the light blue, marbled layer and "600" on the white layer. Each tablet provides 600 mg guaifenesin. US Patent Nos. 6,372,252 B1 and 6,955,821 B2
Shown in Product Identification Guide, page 503

MUCINEX® DM
(Adams Respiratory Therapeutics)
600 mg Guaifenesin and 30 mg Dextromethorphan HBr Extended-Release Bi-Layer Tablets
Expectorant and Cough Suppressant

Drug Facts

Active Ingredients: **Purpose:**
(in each extended-release bi-layer tablet)
Dextromethorphan HBr 30 mg .... Cough suppressant
Guaifenesin 600 mg .... Expectorant

Uses:
• helps loosen phlegm (mucus) and thin bronchial secretions to rid the bronchial passageways of bothersome mucus and make coughs more productive
• temporarily relieves:
cough due to minor throat and bronchial irritation as may occur with the common cold or inhaled irritants
• the intensity of coughing
• the impulse to cough to help you get to sleep

Warnings:
Do not use
• for children under 12 years of age
• if you are now taking a prescription monoamine oxidase inhibitor (MAOI) (certain drugs for depression, psychiatric or emotional conditions, or Parkinson's disease), or for 2 weeks after stopping the MAOI drug. If you do not know if your prescription drug contains a MAOI, ask a doctor or pharmacist before taking this product.
Ask a doctor before use if you have
• persistent or chronic cough such as occurs with smoking, asthma, chronic bronchitis, or emphysema
• cough accompanied by too much phlegm (mucus)
When using this product
• do not use more than directed
Stop use and ask a doctor if
• cough lasts more than 7 days, comes back, or occurs with fever, rash, or persistent headache. These could be signs of a serious illness.
If pregnant or breast-feeding, ask a health professional before use.

Keep out of reach of children. In case of overdose, get medical help or contact a Poison Control Center right away.

Directions:

- do not crush, chew, or break tablet
- take with a full glass of water
- this product can be administered without regard for timing of meals
- adults and children 12 years and older: one or two tablets every 12 hours; not more than 4 tablets in 24 hours
- children under 12 years of age: do not use

Other Information:

- tamper evident: do not use if seal on bottle printed "SEALED for YOUR PROTECTION" is broken or missing
- store at 20–25°C (68–77°F)

Inactive Ingredients: carbomer 934P, NF; D&C yellow #10 aluminum lake; hypromellose, USP; magnesium stearate, NF; microcrystalline cellulose, NF; sodium starch glycolate, NF

How Supplied:
Bottles of 20 tablets (NDC 63824-056-20), 40 tablets (NDC 63824-056-40) and 54 tablets (NDC 63824-056-54).
A modified oval bi-layer tablet debossed with "Adams" on the yellow layer and "600" on the white layer. Each tablet provides 600 mg guaifenesin and 30 mg dextromethorphan HBr. US Patent Nos. 6,372,252 B1 and 6,955,821 B2

Shown in Product Identification Guide, page 503

MUCINEX® D
(Adams Respiratory Therapeutics)
600 mg Guaifenesin and 60 mg Pseudoephedrine HCl Extended-Release Bi-Layer Tablets
Expectorant and Nasal Decongestant

For full product information see page 776.

REFENESEN™ 400
[rĕ-fĕn-ə-sĕn]
NON-DROWSY IMMEDIATE RELEASE EXPECTORANT CAPLETS
(Reese)

REFENESEN™ DM NON-DROWSY IMMEDIATE RELEASE EXPECTORANT & COUGH SUPPRESSANT CAPLETS

REFENESEN™ PE NON-DROWSY IMMEDIATE RELEASE EXPECTORANT & NASAL DECONGESTANT CAPLETS

Expectorant, nasal decongestant, cough suppressant

Description: *Each Refenesen™ 400 caplet contains guaifenesin 400 mg. Each Refenesen™ DM caplet contains guaifenesin 400 mg and dextromethorphan hydrobromide 20 mg. Each Refenesen™ PE caplet contains guaifenesin 400 mg and phenylephrine hydrochloride 10 mg.*

Uses: *Refenesen™ 400* • helps loosen phlegm (mucus) • thin bronchial secretions • helps make coughs more productive; *Refenesen™ DM* • helps loosen phlegm (mucus) • thin bronchial secretions; • relieves cough due to minor throat and bronchial irritation; *Refenesen™ PE* • helps loosen phlegm (mucus) • thin bronchial secretions • loosens and clears nasal congestion • shrinks swollen membranes.

Directions: Refenesen™ 400 Expectorant, Refenesen™ DM Expectorant & Cough Suppressant, and Refenesen™ PE Expectorant & Nasal Decongestant
•do not exceed 6 doses in a 24-hour period or as directed by a doctor

Adults and children 12 years of age and over	Take one caplet every 4 hours as needed
Children 6 to under 12 years of age	Take ½ caplet every 4 hours as needed
Children under 6 years of age	Consult a doctor

How Supplied:
Refenesen 400: Available in 50 and 100 ct.
Refenesen DM: Available in 50 and 100 ct.
Refenesen PE: Available in 50 ct.

ROBITUSSIN Cough & Cold CF Liquid (Wyeth Consumer)
ROBITUSSIN Cough & Cold Pediatric Drops
Cough Suppressant/Expectorant/Nasal decongestant

For full product information see page 735.

ROBITUSSIN® COUGH DM SYRUP
(Wyeth Consumer)
ROBITUSSIN® SUGAR FREE COUGH
ROBITUSSIN® COUGH DM INFANT DROPS
ROBITUSSIN COUGH & CONGESTION
Cough Suppressant, Expectorant

For full product information see page 738.

ROBITUSSIN® Chest Congestion
(Wyeth Consumer)

Active Ingredient: (in each 5 mL tsp) Guaifenesin, USP 100 mg

Use: helps loosen phlegm (mucus) and thin bronchial secretions to make coughs more productive

Warnings:

Ask a doctor before use if you have
- cough that occurs with too much phlegm (mucus)
- cough that lasts or is chronic such as occurs with smoking, asthma, chronic bronchitis, or emphysema

Stop use and ask a doctor if cough lasts more than 7 days, comes back, or is accompanied by fever, rash, or persistent headache. These could be signs of a serious condition.
If pregnant or breast-feeding, ask a health professional before use.
Keep out of reach of children. In case of overdose, get medical help or contact a Poison Control Center right away.

Directions:
- do not take more than 6 doses in any 24-hour period
- adults and children 12 yrs and over: 2–4 tsp every 4 hours
- children 6 to under 12 yrs: 1–2 tsp every 4 hours
- children 2 to under 6 yrs: ½–1 tsp every 4 hours
- children under 2 yrs: ask a doctor

Other Information:
- each teaspoon contains: sodium 2 mg
- store at 20–25°C (68–77°F)
- alcohol-free
- dosage cup provided

Inactive Ingredients: artificial flavor, caramel, citric acid, FD&C red no. 40, glycerin, high fructose corn syrup, liquid glucose, menthol, propylene glycol, purified water, saccharin sodium, sodium benzoate

How Supplied: Bottles of 4 fl oz, 8 fl oz.

ROBITUSSIN® Head & Chest Congestion PE Syrup
(Wyeth Consumer)
Nasal Decongestant, Expectorant

For full product information see page 739.

TYLENOL® Cold Multi-Symptom Daytime Caplets with Cool Burst™ and Gelcaps (McNeil Consumer)

TYLENOL® Cold Multi-Symptom Nighttime Caplets with Cool Burst™

TYLENOL® Cold Multi-Symptom Severe Caplets with Cool Burst™

TYLENOL® Cold Multi-Symptom Daytime Liquid

TYLENOL® Cold Multi-Symptom Nighttime Liquid with Cool Burst™

TYLENOL® Cold Multi-Symptom Severe Daytime Liquid

For full product information see page 752.

TYLENOL® Chest Congestion Caplets with Cool Burst™ (McNeil Consumer)

TYLENOL® Chest Congestion Liquid with Cool Burst™

Product information for all dosage forms of TYLENOL Chest Congestion have been combined under this heading.

Description:
Each *TYLENOL® Chest Congestion Caplet with Cool Burst™* contains acetaminophen 325 mg, and guafenesin 200 mg. *TYLENOL® Chest Congestion Liquid with Cool Burst™* contains acetaminophen 500 mg, and guafenesin 200 mg in each 15 mL (1 tablespoon).

Actions:
TYLENOL® Chest Congestion Caplets and Liquid with Cool Burst™ contain a clinically proven analgesic/antipyretic and an expectorant. Acetaminophen produces analgesia by elevation of the pain threshold and antipyresis through action on the hypothalamic heat regulating center. Acetaminophen is equal to aspirin in analgesic and antipyretic effectiveness and it is unlikely to produce many of the side effects associated with aspirin and aspirin-containing products. Guafenesin is an expectorant which helps loosen phlegm (mucus) and thin bronchial secretions to make coughs more productive.

Uses:
TYLENOL® Chest Congestion Caplets and Liquid
- temporarily relieves:
  - minor aches and pains
  - headache
- temporarily reduces fever
- helps loosen phlegm (mucus) and thin bronchial secretions to make coughs more productive

Directions:
TYLENOL® Chest Congestion Caplets with Cool Burst™
- **do not take more than directed (see overdose warning)**

adults and children 12 years and over	• take 2 caplets every 4–6 hours as needed. • swallow whole - do not crush, chew or dissolve • do not take more than 12 caplets in 24 hours.
children under 12 years	• not intended for use in children under 12; this will provide more than the recommended dose (overdose) and may cause liver damage.

TYLENOL® Chest Congestion Liquid with Cool Burst™
- **do not take more than directed (see overdose warning)**
- use only enclosed measuring cup specifically designed for this product. Do not use any other dosing device.

adults and children 12 years and over	• take 2 tablespoons or 30 mL in dose cup provided every 4–6 hours • do not take more than 8 tablespoons in 24 hours
children under 12 years	• not intended for use in children under 12; this will provide more than the recommended dose (overdose) and may cause liver damage.

Warnings:
Alcohol warning: If you consume 3 or more alcoholic drinks every day, ask your doctor whether you should take acetaminophen or other pain relievers or fever reducers. Acetaminophen may cause liver damage.

Do not use
- with any other product containing acetaminophen

Ask a doctor before use if you have
- persistent or chronic cough such as occurs with smoking, asthma, chronic bronchitis, or emphysema
- cough that occurs with too much phlegm (mucus)

Stop use and ask a doctor if
- pain or cough gets worse or lasts more than 7 days
- fever gets worse or lasts more than 3 days
- redness or swelling is present
- new symptoms occur
- cough comes back or occurs with rash or headache that lasts.

These could be signs of a serious condition.

If pregnant or breast-feeding, ask a health professional before use.

Keep out of reach of children.

Overdose warning: Taking more than the recommended dose (overdose) may cause liver damage. In case of overdose, get medical help or contact a Poison Control Center (1–800–222–1222) right away. Quick medical attention is critical for adults as well as for children even if you do not notice any signs or symptoms.

Other Information:
- each caplet contains: **sodium 3 mg** (*applies to TYLENOL® Chest Congestion Caplets with Cool Burst™ only*)
- each tablespoon contains: **sodium 11 mg** (*applies to TYLENOL® Chest Congestion Liquid with Cool Burst™ only*)
- store between 20–25°C (68–77°F)

PROFESSIONAL INFORMATION: OVERDOSAGE INFORMATION
For overdosage information, please refer to pgs. 696–697.

Inactive Ingredients:
TYLENOL® Chest Congestion Caplets: cellulose, corn starch, croscarmellose sodium, D&C yellow #10, FD&C blue #1, FD&C red #40, flavor, iron oxide, mannitol, polyethylene glycol, polyvinyl alcohol, povidone, silicon dioxide, stearic acid, sucralose, talc, titanium dioxide
TYLENOL® Chest Congestion Liquid: carboxymethylcellulose sodium, citric acid, FD&C blue #1, flavors, polyethylene glycol, propylene glycol, purified water, sodium benzoate, sorbitol, sucralose, sucrose

How Supplied:
TYLENOL® Chest Congestion Caplet with Cool Burst™: Green-colored, imprinted with "Tylenol Chest Cong"—blister packs of 24.
TYLENOL® Chest Congestion Liquid with Cool Burst™: Blue-colored, 8 fl. oz bottle.

Shown in Product Identification Guide, page 511

TYLENOL® COLD
Severe Congestion Non-Drowsy Caplets with Cool Burst™ (McNeil Consumer)

For full product information see page 751.

Respiratory System:
Cough, Cold, and Flu

4-WAY® MENTHOL
(Novartis Consumer Health, Inc.)
Nasal Decongestant

For full product information see page 775.

4-WAY® Fast Acting Nasal Spray
(Novartis Consumer Health, Inc.)
Phenylephrine hydrochloride 1%, nasal decongestant

For full product information see page 775.

4-WAY® SALINE
(Novartis Consumer Health, Inc.)
Moisturizing Mist

For full product information see page 775.

ADVIL® (Wyeth Consumer)
Ibuprofen Tablets, USP
Ibuprofen Caplets (Oval-Shaped Tablets)
Ibuprofen Gel Caplets (Oval-Shaped Gelatin Coated Tablets)
Ibuprofen Liqui-Gel Capsules
Pain reliever/Fever Reducer (NSAID)

For full product information see page 674.

ADVIL® ALLERGY SINUS CAPLETS (Wyeth Consumer)
ADVIL® MULTI-SYMPTOM COLD CAPLETS
Pain Reliever/Fever Reducer (NSAID)
Nasal Decongestant
Antihistamine

For full product information see page 770.

ADVIL® COLD & SINUS
(Wyeth Consumer)
Caplets, and Liqui-Gels
Pain Reliever/Fever Reducer/(NSAID)
Nasal Decongestant

Active Ingredients (in each caplet):
Ibuprofen 200 mg (NSAID)*
Pseudoephedrine HCl 30 mg

*nonsteroidal anti-inflammatory drug

Active Ingredients (in each LiquiGel):
Solubilized Ibuprofen equal to 200 mg ibuprofen (NSAID)* (present as the free acid and potassium salt)
Pseudoephedrine HCl 30 mg

*nonsteroidal anti-inflammatory drug

Uses:
Temporarily relieves these symptoms associated with the common cold, or flu:
- headache
- fever
- nasal congestion
- sinus pressure
- minor body aches and pains

Warnings
Allergy alert: Ibuprofen may cause a severe allergic reaction, especially in people allergic to aspirin. Symptoms may include:
- hives
- facial swelling
- asthma (wheezing)
- shock
- skin reddening
- rash
- blisters

If an allergic reaction occurs, stop use and seek medical help right away.

Stomach bleeding warning: This product contains a nonsteroidal anti-inflammatory drug (NSAID), which may cause stomach bleeding. The chance is higher if you:
- are age 60 or older
- have had stomach ulcers or bleeding problems
- take a blood thinning (anticoagulant) or steroid drug
- take other drugs containing an NSAID [aspirin, ibuprofen, naproxen, or others]
- have 3 or more alcoholic drinks every day while using this product
- take more or for a longer time than directed

Do not use
- if you have ever had an allergic reaction to any other pain reliever/fever reducer
- right before or after heart surgery
- if you are now taking a prescription monoamine oxidase inhibitor (MAOI) (certain drugs for depression, psychiatric, or emotional conditions, or Parkinson's disease), or for 2 weeks after stopping the MAOI drug. If you do not know if your prescription drug contains an MAOI, ask a doctor or pharmacist before taking this product

Ask a doctor before use if you have
- problems or serious side effects from taking pain relievers or fever reducers
- stomach problems that last or come back, such as heartburn, upset stomach, or stomach pain
- ulcers
- bleeding problems
- high blood pressure
- heart or kidney disease
- thyroid disease
- diabetes

- trouble urinating due to an enlarged prostate gland
- taken a diuretic
- reached age 60 or older

Ask a doctor or pharmacist before use if you are
- taking any other drug containing an NSAID (prescription or nonprescription)
- taking a blood thinning (anticoagulant) or steroid drug
- under a doctor's care for any serious condition
- taking any other product that contains pseudoephedrine or any other nasal decongestant
- taking aspirin to prevent heart attack or stroke, because ibuprofen may decrease this benefit of aspirin
- taking any other drug

When using this product
- take with food or milk if stomach upset occurs
- long term continuous use may increase the risk of heart attack or stroke

Stop use and ask a doctor if
- you feel faint, vomit blood, or have bloody or black stools. These are signs of stomach bleeding.
- pain gets worse or lasts more than 10 days
- fever gets worse or lasts more than 3 days
- nasal congestion lasts for more than 7 days
- symptoms continue or get worse
- stomach pain or upset gets worse or lasts
- redness or swelling is present in the painful area
- you get nervous, dizzy, or sleepless
- any new symptoms appear

If pregnant or breast-feeding, ask a health professional before use. It is especially important not to use this product during the last 3 months of pregnancy unless definitely directed to do so by a doctor because it may cause problems in the unborn child or complications during delivery.

Keep out of reach of children. In case of overdose, get medical help or contact a Poison Control Center right away.

Directions:
- **do not take more than directed**
- **the smallest effective dose should be used**
- do not take longer than 10 days, unless directed by a doctor (see Warnings)
- adults and children 12 years of age and over:
  - take 1 caplet or liqui-gel every 4 to 6 hours while symptoms persist. If symptoms do not respond to 1 caplet

Advil Cold & Sinus—Cont.

or liqui-gel, 2 caplets or liqui-gels may be used.

- do not use more than 6 caplets or liqui-gels in any 24-hour period unless directed by a doctor
- children under 12 years of age: consult a doctor

Other Information:

- store at 20–25°C (68–77°F). Avoid excessive heat above 40°C (104°F).
- read all warnings and directions before use. Keep carton.
- **each Liqui-gel contains:** potassium 20 mg

Inactive Ingredients (caplets): carnauba or equivalent wax, croscarmellose sodium, iron oxides, methylparaben, microcrystalline cellulose, propylparaben, silicon dioxide, sodium benzoate, sodium lauryl sulfate, starch, stearic acid, sucrose, titanium dioxide

Inactive Ingredients (liqui-gels): D&C yellow no. 10, FD&C red no. 40, fractionated coconut oil, gelatin, pharmaceutical ink, polyethylene glycol, potassium hydroxide, purified water, sorbitan, sorbitol

How Supplied: Advil® Cold and Sinus is an oval-shaped, tan-colored caplet, or a liqui-gel. The caplet is supplied in blister packs of 20 and 40. The liqui-gel is available in blister packs of 16.

CHILDREN'S ADVIL CHEWABLE TABLETS (Wyeth Consumer)
Fever Reducer/Pain Reliever (NSAID)

For full product information see page 603.

CHILDREN'S ADVIL SUSPENSION (Wyeth Consumer)
Fever Reducer/Pain Reliever (NSAID)

For full product information see page 603.

INFANTS' ADVIL CONCENTRATED DROPS (Wyeth Consumer)
INFANT'S ADVIL WHITE GRAPE CONCENTRATED DROPS (DYE-FREE)
Fever Reducer/Pain Reliever (NSAID)

For full product information see page 604.

JUNIOR STRENGTH ADVIL® SWALLOW TABLETS (Wyeth Consumer)
Fever Reducer/Pain Reliever (NSAID)

For full product information see page 605.

ALAVERT ALLERGY & SINUS D-12 HOUR TABLETS (Wyeth Consumer)
Loratadine/Pseudoephedrine Sulfate Extended Release Tablets
Antihistamine/Nasal Decongestant

For full product information see page 771.

ALEVE CAPLETS (Bayer Healthcare) (NSAID Labeling)
[a-lēv]

For full product information see page 675.

ALEVE COLD & SINUS CAPLETS (Bayer Healthcare) (NSAID Labeling)
[a-lēv]

Drug Facts

Active Ingredients

(in each caplet):	Purposes:
Naproxen sodium 220 mg (naproxen 200 mg) (NSAID)*	Pain reliever/ fever reducer
Pseudoephedrine HCl 120 mg, extended-release	Nasal decongestant

* nonsteroidal anti-inflammatory drug

Uses: temporarily relieves these cold, sinus, and flu symptoms:
- sinus pressure
- minor body aches and pains
- headache
- nasal and sinus congestion (promotes sinus drainage and restores freer breathing through the nose
- fever

Warnings:

Allergy alert: Naproxen sodium may cause a severe allergic reaction, especially in people allergic to aspirin. Symptoms may include:
- hives
- facial swelling
- asthma (wheezing)
- shock
- skin reddening
- rash
- blisters

If an allergic reaction occurs, stop use and seek medical help right away.

Stomach bleeding warning: This product contains a nonsteroidal anti-inflammatory drug (NSAID), which may cause stomach bleeding. The chance is higher if you:
- are age 60 or older
- have had stomach ulcers or bleeding problems
- take a blood thinning (anticoagulant) or steroid drug
- take other drugs containing an NSAID (aspirin, ibuprofen, naproxen, or others)

- have 3 or more alcoholic drinks every day while using this product
- take more or for a longer time than directed

Do not use
- if you have ever had an allergic reaction to any other pain reliever/fever reducer
- right before or after heart surgery
- if you are now taking a prescription monoamine oxidase inhibitor (MAOI) (certain drugs for depression, psychiatric, or emotional conditions, or Parkinson's disease), or for 2 weeks after stopping the MAOI drug. If you do not know if your prescription drug contains an MAOI, ask a doctor or pharmacist before taking this product.

Ask a doctor before use if you have
- problems or serious side effects from taking pain relievers or fever reducers
- stomach problems that last or come back, such as heartburn, upset stomach, or stomach pain
- ulcers
- bleeding problems
- high blood pressure
- heart or kidney disease
- taken a diuretic
- reached age 60 or older
- thyroid disease
- diabetes
- trouble urinating due to an enlarged prostate gland

Ask a doctor or pharmacist before use if you are
- taking any other drug containing an NSAID (prescription or nonprescription)
- taking a blood thinning (anticoagulant) or steroid drug
- under a doctor's care for any serious condition
- using any other product that contains naproxen or pseudoephedrine
- taking any other pain reliever/fever reducer or nasal decongestant
- taking any other drug

When using this product
- take with food or milk if stomach upset occurs
- long term continuous use may increase the risk of heart attack or stroke

Stop use and ask a doctor if
- you feel faint, vomit blood, or have bloody or black stools. These are signs of stomach bleeding.
- pain gets worse or lasts more than 10 days
- fever gets worse or lasts more than 3 days
- stomach pain or upset gets worse or lasts
- redness or swelling is present in the painful area
- any new symptoms appear
- you have difficulty swallowing or the caplet feels stuck in your throat
- you develop heartburn
- you get nervous, dizzy, or sleepless
- nasal congestion lasts more than 7 days

If pregnant or breast-feeding, ask a health professional before use. It is especially important not to use naproxen so-

dium during the last 3 months of pregnancy unless definitely directed to do so by a doctor because it may cause problems in the unborn child or complications during delivery.

Keep out of reach of children. In case of overdose, get medical help or contact a Poison Control Center right away.

Directions:
- **do not take more than directed**
- **the smallest effective dose should be used**
- do not take longer than 10 days, unless directed by a doctor (see Warnings)
- **swallow whole;** do not crush or chew
- **drink a full glass of water with each dose**
- adults and children 12 years and older: **1 caplet every 12 hours;** do not take more than 2 caplets in 24 hours
- children under 12 years; ask a doctor

Other Information:
- **each caplet contains:** sodium 20 mg
- store at 20–25°C (68–77°F).
- store in a dry place

Inactive Ingredients: colloidal silicon dioxide, hypromellose, lactose, magnesium stearate, microcrystalline cellulose, polyethylene glycol, povidone, talc, titanium dioxide

Questions or comments?
1-800-395-0689 (Mon – Fri 9AM – 5PM EST) or www.aleve.com

How Supplied:
Available in 8, 24, 50, 100, 150, 200 and 250 ct.

Shown in Product Identification Guide, page 503

ALEVE GELCAPS
(Bayer Healthcare)
(NSAID Labeling)
[a-lēv]

For full product information see page 675.

ALEVE TABLETS (Bayer Healthcare
(NSAID Labeling))
[a-lēv]

For full product information see page 676.

BC® POWDER
(GlaxoSmithKline Consumer)
ARTHRITIS STRENGTH BC®
POWDER
BC® COLD POWDER LINE

For full product information see page 677.

BUFFERIN®
(Novartis Consumer Health, Inc.)
Regular/Extra Strength
Pain Reliever/Fever Reducer

For full product information see page 678.

CLARITIN-D 12 HOUR
NON-DROWSY
(Schering-Plough Healthcare)
pseudoephedrine sulfate 120 mg/nasal decongestant
Loratadine 5 mg/antihistamine

CLARITIN-D NON-DROWSY
24 HOUR
pseudoephedrine sulfate 240 mg/nasal decongestant
Loratadine 10 mg/antihistamine

For full product information see page 772.

COMTREX®
(Novartis Consumer Health, Inc.)
MAXIMUM STRENGTH
Pain Reliever/Fever Reducer, Cough Suppressant, Nasal Decongestant
Acetaminophon, Dextromethorphan HBr, Phenylephrine HCl
Non-Drowsy Cold & Cough

Fast Relief of:
- Nasal Congestion • headache
- Sore Throat Pain • coughing

Drug Facts
Active Ingredients
(in each caplet):   **Purposes:**
Acetaminophen
   325 mg ..... Pain reliever/fever reducer
Dextromethorphan HBr
   10 mg .... Cough suppressant
Phenylephrine HCl
   5 mg .... Nasal decongestant

Uses:
- for temporary relief of the following symptoms:
  - headache • sore throat pain
  - cough • minor aches and pains
  - nasal congestion
- temporarily reduces fever

Warnings:
Alcohol warning: If you consume 3 or more alcoholic drinks every day, ask your doctor whether you should take acetaminophen or other pain relievers/fever reducers. Acetaminophen may cause liver damage.

Sore throat warning: Severe or persistent sore throat or sore throat accompanied by high fever, headache, nausea, and vomiting may be serious. Ask a doctor right away. Do not use for more than 2 days or give to children under 3 years of age unless directed by a doctor.

Do not use
- for more than 7 days
- if you are now taking a prescription monoamine oxidase inhibitor (MAOI) (certain drugs for depression, psychiatric or emotional conditions, or Parkinson's disease), or for 2 weeks after stopping the MAOI drug. If you do not know if your prescription drug contains an MAOI, ask a doctor or pharmacist before taking this product.
- with any other products containing acetaminophen. Taking more than directed may cause liver damage.

Ask a doctor before use if you have
- heart disease • high blood pressure
- diabetes • thyroid disease
- cough that occurs with too much phlegm (mucus)
- chronic cough that lasts or as occurs with smoking, asthma, or emphysema
- trouble urinating due to an enlarged prostate gland

When using this product • do not use more than directed

Stop use and ask a doctor if
- you get nervous, dizzy, or sleepless
- new symptoms occur
- redness or swelling is present
- fever gets worse or lasts more than 3 days
- pain, cough or nasal congestion gets worse or lasts more than 7 days
- cough comes back, or occurs with rash, or headache that lasts. These could be signs of a serious condition.

If pregnant or breast-feeding, ask a health professional before use.

Keep out of reach of children.

Overdose warning: Taking more than the recommended dose can cause serious health problems. In case of overdose, get medical help or contact a Poison Conrol Center right away. Quick medical attention is critical for adults as well as for children even if you do not notice any signs or symptoms.

Directions:
- do not use more than directed (see overdose warning
- adults and children 12 years of age and over: take 2 caplets every 4 hours, while symptoms persist
- do not use more than 12 caplets in 24 hours
- children under 12 years of age: consult a doctor

Other Information:
- store at room temperature

Inactive Ingredients: benzoic acid, carnauba wax, corn starch, D&C yellow no. 10 lake, FD&C red no. 40 lake, hypromellose, magnesium stearate, microcrystalline cellulose, polyethylene glycol, polysorbate 80, stearic acid, titanium dioxide

Questions or comments?
1-800-468-7746

How Supplied:
Available in cartons of 10 and 20 ct.

Shown in Product Identification Guide, page 513

COMTREX®
(Novartis Consumer Health, Inc.)
MAXIMUM STRENGTH
Day/Night Severe Cold & Sinus
Pain Reliever/Fever Reducer – Nasal Decongestant – Antihistamine*
Acetaminophen, Phenylephrine HCl, Chlorpheniramine Maleate*

Continued on next page

Comtrex—Cont.

Daytime
- Nasal Congestion
- Sinus Pain & Pressure

Nighttime
- Restful Relief of Daytime Symptoms plus Runny Nose & Sneezing

* Antihistamine in nighttime dose only

Drug Facts

Active Ingredients
(in each caplet):   Purposes:

Acetaminophen
325 mg ..... Pain reliever/fever reducer
Chlorpheniramine maleate
2 mg* .... Antihistamine*
Phenylephrine HCl
5 mg .... Nasal decongestant

* antihistamine in nighttime dose only.

Uses:
- **daytime** (orange caplets) — temporarily relieves:
  - minor aches and pains • headaches
  - nasal congestion • sinus congestion & pressure
- **nighttime** (green caplets) — provides the same relief as the daytime caplets plus temporarily relieves:
  - runny nose • sneezing

Warnings:

Alcohol warning: If you consume 3 or more alcoholic drinks every day, ask your doctor whether you should take acetaminophen or other pain relievers/fever reducers. Acetaminophen may cause liver damage.

Do not use
- for more than 7 days
- if you are now taking a prescription monoamine oxidase inhibitor (MAOI) (certain drugs for depression, psychiatric or emotional conditions, or Parkinson's disease), or for 2 weeks after stopping the MAOI drug. If you do not know if your prescription drug contains an MAOI, ask a doctor or pharmacist before taking this product.
- with any other products containing acetaminophen. Taking more than directed may cause liver damage.

Ask a doctor before use if you have
- heart disease • glaucoma • diabetes
- high blood pressure • thyroid disease
- trouble urinating due to an enlarged prostate gland
- a breathing problem such as emphysema or chronic bronchitis

Ask a doctor or pharmacist before use if you are taking sedatives or tranquilizers

When using this product
- **do not use more than directed**

When using nighttime product:
- excitability may occur, especially in children
- may cause drowsiness
- alcohol, sedatives and tranquilizers may increase drowsiness
- avoid alcoholic drinks
- be careful when driving a motor vehicle or operating machinery

Stop use and ask a doctor if
- new symptoms occur
- you get nervous, dizzy, or sleepless
- redness or swelling is present
- pain or nasal congestion gets worse or lasts more than 7 days
- fever gets worse or lasts more than 3 days

If pregnant or breast-feeding, ask a health professional before use.

Keep out of reach of children.

Overdose warning: Taking more than the recommended dose can cause serious health problems. In case of overdose, get medical help or contact a Poison Control Center right away. Quick medical attention is critical for adults as well as for children even if you do not notice any signs or symptoms.

Directions:
- do not use more than directed (see overdose warning)
- children under 12 years of age: ask a doctor
- adults and children 12 years of age and over:
  - **daytime** - take 2 orange caplets every 4 hours, while symptoms persist, not to exceed 8 daytime caplets in 24 hours, or as directed by your doctor.
  - **nighttime** - take 2 green caplets, if needed, to be taken no sooner than 4 hours after the last daytime caplets, not to exceed 4 nighttime caplets in 24 hours, or as directed by your doctor.

Other Information: • store at room temperature

Inactive Ingredients:
- **daytime caplet** - benzoic acid, carnauba wax, corn starch, D&C yellow no. 10 lake, FD&C red no. 40 lake, hypromellose, magnesium stearate, microcrystalline cellulose, polyethylene glycol, polysorbate 80, stearic acid, titanium dioxide
- **nighttime caplet** - benzoic acid, carnauba wax, corn starch, D&C yellow no. 10 lake, FD&C blue no. 1 lake, FD&C red no. 40 lake, hypromellose, magnesium stearate, microcrystalline cellulose, polyethylene glycol, polysorbate 80, stearic acid, titanium dioxide

Questions or comments?
1-800-468-7746

How Supplied:
Available in cartons of 20 ct. caplets.
Shown in Product Identification Guide, page 513

COMTREX® Maximum Strength Day/Night Cold & Cough
(Novartis Consumer Health, Inc.)
Pain Reliever/Fever Reducer

Drug Facts

Active Ingredients: Purpose:
(in each caplet)
Acetaminophen
325 mg .... Pain reliever/fever reducer
Chlorpheniramine maleate
2 mg* .... Antihistamine*
Dextromethorphan HBr
10 mg .... Cough suppressant
Phenylephrine HCl
5 mg .... Nasal decongestant

---

*antihistamine in nighttime dose only

Uses:
- **daytime** (orange caplets) – for temporary relief of the following symptoms:
  - nasal congestion
  - sore throat pain • cough
  - minor aches and pains
  - reduction of fever • headache
- **nighttime** (blue caplets) – provides the same relief as the daytime caplets plus temporarily relieves:
  - runny nose • sneezing

Warnings:
- **Alcohol warning:** If you consume 3 or more alcoholic drinks every day, ask your doctor whether you should take acetaminophen or other pain relievers/fever reducers. Acetaminophen may cause liver damage.
- **Sore throat warning:** Severe or persistent sore throat or sore throat accompanied by high fever, headache, nausea, and vomiting may be serious. Ask a doctor right away. Do not use for more than 2 days or give to children under 3 years of age unless directed by a doctor.

Do not use
- for more than 7 days
- if you are now taking a prescription monoamine oxidase inhibitor (MAOI) (certain drugs for depression, psychiatric or emotional conditions, or Parkinson's disease), or for 2 weeks after stopping the MAOI drug. If you do not know if your prescription drug contains an MAOI, ask a doctor or pharmacist before taking this product.
- with any other products containing acetaminophen. Taking more than directed may cause liver damage.

Ask a doctor before use if you have
- glaucoma • heart disease
- high blood pressure • diabetes
- thyroid disease
- trouble urinating due to an enlarged prostate gland
- cough that occurs with too much phlegm (mucus)
- chronic cough that lasts or as occurs with smoking, asthma or emphysema
- a breathing problem such as emphysema or chronic bronchitis

Ask a doctor or pharmacist before use if you are taking sedatives or tranquilizers

When using this product
- **do not use more than directed**
- when using nighttime product:
  - excitability may occur, especially in children
  - may cause marked drowsiness
  - alcohol, sedatives and tranquilizers may increase drowsiness
  - avoid alcoholic drinks
  - be careful when driving a motor vehicle or operating machinery

Stop use and ask a doctor if
- new symptoms occur
- you get nervous, dizzy, or sleepless
- redness or swelling is present
- fever gets worse or lasts more than 3 days
- pain, cough or nasal congestion gets worse or lasts for more than 7 days
- cough comes back, or occurs with rash, or headache that lasts. These could be signs of a serious condition.

If pregnant or breast-feeding ask a health professional before use.

Keep out of reach of children.

Overdose warning: Taking more than the recommended dose can cause serious health problems. In case of overdose, get medical help or contact a Poison Control Center right away. Quick medical attention is critical for adults as well as for children even if you do not notice any signs or symptoms.

Directions:

do not use more than directed (**see Overdose warning**)
- children under 12 years of age: ask a doctor
- adults and children 12 years of age and over:
  - **daytime** – take 2 orange caplets every 4 hours, while symptoms persist, not to exceed 8 daytime caplets in 24 hours, or as directed by your doctor.
  - **nighttime** – take 2 blue caplets, if needed, to be taken no sooner than 4 hours after the last daytime caplets, not to exceed 4 nighttime caplets in 24 hours, or as directed by your doctor.

Other Information: • store at room temperature

Inactive Ingredients:
- **daytime caplet** – benzoic acid, carnauba wax, corn starch, D&C yellow no. 10 lake, FD&C red no. 40 lake, hypromellose, magnesium stearate, microcrystalline cellulose, polyethylene glycol, polysorbate 80, stearic acid, titanium dioxide
- **nighttime caplet** – benzoic acid, carnauba wax, corn starch, D&C yellow no. 10 lake, FD&C blue no. 1 lake, hypromellose, magnesium stearate, microcrystalline cellulose, polyethylene glycol, stearic acid, titanium dioxide

Questions or comments?
1-800-468-7746

How Supplied: Available in 20 ct. carton.

Shown in Product Identification Guide, page 513

CONTAC® COLD AND FLU DAY AND NIGHT
(GlaxoSmithKline Consumer)

Day-Drug Facts

Active Ingredients: **Purposes:**
(per caplet)

Acetaminophen
   500 mg .... Pain reliever/Fever reducer

Phenylephrine hydrochloride
   5 mg .... Nasal decongestant

Uses:
temporarily relieves these symptoms due to cold or flu
- nasal congestion
- sinus congestion and pressure
- stuffy nose
- headaches
- minor aches and pains
- sore throat
- temporarily reduces fever

Warnings:

Alcohol warning: If you consume 3 or more alcoholic drinks every day, ask your doctor whether you should take acetaminophen or other pain relievers/fever reducers. Acetaminophen may cause liver damage.

Sore throat warning: If sore throat is severe, persists for more than 2 days, is accompanied or followed by fever, headache, rash, nausea, or vomiting, consult a doctor promptly.

Do not use
- with any other product containing acetaminophen
- if you are now taking a prescription monoamine oxidase inhibitor (MAOI) (certain drugs for depression, psychiatric, or emotional conditions, or Parkinson's disease), or for 2 weeks after stopping the MAOI drug. If you do not know if your prescription drug contains an MAOI, ask a doctor or pharmacist before taking this product.

Ask a doctor before use if you have
- heart disease
- high blood pressure
- thyroid disease
- diabetes
- trouble urinating due to an enlarged prostate gland

When using this product do not exceed recommended dosage.

Stop use and ask a doctor if
- new symptoms occur
- redness or swelling is present
- you get nervous, dizzy or sleepless
- pain or nasal congestion gets worse or lasts more than 7 days
- fever gets worse or lasts more than 3 days

If pregnant or breast-feeding, ask a health professional before use.

Keep out of reach of children.

Overdose warning: Taking more than the recommended dose (overdose) can cause serious health problems. In case of overdose, get medical help or contact a Poison Control Center right away. Quick medical attention is crucial for adults as well as for children even if you do not notice any signs or symptoms.

Directions:
- **do not take more than directed** (see overdose warning)
- **adults and children 12 years and over:** take 2 caplets every 4-6 hours as needed. Do not take more than 8 caplets

(whether all day or all night caplets or a combination of each) in 24 hours.
- **children under 12:** ask a doctor

Other Information: store at 20° – 25°C (68° – 77°F).

Inactive Ingredients: hypromellose, microcrystalline cellulose, polyethylene glycol, potassium sorbate, povidone, pregelatinized starch, sodium lauryl sulfate, starch, stearic acid, talc

Questions or comments? call toll-free 1-800-245-1040 (English/Spanish) weekdays

Night-Drug Facts

Active Ingredients: **Purposes:**
(per caplet)

Acetaminophen
   500 mg .... Pain reliever/Fever reducer
Chlorpheniramine maleate
   2 mg .... Antihistamine
Phenylephrine hydrochloride
   5 mg .... Nasal decongestant

Uses:
temporarily relieves these symptoms due to cold or flu
- nasal congestion
- runny nose
- sneezing
- headaches
- sore throat
- minor aches and pains
- temporarily reduces fever

Warnings:

Alcohol warning: If you consume 3 or more alcoholic drinks every day, ask your doctor whether you should take acetaminophen or other pain relievers/fever reducers. Acetaminophen may cause liver damage.

Sore throat warning: If sore throat is severe, persists for more than 2 days, is accompanied or followed by fever, headache, rash, nausea, or vomiting, consult a doctor promptly.

Do not use
- with any other product containing acetaminophen
- if you are now taking a prescription monoamine oxidase inhibitor (MAOI) (certain drugs for depression, psychiatric, or emotional conditions, or Parkinson's disease), or for 2 weeks after stopping the MAOI drug. If you do not know if your prescription drug contains an MAOI, ask a doctor or pharmacist before taking this product.

Ask a doctor before use if you have
- heart disease
- high blood pressure
- thyroid disease
- diabetes
- glaucoma
- a breathing problem such as emphysema or chronic bronchitis
- trouble urinating due to an enlarged prostate gland

Continued on next page

Contac—Cont.

Ask a doctor or pharmacist before use if you are taking sedatives or tranquilizers

When using this product
- **do not exceed recommended dosage**
- drowsiness may occur
- avoid alcoholic drinks
- excitability may occur, especially in children
- alcohol, sedatives, and tranquilizers may increase drowsiness
- be careful when driving a motor vehicle or operating machinery

Stop use and ask a doctor if
- new symptoms occur
- redness or swelling is present
- you get nervous, dizzy, or sleepless
- fever gets worse or lasts more than 3 days
- pain or nasal congestion gets worse or lasts more than 7 days

If pregnant or breast-feeding, ask a health professional before use.

Keep out of reach of children.

Overdose warning: Taking more than the recommended dose (overdose) can cause serious health problems. In case of overdose, get medical help or contact a Poison Control Center right away. Quick medical attention is critical for adults as well as for children even if you do not notice any signs or symptoms.

Directions:
- **do not take more than directed** (see overdose warning)
- **adults and children 12 years and over:** take 2 caplets every 6 hours as needed. Do not take more than 8 caplets (whether all day or all night caplets or a combination of each) in 24 hours.
- **children under 12 years:** ask a doctor

Other Information: store at 20° – 25°C (68° – 77°F)

Inactive Ingredients: carnauba wax, D&C yellow #10 aluminum lake, FD&C yellow #6 aluminum lake, magnesium stearate, microcrystalline cellulose, polyethylene glycol, polyvinyl alcohol, povidone, sodium starch glycolate, starch, stearic acid, talc, titanium dioxide

Questions or comments? call toll-free 1-800-245-1040 (English/Spanish) weekdays

---

CONTAC COLD AND FLU NON-DROWSY MAXIMUM STRENGTH
(GlaxoSmithKline Consumer)

Drug Facts

Active Ingredients: **Purpose:**
(per caplet)

Acetaminophen
   500 mg .... Pain reliever/Fever reducer
Phenylephrine hydrochloride
   5 mg .... Nasal decongestant

Uses:
temporarily relieves these symptoms due to cold or flu
- nasal congestion
- stuffy nose
- minor aches and pains
- sinus congestion and pressure
- headache
- sore throat
- temporarily reduces fever

Warnings:

Alcohol warning: If you consume 3 or more alcoholic drinks every day, ask your doctor whether you should take acetaminophen or other pain relievers/fever reducers. Acetaminophen may cause liver damage.

Sore throat warning: If sore throat is severe, persists for more than 2 days, is accompanied or followed by fever, headache, rash, nausea, or vomiting, ask a doctor.

Do not use
- with any other product containing acetaminophen
- if you are now taking a prescription monoamine oxidase inhibitor (MAOI) (certain drugs for depression, psychiatric, or emotional conditions, or Parkinson's disease), or for 2 weeks after stopping the MAOI drug. If you do not know if your prescription drug contains an MAOI, ask a doctor or pharmacist before taking this product

Ask a doctor before use if you have
- heart disease
- high blood pressure
- thyroid disease
- diabetes
- trouble urinating due to an enlarged prostate gland

When using this product do not exceed recommended dosage.

Stop use and ask a doctor if
- new symptoms occur
- redness or swelling is present
- you get nervous, dizzy or sleepless
- pain or nasal congestion gets worse or lasts more than 7 days
- fever gets worse or lasts more than 3 days

If pregnant or breast-feeding, ask a health professional before use.

Keep out of reach of children. In case of overdose, get medical help or contact a Poison Control Center right away.

Overdose warning: Taking more than the recommended dose (overdose) can cause serious health problems. In case of overdose, get medical help or contact a Poison Control Center right away. Quick medical attention is crucial for adults as well as for children even if you do not notice any signs or symptoms.

Directions:
- **do not take more than directed** (see overdose warning)
- **adults and children 12 years and over:** take 2 caplets every 4–6 hours as

needed. Do not take more than 8 caplets in 24 hours.
- **children under 12:** ask a doctor

Other information: store below 25°C (77°F)

Inactive Ingredients: hypromellose, microcrystalline cellulose, polyethylene glycol, potassium sorbate, povidone, pregelatinized starch, sodium lauryl sulfate, starch, stearic acid, talc

Questions or comments? call toll-free 1-800-245-1040 weekdays

How Supplied: Available in 8ct. and 24ct. boxes.

Shown in Product Identification Guide, page 505

CONTAC® COLD AND FLU MAXIMUM STRENGTH
(GlaxoSmithKline Consumer)

Drug Facts

Active Ingredients: **Purposes:**
(in each caplet)

Acetaminophen
   500 mg ..... Pain reliever/fever reducer
Chlorpheniramine maleate
   2 mg .... Antihistamine
Phenylephrine hydrochloride
   5 mg .... Nasal decongestant

Uses:
- temporarily relieves these symptoms due to cold or flu
  - nasal congestion
  - runny nose
  - sneezing
  - headaches
  - sore throat
  - minor aches and pains
- temporarily reduces fever

Warnings:

Alcohol warning: If you consume 3 or more alcoholic drinks every day, ask your doctor whether you should take acetaminophen or other pain relievers/fever reducers. Acetaminophen may cause liver damage.

Sore throat warning: If sore throat is severe, persists for more than 2 days, is accompanied or followed by fever, headache, rash, nausea, or vomiting, consult a doctor promptly.

Do not use
- with any other product containing acetaminophen
- if you are now taking a prescription monoamine oxidase inhibitor (MAOI) (certain drugs for depression, psychiatric, or emotional conditions, or Parkinson's disease), or for 2 weeks after stopping the MAOI drug. If you do not know if your prescription drug contains an MAOI, ask a doctor or pharmacist before taking this product.

Ask a doctor before use if you have
- heart disease
- high blood pressure

- thyroid disease
- diabetes
- glaucoma
- a breathing problem such as emphysema or chronic bronchitis
- trouble urinating due to an enlarged prostate gland

Ask a doctor or pharmacist before use if you are taking sedatives or tranquilizers

When using this product

- **do not exceed recommended dosage**
- drowsiness may occur
- avoid alcoholic drinks
- excitability may occur, especially in children
- alcohol, sedatives, and tranquilizers may increase drowsiness
- be careful when driving a motor vehicle or operating machinery

Stop use and ask a doctor if

- new symptoms occur
- redness or swelling is present
- you get nervous, dizzy, or sleepless
- fever gets worse or lasts more than 3 days
- pain or nasal congestion gets worse or lasts more than 7 days

If pregnant or breast-feeding, ask a health professional before use.

Keep out of reach of children.

Overdose warning: Taking more than the recommended dose (overdose) can cause serious health problems. In case of overdose, get medical help or contact a Poison Control Center right away. Quick medical attention is critical for adults as well as for children even if you do not notice any signs or symptoms.

Directions:

- **do not take more than directed** (see Overdose warning)
- **adults and children 12 years and over:** take 2 caplets every 6 hours as needed. Do not take more than 8 caplets in 24 hours.
- **children under 12 years:** ask a doctor

Other Information: store at 20 ° – 25°C (68° – 77°F)

Inactive Ingredients: carnauba wax, D&C yellow #10 aluminum lake, FD&C yellow #6 aluminum lake, magnesium stearate, microcrystalline cellulose, polyethylene glycol, polyvinyl alcohol, povidone, sodium starch glycolate, starch, stearic acid, talc, titanium dioxide

Questions or comments? call toll-free **1-800-245-1040** weekdays

How Supplied: Available in 24ct. and 36ct. boxes.

Shown in Product Identification Guide, page 505

CONTAC® Non-Drowsy (GlaxoSmithKline Consumer) Decongestant 12 Hour Cold Caplets

Product Information: Each Maximum Strength Contac 12 Hour Cold Caplet provides up to 12 hours of relief. Part of the caplet goes to work right away for fast relief; the rest is released gradually to provide up to 12 hours of prolonged relief. With just one caplet in the morning and one at bedtime, you feel better all day, sleep better at night, breathing freely without congestion or sinus pressure.

Indications: Temporarily relieves nasal congestion due to the common cold, hay fever or other upper respiratory allergies and associated with sinusitis. Helps decongest sinus openings and passages; temporarily relieves sinus congestion and pressure.

Directions: Adults and children over 12 years of age: One caplet every 12 hours, not to exceed 2 caplets in 24 hours, or as directed by a doctor. Children under 12 years of age: consult a doctor.

TAMPER-EVIDENT PACKAGING FEATURES FOR YOUR PROTECTION:

Each caplet is encased in a plastic cell with a foil back; do not use if cell or foil is broken.

Warnings: Do not exceed the recommended dosage. If nervousness, dizziness, or sleeplessness occur, discontinue use and consult a doctor. If symptoms do not improve within 7 days or are accompanied by high fever, consult a doctor. Do not take this product, unless directed by a doctor, if you have heart disease, high blood pressure, thyroid disease, diabetes, glaucoma or difficulty in urination due to enlargement of the prostate gland. KEEP THIS AND ALL DRUGS OUT OF REACH OF CHILDREN. IN CASE OF ACCIDENTAL OVERDOSE, SEEK PROFESSIONAL ASSISTANCE OR CONTACT A POISON CONTROL CENTER IMMEDIATELY. As with any drug, if you are pregnant or nursing a baby, seek the advice of a health professional before using this product.

Drug Interaction Precaution: Do not use this product if you are now taking a prescription monoamine oxidase inhibitor (MAOI) (certain drugs for depression, psychiatric or emotional conditions, or Parkinson's disease), or for 2 weeks after stopping the MAOI drug. If you are uncertain whether your prescription drug contains an MAOI, consult a health professional before taking this product.

Active Ingredient: Pseudoephedrine Hydrochloride 120 mg. Store at 15° to 25°C (59° to 77°F) in a dry place and protest from light.

Each Caplet Also Contains: Carnauba Wax, Colloidal Silicon Dioxide, Dibasic Calcium Phosphate, Hypromellose, Magnesium Stearate, Microcrystalline Cellulose, Polyethylene Glycol, Polysorbate 80, Titanium Dioxide.

How Supplied: Consumer packages of 10 and 20 caplets.

Note: There are other CONTAC products. Make sure this is the one you are interested in. See the table below for all of the products in the CONTAC line.

Shown in Product Identification Guide, page 505

CONTAC®-D COLD NON-DROWSY DECONGESTANT (GlaxoSmithKline Consumer)

Drug Facts

Active Ingredient: **Purpose:** **(per tablet)**

Phenylephrine hydrochloride 10 mg .... Nasal decongestant

Uses:

temporarily relieves

- nasal congestion
- sinus congestion and pressure
- stuffy nose
- temporarily restores freer breathing through nose
- reduces swelling of nasal passages, shrinks swollen membranes

Warnings:

Do not use if you are now taking a prescription monoamine oxidase inhibitor (MAOI) (certain drugs for depression, psychiatric, or emotional conditions, or Parkinson's disease), or for 2 weeks after stopping the MAOI drug. If you do not know if your prescription drug contains an MAOI, ask a doctor or pharmacist before taking this product.

Ask a doctor before use if you have

- heart disease
- high blood pressure
- thyroid disease
- diabetes
- trouble urinating due to enlargement of the prostate gland

When using this product do not exceed recommended dosage

Stop use and ask a doctor if

- you get nervous, dizzy, or sleepless
- symptoms do not improve within 7 days or are accompanied by fever

If pregnant or breast-feeding, ask a health professional before use.

Keep out of reach of children. In case of overdose, get medical help or contact a Poison Control Center right away.

Directions:

- **adults and children 12 and over:** take 1 tablet every 4 hours as needed. Do not take more than 6 tablets in 24 hours.
- **children under 12:** ask a doctor

Other Information: store at 59°-86°F

Inactive Ingredients: carnauba wax, dibasic calcium phosphate, FD&C red

Continued on next page

Contac—Cont.

#40 aluminum lake, lecithin, magnesium stearate, microcrystalline cellulose, polyethylene glycol, polyvinyl alcohol, silicon dioxide, talc, titanium dioxide

Questions or comments? call toll-free **1-800-245-1040** weekdays

How Supplied: Available in 24ct. and 36ct. boxes.

DELSYM®
(dextromethorphan polistirex)
Extended-Release Suspension
12-Hour Cough Suppressant
(UCB Pharma)

Active Ingredient (in each 5 mL teaspoonful): dextromethorphan polistirex equivalent to 30 mg dextromethorphan hydrobromide.
Purpose: Cough suppressant

Use: Temporarily relieves cough due to minor throat and bronchial irritation as may occur with the common cold or inhaled irritants.

Warnings: Do not use if you are now taking a prescription monoamine oxidase inhibitor (MAOI) (certain drugs for depression, psychiatric or emotional conditions, or Parkinson's disease), or for 2 weeks after stopping the MAOI drug. If you do not know if your prescription drug contains an MAOI, ask a doctor or pharmacist before taking this product.
Ask a doctor before use if you have
• chronic cough that lasts as occurs with smoking, asthma or emphysema
• cough that occurs with too much phlegm (mucus)
Stop use and ask a doctor if cough lasts more than 7 days, cough comes back, or occurs with fever, rash or headache that lasts. These could be signs of a serious condition.
If pregnant or breast-feeding, ask a health professional before use.
Keep out of reach of children. In case of overdose, get medical help or contact a Poison Control Center right away.

Directions:
• **shake bottle well before use**
• dose as follows or as directed by a doctor

adults and children 12 years of age and over	2 teaspoonfuls every 12 hours, not to exceed 4 teaspoonfuls in 24 hours
children 6 to under 12 years of age	1 teaspoonful every 12 hours, not to exceed 2 teaspoonfuls in 24 hours
children 2 to under 6 years of age	½ teaspoonful every 12 hours, not to exceed 1 teaspoonful in 24 hours
children under 2 years of age	consult a doctor

Other Information:
• **each 5 mL teaspoonful contains:** sodium 6 mg
• store at 20°–25°C (68°–77°F)

Inactive Ingredients: citric acid, edetate disodium, ethycellulose, FD&C Yellow No. 6, flavor, high fructose corn syrup, methylparaben, polyethylene glycol 3350, polysorbate 80, propylene glycol, propylparaben, purified water, sucrose, tragacanth, vegetable oil, xanthan gum.

How Supplied:
Delsym® 3 oz. Classic SKU
NDC 53014-463-61
Delsym® 5 oz. Classic SKU
NDC 53014-463-56
Delsym® 3 oz. Children's SKU
NDC 53014-463-43
Delsym® 5 oz. Children's SKU
NDC 53014-463-48
Manufactured by
UCB Manufacturing, Inc.
Rochester, NY 14623 USA
Shown in Product Identification Guide, page 517

CHILDREN'S DIMETAPP® COLD & ALLERGY CHEWABLE TABLETS
(Wyeth Consumer)
Antihistamine/Nasal decongestant

Active Ingredients (in each tablet):
Brompheniramine maleate, USP 1 mg
Phenylephrine HCl, USP 2.5 mg

Uses:
• temporarily relieves nasal congestion due to the common cold, hay fever or other upper respiratory allergies
• temporarily relieves these symptoms due to hay fever (allergic rhinitis) or other upper respiratory allergies:
  • runny nose
  • sneezing
  • itchy, watery eyes
  • itching of the nose or throat
• temporarily restores freer breathing through the nose

Warnings:
Do not use
• in a child under 2 years of age
• in a child who is taking a prescription monoamine oxidase inhibitor (MAOI) (certain drugs for depression, psychiatric, or emotional conditions, or Parkinson's disease), or for 2 weeks after stopping the MAOI drug. If you do not know if your child's prescription drug contains an MAOI, ask a doctor or pharmacist before giving this product.
Ask a doctor before use if the child has
• heart disease
• high blood pressure
• thyroid disease
• diabetes
• glaucoma
• a breathing problem such as emphysema or chronic bronchitis

Ask a doctor or pharmacist before use if the child is taking sedatives or tranquilizers.
When using this product
• **do not use more than directed**
• drowsiness may occur
• sedatives and tranquilizers may increase drowsiness
• excitability may occur, especially in children
Stop use and ask a doctor if
• the child gets nervous, dizzy, or sleepless
• symptoms do not get better within 7 days or are accompanied by fever
Keep out of reach of children. In case of overdose, get medical help or contact a Poison Control Center right away.

Directions:
• do not give more than 6 doses in any 24-hour period

age	dose
children 6 to under 12 years	2 tablets every 4 hours
children 2 to under 6 years	ask a doctor
children under 2 years	do not use

Other Information:
• store at 20–25°C (68–77°F)

Inactive Ingredients: artificial and natural flavors, carmine, carrageenan, croscarmellose sodium, fructose, fumaric acid, glycine, magnesium stearate, maltodextrin, mannitol, microcrystalline cellulose, modified starch, polyethylene oxide, silicon dioxide, sorbitol, sucralose, tribasic calcium phosphate

How Supplied:
Packages of 20 chewable tablets

CHILDREN'S DIMETAPP® Cold & Allergy Elixir (Wyeth Consumer)
Antihistamine, Nasal Decongestant

Active Ingredients:
Each 5 mL (1 teaspoonful) contains:
Brompheniramine Maleate, USP 1 mg
Phenylephrine Hydrochloride, USP 2.5 mg

Uses:
• temporarily relieves nasal congestion due to the common cold, hay fever or other upper respiratory allergies
• temporarily relieves these symptoms due to hay fever (allergic rhinitis):
  • runny nose
  • sneezing
  • itchy, watery eyes
  • itching of the nose or throat
• temporarily restores freer breathing through the nose

Warnings:

Do not use

- in a child under 2 years of age
- if you are now taking a prescription monoamine oxidase inhibitor (MAOI) (certain drugs for depression, psychiatric, or emotional conditions, or Parkinson's disease), or for 2 weeks after stopping the MAOI drug. If you do not know if your prescription drug contains an MAOI, ask a doctor or pharmacist before taking this product.

Ask a doctor before use if you have

- heart disease
- high blood pressure
- thyroid disease
- diabetes
- trouble urinating due to an enlarged prostate gland
- glaucoma
- a breathing problem such as emphysema or chronic bronchitis

Ask a doctor or pharmacist before use if you are taking sedatives or tranquilizers.

When using this product

- **do not use more than directed**
- drowsiness may occur
- avoid alcoholic beverages
- alcohol, sedatives, and tranquilizers may increase drowsiness
- be careful when driving a motor vehicle or operating machinery
- excitability may occur, especially in children

Stop use and ask a doctor if

- you get nervous, dizzy, or sleepless
- symptoms do not get better within 7 days or are accompanied by fever

If pregnant or breast-feeding, ask a health professional before use.

Keep out of reach of children. In case of overdose, get medical help or contact a Poison Control Center right away.

Directions:

- do not take more than 6 doses in any 24-hour period

age	dose
adults and children 12 years and over	4 tsp every 4 hours
children 6 to under 12 years	2 tsp every 4 hours
children 2 to under 6 years	ask a doctor
children under 2 years	do not use

Each teaspoon contains: sodium 3 mg. Store at 20–25°C (68–77°F). Dosage cup provided.

Inactive Ingredients: artificial flavor, citric acid, FD&C blue no. 1, FD&C red no. 40, glycerin, propylene glycol, purified water, sodium benzoate, sodium citrate, sorbitol, sucralose

How Supplied: Purple, grape-flavored liquid in bottles of 4 fl oz, 8 fl oz, and 12 fl oz.

CHILDREN'S DIMETAPP® DM COLD & COUGH Elixir (Wyeth Consumer)
Antihistamine, Cough Suppressant, Nasal Decongestant

Active Ingredients: Each 5 mL (1 teaspoonful) contains

Brompheniramine
    Maleate, USP 1 mg
Dextromethorphan
    Hydrobromide, USP 5 mg
Phenylephrine
    Hydrochloride, USP 2.5 mg

Uses:

- temporarily relieves cough due to minor throat and bronchial irritation occurring with a cold, and nasal congestion due to the common cold, hay fever or other upper respiratory allergies
- temporarily relieves these symptoms due to hay fever (allergic rhinitis):
  - runny nose
  - sneezing
  - itchy, watery eyes
  - itching of the nose or throat
- temporarily restores freer breathing through the nose

Warnings:

Do not use

- in a child under 2 years of age
- if you are now taking a prescription monoamine oxidase inhibitor (MAOI) (certain drugs for depression, psychiatric, or emotional conditions, or Parkinson's disease), or for 2 weeks after stopping the MAOI drug. If you do not know if your prescription drug contains an MAOI, ask a doctor or pharmacist before taking this product.

Ask a doctor before use if you have

- heart disease
- high blood pressure
- thyroid disease
- diabetes
- trouble urinating due to an enlarged prostate gland
- glaucoma
- cough that occurs with too much phlegm (mucus)
- a breathing problem or persistent or chronic cough that lasts such as occurs with smoking, asthma, chronic bronchitis, or emphysema

Ask a doctor or pharmacist before use if you are taking sedatives or tranquilizers.

When using this product

- **do not use more than directed**
- may cause marked drowsiness
- avoid alcoholic beverages
- alcohol, sedatives, and tranquilizers may increase drowsiness
- be careful when driving a motor vehicle or operating machinery
- excitability may occur, especially in children

Stop use and ask a doctor if

- you get nervous, dizzy, or sleepless
- symptoms do not get better within 7 days or are accompanied by fever
- cough lasts more than 7 days, comes back, or is accompanied by fever, rash,

or persistent headache. These could be signs of a serious condition

If pregnant or breast-feeding, ask a health professional before use.

Keep out of reach of children. In case of overdose, get medical help or contact a Poison Control Center right away.

Directions:

- do not take more than 6 doses in any 24-hour period

Age	Dose
adults and children 12 years and over	4 tsp every 4 hours
children 6 to under 12 years	2 tsp every 4 hours
children 2 to under 6 years	ask a doctor
children under 2 years	do not use

Each teaspoon contains: sodium 3 mg Store at 20–25°C (68–77°F). Dosage cup provided.

Inactive Ingredients: artificial flavor, citric acid, FD&C blue no. 1, FD&C red no. 40, glycerin, propylene glycol, purified water, sodium benzoate, sodium citrate, sorbitol, sucralose

How Supplied: Purple, grape-flavored liquid in bottles of 4 fl oz and 8 fl oz.

CHILDREN'S DIMETAPP® LONG ACTING COUGH PLUS COLD SYRUP (Wyeth Consumer)
Cough suppressant/Antihistamine

Active Ingredients (in each 5 mL tsp):

Chlorpheniramine maleate, USP 1.0 mg
Dextromethorphan HBr, USP 7.5 mg

Uses:

- temporarily relieves cough due to minor throat and bronchial irritation as may occur with a cold
- temporarily relieves these symptoms due to hay fever or other upper respiratory allergies:
  - runny nose • sneezing • itchy, watery eyes • itching of the nose or throat

Warnings:

Do not use if you are now taking a prescription monoamine oxidase inhibitor (MAOI) (certain drugs for depression, psychiatric, or emotional conditions, or Parkinson's disease), or for 2 weeks after stopping the MAOI drug. If you do not know if your prescription drug contains an MAOI, ask a doctor or pharmacist before taking this product.

Ask a doctor before use if you have

- trouble urinating due to an enlarged prostate gland
- glaucoma

Continued on next page

Children's Dimetapp—Cont.

- a cough that occurs with too much phlegm (mucus)
- a breathing problem or chronic cough that lasts or as occurs with smoking, asthma, chronic bronchitis or emphysema

Ask a doctor or pharmacist before use if you are taking sedatives or tranquilizers.

When using this product
- **do not use more than directed**
- marked drowsiness may occur • avoid alcoholic drinks
- alcohol, sedatives, and tranquilizers may increase drowsiness
- be careful when driving a motor vehicle or operating machinery
- excitability may occur, especially in children

Stop use and ask a doctor if cough lasts more than 7 days, comes back, or is accompanied by fever, rash, or persistent headache. These could be signs of a serious condition.

If pregnant or breast-feeding, ask a health professional before use.

Keep out of reach of children. In case of overdose, get medical help or contact a Poison Control Center right away.

Directions:
- do not take more than 4 doses in any 24-hour period

age	dose
12 years and older	4 tsp every 6 hours
6 to under 12 years	2 tsp every 6 hours
under 6 years	ask a doctor

Other Information: • **each teaspoon contains:** sodium 3 mg
- store at 20–25°C (68–77°F)
- dosage cup provided

Inactive Ingredients: artificial flavor, anhydrous citric acid, FD&C blue no. 1, FD&C red no. 40, glycerin, propylene glycol, purified water, sodium benzoate, sodium citrate, sorbitol, sucralose

How Supplied: Bottles of 4 fl. oz.

TODDLER'S DIMETAPP COLD AND COUGH DROPS (Wyeth Consumer)
Cough suppressant/Nasal decongestant

Active Ingredients: Each 0.8 mL contains: 2.5 mg Dextromethorphan Hydrobromide, USP; 1.25 mg Phenylephrine Hydrochloride, USP.

Indications: Temporarily relieves cough occurring with the common cold and temporarily relieves nasal congestion due to the common cold, hay fever, or other upper respiratory allergies

Warnings:
Do not use
- in a child under 2 years of age
- in a child who is taking a prescription monoamine oxidase inhibitor (MAOI) (certain drugs for depression, psychiatric, or emotional conditions, or Parkinson's disease), or for 2 weeks after stopping the MAOI drug. If you do not know if your child's prescription drug contains an MAOI, ask a doctor or pharmacist before giving this product.

Ask a doctor before use if the child has
- heart disease
- high blood pressure
- thyroid disease
- diabetes
- cough that occurs with too much phlegm (mucus)
- cough that lasts or is chronic such as occurs with asthma

When using this product do not use more than directed

Stop use and ask a doctor if
- the child gets nervous, dizzy, or sleepless
- symptoms do not get better within 7 days or are accompanied by fever
- cough lasts more than 7 days, comes back, or is accompanied by fever, rash, or persistent headache. These could be signs of a serious condition.

Keep out of reach of children. In case of overdose, get medical help or contact a Poison Control Center right away.

Directions: do not give more than 6 doses in any 24-hour period
- repeat every 4 hours or as directed by a physician
- measure with the dosing device provided. Do not use with any other device.

age	dose
under 2 years	do not use
2 to under 6 years	1.6 mL

Other Information: • store at 20–25°C (68–77°F) • oral dosing device enclosed

Inactive Ingredients: anhydrous citric acid, artificial flavor, glycerin, propylene glycol, purified water, sodium benzoate, sorbitol solution, sucralose

How Supplied: ½ oz bottle with oral dosing device.

EXCEDRIN® EXTRA STRENGTH (Novartis Consumer Health, Inc.)
PAIN RELIEVER

For full product information see page 684.

GOODY'S®
(GlaxoSmithKline Consumer)
Extra Strength Pain Relief Tablets

For full product information see page 685.

HUMIBID® (Adams Respiratory Therapeutics)
1200 mg Guaifenesin Extended-Release Bi-Layer Tablets
Expectorant

For full product information see page 720.

HYLAND'S COMPLETE FLU CARE 4 KIDS (Standard Homeopathic)

Active Ingredients: EUPATORIUM PERFOLIATUM 3X HPUS, BRYONIA 3X HPUS, GELSEMIUM SEMPERVIRENS 3X HPUS EUPHARSIA OFFICINALIS 3X HPUS, KALI IODATUM 3X HPUS ANAS BARBARIAE HEPATIS ET CORDIS EXTRACTUM 200C HPUS

Inactive Ingredients: Lactose, N.F.

Indications: Temporarily relieves the symptoms of fever, chills, body aches, headache, cough and congestion from the flu or common cold

Directions: Children ages 2-5: Dissolve 2 tablets under tongue every 15 minutes for up to 8 doses until relieved; Then every 4 hours as required.
Children ages 6-11: Dissolve 3 tablets under tongue Every 15 minutes for up to 8 doses until relieved; Then every 4 hours as required.
Children 12 years and over: Dissolve 4 tablets under tongue every 15 minutes for up to 8 does until relieved; then every 4 hours as are required or as recommended by a health care professional

Warnings: Ask a doctor before use if: pregnant or nursing, consult a physician if symptoms persist for more than 7 days. Keep this and all medications out of reach of children.
Do not use if imprinted tamper band is broken or missing. In case of accidental overdose, contact a poison control center immediately. In case of emergency, the manufacturer may be contacted 24 hours a day, 7 days a week at 800/624-9659.

How Supplied: Bottles of 125 1 grain Tablets (NDC 54973-3016-01). Store at room temperature.

HYLAND'S SNIFFLES'N SNEEZES 4 KIDS (Standard Homeopathic)

Active Ingredients: ACONITUM NAPELLUS 6X HPUS, ALLIUM CEPA 6X HPUS, ZINCUM GLUCONICUM 2X HPUS, GELSENIUM SEMPERVIRENS 6X HPUS.

Inactive Ingredients: Lactose, N.F.

Indications: Temporarily relieves the symptoms of the common cold.

Directions: Children ages 2-5: dissolve 2 tablets under tongue every 15 minutes for up to 8 doses until relieved; then every 4 hours as required. Children ages 6-11:

dissolve 3 tablets under tongue every 15 minutes for up to 8 doses until relieved; then every 4 hours as required. Children 12 years and older: dissolve 4 tablets under tongue every 15 minutes for up to 8 doses until relieved; then every 4 hours as required or as recommended by a health care professional.

Warnings: Ask a doctor before use if pregnant or nursing. Consult a physician if: symptoms persist for more than 7 days or worsen. Inflammation, fever or infection develops. Symptoms are accompanied by high fever. (over 101 ° F) Keep this and all medications out of the reach of children. Do not use if imprinted tamper band is broken or missing. In case of accidental overdose, contact a poison control center immediately. In case of emergency, the manufacturer may be contacted 24 hours a day, 7 days a week at 800/624-9659.

How Supplied: Bottles of 125 1 grain tablets (NDC 54973-7519-1). Store at room temperature.

CHILDREN'S MOTRIN® Cold
(McNeil Consumer)
ibuprofen/pseudoephedrine HCl
Oral Suspension

Description:

Children's MOTRIN® Cold Oral Suspension is an alcohol-free berry-flavored suspension. Each 5 mL (teaspoonful) contains the pain reliever/fever reducer ibuprofen 100 mg and the nasal decongestant pseudoephedrine HCl 15 mg.

Uses:
- temporarily relieves these cold, sinus and flu symptoms:
  - nasal and sinus congestion
  - stuffy nose • headache • sore throat
  - minor body aches and pains • fever

Directions:

See Table 2: Children's Motrin Dosing Chart on pg. 734.

Warnings:
Allergy alert: Ibuprofen may cause a severe allergic reaction, especially in people allergic to aspirin.
Symptoms may include:
- hives • facial swelling • asthma (wheezing) • shock • skin reddening • rash • blisters
If an allergic reaction occurs, stop use and seek medical help right away.
Stomach bleeding warning: This product contains a nonsteroidal anti-inflammatory drug (NSAID), which may cause stomach bleeding. The chance is higher if the child:
- has had stomach ulcers or bleeding problems
- takes a blood thinning (anticoagulant) or steroid drug

- takes other drugs containing an NSAID (aspirin, ibuprofen, naproxen, or others)
- takes more or for a longer time than directed

Sore throat warning: Severe or persistent sore throat or sore throat accompanied by high fever, headache, nausea, and vomiting may be serious. Consult doctor promptly. Do not use more than 2 days or administer to children under 3 years of age unless directed by doctor.
Do not use
- if the child has ever had an allergic reaction to any other pain reliever/fever reducer and/or nasal decongestant
- right before or after heart surgery
- in a child who is taking a prescription monoamine oxidase inhibitor [MAOI] (certain drugs for depression, psychiatric or emotional conditions, or Parkinson's disease), or for 2 weeks after stopping the MAOI drug. If you do not know if your child's prescription drug contains an MAOI, ask a doctor or pharmacist before giving this product.

Ask a doctor before use if the child has
- problems or serious side effects from taking pain relievers, fever reducers, or nasal decongestants
- stomach problems that last or come back, such as heartburn, upset stomach, or stomach pain
- ulcers
- bleeding problems
- not been drinking fluids
- lost a lot of fluid due to vomiting or diarrhea
- high blood pressure
- heart or kidney disease
- thyroid disease
- diabetes
- taken a diuretic

Ask a doctor before use if the child is
- taking any other drug containing an NSAID (prescription or nonprescription) and/or pseudoephedrine or any other nasal decongestant
- taking a blood thinning (anticoagulant) or steroid drug
- under a doctor's care for any serious condition
- taking any other drug

When using this product
- **do not exceed recommended dosage**
- take with food or milk if stomach upset occurs
- long term continuous use may increase the risk of heart attack or stroke

Stop use and ask a doctor if
- the child feels faint, vomits blood, or has bloody or black stools. These are signs of stomach bleeding.
- stomach pain or upset gets worse or lasts
- the child does not get any relief within first day (24 hours) of treatment
- fever, pain, or nasal congestion gets worse or lasts more than 3 days
- redness or swelling is present in the painful area
- any new symptoms appear

- the child gets nervous, dizzy, or sleepless

Keep out of reach of children. In case of overdose, get medical help or contact a Poison Control Center right away. (1-800-222-1222)

Other Information:
- store between 20–25°C (68–77°F)

PROFESSIONAL INFORMATION: OVERDOSAGE INFORMATION

For overdosage information, please refer to pg. 680.

Inactive Ingredients:

acesulfame potassium, citric acid, corn starch, D&C yellow #10, FD&C red #40, flavors, glycerin, polysorbate 80, purified water, sodium benzoate, sucrose, xanthan gum.

How Supplied:

Berry-flavored, pink-colored liquid in child resistant tamper-evident bottles of 4 fl. oz.

Shown in Product Identification Guide, page 508

CHILDREN'S MOTRIN®
Dosing Chart
(McNeil Consumer)

[See table on next page]

MUCINEX®
(Adams Respiratory Therapeutics)
600 mg Guaifenesin Extended-Release Bi-Layer Tablets
Expectorant

For full product information see page 720.

MUCINEX® DM
(Adams Respiratory Therapeutics)
600 mg Guaifenesin and 30 mg Dextromethorphan HBr Extended-Release Bi-Layer Tablets
Expectorant and Cough Suppressant

For full product information see page 720.

NASAL COMFORT™ (Matrixx)
Moisture Therapy

Scented:

Ingredients: Purified water, high purity sodium chloride, spearmint oil (no preservatives).

Unscented:

Ingredients: Purified water, high purity sodium chloride, aloe vera (no preservatives).

Continued on page 735

Table 2. Children's Motrin Dosing Chart

AGE GROUP*	0-5 mos*	6-11 mos	12-23 mos	2-3 yrs	4-5 yrs	6-8 yrs	9-10 yrs	11 yrs	Maximum doses/ 24 hrs
WEIGHT	6-11 lbs	12-17 lbs	18-23 lbs	24-35 lbs	36-47 lbs	48-59 lbs	60-71 lbs	72-95 lbs	
PRODUCT FORM / INGREDIENTS	Dose to be administered based on weight or age†								
Infants' Drops	Per 1.25 mL								
Infants' Motrin Concentrated Drops — Ibuprofen 50 mg		1.25 mL	1.875 mL	—	—	—	—	—	4 times in 24 hrs
Children's Liquid	Per 5 mL = 1 teaspoonful (TSP)								
Children's Motrin Suspension — Ibuprofen 100 mg		—	—	1 TSP or 5 mL	1 ½ TSP or 7.5 mL	2 TSP or 10 mL	2 ½ TSP or 12.5 mL	3 TSP or 15 mL	4 times in 24 hrs
Children's Motrin Cold Suspension Liquid† — Ibuprofen 100 mg, Pseudoephedrine HCl 15 mg		—	—	1 TSP or 5 mL	1 TSP or 5 mL	2 TSP or 10 mL	2 TSP or 10 mL	2 TSP or 10 mL	4 times in 24 hrs
Junior Strength Tablets & Caplets	Per tablet/ caplet								
Junior Strength Motrin Chewable Tablets — Ibuprofen 100 mg		—	—	—	—	2 tablets	2 ½ tablets	3 tablets	4 times in 24 hrs
Junior Strength Motrin Caplets — Ibuprofen 100 mg		—	—	—	—	2 caplets	2 ½ caplets	3 caplets	4 times in 24 hrs

†Do not give more than directed. If needed, repeat dose every 6-8 hours; except for Children's Motrin Cold which is every 6 hours.

* Under 6 mos, ask a doctor.

- Infants' drops: Shake well before using. Dispense liquid slowly into the child's mouth, toward the inner cheek.
- Infants' Motrin Drops are more concentrated than Children's Motrin Liquids. The Infants' Concentrated Drops have been specifically designed for use only with enclosed dosing device. Do not use any other dosing device with this product.
- Children's Motrin Liquids are less concentrated than Infants' Motrin Drops. The Children's Motrin Liquids have been specifically designed for use with the enclosed measuring cup. Use only enclosed measuring cup to dose this product. Shake well before using.
- Children's Motrin Suspensions (including cold)—replace original bottle cap to maintain child resistance
- Do not give longer than 10 days, unless directed by a doctor (see WARNINGS).

Description:

Makes Breathing Easier

Dry heated rooms, air conditioning, allergens, colds, certain medications and environmental pollutants all contribute to the irritation and dehydration of nasal passages. Nasal Comfort™ Moisture Therapy not only soothes and moisturizes sensitive nasal membranes, but also helps your nose cleanse and filter the air you breathe. Used twice a day, our pure hypertonic formula provides refreshing relief from dryness, irritation and conditions that can lead to congestion.

- Safe to use with all medications
- Non-habit forming
- *Preservative Free* and so pure you can use it as often as you need it
- Spearmint oil is light, refreshing and soothes nasal passages
- Patented *Micro-Filtration Sprayer* prevents product contamination and is easy to use

Discover easier, more comfortable breathing. Make Nasal Comfort™ Moisture Therapy part of your daily routine.

Instructions: Shake well before every use. Before first use, prime sprayer until the fine mist is delivered. Use twice daily (before bed and in the morning), or as often as needed. One spray per nostril. Wipe nozzle clean after each use. For more information, see enclosed insert. 1 oz bottle lasts 45 days when used twice daily.

Other Information:

Do not share sprayer with others as this may spread germs.
Keep out of reach of children.

How Supplied: 1 FL. OZ.

Shown in Product Identification Guide, page 507

REFENESEN™ 400 NON-DROWSY
[rĕ-fĕn-ə-sĕn]
IMMEDIATE RELEASE
EXPECTORANT CAPLETS
(Reese)

REFENESEN™ DM NON-DROWSY
IMMEDIATE RELEASE
EXPECTORANT & COUGH
SUPPRESSANT CAPLETS

REFENESEN™ PE NON-DROWSY
IMMEDIATE RELEASE
EXPECTORANT & NASAL
DECONGESTANT CAPLETS

Expectorant, nasal decongestant, cough suppressant

For full product information see page 721.

ROBITUSSIN Cough & Cold CF
Liquid (Wyeth Consumer)
ROBITUSSIN Cough & Cold
Pediatric Drops
Cough Suppressant/Expectorant/
Nasal decongestant

Active Ingredients: (in each 5 mL tsp Robitussin Cough & Cold CF)

Dextromethorphan HBr, USP ...... 10 mg
Guaifenesin, USP .... 100 mg
Phenylephrine, HCl .... 5 mg
(in each 2.5mL Robitussin Cough & Cold Pediatric Drops)
Dextromethorphan HBr, USP .... 5 mg
Guaifenesin, USP .... 100 mg
Phenylephrine HCl .... 2.5 mg

Uses:

- temporarily relieves these symptoms occurring with a cold:
  - nasal congestion
  - cough due to minor throat and bronchial irritation
- helps loosen phlegm (mucus) and thin bronchial secretions to drain bronchial tubes

Warnings:

Do not use:

- in a child under 2 years of age
- if you or your child are taking a prescription monoamine oxidase inhibitor (MAOI) (certain drugs for depression, psychiatric, or emotional conditions, or Parkinson's disease), or for 2 weeks after stopping the MAOI drug. If you do not know if your child's or your prescription drug contains an MAOI, ask a doctor or pharmacist before taking this product or giving it to your child.

Ask a doctor before use if you or your child has

- heart disease
- high blood pressure
- thyroid disease
- diabetes
- trouble urinating due to an enlarged prostate gland
- cough that occurs with too much phlegm (mucus)
- cough that lasts or is chronic such as occurs with smoking, asthma, chronic bronchitis or emphysema

When using this product do not use more than directed.

Stop use and ask a doctor if

- you or your child gets nervous, dizzy, or sleepless
- symptoms do not get better within 7 days or are accompanied by fever
- cough lasts more than 7 days, comes back, or is accompanied by fever, rash, or persistent headache. These could be signs of a serious condition.

If pregnant or breast-feeding, ask a health professional before use.

Keep out of reach of children. In case of overdose, get medical help or contact a Poison Control Center right away.

Directions: (Robitussin Cough & Cold CF):

- do not take more than 6 doses in any 24-hour period
- adults and children 12 yrs and over: 2 tsp every 4 hours
- children 6 to under 12 yrs: 1 tsp every 4 hours
- children 2 to under 6 yrs: ½ tsp or 2.5 mL every 4 hours

- children under 2 yrs: do not use

Directions: (Robitussin Cough & Cold Pediatric Drops):

- do not use more than 6 doses in any 24-hour period
- repeat every 4 hours
- choose dosage by weight (if weight is not known, choose by age)
- measure with the dosing device provided. Do not use with any other device.
- 24–47 lbs (2 to under 6 yrs): 2.5 mL
- under 24 lbs (under 2 yrs): do not use

Other Information:

- store at 20–25°C (68–77°F)
- alcohol-free
- dosage cup or oral dosing device provided

Inactive Ingredients: (Robitussin Cough & Cold CF) artificial and natural flavor, citric acid, FD&C red no. 40, glycerin, lactic acid, menthol, propylene glycol, purified water, sodium benzoate, sorbitol, sucralose
(Robitussin Cough & Cold Pediatric Drops) anhydrous citric acid, artificial & natural flavor, FD&C red no. 40, glycerin, lactic acid, polyethylene glycol, propylene glycol, purified water, sodium benzoate, sodium citrate, sorbitol solution, sucralose

How Supplied: Robitussin Cough & Cold CF (red-colored) in bottles of 4, 8, and 12 fl oz. Robitussin Cough & Cold Pediatric Drops in 1 fl oz bottles

---

ROBITUSSIN® Cough & Cold
(Wyeth Consumer)
Long-Acting
ROBITUSSIN® Pediatric Cough &
Cold Long-Acting
Cough Suppressant, Antihistamine

Active Ingredients (in each 5 mL tsp Robitussin Cough & Cold Long Acting):

Dextromethorphan HBr, USP 15 mg
Chlorpheniramine maleate, USP 2 mg
(in each 5 mL tsp Robitussin Pediatric Cough & Cold Long Acting):
Dextromethorphan HBr, USP 7.5 mg
Chlorpheniramine maleate, USP 1 mg

Uses:

- temporarily relieves cough due to minor throat and bronchial irritation as may occur with a cold
- temporarily relieves these symptoms due to hay fever or other upper respiratory allergies:
  - runny nose
  - sneezing
  - itchy, watery eyes
  - itching of the nose or throat

Warnings:

Do not use if you are now taking a prescription monoamine oxidase inhibitor (MAOI) (certain drugs for depression,

Continued on next page

Robitussin Cough & Cold—Cont.

psychiatric, or emotional conditions, or Parkinson's disease), or for 2 weeks after stopping the MAOI drug. If you do not know if your prescription drug contains an MAOI, ask a doctor or pharmacist before taking this product.

Ask a doctor before use if you have

- trouble urinating due to an enlarged prostate gland
- glaucoma
- a cough that occurs with too much phlegm (mucus)
- a breathing problem or chronic cough that lasts or as occurs with smoking, asthma, chronic bronchitis or emphysema

When using this product

- **do not use more than directed**
- marked drowsiness may occur
- avoid alcoholic drinks
- alcohol, sedatives and tranquilizers may increase drowsiness
- be careful when driving a motor vehicle or operating machinery
- excitability may occur, especially in children

Stop use and ask a doctor if cough lasts more than 7 days, comes back, or is accompanied by fever, rash, or persistent headache. These could be signs of a serious condition.

If pregnant or breast-feeding, ask a health professional before use. **Keep out of reach of children.** In case of overdose, get medical help or contact a Poison Control Center right away.

Directions:

- repeat dose every 6 hrs, as needed.
- do not take more than 4 doses in any 24-hour period

Robitussin® Cough & Cold Long-Acting:

- adults and children 12 years and over: 2 tsps
- children under 12 years: ask a doctor

Robitussin® Pediatric Cough & Cold Long-Acting:

- choose dosage by weight (if weight is not known, choose by age)
- under 48 lbs (under 6 yrs): ask a doctor
- 48–95 lbs (6 to under 12 yrs): 2 tsp
- 96 lbs and over (12 yrs and older): 4 tsp

Other Information: • store at 20–25°C (68–77°F) • dosage cup provided

Inactive Ingredients (Robitussin Cough & Cold Long Acting): artificial & natural flavor, citric acid, FD&C red no. 40, glycerin, lactic acid, menthol, propylene glycol, purified water, sodium benzoate, sodium citrate, sorbitol, sucralose

Inactive Ingredients (Robitussin Pediatric Cough & Cold Long Acting): artificial & natural flavor, citric acid, FD&C red no. 40, glycerin, lactic acid, propylene glycol, purified water, sodium benzoate, sodium citrate, sorbitol, sucralose

- **each teaspoon contains:** sodium 3 mg

How Supplied:

Robitussin Cough & Cold Long Acting: Red syrup in bottles of 4 fl oz
Robitussin Pediatric Cough & Cold Long Acting: (bright red) in bottles of 4 fl oz

---

ROBITUSSIN® Cough & Cold Nighttime (Wyeth Consumer)
ROBITUSSIN® Pediatric Cough & Cold Nighttime
ROBITUSSIN® Cough & Allergy
Nasal Decongestant, Cough Suppressant, Antihistamine

Active Ingredients: (in each 5 mL tsp Robitussin® Cough & Cold Nighttime and Robitussin® Pediatric Cough & Cold Nighttime)
Chlorpheniramine maleate, USP 1 mg
Dextromethorphan HBr, USP 5 mg
Phenylephrine HCl, USP 2.5 mg

Active Ingredients: (in each 5mL tsp Robitussin® Cough & Allergy)
Chlorpheniramine maleate, USP 2 mg
Dextromethorphan HBr, USP 10 mg
Phenylephrine HCl, USP 5 mg

Uses: (for Robitussin® Cough & Cold Nighttime and Robitussin® Pediatric Cough & Cold Nighttime)

- temporarily relieves these symptoms occurring with a cold:
  - cough due to minor throat and bronchial irritation
  - nasal congestion
- temporarily relieves these symptoms due to hay fever or other upper respiratory allergies:
  - runny nose
  - sneezing • itchy, watery eyes
  - itching of the nose or throat

Uses: (for Robitussin® Cough & Allergy)

- temporarily relieves these symptoms due to hay fever (allergic rhinitis):
  - runny nose
  - sneezing
  - itchy, watery eyes
  - itching of the nose or throat
  - nasal congestion
- temporarily controls cough due to minor throat and bronchial irritation associated with inhaled irritants
- temporarily restores freer breathing through the nose

Warnings:

Do not use • in a child under 2 years of age • if you are now taking a prescription monoamine oxidase inhibitor (MAOI) (certain drugs for depression, psychiatric, or emotional conditions, or Parkinson's disease), or for 2 weeks after stopping the MAOI drug. If you do not know if your prescription drug contains an MAOI, ask a doctor or pharmacist before taking this product.

Ask a doctor before use if you have:

- heart disease
- high blood pressure
- thyroid disease
- diabetes
- trouble urinating due to an enlarged prostate gland
- glaucoma
- a cough that occurs with too much phlegm (mucus)
- a breathing problem or chronic cough that lasts or as occurs with smoking, asthma, chronic bronchitis, or emphysema

Ask a doctor or pharmacist before use if you are taking sedatives or tranquilizers.

When using this product:

- **do not use more than directed**
- marked drowsiness may occur
- avoid alcoholic drinks
- alcohol, sedatives, and tranquilizers may increase drowsiness
- be careful when driving a motor vehicle or operating machinery
- excitability may occur, especially in children

Stop use and ask a doctor if:

- you get nervous, dizzy, or sleepless
- symptoms do not get better within 7 days or are accompanied by fever
- cough lasts more than 7 days, comes back, or is accompanied by fever, rash, or persistent headache. These could be signs of a serious condition.

If pregnant or breast-feeding, ask a health professional before use.

Keep out of reach of children. In case of overdose, get medical help or contact a Poison Control Center right away.

Directions:

- repeat dose every 4 hours
- do not take more than 6 doses in any 24-hour period

Robitussin® Cough & Cold Nighttime

- adults and children 12 years and over: 4 tsp
- children 6 to under 12 years: 2 tsp
- children 2 to under 6 years: ask a doctor
- children under 2 years: do not use

Robitussin® Pediatric Cough & Cold Nighttime

- choose dosage by weight (if weight is not known, choose by age)
- under 24 lbs (under 2 years): do not use
- 24–47 lbs (2 to under 6 yrs): ask a doctor
- 48–95 lbs (6 to under 12 yrs): 2 tsp
- 96 lbs and over (12 yrs and older): 4 tsp

Robitussin® Cough & Allergy

- adults and children 12 years and over: 2 tsp
- children 6 to under 12 years: 1 tsp
- children 2 to under 6 years: ask a doctor
- children under 2 years: do not use

Other Information:

- **each teaspoon contains:** sodium 3 mg
- store at 20–25°C (68–77°F)
- dosage cup provided

Inactive Ingredients:

Robitussin® Cough & Cold Nighttime

artificial and natural flavor, citric acid, FD&C red no. 40, glycerin, lactic acid, menthol, propylene glycol, purified water,

sodium benzoate, sodium citrate, sorbitol, sucralose

Robitussin® Pediatric Cough & Cold Nighttime

artificial and natural flavor, citric acid, FD&C red no. 40, glycerin, lactic acid, propylene glycol, purified water, sodium benzoate, sodium citrate, sorbitol, sucralose

Robitussin® Cough & Allergy

anhydrous citric acid, artificial and natural flavor, FD&C red no. 40, glycerin, lactic acid, menthol, propylene glycol, purified water, sodium benzoate, sodium citrate, sorbitol solution, sucralose

How Supplied:
Bottles of 4 fl. oz.

ROBITUSSIN® COUGH DROPS
(Wyeth Consumer)
Menthol Eucalyptus, Cherry and Honey-Lemon Flavors

ROBITUSSIN® HONEY COUGH DROPS
Honey-Lemon Tea, Natural Honey Center

ROBITUSSIN® SUGAR FREE Throat Drops
Natural Citrus

Active Ingredients:
Robitussin Cough Drops: (in each drop)
Menthol Eucalyptus:
Menthol, USP 10 mg
Cherry and Honey-Lemon:
Menthol, USP 5 mg
Robitussin Honey Cough Drops: (in each drop)
Natural Honey Center and *Honey Lemon Tea*
Menthol, USP 5 mg
Robitussin Sugar Free Throat Drops: (in each drop)
Menthol, USP 2.5 mg

Uses:
• temporarily relieves
 • occasional minor irritation, pain sore mouth, and sore throat
 • cough associated with a cold or inhaled irritants

Warnings:
Sore throat warning: Severe or persistent sore throat or sore throat accompanied by high fever, headache, nausea, and vomiting may be serious. Consult a doctor right away. Do not use more than 2 days or give to children under 3 years of age unless directed by a doctor.
Ask a doctor before use if you have
• cough that occurs with too much phlegm (mucus)
• cough that lasts or is chronic such as occurs with smoking, asthma, or emphysema

For ROBITUSSIN® SUGAR FREE Throat Drops:
When using this product excessive use may have a laxative effect.

For All ROBITUSSIN® Cough and Throat Drops:
Stop use and ask a doctor if cough lasts more than 7 days, comes back, or is accompanied by fever, rash, or persistent headache. These could signs of a serious condition.
If pregnant or breast-feeding, ask a health professional before use.
Keep out of reach of children.

Directions:
ROBITUSSIN® Cough Drops:
• adults and children 4 years and over: allow 1 drop to dissolve slowly in the mouth
• for sore throat: may be repeated every 2 hours, as needed, or as directed by a doctor
• for cough: may be repeated every 2 hours, as needed, or as directed by a doctor
• children under 4 years of age: ask a doctor

ROBITUSSIN® Honey Cough Drops:
• adults and children 4 years and over:
• for cough or sore throat: *Honey Lemon Tea and Natural Honey center--allow 1 drop to dissolve slowly in mouth.*
 May be repeated every 2 hours, as needed, or as directed by a doctor
• children under 4 years: ask a doctor

ROBITUSSIN® Sugar Free Throat Drops:
• adults and children 4 years and over: allow 2 drops to dissolve slowly in the mouth
• for sore throat: may be repeated every 2 hours, as needed, up to 9 drops per day, or as directed by a doctor
• for cough: may be repeated every 2 hours, as needed, up to 9 drops per day, or as directed by a doctor
• children under 4 years of age: ask a doctor

For ROBITUSSIN® Sugar Free Throat Drops:
• **phenylketonurics:** contains phenylalanine 3.37 mg per drop
• does not promote tooth decay
• product may be useful in a diabetic's diet on the advice of a doctor.
  3 Drops = FREE Exchange
  9 Drops = 1 Fruit
* The dietary exchanges are based on Exchange Lists for Meal Planning. Copyright 1995 by the American Diabetes Association Inc. and the American Dietetic Association.

Other Information:
Store at 20–25°C (68–77°F).

Inactive Ingredients:
ROBITUSSIN® Cough Drops:
Menthol Eucalyptus: corn syrup, eucalyptus oil, flavor, sucrose

Cherry: corn syrup, FD&C red no. 40, flavor, methylparaben, propylparaben, sodium benzoate, sucrose
Honey-Lemon: citric acid, corn syrup, D&C yellow no. 10, FD&C yellow no. 6, honey, lemon oil, methylparaben, povidone, propylparaben, sodium benzoate, sucrose

ROBITUSSIN® Honey Cough Drops:
Natural Honey Center: caramel, corn syrup, glycerin, high fructose corn syrup, honey, natural herbal flavor, sorbitol, sucrose
Honey Lemon Tea: caramel, citric acid, corn syrup, honey, natural flavor, sucrose, tea extract

ROBITUSSIN® Sugar Free Throat Drops: aspartame, canola oil, citric acid, D&C yellow no. 10 aluminum lake, FD&C blue no. 1, isomalt, maltitol, natural flavor

How Supplied:
ROBITUSSIN® Cough Drops:
All 3 flavors of Robitussin Cough Drops are available in bags of 25 drops.

ROBITUSSIN® Honey Cough Drops:
Honey Lemon Tea in bags of 25 drops. Natural Honey Center in bags of 20 drops.

ROBITUSSIN® Sugar Free Throat Drops:
Packages of 18 drops.

ROBITUSSIN® CoughGels
(Wyeth Consumer)
Long-Acting
Cough Suppressant

Active Ingredient (in each liquid-filled capsule):
Dextromethorphan HBr, USP 15 mg

Uses:
temporarily relieves cough due to minor throat and bronchial irritation as may occur with a cold.

Warnings:
Do not use if you are now taking a prescription monoamine oxidase inhibitor (MAOI) (certain drugs for depression, psychiatric, or emotional conditions, or Parkinson's disease), or for 2 weeks after stopping the MAOI drug. If you do not know if your prescription drug contains an MAOI, ask a doctor or pharmacist before taking this product.
Ask a doctor before use if you have
• a cough that occurs with too much phlegm (mucus)
• a cough that lasts or is chronic as occurs with smoking, asthma, or emphysema
Stop use and ask a doctor if cough lasts for more than 7 days, comes back, or is accompanied by fever, rash, or persistent headache. These could be signs of a serious condition.

Continued on next page

Robitussin—Cont.

If pregnant or breast-feeding, ask a health professional before use.

Keep out of reach of children. In case of overdose, get medical help or contact a Poison Control Center right away.

Directions:

- do not take more than 8 capsules in any 24-hour period
- adults and children 12 years and over: take 2 capsules every 6 to 8 hours, as needed
- children under 12 years: ask a doctor

Other Information:

- store at 20–25°C (68–77°F)
- avoid excessive heat above 40°C (104°F)
- protect from light

Inactive Ingredients:

FD&C blue no. 1, FD&C red no. 40, fractionated coconut oil, gelatin, glycerin, mannitol, pharmaceutical ink, polyethylene glycol, povidone, propyl gallate, propylene glycol, purified water, sorbitol, sorbitol anhydrides

How Supplied:

Packages of 20 liquid-filled capsules

ROBITUSSIN® COUGH DM SYRUP (Wyeth Consumer)

ROBITUSSIN® SUGAR FREE COUGH

ROBITUSSIN® COUGH DM INFANT DROPS

ROBITUSSIN COUGH & CONGESTION
Cough Suppressant, Expectorant

Active Ingredients: (in each 5 mL tsp: Robitussin Cough DM, Robitussin Sugar Free Cough)
Dextromethorphan HBr, USP 10 mg
Guaifenesin, USP 100 mg

Active Ingredients: (in each 2.5 mL Robitussin Cough DM Infant Drops)
Dextromethorphan HBr, USP 5 mg
Guaifenesin, USP 100 mg

Active Ingredients: (in each 5 mL Robitussin Cough & Congestion)
Dextromethorphan HBr, USP 10 mg
Guaifenesin, USP 200 mg

Uses:

- temporarily relieves cough due to minor throat and bronchial irritation as may occur with a cold
- helps loosen phlegm (mucus) and thin bronchial secretions to drain bronchial tubes

Warnings:

Do not use if you or your child are now taking a prescription monoamine oxidase inhibitor (MAOI) (certain drugs for depression, psychiatric, or emotional conditions, or Parkinson's disease), or for 2 weeks after stopping the MAOI drug. If you do not know if your child's or your prescription drug contains an MAOI, ask a doctor or pharmacist before taking this product or giving it to your child.

Ask a doctor before use if you or your child has

- cough that occurs with too much phlegm (mucus)
- cough that lasts or is chronic such as occurs with smoking, asthma, chronic bronchitis, or emphysema

Stop use and ask a doctor if cough lasts more than 7 days, comes back, or is accompanied by fever, rash, or persistent headache. These could be signs of a serious condition.

If pregnant or breast-feeding, ask a health professional before use.

Keep out of reach of children. In case of overdose, get medical help or contact a Poison Control Center right away.

Directions: (Robitussin Cough DM, Robitussin Sugar Free Cough, Robitussin Cough & Congestion):

- do not take more than 6 doses in any 24-hour period
- adults and children 12 yrs and over: 2 tsp every 4 hours
- children 6 to under 12 yrs: 1 tsp every 4 hours
- children 2 to under 6 yrs: ½ tsp every 4 hours
- children under 2 yrs: ask a doctor
- shake well before use (Robitussin Cough & Congestion)

Directions: (Robitussin Cough DM Infant Drops):

- repeat every 4 hrs
- do not use more than 6 doses in any 24-hr period
- choose by weight (if weight not known, choose by age)
- measure with the dosing device provided. Do not use with any other device.
- 24–47 lbs (2 to under 6 yrs): 2.5 mL
- under 24 lbs (under 2 yrs): ask a doctor

Inactive Ingredients: (Robitussin Cough DM): citric acid, FD&C red no. 40, flavors, glucose, glycerin, high fructose corn syrup, menthol, saccharin sodium, sodium benzoate, water

Inactive Ingredients: (Robitussin Sugar Free Cough): acesulfame potassium, citric acid, flavors, glycerin, methylparaben, polyethylene glycol, povidone, propylene glycol, saccharin sodium, sodium benzoate, water

Inactive Ingredients: (Robitussin Cough DM Infant Drops): artificial flavors, citric acid, FD&C red no. 40, glycerin, high fructose corn syrup, magnasweet, maltitol solution, maltol, polyethylene glycol, povidone, propylene glycol, purified water, saccharin sodium, sodium benzoate, sodium chloride, sodium citrate

Inactive Ingredients: (Robitussin Cough & Congestion): Carboxymethylcellulose sodium, citric acid, D&C red no. 33, FD&C red no. 40, glycerin, high fructose corn syrup, menthol, microcrystalline cellulose, natural and artificial flavors, polyethylene glycol, povidone, propylene glycol, purified water, saccharin sodium, sodium benzoate, sorbitol solution, xanthan gum

Other Information:

- **each 2.5 mL contains:** sodium 5 mg (Robitussin Cough DM Infant Drops)
- **each teaspoon contains:** sodium 5 mg (Robitussin Cough & Congestion)
- store at 20–25°C (68–77°F)
- alcohol-free
- dosage cup or oral dosing device provided

How Supplied: Robitussin DM (cherry-colored) in bottles of 4, 8 and 12 fl oz, and single doses (premeasured doses 1/3 fl oz each)
Robitussin Sugar Free Cough in bottles of 4 fl oz
Robitussin DM Infant Drops in 1 fl oz bottles

ROBITUSSIN COUGH, COLD & FLU NIGHTTIME (Wyeth Consumer)
Pain Reliever/Fever Reducer, Nasal Decongestant, Cough Suppressant, Antihistamine

Active Ingredients: (in each 5 mL tsp)
Acetaminophen, USP 160 mg
Chlorpheniramine maleate, USP 1 mg
Dextromethorphan HBr, USP 5 mg
Phenylephrine HCl, USP 2.5 mg

Uses:

- temporarily relieves these symptoms occurring with a cold or flu, hay fever, or other upper respiratory allergies:
  - headache • cough • runny nose • itching of the nose or throat • nasal congestion • sneezing • minor aches and pains • itchy, watery eyes • fever

Warnings:

Alcohol warning: If you consume 3 or more alcoholic drinks every day, ask your doctor whether you should take acetaminophen or other pain relievers/fever reducers. Acetaminophen may cause liver damage.

Taking more than the recommended dose (overdose) may cause serious liver damage.

Sore throat warning: If sore throat is severe, persists for more than 2 days, is accompanied or followed by fever, headache, rash, nausea, or vomiting, consult a doctor promptly.

Do not use:

- in a child under 2 years of age
- if you are now taking a prescription monoamine oxidase inhibitor (MAOI) (certain drugs for depression, psychiatric, or emotional conditions, or Parkinson's disease), or for 2 weeks after stopping the MAOI drug. If you do not know if your prescription drug contains an MAOI, ask a doctor or pharmacist before taking this product.
- with any other product containing acetaminophen as this may lead to an overdose. Overdose requires prompt

medical attention even if you do not notice any signs or symptoms.

Ask a doctor before use if you have
- heart disease • high blood pressure
- thyroid disease
- trouble urinating due to an enlarged prostate gland • diabetes
- cough that occurs with too much phlegm (mucus) • glaucoma
- a breathing problem or chronic cough that lasts or as occurs with smoking, asthma, chronic bronchitis, or emphysema

Ask a doctor or pharmacist before use if you are • taking any other product containing acetaminophen, or any other pain reliever/fever reducer
- taking sedatives or tranquilizers

When using this product
- **do not use more than directed**
- marked drowsiness may occur
- avoid alcoholic drinks
- alcohol, sedatives, and tranquilizers may increase drowsiness
- be careful when driving a motor vehicle or operating machinery
- excitability may occur, especially in children

Stop use and ask a doctor if
- you get nervous, dizzy, or sleepless
- pain, cough, or nasal congestion gets worse or lasts more than 5 days (children) or 7 days (adults)
- fever gets worse or lasts more than 3 days
- redness or swelling is present
- cough comes back or occurs with rash or headache that lasts. These could be signs of a serious condition.
- new symptoms occur

If pregnant or breast-feeding, ask a health professional before use.

Keep out of reach of children. In case of overdose, get medical help or contact a Poison Control Center right away. Prompt medical attention is critical for adults as well as for children, even if you do not notice any signs or symptoms.

Directions:
- do not take more than 5 doses in any 24-hour period
- do not exceed recommended dosage. Taking more than the recommended dose (overdose) may cause serious liver damage.
- adults and children 12 years and over: 4 teaspoons every 4 hours
- children 6 to under 12 years: 2 teaspoons every 4 hours
- children 2 to under 6 years: ask a doctor
- children under 2 years: do not use

Other Information:
- **each teaspoon contains:** sodium 2 mg
- store at 20–25°C (68–77°F)

Inactive Ingredients:
artificial flavor, citric acid, FD&C red no. 40, glycerin, lactic acid, menthol, natural flavor, polyethylene glycol, propyl gallate, propylene glycol, purified water, sodium benzoate, sodium citrate, sorbitol solution, sucralose

How Supplied:
Bottles of 4 fl. oz.

ROBITUSSIN® COUGH Long Acting (Wyeth Consumer)
ROBITUSSIN® PEDIATRIC COUGH Long Acting
Cough Suppressant

Active Ingredients **(in each 5 mL tsp Robitussin Cough Long Acting):**
Dextromethorphan HBr, USP 15 mg
(in each 5 mL tsp Robitussin Pediatric Cough Long Acting):
Dextromethorphan HBr, USP 7.5 mg

Use: temporarily relieves cough due to minor throat and bronchial irritation as may occur with a cold

Warnings:
Do not use if you are now taking a prescription monoamine oxidase inhibitor (MAOI) (certain drugs for depression, psychiatric, or emotional conditions, or Parkinson's disease), or for 2 weeks after stopping the MAOI drug. If you do not know if your prescription drug contains an MAOI, ask a doctor or pharmacist before taking this product.

Ask a doctor before use if you have
- cough that occurs with too much phlegm (mucus)
- cough that lasts or is chronic such as occurs with smoking, asthma, or emphysema

Stop use and ask a doctor if cough lasts more than 7 days, comes back, or is accompanied by fever, rash, or persistent headache. These could be signs of a serious condition.

If pregnant or breast-feeding, ask a health professional before use.

Keep out of reach of children. In case of overdose, get medical help or contact a Poison Control Center right away.

Directions:
- do not take more than 4 doses in any 24-hr period

Robitussin Cough Long Acting
- adults and children 12 yrs and over: 2 tsp every 6 to 8 hours, as needed
- children under 12 yrs: ask a doctor

Robitussin Pediatric Cough Long Acting
- choose dosage by weight (if weight is not known, choose by age)
  - under 24 lbs (under 2 yrs): ask a doctor
  - 24–47 lbs (2 to under 6 yrs): 1 tsp every 6 to 8 hours
  - 48–95 lbs (6–under 12 yrs): 2 tsp every 6 to 8 hours
  - 96 lbs and over (12 yrs and older): 4 tsp every 6 to 8 hours

Other Information:
- store at 20–25°C (68–77°F)
- dosage cup provided

Inactive Ingredients: (Robitussin Cough Long Acting): alcohol, citric acid, FD&C red no. 40, flavors, glucose, glycerin, high fructose corn syrup, menthol, saccharin sodium, sodium benzoate, water

(Robitussin Pediatric Cough Long Acting): artificial flavor, citric acid,

FD&C red no. 40, glycerin, high fructose corn syrup, propylene glycol, purified water, saccharin sodium, sodium benzoate, sodium chloride, sodium citrate
- **each teaspoon contains:** sodium 5 mg

How Supplied:
Robitussin Cough Long Acting (dark red-colored) in bottles of 4 fl oz.
Robitussin Pediatric (cherry-colored) in bottles of 4 fl oz.

ROBITUSSIN® Head & Chest Congestion PE Syrup
(Wyeth Consumer)
Nasal Decongestant, Expectorant

Active Ingredients:
(in each 5 mL tsp):
Guaifenesin, USP 100 mg
Phenylephrine HCl, USP 5 mg

Uses: • helps loosen phlegm (mucus) and thin bronchial secretions to make coughs more productive • temporarily relieves nasal congestion due to a cold.

Warnings:
Do not use
- in a child under 2 years of age
- if you are now taking a prescription monoamine oxidase inhibitor (MAOI) (certain drugs for depression, psychiatric, or emotional conditions, or Parkinson's disease), or for 2 weeks after stopping the MAOI drug. If you do not know if your prescription drug contains an MAOI, ask a doctor or pharmacist before taking this product.

Ask a doctor before use if you have
- heart disease • high blood pressure
- thyroid disease • diabetes
- trouble urinating due to an enlarged prostate gland
- cough that occurs with too much phlegm (mucus)
- cough that lasts or is chronic such as occurs with smoking, asthma, chronic bronchitis, or emphysema

When using this product do not use more than directed.

Stop use and ask a doctor if
- you get nervous, dizzy, or sleepless
- symptoms do not get better within 7 days or are accompanied by fever
- cough lasts more than 7 days, comes back, or is accompanied by fever, rash, or persistent headache. These could be signs of a serious condition.

If pregnant or breast-feeding, ask a health professional before use.

Keep out of reach of children. In case of overdose, get medical help or contact a Poison Control Center right away.

Directions:
- do not take more than 6 doses in any 24-hr period
- adults and children 12 yrs and over: 2 tsp every 4 hours

Continued on next page

Robitussin Head & Chest—Cont.

- children 6 to under 12 yrs: 1 tsp every 4 hours
- children 2 to under 6 yrs: ½ tsp every 4 hours
- children under 2 yrs: do not use

Other Information:
- store at 20–25°C (68–77°F)
- alcohol-free
- dosage cup provided

Inactive Ingredients:
artificial & natural flavor, citric acid, FD&C red no. 40, glycerin, lactic acid, menthol, propylene glycol, purified water, sodium benzoate, sorbitol, sucralose

How Supplied: Bottles of 4 fl oz

THERAFLU® Nighttime Severe Cold
(Novartis Consumer Health, Inc.)
Pain Reliever-Fever Reducer (Acetaminophen)
Antihistamine (Pheniramine maleate)
Nasal Decongestant (Phenylephrine HCl)

Drug Facts

Active Ingredient: **Purpose:**
(in each packet)
Acetaminophen
   650 mg .... Pain reliever/
                                   Fever reducer
Pheniramine maleate
   20 mg .... Antihistamine
Phenylephrine hydrochloride
   10 mg .... Nasal decongestant

Uses:
- temporarily relieves these symptoms due to a cold:
  - minor aches and pains • headache
  - minor sore throat pain • nasal congestion • temporarily reduces fever
- temporarily relieves these symptoms due to hay fever or other upper respiratory allergies:
  - runny nose • sneezing • itchy nose and throat • itchy, watery eyes

Warnings:
Alcohol Warning: If you consume 3 or more alcoholic drinks every day, ask your doctor whether you should take acetaminophen or other pain relievers/fever reducers. Acetaminophen may cause liver damage.

Do not use • if you are now taking a prescription monoamine oxidase inhibitor (MAOI) (certain drugs for depression, psychiatric, or emotional conditions, or Parkinson's disease), or for 2 weeks after stopping the MAOI drug. If you do not know if your prescription drug contains an MAOI, ask a doctor or pharmacist before taking this product.
• with any other product containing acetaminophen (**see Overdose Warning**)
Ask a doctor before use if you have
- heart disease • high blood pressure
- thyroid disease • diabetes • glaucoma

- a breathing problem such as emphysema, asthma, or chronic bronchitis
- trouble urinating due to an enlarged prostate gland
- a sodium-restricted diet

Ask a doctor or pharmacist before use if you are taking sedatives or tranquilizers.
When using this product • do not exceed recommended dosage • avoid alcoholic drinks
- may cause drowsiness • alcohol, sedatives, and tranquilizers may increase drowsiness
- be careful when driving a motor vehicle or operating machinery
- excitability may occur, especially in children

Stop use and ask a doctor if • nervousness, dizziness, or sleeplessness occur
- pain or nasal congestion gets worse or lasts more than 7 days
- fever gets worse or lasts more than 3 days
- redness or swelling is present
- new symptoms occur
- sore throat is severe, persists for more than 2 days, is accompanied or followed by fever, headache, rash, nausea, or vomiting. These could be signs of a serious condition.

If pregnant or breast-feeding, ask a health care professional before use.
Keep out of reach of children.
Overdose Warning: Taking more than the recommended dose can cause serious health problems, including serious liver damage. In case of overdose, get medical help or contact a poison control center right away. Prompt medical attention is critical for adults as well as for children even if you do not notice any signs or symptoms.

Directions:
- do not use more than directed (see **Overdose Warning**)
- take every 4 hours; not to exceed 6 packets in 24 hours or as directed by a doctor
- adults and children 12 years of age and over: dissolve contents of one packet into 8 oz. hot water; sip while hot. Consume entire drink within 10–15 minutes.
- children under 12 years of age: consult a doctor.
- If using a microwave, add contents of one packet to 8 oz. of cool water; stir briskly before and after heating. Do not overheat.

Other Information:
- each packet contains: **sodium 44 mg**
- store at controlled room temperature 20-25°C (68-77°F)

How Supplied: 6 packets in a carton

Inactive Ingredients: acesulfame K, citric acid, D&C Yellow 10, FD&C Yellow 6, lecithin, maltodextrin, natural flavors, silicon dioxide, sodium citrate, sucrose, tribasic calcium phosphate
Questions? call 1-800-452-0051
24 hours a day, 7 days a week.

Shown in Product Identification Guide, page 515

THERAFLU® Cold & Cough
(Novartis Consumer Health, Inc.)
Cough Suppressant (Dextromethorphan HBr)
Antihistamine (Pheniramine maleate)
Nasal Decongestant (Phenylephrine HCl)

Drug Facts

Active Ingredients: **Purpose:**
(in each packet)
Dextromethorphan hydrobromide
20 mg .... Cough suppressant
Pheniramine maleate
20 mg .... Antihistamine
Phenylephrine hydrochloride
10 mg .... Nasal decongestant

Uses:
- temporarily relieves these symptoms due to a cold:
  - nasal and sinus congestion
  - cough due to minor throat and bronchial irritation
- temporarily relieves these symptoms due to hay fever or other upper respiratory allergies:
  - runny nose • sneezing • itchy nose and throat
  - itchy, watery eyes

Warnings:
Do not use • if you are now taking a prescription monoamine oxidase inhibitor (MAOI) (certain drugs for depression, psychiatric, or emotional conditions, or Parkinson's disease), or for 2 weeks after stopping the MAOI drug. If you do not know if your prescription drug contains an MAOI, ask a doctor or pharmacist before taking this product.

Ask a doctor before use if you have
- heart disease • high blood pressure
- thyroid disease • diabetes • glaucoma
- a breathing problem such as emphysema, asthma, or chronic bronchitis
- trouble urinating due to an enlarged prostate gland • cough that occurs with smoking, too much phlegm (mucus) or chronic cough that lasts
- a sodium-restricted diet

Ask a doctor or pharmacist before use if you are taking sedatives or tranquilizers.

When using this product • do not exceed recommended dosage • avoid alcoholic drinks • may cause marked drowsiness • alcohol, sedatives, and tranquilizers may increase drowsiness • be careful when driving a motor vehicle or operating machinery • excitability may occur, especially in children

Stop use and ask a doctor if
- nervousness, dizziness, or sleeplessness occur
- symptoms do not improve within 7 days or occur with a fever
- cough persists for more than 7 days, comes back or occurs with a fever, rash, or persistent headache. These could be signs of a serious condition.

If pregnant or breast-feeding, ask a health care professional before use.

Keep out of reach of children. In case of overdose, get medical help or contact a poison control center right away.

Directions:
- take every 4 hours; not to exceed 6 packets in 24 hours or as directed by a doctor.
- adults and children 12 years of age and over: dissolve contents of one packet in 8 oz. hot water; sip while hot. Consume entire drink within 10–15 minutes.
- children under 12 years of age: consult a doctor.
- If using a microwave, add contents of one packet to 8 oz. of cool water; stir briskly before and after heating. Do not overheat.

Other Information:
- each packet contains: **sodium 46 mg**
- store at controlled room temperature 20-25°C (68-77°F)

How Supplied: 6 packets in a carton.

Inactive Ingredients: acesulfame K, citric acid, D&C yellow 10, FD&C Yellow 6, lecithin, magnesium stearate, maltodextrin, natural flavors, silicon dioxide, sodium citrate, sucrose, tribasic calcium phosphate

Questions? call **1-800-452-0051** 24 hours a day, 7 days a week.

Shown in Product Identification Guide, page 515

THERAFLU® Cold & Sore Throat (Novartis Consumer Health, Inc.)
Pain Reliever-Fever Reducer (Acetaminophen)
Antihistamine (Pheniramine maleate)
Nasal Decongestant (Phenylephrine HCl)

Drug Facts

Active Ingredient: **Purpose:**
(in each packet)
Acetaminophen
325 mg .... Pain reliever/
                                 Fever reducer
Pheniramine maleate
20 mg .... Antihistamine
Phenylephrine hydrochloride
10 mg .... Nasal decongestant

Uses:
- temporarily relieves these symptoms due to a cold:
  - minor aches and pains • headache
  - minor sore throat pain • nasal congestion • temporarily reduces fever
- temporarily relieves these symptoms due to hay fever or other upper respiratory allergies:
  - runny nose • sneezing • itchy nose and throat • itchy, watery eyes

Warnings:

Alcohol Warning: If you consume 3 or more alcoholic drinks every day, ask your doctor whether you should take acetaminophen or other pain relievers/fever re-

ducers. Acetaminophen may cause liver damage.
Do not use • if you are now taking a prescription monoamine oxidase inhibitor (MAOI) (certain drugs for depression, psychiatric, or emotional conditions, or Parkinson's disease), or for 2 weeks after stopping the MAOI drug. If you do not know if your prescription drug contains an MAOI, ask a doctor or pharmacist before taking this product.
- with any other product containing acetaminophen **(see Overdose Warning)**
Ask a doctor before use if you have
- heart disease • high blood pressure
- thyroid disease • diabetes • glaucoma
- a breathing problem such as emphysema or chronic bronchitis
- trouble urinating due to an enlarged prostate gland
- a sodium-restricted diet
Ask a doctor or pharmacist before use if you are taking sedatives or tranquilizers.
When using this product • do not exceed recommended dosage • avoid alcoholic drinks • may cause drowsiness • alcohol, sedatives, and tranquilizers may increase drowsiness • be careful when driving a motor vehicle or operating machinery • excitability may occur, especially in children
Stop use and ask a doctor if • nervousness, dizziness, or sleeplessness occur
- pain or nasal congestion gets worse or lasts more than 7 days
- fever gets worse or lasts more than 3 days
- redness or swelling is present
- new symptoms occur
- sore throat is severe, persists for more than 2 days, is accompanied or followed by fever, headache, rash, nausea, or vomiting. These could be signs of a serious condition.
If pregnant or breast-feeding, ask a health care professional before use.
Keep out of reach of children.
Overdose Warning: Taking more than the recommended dose can cause serious health problems, including serious liver damage. In case of overdose, get medical help or contact a poison control center right away. Prompt medical attention is critical for adults as well as for children even if you do not notice any signs or symptoms.

Directions:
- do not use more than directed **(see Overdose Warning)**
- take every 4 hours; not to exceed 6 packets in 24 hours or as directed by a doctor.
- adults and children 12 years of age and over: dissolve contents of one packet into 8 oz. hot water; sip while hot. Consume entire drink within 10–15 minutes.
- children under 12 years of age: consult a doctor.
- If using a microwave, add contents of one packet to 8 oz. of cool water; stir briskly before and after heating. Do not overheat.

Other Information:
- each packet contains: **sodium 44 mg**
- store at controlled room temperature 20-25°C (68-77°F)

How Supplied: 6 packets in a carton.

Inactive Ingredients: acesulfame K, citric acid, D&C Yellow 10, FD&C Yellow 6, lecithin, magnesium stearate, maltodextrin, natural flavors, silicon dioxide, sodium citrate, sucrose, tribasic calcium phosphate
Questions? call **1-800-452-0051** 24 hours a day, 7 days a week.

Shown in Product Identification Guide, page 515

THERAFLU® Flu & Chest Congestion
(Novartis Consumer Health, Inc.)
Pain Reliever-Fever Reducer (Acetaminophen)
Expectorant (Guaifenesin)

Drug Facts

Active Ingredient: **Purpose:**
(in each packet):
Acetaminophen
1000 mg .... Pain reliever/
                                 Fever reducer
Guaifenesin
400 mg .... Expectorant

Uses: • temporarily relieves these symptoms due to a cold:
- minor aches and pains • headache
- minor sore throat pain
- helps loosen phlegm (mucus) and thin bronchial secretions to drain bronchial tubes and make coughs more productive
- temporarily reduces fever

Warnings: **Alcohol Warning:** If you consume 3 or more alcoholic drinks every day, ask your doctor whether you should take acetaminophen or other pain relievers/fever reducers. Acetaminophen may cause liver damage.
Do not use • with any other product containing acetaminophen **(see Overdose Warning)**
Ask a doctor before use if you have
- a breathing problem such as emphysema or chronic bronchitis
- cough that occurs with smoking, too much phlegm (mucus) or chronic cough that lasts
Stop use and ask a doctor if
- pain or cough gets worse or lasts more than 7 days
- fever gets worse or lasts more than 3 days
- redness or swelling is present
- new symptoms occur
- cough comes back or occurs with rash or headache that lasts. These could be signs of a serious condition.
- sore throat is severe, persists for more than 2 days, is accompanied or followed

Continued on next page

Theraflu Chest Congestion—Cont.

by fever, headache, rash, nausea, or vomiting

If pregnant or breast-feeding, ask a health care professional before use.
Keep out of reach of children.
Overdose Warning: Taking more than the recommended dose can cause serious health problems, including serious liver damage. In case of overdose, get medical help or contact a poison control center right away. Prompt medical attention is critical for adults as well as for children even if you do not notice any signs or symptoms.

Directions:

- do not use more than directed (**see Overdose Warning**)
- take every 6 hours; not to exceed 4 packets in 24 hours or as directed by a doctor.
- adults and children 12 years of age and over: dissolve contents of one packet into 8 oz. hot water; sip while hot. Consume entire drink within 10–15 minutes.
- children under 12 years of age: consult a doctor.
- If using a microwave, add contents of one packet to 8 oz. of cool water; stir briskly before and after heating. Do not overheat.

Other Information:

- Phenylketonurics: Contains Phenylalanine 24 mg per packet
- each packet contains: **sodium 15 mg**
- each packet contains: **potassium 10 mg**
- store at controlled room temperature 20-25°C (68-77°F)

How Supplied: 6 packets in a carton.

Inactive Ingredients: acesulfame K, aspartame, citric acid, D&C Yellow 10, FD&C Red 40, maltodextrin, natural flavors, silicon dioxide, sodium citrate, sucrose, tribasic calcium phosphate
Questions? call **1-800-452-0051** 24 hours a day, 7 days a week.

Shown in Product Identification Guide, page 515

THERAFLU® Flu & Sore Throat
(Novartis Consumer Health, Inc.)
Pain Reliever-Fever Reducer (Acetaminophen)
Antihistamine (Pheniramine maleate)
Nasal Decongestant (Phenylephrine HCl)

Drug Facts

Active Ingredient: (in each packet)	Purpose:
Acetaminophen 650 mg	Pain reliever/ Fever reducer
Pheniramine maleate 20 mg	Antihistamine
Phenylephrine hydrochloride 10 mg	Nasal decongestant

Uses:

- temporarily relieves these symptoms due to a cold:
  - minor aches and pains • headache
  - minor sore throat pain • nasal congestion • temporarily reduces fever
- temporarily relieves these symptoms due to hay fever or other upper respiratory allergies:
  - runny nose • sneezing • itchy nose and throat • itchy, watery eyes

Warnings:

Alcohol Warning: If you consume 3 or more alcoholic drinks every day, ask your doctor whether you should take acetaminophen or other pain relievers/fever reducers. Acetaminophen may cause liver damage.
Do not use • if you are now taking a prescription monoamine oxidase inhibitor (MAOI) (certain drugs for depression, psychiatric, or emotional conditions, or Parkinson's disease), or for 2 weeks after stopping the MAOI drug. If you do not know if your prescription drug contains an MAOI, ask a doctor or pharmacist before taking this product.
• with any other product containing acetaminophen (**see Overdose Warning**)
Ask a doctor before use if you have
- heart disease • high blood pressure
- thyroid disease • diabetes • glaucoma
- a breathing problem such as emphysema, asthma or chronic bronchitis
- trouble urinating due to an enlarged prostate gland
- a sodium-restricted diet
Ask a doctor or pharmacist before use if you are taking sedatives or tranquilizers.
When using this product • do not exceed recommended dosage • avoid alcoholic drinks • may cause drowsiness • alcohol, sedatives, and tranquilizers may increase drowsiness • be careful when driving a motor vehicle or operating machinery • excitability may occur, especially in children
Stop use and ask a doctor if • nervousness, dizziness, or sleeplessness occur
- pain or nasal congestion gets worse or lasts more than 7 days
- fever gets worse or lasts more than 3 days
- redness or swelling is present
- new symptoms occur
- sore throat is severe, persists for more than 2 days, is accompanied or followed by fever, headache, rash, nausea, or vomiting. These could be signs of a serious condition.
If pregnant or breast-feeding, ask a health care professional before use.
Keep out of reach of children.
Overdose Warning: Taking more than the recommended dose can cause serious health problems, including serious liver damage. In case of overdose, get medical help or contact a poison control center right away. Prompt medical attention is critical for adults as well as for children even if you do not notice any signs or symptoms.

Directions:

- do not use more than directed (**see Overdose Warning**)
- take every 4 hours; not to exceed 6 packets in 24 hours or as directed by a doctor.
- adults and children 12 years of age and over: dissolve contents of one packet in 8 oz. hot water; sip while hot. Consume entire drink within 10–15 minutes.
- children under 12 years of age: consult a doctor.
- If using a microwave, add contents of one packet to 8 oz. of cool water; stir briskly before and after heating. Do not overheat.

Other Information:

- each packet contains: **sodium 51 mg**
- each packet contains: **potassium 10 mg**
- store at controlled room temperature 20-25°C (68-77°F)

How Supplied: 6 packets in a carton.

Inactive Ingredients: acesulfame K, citric acid, D&C Yellow 10, FD&C Blue 1, FD&C Red 40, lecithin, maltodextrin, medium chain triglycerides, natural flavors, silicon dioxide, sodium chloride, sodium citrate, sucrose, triacetin, tribasic calcium phosphate
Questions? call **1-800-452-0051** 24 hours a day, 7 days a week.

Shown in Product Identification Guide, page 515

THERAFLU® Daytime Severe Cold
(Novartis Consumer Health, Inc.)
Pain Reliever-Fever Reducer (Acetaminophen)
Nasal Decongestant (Phenylephrine HCl)

Drug Facts

Active Ingredient: (in each packet)	Purpose:
Acetaminophen 650 mg	Pain reliever/ Fever reducer
Phenylephrine hydrochloride 10 mg	Nasal decongestant

Uses: • temporarily relieves these symptoms due to a cold:
- headache
- minor aches and pains
- minor sore throat pain
- nasal and sinus congestion
- temporarily reduces fever

Warnings:

Alcohol Warning: If you consume 3 or more alcoholic drinks every day, ask your doctor whether you should take acetaminophen or other pain relievers/fever reducers. Acetaminophen may cause liver damage.
Do not use • if you are now taking a prescription monoamine oxidase inhibitor (MAOI) (certain drugs for depression, psychiatric, or emotional conditions, or Parkinson's disease), or for 2 weeks after stopping the MAOI drug. If you do not

know if your prescription drug contains an MAOI, ask a doctor or pharmacist before taking this product.
- with any other product containing acetaminophen (**see Overdose Warning**)

Ask a doctor before use if you have
- heart disease • high blood pressure
- thyroid disease • diabetes
- trouble urinating due to an enlarged prostate gland
- a sodium-restricted diet

When using this product • do not exceed recommended dosage

Stop use and ask a doctor if • nervousness, dizziness, or sleeplessness occur
- pain or nasal congestion gets worse or lasts more than 7 days
- fever gets worse or lasts more than 3 days
- redness or swelling is present
- new symptoms occur
- sore throat is severe, persists for more than 2 days, is accompanied or followed by fever, headache, rash, nausea, or vomiting. These could be signs of a serious condition.

If pregnant or breast-feeding, ask a health care professional before use.

Keep out of reach of children.

Overdose Warning: Taking more than the recommended dose can cause serious health problems, including serious liver damage. In case of overdose, get medical help or contact a poison control center right away. Prompt medical attention is critical for adults as well as for children even if you do not notice any signs or symptoms.

Directions:
- do not use more than directed (**see Overdose Warning**)
- take every 4 hours; not to exceed 6 packets in 24 hours or as directed by a doctor
- adults and children 12 years of age and over: dissolve contents of one packet in 8 oz. hot water; sip while hot. Consume entire drink within 10–15 minutes.
- children under 12 years of age: consult a doctor.
- If using a microwave, add contents of one packet to 8 oz. of cool water; stir briskly before and after heating. Do not overheat.

Other Information:
- each packet contains: **sodium 44 mg**
- store at controlled room temperature 20-25°C (68-77°F)

How Supplied: 6 packets in a carton.

Inactive Ingredients: acesulfame K, citric acid, D&C Yellow 10, FD&C Yellow 6, lecithin, maltodextrin, natural flavors, silicon dioxide, sodium citrate, sucrose, tribasic calcium phosphate

Questions? call **1-800-452-0051**
24 hours a day, 7 days a week.

Shown in Product Identification Guide, page 515

THERAFLU® WARMING RELIEF DAYTIME SEVERE COLD
(Novartis Consumer Health, Inc.)
Pain Reliever/Fever Reducer/Cough Suppressant/Nasal Decongestant

Drug Facts

Active Ingredients: **Purpose:**
(in each 15 mL tablespoonful)
Acetaminophen
325 mg .... Pain reliever/fever reducer
Dextromethorphan HBr
10 mg .... Cough suppressant
Phenylephrine HCl
5 mg .... Nasal decongestant

Uses:
- temporarily relieves
  - minor aches and pains • headache
  - minor sore throat pain
  - nasal congestion
  - cough due to minor throat and bronchial irritation
- temporarily reduces fever

Warnings:

Alcohol Warning: If you consume 3 or more alcoholic drinks every day, ask your doctor whether you should take acetaminophen or other pain relievers/fever reducers. Acetaminophen may cause liver damage.

Do not use
- if you are now taking a prescription monoamine oxidase inhibitor (MAOI) (certain drugs for depression, psychiatric, or emotional conditions, or Parkinson's disease), or for 2 weeks after stopping the MAOI drug. If you do not know if your prescription drug contains an MAOI, ask a doctor or pharmacist before taking this product.
- with any other product containing acetaminophen (**see Overdose Warning**)

Ask a doctor before use if you have
- heart disease • high blood pressure
- thyroid disease • diabetes
- cough that occurs with too much phlegm (mucus)
- trouble urinating due to an enlarged prostate gland
- cough that lasts or is chronic such as occurs with smoking, asthma or emphysema

When using this product
- **do not exceed recommended dosage**

Stop use and ask a doctor if
- nervousness, dizziness, or sleeplessness occurs
- pain, cough or nasal congestion gets worse or lasts more than 7 days
- fever gets worse or lasts more than 3 days
- redness or swelling is present
- new symptoms occur
- sore throat is severe, persists for more than 2 days, is accompanied or followed by fever, headache, rash, nausea, or vomiting.
- cough comes back or occurs with rash or headache that lasts. These could be signs of a serious condition.

If pregnant or breast-feeding, ask a health care professional before use.

Keep out of reach of children.

Overdose Warning: Taking more than the recommended dose can cause serious health problems, including serious liver damage. In case of overdose, get medical help or contact a poison control center right away. Prompt medical attention is critical for adults as well as for children even if you do not notice any signs or symptoms.

Directions:
- do not use more than directed (**see Overdose Warning**)
- adults and children 12 years of age and over: take 2 tablespoons (30 mL) in dose cup provided, every 4 hours as needed
- do not take more than 6 doses (12 tablespoons) in 24 hours
- Consult a physician for use in children under 12 years of age

Other Information:
- each tablespoon contains: **sodium 8 mg**
- store at controlled room temperature 20-25°C (68-77°F)

Inactive Ingredients:
acesulfame potassium, alcohol, citric acid, edetate disodium, FD&C blue 1, FD&C red 40, flavors, glycerin, maltitol solution, propylene glycol, purified water, sodium benzoate, sodium citrate
Alcohol content: 10%

Questions? call **1-800-452-0051**
24 hours a day, 7 days a week.

How Supplied:
Available in 8.3 fl oz bottles. Cherry Flavor.

THERAFLU® WARMING RELIEF NIGHTTIME SEVERE COLD
(Novartis Consumer Health, Inc.)
Cough Suppressant/Antihistamine/Pain Reliever/Fever Reducer/Nasal Decongestant

Drug Facts

Active Ingredients: **Purpose:**
(in each 15 mL tablespoonful)
Acetaminophen
325 mg .... Pain reliever/fever reducer
Diphenhydramine HCl
12.5 mg .... Antihistamine/
                               Cough suppressant
Phenylephrine HCl
5 mg .... Nasal decongestant

Uses:
- temporarily relieves
  - minor aches and pains • headache
  - runny nose • sneezing
  - itchy nose or throat
  - itchy, watery eyes
  - minor sore throat pain
  - nasal and sinus congestion
  - cough due to minor throat and bronchial irritation
- temporarily reduces fever

Continued on next page

Theraflu Warming Relief—Cont.

Warnings:

Alcohol Warning: If you consume 3 or more alcoholic drinks every day, ask your doctor whether you should take acetaminophen or other pain relievers/fever reducers. Acetaminophen may cause liver damage.

Do not use
- if you are now taking a prescription monoamine oxidase inhibitor (MAOI) (certain drugs for depression, psychiatric, or emotional conditions, or Parkinson's disease), or for 2 weeks after stopping the MAOI drug. If you do not know if your prescription drug contains an MAOI, ask a doctor or pharmacist before taking this product.
- with any other product containing diphenhydramine, even one used on skin
- with any other product containing acetaminophen **(see Overdose Warning)**

Ask a doctor before use if you have
- heart disease • high blood pressure
- thyroid disease • diabetes • glaucoma
- a breathing problem such as emphysema or chronic bronchitis
- trouble urinating due to an enlarged prostate gland
- cough that occurs with too much phlegm (mucus)
- cough that lasts or is chronic such as occurs with smoking, asthma or emphysema

Ask a doctor or pharmacist before use if you are taking sedatives or tranquilizers.

When using this product
- **do not exceed recommended dosage**
- avoid alcoholic drinks
- may cause marked drowsiness
- alcohol, sedatives, and tranquilizers may increase drowsiness
- be careful when driving a motor vehicle or operating machinery
- excitability may occur, especially in children

Stop use and ask a doctor If
- nervousness, dizziness, or sleeplessness occurs
- pain, cough or nasal congestion gets worse or lasts more than 7 days
- fever gets worse or lasts more than 3 days
- redness or swelling is present
- new symptoms occur
- sore throat is severe, persists for more than 2 days, is accompanied or followed by fever, headache, rash, nausea, or vomiting
- cough comes back or occurs with rash or headache that lasts. These could be signs of a serious condition.

If pregnant or breast-feeding, ask a health care professional before use.

Keep out of reach of children.

Overdose Warning: Taking more than the recommended dose can cause serious health problems, including serious liver damage. In case of overdose, get medical help or contact a poison control center

right away. Prompt medical attention is critical for adults as well as for children even if you do not notice any signs or symptoms.

Directions:
- do not use more than directed **(see Overdose Warning)**
- adults and children 12 years of age and over: take 2 tablespoons (30 mL) in dose cup provided, every 4 hours as needed
- do not take more than 6 doses (12 tablespoons) in 24 hours
- Consult a physician for use in children under 12 years of age

Other Information:
- each tablespoon contains: **sodium 7 mg**
- each tablespoon contains: **potassium 5 mg**
- store at controlled room temperature 20-25°C (68-77°F)

Inactive Ingredients:
acesulfame potassium, alcohol, citric acid, edetate disodium, FD&C blue 1, FD&C red 40, flavors, glycerin, maltitol solution, propylene glycol, purified water, sodium benzoate, sodium citrate
Alcohol content: 10%

Questions? call **1-800-452-0051** 24 hours a day, 7 days a week.

How Supplied:
Available in 8.3 fl oz bottles. Cherry Flavor.

Shown in Product Identification Guide, page 515

THERAFLU® THIN STRIPS® LONG ACTING COUGH
(Novartis Consumer Health, Inc.)
Cough Suppressant
(Dextromethorphen HBr)

Drug Facts:

Active Ingredient:

(in each strip)	**Purpose:**

Dextromethorphan 11 mg (equivalent to 15 mg dextromethorphan HBr) ... Cough suppressant

Uses: • temporarily relieves cough due to minor throat and bronchial irritation as may occur with a cold

Warnings:

Do not use if you are now taking a prescription monoamine oxidase inhibitor (MAOI) (certain drugs for depression, psychiatric, or emotional conditions, or Parkinson's disease), or for 2 weeks after stopping the MAOI drug. If you do not know if your prescription drug contains an MAOI, ask a doctor or pharmacist before taking this product.

Ask a doctor before use if you have
- a cough that occurs with too much phlegm (mucus)
- a cough that lasts or is chronic such as occurs with smoking, asthma, or emphysema

When using this product • do not use more than directed

Stop use and ask a doctor if
- cough lasts more than 7 days, comes back, or is accompanied by fever, rash, or persistent headache. These could be signs of a serious condition.

If pregnant or breast-feeding, ask a health care professional before use.

Keep out of reach of children. In case of overdose, get medical help or contact a Poison Control Center right away.

Directions:
- adults and children 12 years of age and over: allow 2 strips to dissolve on your tongue every 6 to 8 hours as needed, not to exceed 8 strips in 24 hours or as directed by a doctor
- children under 12 years of age: ask a doctor

Other Information:
- store at controlled room temperature 20–25° (68–77° F)

Inactive Ingredients: acetone, alcohol, dibasic sodium phosphate, FD&C Red 40, flavors, hydroxypropyl cellulose, hypromellose, maltodextrin, microcrystalline cellulose, polacrilin, polyethylene glycol, pregelatinized starch, propylene glycol, purified water, sorbitol, sucralose, titanium dioxide
Cherry Flavor. Alcohol: less than 5%

How Supplied: Available in 12 ct. cartons
Questions? call **1-800-452-0051** 24 hours a day, 7 days a week.

Shown in Product Identification Guide, page 515

THERAFLU® THIN STRIPS®-MULTISYMPTOM
(Novartis Consumer Health, Inc.)
Antihistamine/Cough Suppressant
(Diphenhydramine HCl)

Drug Facts

Active Ingredient

(in each strip):	**Purpose:**

Diphenhydramine HCl 25 mg ... Antihistamine/Cough Suppressant

Uses: • temporarily relieves
- cough due to minor throat and bronchial irritation occurring with a cold
- runny nose • sneezing • itchy nose or throat • itchy, watery eyes due to hay fever

Warnings:

Do not use • with any other product containing diphenhydramine, even one used on skin

Ask a doctor before use if you have
- glaucoma
- a breathing problem such as emphysema, asthma or chronic bronchitis
- a cough that occurs with smoking, too much phlegm (mucus) or chronic cough that lasts
- trouble urinating due to an enlarged prostate gland

Ask a doctor or pharmacist before use if you are • taking sedatives or tranquilizers

When using this product • do not take more than directed • avoid alcoholic drinks
• marked drowsiness may occur • alcohol, sedatives, and tranquilizers may increase drowsiness
• be careful when driving a motor vehicle or operating machinery
• excitability may occur, especially in children

Stop use and ask a doctor if
• cough lasts more than 7 days, comes back, or is accompanied by fever, rash, or persistent headache. These could be signs of a serious condition.

If pregnant or breast-feeding, ask a health care professional before use.

Keep out of reach of children. In case of overdose, get medical help or contact a Poison Control Center right away.

Directions:
• adults and children 12 years of age and over: allow 1 strip to dissolve on tongue every 4 hours, not to exceed 6 strips in 24 hours, or as directed by a doctor
• children under 12 years of age: ask a doctor

Other Information:
• store at controlled room temperature 20–25° (68–77° F)

Inactive Ingredients: acetone, alcohol, FD&C Red 40, flavors, hydroxypropyl cellulose, hypromellose, maltodextrin, microcrystalline cellulose, polyethylene glycol, pregelatinized starch, propylene glycol, purified water, sodium polystyrene sulfonate, sorbitol, sucralose, titanium dioxide

Questions? call **1-800-452-0051** 24 hours a day, 7 days a week.
Cherry Flavor. Alcohol: less than 5%

How Supplied: Available in 12 ct. cartons
Shown in Product Identification Guide, page 515

THERAFLU® VAPOR PATCH®
(Novartis Consumer Health, Inc.)
8 Hour Cough
Cough Suppressant (Menthol)

Drug Facts

Active Ingredient: **Purpose:**
(in each patch):

Menthol 2.6% .... Cough suppressant

Uses:
• temporarily relieves cough due to
• a cold
• minor throat and bronchial irritation to help you sleep

Warnings:
For external use only.
Do not take by mouth or place in nostrils.
Combustible: Keep away from fire or flame.

Ask a doctor before use if you have
• a persistent or chronic cough such as occurs with smoking, asthma or emphysema
• cough that occurs with too much phlegm (mucus)
• a history of skin sensitivity, including to any of the ingredients in the product or to skin adhesives

When using this product do not
• **heat**
• **microwave**
• **use near an open flame**
• **add to water or any container where heating water. May cause splattering and result in burns.**

Stop use and ask a doctor if
• cough persists for more than 7 days, comes back or occurs with a fever, rash or persistent headache. These could be signs of a serious condition
• skin irritation occurs or gets worse

Keep out of reach of children.
If swallowed, get medical help or contact a poison control center right away.

Directions:
• **see important warnings under When Using this product**
• adults and children 12 years of age and over:
  • remove plastic packing
  • apply patch on the throat or chest. More than one patch can be applied
  • clothing should be loose about the throat and chest to help the vapors reach the nose and mouth
  • discard old and apply a new patch or patches up to three times daily or as directed by a doctor
• children under 12 years of age: ask a doctor

Other Information:
• store at controlled room temperature 20–25°C (68–77°F)
• protect from excessive heat

Inactive Ingredients: acrylic ester copolymer, aloe vera gel, camphor, eucalyptus oil, glycerin, karaya, spirits of turpentine

Questions?
call **1-800-452-0051** 24 hours a day, 7 days a week.

How Supplied: Menthol Scent, in cartons of 6 patches.

TRIAMINIC® Day Time Cold & Cough
(Novartis Consumer Health, Inc.)
Cough Suppressant, Nasal Decongestant
Cherry Flavor

Drug Facts

Active Ingredients: **Purpose:**
(in each 5 mL, 1 teaspoon)
Dextromethorphan HBr,
  USP, 5 mg .... Cough suppressant

Phenylephrine HCl,
  USP, 2.5 mg .... Nasal decongastant

Uses:
• temporarily relieves
• nasal and sinus congestion
• cough due to minor throat and bronchial irritation

Warnings:
Do not use
• in a child who is taking a prescription monoamine oxidase inhibitor (MAOI) (certain drugs for depression, psychiatric or emotional conditions, or Parkinson's disease), or for 2 weeks after stopping the MAOI drug. If you do not know if the child's prescription drug contains an MAOI, ask a doctor or pharmacist before giving this product.

Ask a doctor before use if the child has
• heart disease • high blood pressure
• thyroid disease • diabetes
• a breathing problem such as asthma or chronic bronchitis
• cough that occurs with too much phlegm (mucus) or chronic cough that lasts

When using this product
• **do not exceed recommended dosage**
Stop use and ask a doctor if
• nervousness, dizziness or sleeplessness occurs
• symptoms do not improve within 7 days or occur with a fever
• cough persists for more than 7 days, comes back or occurs with a fever, rash or persistent headache. These could be signs of a serious condition.

Keep out of reach of children. In case of overdose, get medical help or contact a poison control center right away.

Directions:
• take every 4 hours not to exceed 6 doses in 24 hours or as directed by a doctor

children 6 to under 12 years of age	2 teaspoons
children 2 to under 6 years of age	1 teaspoon
children under 2 years of age	ask a doctor

Other Information:
• each teaspoon contains: **sodium 2 mg**
• contains no aspirin
• store at controlled room temperature 20–25°C (68–77°F)

Inactive Ingredients: acesulfame K, benzoic acid, citric acid, edetate disodium, FD&C Red 40, flavors, maltitol solution, propylene glycol, purified water, sodium citrate

Questions? call **1-800-452-0051**
24 hours a day, 7 days a week.

How Supplied: Available in cartons of 4 FL oz and 8 FL oz bottles.

Shown in Product Identification Guide, page 515

TRIAMINIC® NIGHT TIME Cold & Cough

(Novartis Consumer Health, Inc.)
Antihistamine/Cough Suppressant, Nasal Decongestant
Grape Flavor

Drug Facts

Active Ingredients:	Purpose:
(in each 5 mL, 1 teaspoon)	
Diphenhydramine HCl, USP, 6.25 mg	Antihistamine/Cough suppressant
Phenylephrine HCl, USP, 2.5 mg	Nasal decongestant

Uses:
- temporarily relieves
- sneezing
- itchy nose or throat
- runny nose
- itchy, watery eyes due to hay fever
- nasal and sinus congestion
- cough due to minor throat and bronchial irritation

Warnings:

Do not use
- in a child who is taking a prescription monoamine oxidase inhibitor (MAOI) (certain drugs for depression, psychiatric or emotional conditions, or Parkinson's disease), or for 2 weeks after stopping the MAOI drug. If you do not know if the child's prescription drug contains an MAOI, ask a doctor or pharmacist before giving this product.
- with any other product containing diphenhydramine, even one used on skin

Ask a doctor before use if the child has
- heart disease • high blood pressure
- thyroid disease • diabetes • glaucoma
- a breathing problem such as asthma or chronic bronchitis
- cough that occurs with too much phlegm (mucus) or chronic cough that lasts

Ask a doctor or pharmacist before use if the child is taking sedatives or tranquilizers

When using this product
- **do not exceed recommended dosage**
- may cause marked drowsiness
- sedatives and tranquilizers may increase drowsiness
- excitability may occur, especially in children

Stop use and ask a doctor if
- nervousness, dizziness or sleeplessness occurs
- symptoms do not improve within 7 days or occur with a fever
- cough persists for more than 7 days, comes back or occurs with a fever, rash, or persistent headache. These could be signs of a serious condition

Keep out of reach of children. In case of overdose, get medical help or contact a poison control center right away

Directions:
- take every 4 hours; not to exceed 6 doses in 24 hours or as directed by a doctor

children 6 to under 12 years of age	2 teaspoons
children under 6 years of age	ask a doctor

Other Information:
- each teaspoon contains **sodium 6 mg**
- contains no aspirin
- store at controlled room temperature 20–25°C (68–77°F)

Inactive Ingredients: acesulfame K, benzoic acid, citric acid, edetate disodium, FD&C Blue 1, FD&C Red 40, flavor, maltitol solution, propylene glycol, purified water, sodium citrate

Questions? call 1-800-452-0051
24 hours a day, 7 days a week.

How Supplied:
Available in cartons of 4 FL oz and 8 FL oz bottles

Shown in Product Identification Guide, page 515

TRIAMINIC® CHEST & NASAL CONGESTION

(Novartis Consumer Health, Inc.)
Expectorant, Nasal Decongestant

Drug Facts

Active Ingredients:	Purpose:
(in each 5 mL, 1 teaspoon)	
Guaifenesin, USP, 50 mg	Expectorant
Phenylephrine HCl, USP, 2.5 mg	Nasal decongestant

Uses:
- temporarily relieves
- chest congestion by loosening phlegm (mucus) to help clear bronchial passageways
- nasal and sinus congestion

Warnings:

Do not use
- in a child who is taking a prescription monoamine oxidase inhibitor (MAOI) (certain drugs for depression, psychiatric or emotional conditions, or Parkinson's disease), or for 2 weeks after stopping the MAOI drug. If you do not know if the child's prescription drug contains an MAOI, ask a doctor or pharmacist before giving this product.

Ask a doctor before use if the child has
- heart disease • high blood pressure
- thyroid disease • diabetes
- cough that occurs with too much phlegm (mucus)
- chronic cough that lasts or as occurs with asthma

When using this product
- **do not exceed recommended dosage**

Stop use and ask a doctor if
- nervousness, dizziness, or sleeplessness occurs
- symptoms do not improve within 7 days or occur with a fever
- cough persists for more than 7 days, comes back or occurs with a fever, rash, or persistent headache. These could be signs of a serious condition.

Keep out of reach of children. In case of overdose, get medical help or contact a poison control center right away.

Directions:
- take every 4 hours; not to exceed 6 doses in 24 hours or as directed by a doctor

children 6 to under 12 years of age	2 teaspoons
children 2 to under 6 years of age	1 teaspoon
children under 2 years of age	ask a doctor

Other Information:
- each teaspoon contains: **sodium 3 mg**
- contains no aspirin
- store at controlled room temperature 20-25°C (68-77°F)

Inactive Ingredients: acesulfame K, benzoic acid, citric acid, D&C Yellow 10, edetate disodium, FD&C Yellow 6, flavors, maltitol solution, propylene glycol, purified water, sodium citrate

Questions? call **1-800-452-0051**
24 hours a day, 7 days a week.

How Supplied: Available in cartons of 4 fl oz bottles. Tropical Flavor.

TRIAMINIC® COLD & ALLERGY

(Novartis Consumer Health, Inc.)
Antihistamine, Nasal Decongestant
Orange Flavor

Drug Facts

Active Ingredients:	Purpose:
Chlorpheniramine maleate, USP, 1 mg	Antihistamine
Phenylephrine HCl, USP, 2.5 mg	Nasal decongestant

Uses:
- temporarily relieves
  - itchy, watery eyes • runny nose
  - itchy nose or throat • sneezing
  - nasal and sinus congestion

Warnings:

Do not use • in a child who is taking a prescription monoamine oxidase inhibitor (MAOI) (certain drugs for depression, psychiatric or emotional conditions, or Parkinson's disease), or for 2 weeks after stopping the MAOI drug. If you do not know if the child's prescription drug contains an MAOI, ask a doctor or pharmacist before giving this product.

Ask a doctor before use if the child has
- heart disease • high blood pressure

• thyroid disease • diabetes • glaucoma
• a breathing problem such as asthma or chronic bronchitis

Ask a doctor or pharmacist before use if the child is taking sedatives or tranquilizers

When using this product
• **do not exceed recommended dosage**
• may cause drowsiness
• sedatives and tranquilizers may increase drowsiness
• excitability may occur, especially in children

Stop use and ask a doctor if
• nervousness, dizziness or sleeplessness occurs
• symptoms do not improve within 7 days or occur with a fever. These could be signs of a serious condition.

Keep out of reach of children. In case of overdose, get medical help or contact a poison control center right away.

Directions: take every 4 hours; not to exceed 6 doses in 24 hours or as directed by a doctor

children 6 to under 12 years of age	2 teaspoons
children under 6 years of age	ask a doctor

Other Information:
• each teaspoon contains: **sodium 3 mg**
• contains no aspirin
• store at controlled room temperature 20-25°C (68-77°F)

Inactive Ingredients: acesulfame K, benzoic acid, citric acid, edetate disodium, FD&C Yellow 6, flavors, maltitol solution, purified water, sodium citrate

Questions? call 1-800-452-0051 24 hours a day, 7 days a week.

How Supplied: 4 fl oz bottle in a carton.

Shown in Product Identification Guide, page 515

TRIAMINIC® COUGH & SORE THROAT

(Novartis Consumer Health, Inc.)
Pain Reliever/Fever Reducer/Cough Suppressant

Drug Facts

Active Ingredients: **Purpose:**
(in each 5 mL, 1 teaspoon)
Cough & Sore Throat
Acetaminophen,
USP, 160 mg .... Pain reliever/
Fever reducer
Dextromethorphan HBr,
USP, 5 mg .... Cough suppressant

Uses:
• temporarily relieves
• minor aches and pains
• headache
• minor sore throat pain

• cough due to minor throat and bronchial irritation
• temporarily reduces fever

Warnings:
Do not use • in a child who is taking a prescription monoamine oxidase inhibitor (MAOI) (certain drugs for depression, psychiatric or emotional conditions, or Parkinson's disease), or for 2 weeks after stopping the MAOI drug. If you do not know if the child's prescription drug contains an MAOI, ask a doctor or pharmacist before giving this product.
• with any other product containing acetaminophen **(see Overdose Warning)**

Ask a doctor before use if the child has
• cough that occurs with too much phlegm (mucus)
• chronic cough that lasts, or as occurs with asthma

Stop use and ask a doctor if
• pain or cough gets worse or lasts more than 5 days
• fever gets worse or lasts more than 3 days
• redness or swelling is present
• new symptoms occur
• sore throat is severe, persists for more than 2 days or occurs with fever, headache, rash, nausea or vomiting
• cough comes back or occurs with a fever, rash or persistent headache. These could be signs of a serious condition.

Keep out of reach of children.
Overdose Warning: Taking more than the recommended dose can cause serious health problems, including serious liver damage. In case of overdose, get medical help or contact a poison control center right away. Prompt medical attention is critical for adults as well as for children even if you do not notice any signs or symptoms.

Directions:
• do not use more than directed **(see Overdose Warning)**
• take every 4 hours; not to exceed 5 doses in 24 hours or as directed by a doctor

children 6 to under 12 years of age	2 teaspoons
children 2 to under 6 years of age	1 teaspoon
children under 2 years of age	ask a doctor

Other Information:
• each teaspoon contains: **sodium 5 mg**
• contains no aspirin
• store at controlled room temperature 20-25°C (68-77°F)

Inactive Ingredients:
citric acid, edetate disodium, FD&C Blue 1, FD&C Red 40, flavor, glycerin, poly-

ethylene glycol, purified water, sodium benzoate, sodium citrate, sorbitol, sucrose

Questions? call 1-800-452-0051 24 hours a day, 7 days a week.

How Supplied: Available in 4 fl oz cartons, Grape Flavor.

INFANT TRIAMINIC THIN STRIPS®
(Novartis Consumer Health, Inc.)
Decongestant
Nasal Decongestant
Decongestant Plus Cough
Nasal Decongestant, Cough Suppressant

Drug Facts
Decongestant:
Active Ingredients: **Purpose:**
(in each strip)
Phenylephrine HCl
1.25 mg .... Nasal decongestant

Decongestant plus Cough:
Active Ingredients: **Purpose:**
(in each strip)
Dextromethorphan 1.83 mg (equivalent to 2.5 mg dextromethorphan HBr) .... Cough suppressant
Phenylephrine
HCl 1.25 mg .... Nasal decongestant

Uses:
Decongestant:
• temporarily relieves
• nasal and sinus congestion due to a cold

Decongestant plus Cough:
• temporarily relieves
• nasal and sinus congestion due to a cold
• cough due to minor throat and bronchial irritation

Warnings:
Do not use
• in a child who is taking a prescription monoamine oxidase inhibitor (MAOI) (certain drugs for depression, psychiatric, or emotional conditions, or Parkinson's disease), or for 2 weeks after stopping the MAOI drug. If you do not know if the child's prescription drug contains an MAOI, ask a doctor or pharmacist before giving this product.

Ask a doctor before use if the child has
• heart disease • high blood pressure
• thyroid disease • diabetes

Decongestant plus Cough:
• chronic cough that lasts, or as occurs with asthma
• cough that occurs with too much phlegm (mucus)

When using this product
• **do not exceed recommended dosage**
Stop use and ask a doctor if

Continued on next page

Triaminic Infant Thin Strips—Cont.

- nervousness, dizziness or sleeplessness occurs
- symptoms do not improve within 7 days or occur with a fever

Decongestant plus Cough:

- cough persists for more than 7 days, comes back or occurs with a fever, rash or persistent headache. These could be signs of a serious condition.

Keep out of reach of children. In case of overdose, get medical help or contact a poison control center right away.

Directions:

- take every 4 hours; not to exceed 6 doses in 24 hours or as directed by a doctor

children 2 to 3 years of age	allow 2 strips to dissolve on tongue
children under 2 years of age	ask a doctor

Other Information:

- contains no aspirin
- store at controlled room temperature 20-25°C (68-77°F)

Decongestant:

Inactive Ingredients: acetone, alcohol, FD&C Blue 1, FD&C Red 40, flavor, hypromellose, maltodextrin, microcrystalline cellulose, polyethylene glycol, propylene glycol, purified water, sodium polystyrene sulfonate, sucralose, titanium dioxide

Decongestant plus Cough:

Inactive Ingredients: acetone, alcohol, FD&C Blue 1, FD&C Red 40, flavor, hypromellose, microcrystalline cellulose, polacrilin, polyethylene glycol, propylene glycol, purified water, sodium polystyrene sulfonate, sucralose, titanium dioxide

Questions? call **1-800-452-0051** 24 hours a day, 7 days a week.

Alcohol: less than 0.5%

How Supplied: 16 Mixed Berry Medicated Strips in a carton.

Shown in Product Identification Guide, page 515

TRIAMINIC® Softchews®
(Novartis Consumer Health, Inc.)
Cough & Runny Nose
Antihistamine, Cough Suppressant
Cherry Flavor

Drug Facts

Active Ingredients: **Purpose:**
(in each tablet)
Chlorpheniramine maleate, USP,
1 mg .... Antihistamine
Dextromethorphan HBr, USP,
5 mg .... Cough Suppressant

Uses: • temporarily relieves • sneezing • itchy nose or throat • runny nose

- itchy, watery eyes due to hay fever
- cough due to minor throat and bronchial irritation

Warnings:

Do not use • in a child who is taking a prescription monoamine oxidase inhibitor (MAOI) (certain drugs for depression, psychiatric, or emotional conditions, or Parkinson's disease), or for 2 weeks after stopping the MAOI drug. If you do not know if the child's prescription drug contains an MAOI, ask a doctor or pharmacist before giving this product.

Ask a doctor before use if the child has

- glaucoma
- a breathing problem such as asthma or chronic bronchitis
- cough that occurs with too much phlegm (mucus) or chronic cough that lasts

Ask a doctor or pharmacist before use if the child is taking sedatives or tranquilizers.

When using this product • do not use more than directed • may cause marked drowsiness • sedatives and tranquilizers may increase drowsiness • excitability may occur, especially in children

Stop use and ask a doctor if • symptoms do not improve within 7 days or occurs with a fever • cough persists for more than 7 days, comes back or occurs with a fever, rash, or persistent headache. These could be signs of a serious condition.

Keep out of reach of children. In case of overdose, get medical help or contact a poison control center right away.

Directions: • Let Softchews® tablet dissolve in mouth or chew Softchews® tablet before swallowing, whichever is preferred • take every 4 to 6 hours; not to exceed 6 doses in 24 hours or as directed by a doctor

children 6 to under 12 years of age	2 tablets
children under 6 years of age	ask a doctor

Other Information:

- each Softchews® tablet contains: **sodium 5 mg**
- Phenylketonurics: Contains **Phenylalanine, 17.6 mg** per Softchews® tablet
- contains no aspirin • store at controlled room temperature 20–25°C (68–77°F)
- protect from light.

Inactive Ingredients: aspartame, carnauba wax, citric acid, crospovidone, D&C Red 27 aluminum lake, D&C Red 30 aluminum lake, ethylcellulose, FD&C Blue 2 aluminum lake, flavors, fractionated coconut oil, gum arabic, hypromellose, magnesium stearate, maltodextrin, mannitol, microcrystalline cellulose, mono- and di-glycerides, oleic acid, povidone, silicon dioxide, sodium bicarbonate, sodium chloride, sorbitol, starch, sucrose, triethyl citrate

Questions? call **1-800-452-0051** 24 hours a day, 7 days a week.

How Supplied: 18 Softchews® Tablets in a carton.

TRIAMINIC THIN STRIPS®
Cold & Cough
(Novartis Consumer Health, Inc.)
Cough Suppressant, Nasal Decongestant

For full product information see page 778.

TRIAMINIC THIN STRIPS®
COLD
(Novartis Consumer Health, Inc.)
Nasal Decongestant

Drug Facts

Active Ingredient: **Purpose:**
(in each strip)
Phenylephrine HCl,
2.5 mg .... Nasal decongestant

Uses:

- temporarily relieves
- nasal and sinus congestion due to a cold

Warnings:

Do not use • in a child who is taking a prescription monoamine oxidase inhibitor (MAOI) (certain drugs for depression, psychiatric, or emotional conditions, or Parkinson's disease), or for 2 weeks after stopping the MAOI drug. If you do not know if the child's prescription drug contains an MAOI, ask a doctor or pharmacist before giving this product.

Ask a doctor before use if the child has

- heart disease
- thyroid disease
- high blood pressure
- diabetes

When using this product

- **do not exceed recommended dosage**

Stop use and ask a doctor if

- nervousness, dizziness, or sleeplessness occur
- symptoms do not improve within 7 days or occur with a fever. These could be signs of a serious condition.

Keep out of reach of children.

In case of overdose, get medical help or contact a poison control center right away.

Directions:

- take every 4 hours; not to exceed 6 doses in 24 hours or as directed by a doctor

children 6 to under 12 years of age:	allow 2 strips to dissolve on tongue
children 2 to under 6 years of age:	allow 1 strip to dissolve on tongue
children under 2 years of age:	ask a doctor

Other Information:
• contains no aspirin
• store at controlled room temperature 20-25°C (68-77°F)

Inactive Ingredients:
acetone, FD&C Blue 1, FD&C Red 40, flavors, hypromellose, maltodextrin, microcrystalline cellulose, polyethylene glycol, purified water, sodium polystyrene sulfonate, sucralose, titanium dioxide

Questions? call **1-800-452-0051** 24 hours a day, 7 days a week.

How Supplied: 16 Raspberry Flavored Medicated Strips in a carton.
Shown in Product Identification Guide, page 515

**TRIAMINIC THIN STRIPS®
COUGH & RUNNY NOSE
(Novartis Consumer Health, Inc.)**

Drug Facts

Active ingredient:	Purpose:
(in each strip)	

Diphenhydramine HCl
12.5 mg .... Cough suppressant/Antihistamine

Uses:
• temporarily relieves
  • runny nose • sneezing
  • itchy nose or throat
  • itchy, watery eyes due to hay fever
  • cough due to minor throat and bronchial irritation occurring with a cold

Warnings:
Do not use
• with any other product containing diphenhydramine, even one used on skin
Ask a doctor before use if the child has
• glaucoma
• cough that occurs with too much phlegm (mucus)
• cough that lasts or is chronic such as occurs with asthma or chronic bronchitis
Ask a doctor or pharmacist before use if the child is
• taking sedatives or tranquilizers
When using this product
• do not use more than directed
• marked drowsiness may occur. Sedatives and tranquilizers may increase the drowsiness effect.
• excitability may occur, especially in children
Stop use and ask a doctor if
• cough lasts more than 7 days, comes back, or is accompanied by fever, rash, or persistent headache. These could be signs of a serious condition.
Keep out of reach of children. In case of overdose, get medical help or contact a Poison Control Center right away.

Directions:
• children 6 to under 12 years of age: allow 1 strip to dissolve on tongue. May be taken every 4 hours.

• do not exceed 6 strips in 24 hours, or as directed by a doctor
• children under 6 years of age: ask a doctor

Other Information:
• store at controlled room temperature 20-25°C (68-77°F)

Inactive Ingredients:
acetone, alcohol, FD&C Blue 1, FD&C Red 40, flavors, hydroxypropyl cellulose, hypromellose, maltodextrin, microcrystalline cellulose, polyethylene glycol, pregelatinized starch, propylene glycol, purified water, sodium polystyrene sulfonate, sorbitol, sucralose, titanium dioxide
Alcohol: less than 5%

Questions? call **1-800-452-0051** 24 hours a day, 7 days a week.

How Supplied:
16 Grape Flavored medicated strips in a carton.
Shown in Product Identification Guide, page 515

**TRIAMINIC® Vapor Patch® Cough
(Novartis Consumer Health, Inc.)**
Menthol Cough Suppressant
Menthol Scent
Mentholated Cherry Scent

Drug Facts

Active Ingredient	Purpose:
(in each patch):	

Menthol 2.6% .... Cough suppressant

Uses:
• temporarily relieves cough due to
  • a cold
  • minor throat and bronchial irritation to help you sleep

Warnings:
For external use only. Do not take by mouth or place in nostrils.
Combustible: Keep away from fire or flame (for Menthol Scent only).
Ask a doctor before use if the child has
• a persistent or chronic cough such as occurs with asthma
• cough that occurs with too much phlegm (mucus)
• a history of skin sensitivity, including to any of the ingredients in this product or to skin adhesives
When using this product do not
• heat
• microwave
• use near an open flame (for Menthol Scent only)
• add to hot water or any container where heating water.
May cause splattering and result in burns.
Stop use and ask a doctor if
• cough persists for more than 7 days, comes back or occurs with a fever, rash or persistent headache. These could be signs of a serious condition

• too much skin irritation occurs or gets worse
Keep out of reach of children. If swallowed, get medical help or contact a poison control center right away.

Directions:
• **see important warnings under 'When Using this product'**
• children 2 to under 12 years of age:
  • remove plastic packing
  • apply patch on the throat or chest. More than one patch can be applied.
  • clothing should be loose about the throat and chest to help vapors reach the nose and mouth
  • discard old and apply a new patch or patches up to three times daily or as directed by a doctor
• children under 2 years of age: Ask a doctor
• may use with other cough suppressant products.
Other Information:
• store at controlled room temperature 20–25° C (68–77° F)
• protect from excessive heat (for Menthol Scent only)

Menthol Scent:
Inactive Ingredients:
acrylic ester copolymer, aloe vera gel, camphor, eucalyptus oil, glycerin, karaya, turpentine spirits

Mentholated Cherry Scent:
Inactive Ingredients
acrylic ester copolymer, aloe vera gel, camphor, eucalyptus oil, glycerin, karaya, propylene glycol, purified water, wild cherry fragrance

Questions?
Call 1-800-452-0051
24 hours a day, 7 days a week.

How Supplied:
Available in 6 ct. Chest Patch cartons.

CHILDREN'S TYLENOL® Plus Cold & Allergy (McNeil Consumer)

For full product information see page 716.

CHILDREN'S TYLENOL® Plus Flu (McNeil Consumer)

Description:
Children's TYLENOL® Plus Flu Suspension Liquid is Bubble Gum flavored and contains no alcohol or aspirin. Each teaspoon (5 mL) contains acetaminophen 160 mg, chlorpheniramine maleate 1 mg, dextromethorphan HBr 5 mg and phenylephrine HCl 2.5 mg.

Continued on next page

Tylenol Children's Plus Flu—Cont.

Actions:

Children's TYLENOL® Plus Flu Suspension Liquid combines the analgesic-antipyretic acetaminophen with the decongestant phenylephrine hydrochloride, the cough suppressant dextromethorphan hydrobromide and the antihistamine chlorpheniramine maleate to provide fast, effective, temporary relief of all your child's symptoms associated with flu including fever, body aches, headache, stuffy nose, runny nose, sore throat and coughs. Acetaminophen is equal to aspirin in analgesic and antipyretic effectiveness and it is unlikely to produce the side effects often associated with aspirin or aspirin-containing products.

Uses:

temporarily relieves the following cold/flu symptoms:
- minor aches and pains
- headache • sore throat
- cough • stuffy nose • sneezing and runny nose
- temporarily reduces fever

Directions:

See Table 1: Children's Tylenol Dosing Chart on pgs. 757–758.

Warnings:

Sore throat warning: If sore throat is severe, persists for more than 2 days, is accompanied or followed by fever, headache, rash, nausea or vomiting, consult a doctor promptly.

Do not use
- with any other product containing acetaminophen
- in a child who is taking a prescription monoamine oxidase inhibitor (MAOI) (certain drugs for depression, psychiatric or emotional conditions, or Parkinson's disease), or for 2 weeks after stopping the MAOI drug. If you do not know if your child's prescription drug contains an MAOI, ask a doctor or pharmacist before giving this product.

Ask a doctor before use if the child has
- heart disease
- high blood pressure
- thyroid disease
- diabetes
- persistent or chronic cough such as occurs with asthma
- cough that occurs with too much phlegm (mucus)
- a breathing problem such as chronic bronchitis
- glaucoma

Ask a doctor or pharmacist before use if the child is taking sedatives or tranquilizers

When using this product
- **do not exceed recommended dosage (see overdose warning)**
- excitability may occur, especially in children
- marked drowsiness may occur
- sedatives and tranquilizers may increase the drowsiness effect

Stop use and ask a doctor if
- nervousness, dizziness or sleeplessness occur

- pain, nasal congestion or cough gets worse or lasts for more than 5 days
- fever gets worse or lasts for more than 3 days
- redness or swelling is present
- new symptoms occur
- cough comes back or occurs with rash or headache that lasts

These could be signs of a serious condition.

Keep out of reach of children.

Overdose warning: Taking more than the recommended dose (overdose) may cause liver damage. In case of overdose, get medical help or contact a Poison Control Center right away (1-800-222-1222). Quick medical attention is critical for adults as well as for children even if you do not notice any signs or symptoms.

Other Information:

- store between 20–25°C (68–77°F).

PROFESSIONAL INFORMATION: OVERDOSAGE INFORMATION

For overdosage information, please refer to pg. 680.

Inactive Ingredients: carboxymethylcellulose sodium, cellulose, citric acid, D&C red #33, FD&C red #40, flavors, glycerin, purified water, sodium benzoate, sorbitol, sucrose, xanthan gum.

How Supplied:

Pink colored, Bubble Gum flavored liquid in child resistant tamper-evident bottle of 4 fl. oz.

Shown in Product Identification Guide, page 510

TYLENOL® Cold Head Congestion Daytime Caplets with Cool Burst™ and Gelcaps (McNeil Consumer)

TYLENOL® Cold Head Congestion Nighttime Caplets with Cool Burst™

TYLENOL® Cold Head Congestion Severe Caplets with Cool Burst™

Product information for all dosage forms of TYLENOL® Cold Head Congestion have been combined under this heading.

Description:

Each *TYLENOL® Cold Head Congestion Daytime Caplet with Cool Burst*™ and *Gelcap* contains acetaminophen 325 mg, dextromethorphan HBr 10 mg, and phenylephrine HCl 5 mg. Each *TYLENOL® Cold Head Congestion Nighttime Caplet with Cool Burst*™ contains acetaminophen 325 mg, chlorpheniramine maleate 2 mg, dextromethorphan HBr 10 mg, and phenylephrine HCl 5 mg. Each *TYLENOL® Cold Head Congestion Severe Caplet with Cool Burst*™ contains acetaminophen 325 mg, dextromethorphan HBr 10 mg, guaifenesin 200 mg and phenylephrine HCl 5 mg.

Actions:

TYLENOL® Cold Head Congestion Daytime contains a clinically proven analgesic/antipyretic, a decongestant and a cough suppressant. Acetaminophen produces analgesia by elevation of the pain threshold and antipyresis through action on the hypothalamic heat regulating center. Acetaminophen is equal to aspirin in analgesic and antipyretic effectiveness and it is unlikely to produce many of the side effects associated with aspirin and aspirin-containing products. Phenylephrine is a sympathomimetic amine which provides temporary relief of nasal congestion. Dextromethorphan is a cough suppressant which provides temporary relief of coughs due to minor throat irritations that may occur with the common cold. *TYLENOL® Cold Head Congestion Nighttime* contains, in addition to the above ingredients, an antihistamine. Chlorpheniramine is an antihistamine which helps provide temporary relief of runny nose, sneezing and watery and itchy eyes. *TYLENOL® Cold Head Congestion Severe* contains, in addition to the above ingredients, an expectorant. Guafenesin is an expectorant which helps loosen phlegm (mucus) and thin bronchial secretions to make coughs more productive.

Uses:

TYLENOL® Cold Head Congestion Daytime
- temporarily relieves these common cold symptoms:
  - minor aches and pains • headache
  - sore throat • nasal congestion • cough
  - sinus congestion and pressure
- helps clear nasal passages

TYLENOL® Cold Head Congestion Nighttime
- temporarily relieves these common cold symptoms:
  - minor aches and pains • headache
  - sore throat • nasal congestion • cough
  - sinus congestion and pressure
  - sneezing and runny nose
- helps clear nasal passages
- relieves cough to help you sleep

TYLENOL® Cold Head Congestion Severe
- for the temporary relief of the following cold/flu symptoms:
  - minor aches and pains • headache
  - sore throat • nasal congestion • cough
  - impulse to cough
- helps loosen phlegm (mucus) and thin bronchial secretions to make coughs more productive
- temporarily reduces fever

Directions:

TYLENOL® Cold Head Congestion Daytime Gelcaps
- **do not take more than directed (see overdose warning)**

adults and children 12 years and over	• take 2 gelcaps every 4 hours • do not take more than 12 gelcaps in 24 hours

children under 12 years	• do not use this adult product in children under 12 years of age; this will provide more than the recommended dose (overdose) and may cause liver damage.

TYLENOL® Cold Head Congestion Daytime, Nighttime and Severe Caplets with Cool Burst™
- **do not take more than directed (see overdose warning)**

adults and children 12 years and over	• take 2 caplets every 4 hours • swallow whole – do not crush, chew or dissolve • do not take more than 12 caplets in 24 hours
children under 12 years	• do not use this adult product in children under 12 years of age; this will provide more than the recommended dose (overdose) and may cause liver damage.

Warnings:

Alcohol warning: If you consume 3 or more alcoholic drinks every day, ask your doctor whether you should take acetaminophen or other pain relievers or fever reducers. Acetaminophen may cause liver damage.

Sore throat warning: If sore throat is severe, persists for more than 2 days, is accompanied or followed by fever, headache, rash, nausea, or vomiting, consult a doctor promptly.

Do not use
- with any other product containing acetaminophen
- if you are now taking a prescription monoamine oxidase inhibitor (MAOI) (certain drugs for depression, psychiatric or emotional conditions, or Parkinson's disease), or for 2 weeks after stopping the MAOI drug. If you do not know if your prescription drug contains an MAOI, ask a doctor or pharmacist before taking this product.

TYLENOL® Cold Head Congestion Daytime Gelcaps and Caplets and Severe Caplets with Cool Burst™
Ask a doctor before use if you have
- heart disease • high blood pressure
- thyroid disease • diabetes
- trouble urinating due to an enlarged prostate gland
- persistent or chronic cough such as occurs with smoking, asthma or emphysema (applies to *TYLENOL® Cold Head Congestion Daytime Gelcaps and Caplets only*)
- cough that occurs with too much phlegm (mucus)
- persistent or chronic cough such as occurs with smoking, asthma, chronic

bronchitis or emphysema (*applies to TYLENOL® Cold Head Congestion Severe Caplets with Cool Burst*™ only)
When using this product do not exceed recommended dosage
TYLENOL® Cold Head Congestion Nighttime Caplets with Cool Burst™
Ask a doctor before use if you have
- heart disease • high blood pressure
- thyroid disease • diabetes
- trouble urinating due to an enlarged prostate gland
- persistent or chronic cough such as occurs with smoking, asthma or emphysema
- cough that occurs with too much phlegm (mucus)
- a breathing problem such as emphysema or chronic bronchitis
- glaucoma

Ask a doctor or pharmacist before use if you are taking sedatives or tranquilizers
When using this product
- **do not exceed recommended dosage**
- excitability may occur, especially in children
- marked drowsiness may occur
- alcohol, sedatives and tranquilizers may increase the drowsiness effect
- avoid alcoholic drinks
- be careful when driving a motor vehicle or operating machinery

Stop use and ask a doctor if
- nervousness, dizziness, or sleeplessness occur
- pain, nasal congestion or cough gets worse or lasts for more than 7 days
- fever gets worse or lasts for more than 3 days
- redness or swelling is present
- new symptoms occur
- cough comes back or occurs with rash or headache that lasts

These could be signs of a serious condition.

If pregnant or breast-feeding, ask a health professional before use.

Keep out of reach of children.

Overdose warning: Taking more than the recommended dose (overdose) may cause liver damage. In case of overdose, get medical help or contact a Poison Control Center right away (1-800-222-1222). Quick medical attention is critical for adults as well as for children even if you do not notice any signs or symptoms.

Other information:
- each caplet contains: **sodium 3 mg** (*applies to TYLENOL® Cold Head Congestion Severe Caplets with Cool Burst*™ *only*)
- store between 20-25°C (68-77°F)
- avoid high humidity (*applies to TYLENOL® Cold Head Congestion Daytime Gelcaps only*)

PROFESSIONAL INFORMATION: OVERDOSAGE INFORMATION
For overdosage information, please refer to pgs. 696–697.

Inactive Ingredients:
TYLENOL® Cold Head Congestion Daytime Caplets: carnauba wax, castor

oil, cellulose, corn starch, flavors, hypromellose, iron oxide, silicon dioxide, sodium starch glycolate, stearic acid, sucralose

Gelcaps: benzyl alcohol, butylparaben, castor oil, cellulose, corn starch, edetate calcium disodium, FD&C blue #1, FD&C red #40, gelatin, hypromellose, iron oxide, methylparaben, propylparaben, silicon dioxide, sodium lauryl sulfate, sodium propionate, sodium starch glycolate, stearic acid, titanium dioxide
TYLENOL® Cold Head Congestion Nighttime Caplets: carnauba wax, cellulose, corn starch, FD&C blue #1, flavors, hypromellose, iron oxide, polyethylene glycol, polysorbate 80, silicon dioxide, sodium starch glycolate, stearic acid, sucralose, titanium dioxide
TYLENOL® Cold Head Congestion Severe Caplets: carnauba wax, cellulose, corn starch, croscarmellose sodium, D&C yellow #10, flavors, hydroxypropyl cellulose, hypromellose, iron oxide, mannitol, silicon dioxide, stearic acid, sucralose

How Supplied:
TYLENOL® Cold Head Congestion Daytime Caplet with Cool Burst™: White-colored, imprinted with "TY C1078"—blister packs of 24.
TYLENOL® Cold Head Congestion Daytime Gelcaps: Red- and white-colored, imprinted with "TY C1079"—blister packs of 24.
TYLENOL® Cold Head Congestion Nighttime Caplet with Cool Burst™: Light blue-colored, imprinted with "TY C1075"—blister packs 24.
TYLENOL® Cold Head Congestion Severe Caplet with Cool Burst™: Yellow-colored, imprinted with "TY MS C1071"—blister packs of 24.
Shown in Product Identification Guide, page 511 & 512

TYLENOL® COLD
Severe Congestion Non-Drowsy
Caplets with Cool Burst™
(McNeil Consumer)

Description:
Each *TYLENOL® Cold Severe Congestion Non-Drowsy Caplet with Cool Burst*™ contains acetaminophen 325 mg, dextromethorphan HBr 15 mg, guaifenesin 200 mg and pseudoephedrine HCl 30 mg.

Actions:
TYLENOL® Cold Severe Congestion Non-Drowsy Caplets with Cool Burst™ contain a clinically proven analgesic-antipyretic, decongestant, expectorant and cough suppressant. Acetaminophen produces analgesia by elevation of the pain threshold and antipyresis through action on the hypothalamic heat regulating center. Acetaminophen is equal to aspirin in analgesic and antipyretic effec-

Continued on next page

Tylenol Cold Severe—Cont.

tiveness and is unlikely to produce many of the side effects associated with aspirin and aspirin-containing products. Pseudoephedrine is a sympathomimetic amine which provides temporary relief of nasal congestion. Guaifenesin is an expectorant which helps loosen phlegm (mucus) and thin bronchial secretions to make coughs more productive. Dextromethorphan is a cough suppressant which provides temporary relief of coughs due to minor throat irritations that may occur with the common cold.

Uses:

temporarily relieves:
- cough • sore throat • minor aches and pains • headache • nasal congestion
- helps loosen phlegm (mucus) and thin bronchial secretions to make coughs more productive
- temporarily reduces fever

Directions:

- **do not take more than directed (see overdose warning)**

adults and children 12 years and over	• take 2 caplets every 6 hours as needed • swallow whole – do not crush, chew or dissolve • do not take more than 8 caplets in 24 hours
children under 12 years	• do not use this adult product in children under 12 years of age; this will provide more than the recommended dose (overdose) and may cause liver damage.

Warnings:

Alcohol warning: If you consume 3 or more alcoholic drinks every day, ask your doctor whether you should take acetaminophen or other pain relievers/fever reducers. Acetaminophen may cause liver damage.

Sore throat warning: If sore throat is severe, persists for more than 2 days, is accompanied or followed by fever, headache, rash, nausea or vomiting, consult a doctor promptly.

Do not use

- if you are now taking a prescription monoamine oxidase inhibitor (MAOI) (certain drugs for depression, psychiatric or emotional conditions, or Parkinson's disease), or for 2 weeks after stopping the MAOI drug. If you do not know if your prescription drug contains an MAOI, ask a doctor or pharmacist before taking this product.
- with any other product containing acetaminophen

Ask a doctor before use if you have

- heart disease • diabetes • thyroid disease • cough that occurs with too much phlegm (mucus) • high blood pressure

• trouble urinating due to an enlarged prostate gland • chronic cough that lasts as occurs with smoking, asthma or emphysema

When using this product

- **do not exceed recommended dosage**

Stop use and ask a doctor if

- pain, nasal congestion or cough gets worse or lasts for more than 7 days
- fever gets worse or lasts for more than 3 days
- redness or swelling is present
- new symptoms occur
- you get nervous, dizzy or sleepless
- cough comes back or occurs with rash or headache that lasts.

These could be signs of a serious condition.

If pregnant or breast-feeding, ask a health professional before use.

Keep out of reach of children.

Overdose warning: Taking more than the recommended dose (overdose) may cause liver damage. In case of overdose, get medical help or contact a Poison Control Center (1-800-222-1222) right away. Quick medical attention is critical for adults as well as for children even if you do not notice any signs or symptoms.

Other Information:

- each caplet contains: **sodium 3 mg**
- store at 20–25°C (68–77°F)

PROFESSIONAL INFORMATION: OVERDOSAGE INFORMATION

For overdosage information, please refer to pgs. 696–697.

Inactive Ingredients: carnauba wax, cellulose, corn starch, croscarmellose sodium, FD&C Blue #1, flavor, hypromellose, mannitol, povidone, silicon dioxide, stearic acid, sucralose, titanium dioxide

How Supplied:

Caplets: White-colored, imprinted with "TYLENOL COLD SC" in blue ink—blister packs of 24.

Shown in Product Identification Guide, page 512

TYLENOL® Cold Multi-Symptom Daytime Caplets with Cool Burst™ and Gelcaps (McNeil Consumer)

TYLENOL® Cold Multi-Symptom Nighttime Caplets with Cool Burst™

TYLENOL® Cold Multi-Symptom Severe Caplets with Cool Burst™

TYLENOL® Cold Multi-Symptom Daytime Liquid

TYLENOL® Cold Multi-Symptom Nighttime Liquid with Cool Burst™

TYLENOL® Cold Multi-Symptom Severe Daytime Liquid

Patient information for all dosage forms of TYLENOL® Cold Multi-Symptom have been combined under this heading.

Description:

Each *TYLENOL® Cold Multi-Symptom Daytime Caplet with Cool Burst™ and Gelcap* contains acetaminophen 325 mg, dextromethorphan HBr 10 mg and phenylephrine HCl 5 mg. Each *TYLENOL® Cold Multi-Symptom Nighttime Caplet with Cool Burst™* contains acetaminophen 325 mg, chlorpheniramine maleate 2 mg, dextromethorphan HBr 10 mg and phenylephrine HCl 5 mg. Each *TYLENOL® Cold Multi-Symptom Severe Caplet with Cool Burst™* contains acetaminophen 325 mg, dextromethorphan HBr 10 mg, guaifensin 200 mg and phenylephrine HCl 5 mg. *TYLENOL® Cold Multi-Symptom Daytime Liquid:* Each 15 mL (1 tablespoon) contains acetaminophen 325 mg, dextromethorphan HBr 10 mg and phenylephrine HCl 5 mg. *TYLENOL® Cold Multi-Symptom Nighttime Liquid with Cool Burst™:* Each 15 mL (1 tablespoon) contains acetaminophen 325 mg, dextromethorphan HBr 10 mg, doxylamine succinate 6.25 mg and phenylephrine HCl 5 mg. *TYLENOL® Cold Multi-Symptom Severe Daytime Liquid:* Each 15 mL (1 tablespoon) contains acetaminophen 325 mg, dextromethorphan HBr 10 mg, guaifenesin 200 mg and phenylephrine HCl 5 mg.

Actions:

TYLENOL® Cold Multi-Symptom Daytime Caplets with Cool Burst™ and Gelcaps contain a clinically proven analgesic/antipyretic, a decongestant and a cough suppressant. Acetaminophen produces analgesia by elevation of the pain threshold and antipyresis through action on the hypothalamic heat regulating center. Acetaminophen is equal to aspirin in analgesic and antipyretic effectiveness and it is unlikely to produce many of the side effects associated with aspirin and aspirin-containing products. Phenylephrine hydrochloride is a sympathomimetic amine which provides temporary relief of nasal congestion. Dextromethorphan is a cough suppressant which provides temporary relief of coughs due to minor throat irritations that may occur with the common cold. *TYLENOL® Cold Multi-Symptom Nighttime Caplets with Cool Burst™* contain the same clinically proven analgesic/antipyretic, decongestant and cough suppressant as *TYLENOL® Cold Multi-Symptom Daytime Caplets with Cool Burst™ and Gelcaps* along with an antihistamine. Chlorpheniramine maleate is an antihistamine that helps provide temporary relief of runny nose and sneezing. *TYLENOL® Cold Multi-Symptom Severe Caplets with Cool Burst™* contain the same clinically proven analgesic/antipyretic, decongestant and cough suppressant as *TYLENOL® Cold Multi-Symptom Caplets with Cool Burst™ and Gelcaps* along with an expectorant. Guaifenesin is an expectorant that helps loosen phlegm (mucus) and thin bronchial

secretions to make coughs more productive. *TYLENOL® Cold Multi-Symptom Daytime Liquid* contains the same clinically proven analgesic/antipyretic, cough suppressant and decongestant as *TYLENOL® Cold Multi-Symptom Daytime Caplets with Cool Burst™ and Gelcaps.*

TYLENOL® Cold Multi-Symptom Nighttime Liquid with Cool Burst™ contains the same clinically proven analgesic/ antipyretic, cough suppressant and decongestant as *TYLENOL® Cold Multi-Symptom Daytime Liquid* along with an antihistamine, doxylamine succinate. Doxylamine succinate is an antihistamine that helps provide temporary relief of runny nose and sneezing.

TYLENOL® Cold Multi-Symptom Severe Daytime Liquid contains the same clinically proven analgesic/antipyretic, cough suppressant, expectorant and decongestant as *TYLENOL® Cold Multi-Symptom Severe Caplets with Cool Burst™.*

Uses:

TYLENOL® Cold Multi-Symptom Daytime Caplets with Cool Burst™ and Gelcaps:
• temporarily relieves these common cold symptoms:
  • minor aches and pains • headache
  • sore throat • nasal congestion • cough
• helps clear nasal passages
• temporarily reduces fever
TYLENOL® Cold Multi-Symptom Nighttime Caplets with Cool Burst™:
• temporarily relieves these common cold symptoms:
  • minor aches and pains • headache
  • sore throat • nasal congestion • cough
  • sneezing and runny nose
• helps clear nasal passages
• relieves cough to help you sleep
TYLENOL® Cold Multi-Symptom Severe Caplets with Cool Burst™:
• for the temporary relief of the following cold/flu symptoms:
  • minor aches and pains • headache
  • sore throat • nasal congestion • cough
  • impulse to cough
• helps loosen phlegm (mucus) and thin bronchial secretions to make coughs more productive
• temporarily reduces fever
TYLENOL® Cold Multi-Symptom Daytime Liquid:
• temporarily relieves these common cold symptoms:
  • minor aches and pains • headache
  • sore throat • nasal congestion • cough
  • sinus congestion and pressure
• helps clear nasal passages
TYLENOL® Cold Multi-Symptom Nighttime Liquid with Cool Burst™:
• temporarily relieves these common cold symptoms:
  • minor aches and pains • headache
  • sore throat • nasal congestion • runny nose and sneezing • cough
• relieves cough to help you get rest
• temporarily reduces fever

TYLENOL® Cold Multi-Symptom Severe Daytime Liquid:
• for the temporary relief of the following cold symptoms:
  • minor aches and pains • headache
  • sore throat • nasal congestion • cough
• helps loosen phlegm (mucus) and thin bronchial secretions to make coughs more productive
• temporarily reduces fever

Directions:
• **do not take more than directed (see overdose warning)**
TYLENOL® Cold Multi-Symptom Daytime Caplets with Cool Burst™ and Gelcaps:

adults and children 12 years and over	• take 2 caplets or gelcaps every 4 hours • swallow whole – do not crush, chew or dissolve (caplets only) • do not take more than 12 caplets or gelcaps in 24 hours
children under 12 years	• do not use this adult product in children under 12 years of age; this will provide more than the recommended dose (overdose) and may cause liver damage.

TYLENOL® Cold Multi-Symptom Nighttime Caplets with Cool Burst™ and TYLENOL® Cold Multi-Symptom Severe Caplets with Cool Burst™:
• **do not take more than directed (see overdose warning)**

adults and children 12 years and over	• take 2 caplets every 4 hours • swallow whole – do not crush, chew or dissolve • do not take more than 12 caplets in 24 hours
children under 12 years	• do not use this adult product in children under 12 years of age; this will provide more than the recommended dose (overdose) and may cause liver damage.

TYLENOL® Cold Multi-Symptom Daytime Liquid and TYLENOL® Cold Multi-Symptom Severe Daytime Liquid
• **do not take more than directed (see overdose warning)**
• use only enclosed measuring cup designed for use with this product. Do not use any other dosing device.

adults and children 12 years and over	• take 2 tablespoons (tbsp) or 1 oz every 4 hours • do not take more than 12 tablespoons (tbsp) or 6 oz in 24 hours

children under 12 years	• do not use this adult product in children under 12 years of age; this will provide more than the recommended dose (overdose) and may cause liver damage.

TYLENOL® Cold Multi-Symptom Nighttime Liquid with Cool Burst™:
• **do not take more than directed (see overdose warning)**
• only use enclosed measuring cup designed for use with this product

adults and children 12 years and over	• take 2 tablespoons (Tbsp) or 30 mL every 4 hours • do not take more than 12 tablespoons (Tbsp) or 180 mL in 24 hours
children under 12 years	• do not use this adult product in children under 12 years of age; this will provide more than the recommended dose (overdose) and may cause liver damage.

WARNINGS

Alcohol warning: If you consume 3 or more alcoholic drinks every day, ask your doctor whether you should take acetaminophen or other pain relievers or fever reducers. Acetaminophen may cause liver damage.

Sore throat warning: If sore throat is severe, persists for more than 2 days, is accompanied or followed by fever, headache, rash, nausea, or vomiting, consult a doctor promptly.

Do not use
• with any other product containing acetaminophen
• if you are now taking a prescription monoamine oxidase inhibitor (MAOI) (certain drugs for depression, psychiatric or emotional conditions, or Parkinson's disease), or for 2 weeks after stopping the MAOI drug. If you do not know if your prescription drug contains an MAOI, ask a doctor or pharmacist before taking this product.

Ask a doctor before use if you have
TYLENOL® Cold Multi-Symptom Daytime Caplets with Cool Burst™ and Gelcaps and TYLENOL® Cold Multi-Symptom Daytime Liquid
• heart disease • high blood pressure
• thyroid disease • diabetes
• trouble urinating due to an enlarged prostate gland
• persistent or chronic cough such as occurs with smoking, asthma or emphysema
• cough that occurs with too much phlegm (mucus)

Continued on next page

Tylenol—Cont.

TYLENOL® Cold Multi-Symptom Night-time Caplets with Cool Burst™ and TYLENOL® Cold Multi-Symptom Nighttime Liquid

- heart disease • high blood pressure
- thyroid disease • diabetes
- trouble urinating due to an enlarged prostate gland
- persistent or chronic cough such as occurs with smoking, asthma or emphysema
- cough that occurs with too much phlegm (mucus)
- a breathing problem such as emphysema or chronic bronchitis
- glaucoma

TYLENOL® Cold Multi-Symptom Severe Caplets with Cool Burst™ and TYLENOL® Cold Multi-Symptom Severe Daytime Liquid

- heart disease • high blood pressure
- thyroid disease • diabetes
- trouble urinating due to an enlarged prostate gland
- persistent or chronic cough such as occurs with smoking, asthma, chronic bronchitis or emphysema
- cough that occurs with too much phlegm (mucus)

Ask a doctor or pharmacist before use if you are taking sedatives or tranquilizers (applies to *TYLENOL® Cold Multi-Symptom Nighttime Caplets with Cool Burst™ and TYLENOL® Cold Multi-Symptom Nighttime Liquid with Cool Burst™ only*)

When using this product

- **do not exceed recommended dosage** *(all products)*

(the following applies to *TYLENOL® Cold Multi-Symptom Nighttime Caplets with Cool Burst™ and TYLENOL® Cold Multi-Symptom Nighttime Liquid with Cool Burst™ only*)

- excitability may occur, especially in children
- marked drowsiness may occur
- alcohol, sedatives and tranquilizers may increase the drowsiness effect
- avoid alcoholic drinks
- be careful when driving a motor vehicle or operating machinery

Stop use and ask a doctor if

- nervousness, dizziness, or sleeplessness occur
- pain, nasal congestion or cough gets worse or lasts for more than 7 days
- fever gets worse or lasts for more than 3 days
- redness or swelling is present
- new symptoms occur
- cough comes back or occurs with rash or headache that lasts.

These could be signs of a serious condition.

If pregnant or breast-feeding, ask a health professional before use.

Keep out of reach of children.

Overdose Warning: Taking more than the recommended dose (overdose) may cause liver damage. In case of overdose, get medical help or contact a Poison Control Center right away (1-800-222-1222). Quick medical attention is critical for adults as well as for children even if you do not notice any signs or symptoms.

Other Information:

TYLENOL® Cold Multi-Symptom Severe Caplets with Cool Burst™

- each caplet contains: **sodium 3 mg**

TYLENOL® Cold Multi-Symptom Daytime Liquid, TYLENOL® Cold Multi-Symptom Nighttime Liquid with Cool Burst™ and TYLENOL® Cold Multi-Symptom Severe Daytime Liquid

- each tablespoon contains: **sodium 5 mg**

TYLENOL® Cold Multi-Symptom Daytime Caplets with Cool Burst™, TYLENOL® Cold Multi-Symptom Nighttime Caplets with Cool Burst™, TYLENOL® Cold Multi-Symptom Severe Caplets with Cool Burst™, TYLENOL® Cold Multi-Symptom Daytime Liquid, TYLENOL® Cold Multi-Symptom Nighttime Liquid with Cool Burst™, TYLENOL® Cold Multi-Symptom Severe Daytime Liquid:

- store between 20-25° C (68-77° F)

TYLENOL® Cold Multi-Symptom Daytime Gelcaps

- store between 20-25° C (68-77° F). Avoid high humidity.

PROFESSIONAL INFORMATION:

Overdosage Information:

For overdosage information, please refer to pgs. 696–697.

Inactive Ingredients: *TYLENOL® Cold Multi-Symptom Daytime:* **Caplets with Cool Burst™:** carnauba wax, castor oil, cellulose, corn starch, flavors, hypromellose, iron oxide, silicon dioxide, sodium starch glycolate, stearic acid, sucralose **Gelcaps:** benzyl alcohol, butylparaben, castor oil, cellulose, corn starch, edetate calcium disodium, FD&C blue #1, FD&C red #40, gelatin, hypromellose, iron oxide, methylparaben, propylparaben, silicon dioxide, sodium lauryl sulfate, sodium propionate, sodium starch glycolate, stearic acid, titanium dioxide *TYLENOL® Cold Multi-Symptom Nighttime Caplets with Cool Burst™:* carnauba wax, cellulose, corn starch, FD&C blue #1, flavors, hypromellose, iron oxide, polyethylene glycol, polysorbate 80, silicon dioxide, sodium starch glycolate, stearic acid, sucralose, titanium dioxide *TYLENOL® Cold Multi-Symptom Severe Caplets with Cool Burst™:* carnauba wax, cellulose, corn starch, croscarmellose sodium, D&C yellow #10, flavors, hydroxypropyl cellulose, hypromellose, iron oxide, mannitol, silicon dioxide, stearic acid, sucralose *TYLENOL® Cold Multi-Symptom Daytime Liquid and TYLENOL® Cold Multi-Symptom Severe Daytime Liquid:* critic acid, ethyl alcohol, FD&C yellow #6, flavors, glycerin, propylene glycol, purified water, sodium benzoate, sorbitol, sucralose *TYLENOL® Cold Multi-Symptom Nighttime Liquid with Cool Burst™:* citric acid, FD&C blue #1, flavors, glycerin, propylene glycol, purified water, sodium benzoate, sorbitol, sucralose

How Supplied:

TYLENOL® Cold Multi-Sympiom Daytime Caplets with Cool Burst™: clear (white) caplet, imprinted with "TY C1078" – blister packs of 24. *Gelcaps:* red and white colored gelcap, imprinted with "TY C1079" – blister packs of 24.

TYLENOL® Cold Multi-Symptom Nighttime Caplets with Cool Burst™: light blue, imprinted with "TY C1075" – blister packs of 24.

TYLENOL® Cold Multi-Symptom Severe Caplets with Cool Burst™: yellow, imprinted with "TY MS C1071" – blister packs of 24 and 48.

TYLENOL® Cold Multi-Symptom Daytime Liquid and TYLENOL® Cold Multi-Symptom Severe Daytime Liquid: Citrus Burst Liquid, orange colored – bottles of 8 fl. Oz.

TYLENOL® Cold Multi-Symptom Nighttime Liquid with Cool Burst™: Cool Burst flavor, blue colored – bottles of 8 fl. oz.

Shown in Product Identification Guide, page 511

TYLENOL® Sore Throat Daytime Liquid with Cool Burst™ (McNeil Consumer)

TYLENOL® Sore Throat Nighttime Liquid with Cool Burst™

TYLENOL® Cough & Sore Throat Daytime Liquid with Cool Burst™

TYLENOL® Cough & Sore Throat Nighttime Liquid with Cool Burst™

For full product information see page 790.

CONCENTRATED TYLENOL® Infants' Drops Plus Cold Nasal Decongestant, Fever Reducer & Pain Reliever (McNeil Consumer)

CONCENTRATED TYLENOL® Infants' Drops Plus Cold & Cough Nasal Decongestant, Fever Reducer & Pain Reliever, Cough Suppressant

CHILDREN'S TYLENOL® Plus Cough & Sore Throat Suspension Liquid

CHILDREN'S TYLENOL® Plus Cough & Runny Nose Suspension Liquid

CHILDREN'S TYLENOL® Plus Multi-Symptom Cold Suspension Liquid

CHILDREN'S TYLENOL® Plus Cold Suspension Liquid

Description:

Concentrated TYLENOL® Infants' Drops Plus Cold are alcohol-free, aspirin-free,

BubbleGum-flavored and red in color. Each 0.8 mL contains acetaminophen 80 mg and phenylephrine HCl 1.25 mg.

Concentrated TYLENOL® Infants' Drops Plus Cold & Cough are alcohol-free, aspirin-free, Cherry-flavored and red in color. Each 0.8 mL contains acetaminophen 80 mg, dextromethorphan HBr 2.5 mg, and phenlyephrine HCl 1.25 mg.

Children's TYLENOL® Plus Cough & Sore Throat Suspension Liquid is Cherry-flavored and contains no alcohol or aspirin. Each teaspoon (5 mL) contains acetaminophen 160 mg and dextromethorphan HBr 5 mg.

Children's TYLENOL® Plus Cough & Runny Nose Suspension Liquid is Cherry-flavored and contains no alcohol or aspirin. Each teaspoon (5 mL) contains acetaminophen 160 mg, chlorpheniramine maleate 1 mg and dextromethorphan HBr 5 mg.

Children's TYLENOL® Plus Multi-Symptom Cold Suspension Liquid is Grape-flavored and contains no alcohol or aspirin. Each teaspoonful (5 mL) contains acetaminophen 160 mg, chlorpheniramine maleate 1 mg, dextromethorphan HBr 5 mg and phenylephrine HCl 2.5 mg.

Children's TYLENOL® Plus Cold Suspension Liquid is Grape-flavored and contains no alcohol or aspirin. Each teaspoon (5 mL) contains acetaminophen 160 mg, chlorpheniramine maleate 1 mg, and phenylephrine HCl 2.5 mg.

Actions:

Acetaminophen is a clinically proven analgesic/antipyretic. Acetaminophen produces analgesia by elevation of the pain threshold and antipyresis through action on the hypothalamic heat-regulating center. Acetaminophen is equal to aspirin in analgesic and antipyretic effectiveness and it is unlikely to produce many of the side effects associated with aspirin and aspirin-containing products. Phenylephrine hydrochloride is a sympathomimetic amine which provides temporary relief of nasal cogestion. Chlorpheniramine maleate is an antihistamine that provides temporary relief of runny nose, sneezing and watery and itchy eyes. Dextromethorphan hydrobromide is a cough suppressant which helps relieve coughs.

Uses:

Concentrated TYLENOL® Infants' Drops Plus Cold
- for the temporary relief of the following cold symptoms
  - minor aches and pains • headache
  - sore throat • stuffy nose
- temporarily reduces fever

Concentrated TYLENOL® Infants' Drops Plus Cold & Cough
- temporarily relieves the following cold/flu symptoms:
  - minor aches and pains • headache
  - sore throat • cough • stuffy nose
- temporarily reduces fever

Children's TYLENOL® Plus Cough & Sore Throat
- temporarily relieves the following cold/flu symptoms:
  - minor aches and pains • headache
  - sore throat • cough
- temporarily reduces fever

Children's TYLENOL® Plus Cough & Runny Nose
- temporarily relieves the following cold/flu symptoms:
  - minor aches and pains • headache
  - sore throat • sneezing and runny nose
  - cough
- temporarily reduces fever

TYLENOL® Plus Multi-Symptom Cold
- temporarily relieves the following cold/flu symptoms:
  - minor aches and pains • headache
  - sore throat • cough • stuffy nose
  - sneezing and runny nose
- temporarily reduces fever

Children's TYLENOL® Plus Cold
- temporarily relieves the following cold/flu symptoms:
  - minor aches and pains • headache
  - sore throat • stuffy nose • sneezing and runny nose
- temporarily reduces fever

Directions:

See Table 1: Children's Tylenol Dosing Chart on pgs. 757–758.

Warnings:

Sore throat warning: If sore throat is severe, persists for more than 2 days, is accompanied by or followed by fever, headache, rash, nausea, or vomiting, consult a doctor promptly.

Do not use
- with any other product containing acetaminophen
- in a child who is taking a prescription monoamine oxidase inhibitor (MAOI) (certain drugs for depression, psychiatric or emotional conditions, or Parkinson's disease), or for 2 weeks after stopping the MAOI drug. If you do not know if your child's prescription drug contains an MAOI, ask a doctor or pharmacist before giving this product.

Ask a doctor before use if the child has

Concentrated TYLENOL® Infants' Drops Plus Cold
- heart disease • high blood pressure
- thyroid disease • diabetes

Concentrated TYLENOL® Infants' Drops Plus Cold & Cough
- heart disease • high blood pressure
- thyroid disease • diabetes
- persistent or chronic cough such as occurs with asthma
- cough that occurs with too much phlegm (mucus)

Children's TYLENOL® Plus Cough & Sore Throat
- a persistent or chronic cough such as occurs with asthma
- a cough that occurs with too much phlegm (mucus)

Children's TYLENOL® Plus Cough & Runny Nose
- a breathing problem such as chronic bronchitis
- glaucoma
- persistent or chronic cough such as occurs with asthma
- cough that occurs with too much phlegm (mucus)

Children's TYLENOL® Plus Multi-Symptom Cold
- heart disease • high blood pressure
- thyroid disease • diabetes
- persistent or chronic cough such as occurs with asthma
- cough that occurs with too much phlegm (mucus)
- a breathing problem such as chronic bronchitis
- glaucoma

Children's TYLENOL® Plus Cold
- heart disease • high blood pressure
- thyroid disease • diabetes
- a breathing problem such as chronic bronchitis
- glaucoma

Ask a doctor or pharmacist before use if the child is taking sedatives or tranquilizers *(applies to Children's TYLENOL® Cough & Runny Nose, Children's TYLENOL® Plus Multi-Symptom Cold, and Children's TYLENOL® Plus Cold)*

When using this product
- **do not exceed recommended dosage (see overdose warning)**

Children's TYLENOL® Plus Cold
- excitability may occur, especially in children
- drowsiness may occur
- sedatives and tranquilizers may increase the drowsiness effect

Children's TYLENOL® Plus Cough & Runny Nose and Children's TYLENOL® Plus Multi-Symptom Cold
- excitability may occur, especially in children
- marked drowsiness may occur
- sedatives and tranquilizers may increase the drowsiness effect

Stop use and ask a doctor if

Concentrated TYLENOL® Infants' Drops Plus Cold and Children's TYLENOL® Plus Cold
- nervousness, dizziness or sleeplessness occur
- pain or nasal congestion gets worse or lasts for more than 5 days
- fever gets worse or lasts for more than 3 days
- new symptoms occur
- redness or swelling is present

These could be signs of a serious condition.

Concentrated TYLENOL® Infants' Drops Plus Cold & Cough and Children's TYLENOL® Plus Multi-Symptom Cold
- nervousness, dizziness or sleeplessness occur
- pain, nasal congestion or cough gets worse or lasts for more than 5 days
- fever gets worse or lasts for more than 3 days
- new symptoms occur
- redness or swelling is present
- cough comes back or occurs with rash or headache that lasts

These could be signs of a serious condition.

Children's TYLENOL® Plus Cough & Sore Throat and Children's TYLENOL® Plus Cough & Runny Nose

Continued on next page

Tylenol—Cont.

- pain or cough gets worse or lasts for more than 5 days
- fever gets worse or lasts for more than 3 days
- redness or swelling is present
- new symptoms occur
- cough comes back or occurs with rash or headache that lasts

These could be signs of a serious condition.

Keep out of reach of children

Overdose warning: Taking more than the recommended dose (overdose) may cause liver damage. In case of overdose, get medical help or contact a Poison Control Center right away (1-800-222-1222). Quick medical attention is critical for adults as well as for children even if you do not notice any signs or symptoms.

Other Information:
- store between 20-25° C (68-77° F)

PROFESSIONAL INFORMATION: OVERDOSAGE INFORMATION

For overdosage information, please refer to pg. 680.

Inactive Ingredients:
Concentrated TYLENOL® Infants' Drops Plus Cold: carboxymethylcellulose sodium, cellulose, citric acid, D&C red #33, FD&C red #40, flavors, glycerin, purified water, sodium benzoate, sorbitol, sucralose, xanthan gum

Concentrated TYLENOL® Infants' Drops Plus Cold & Cough: carboxymethylcellulose sodium, cellulose, citric acid, FD&C red #40, flavors, glycerin, purified water, sodium benzoate, sorbitol, sucralose, xanthan gum

Children's TYLENOL® Plus Cough & Sore Throat: acesulfame potassium, carboxymethylcellulose sodium, cellulose, citric acid, corn syrup, D&C red #33, FD&C red #40, flavors, glycerin, purified water, sodium benzoate, sorbitol, xanthan gum

Children's TYLENOL® Plus Cough & Runny Nose: acesulfame potassium, carboxymethylcellulose sodium, cellulose, citric acid, corn syrup, D&C red #33, FD&C red #40, flavors, glycerin, purified water, sodium benzoate, sorbitol, xanthan gum

Children's TYLENOL® Plus Multi-Symptom Cold: carboxymethylcellulose sodium, cellulose, citric acid, D&C red #33, FD&C blue #1, FD&C red #40, flavors, glycerin, purified water, sodium benzoate, sorbitol, sucrose, xanthan gum

Children's TYLENOL® Plus Cold: carboxymethylcellulose sodium, cellulose, citric acid, D&C red #33, FD&C blue #1, FD&C red #40, flavors, glycerin, purified water, sodium benzoate, sorbitol, sucrose, xanthan gum

How Supplied:
Concentrated TYLENOL® Infants' Drops Plus Cold: Pink colored, Bubble Gum flavored drops in child resistant tamper-evident bottles of ½ fl. oz.

Concentrated TYLENOL® Infants' Drops Plus Cold & Cough: Red colored, Cherry flavored drops in child resistant tamper-evident bottles of ½ fl. oz.

Children's TYLENOL® Plus Cough & Sore Throat: Red colored, Cherry flavored liquid in child resistant tamper-evident bottles of 4 fl. oz.

Children's TYLENOL® Plus Cough & Runny Nose: Red colored, Cherry flavored liquid in child resistant tamper-evident bottles of 4 fl. oz.

Children's TYLENOL® Plus Multi-Symptom Cold: Purple colored, Grape flavored liquid in child resistant tamper-evident bottles of 4 fl. oz.

Children's TYLENOL® Plus Cold: Purple colored, Grape flavored liquid in child resistant tamper-evident bottles of 4 fl. oz.

Shown in Product Identification Guide, page 510

CHILDREN'S TYLENOL® Dosing Chart (McNeil Consumer)

[See table on pages 757 & 758]

CHILDREN'S VICKS® NYQUIL® (Procter & Gamble)
Antihistamine/Cough Suppressant

Children's NyQuil was specially formulated with three effective ingredients to relieve nighttime cough and runny nose so children can rest. Children's NyQuil® is alcohol free and analgesic free and has a peasant cherry flavor.

Drug Facts
Active Ingredients:
(in each 15 ml tablespoon)   Purposes:
Chlorpheniramine maleate
    2 mg .... Antihistamine
Dextromethorphan HBr
    15 mg .... Cough suppressant

Uses: temporarily relieves cold symptoms:
- cough due to minor throat and bronchial irritation
- sneezing
- runny nose

Warnings:
Do not use if you are now taking a prescription monoamine oxidase inhibitor (MAOI) (certain drugs for depression, psychiatric or emotional conditions, or Parkinson's disease), or for 2 weeks after stopping the MAOI drug. If you do not know if your prescription drug contains an MAOI, ask a doctor or pharmacist before taking this product.

Ask a doctor before use if you have
- glaucoma
- cough that occurs with too much phlegm (mucus)
- a breathing problem or chronic cough that lasts or as occurs with smoking, asthma, chronic bronchitis, or emphysema

- trouble urinating due to enlarged prostate gland
- a sodium-restricted diet

Ask a doctor or pharmacist before use if you are taking sedatives or tranquilizers.

When using this product
- do not use more than directed
- excitability may occors, especially in children
- marked drowsiness may occur
- avoid alcoholic drinks
- be careful when driving a motor vehicle or operating machinery
- alcohol, sedatives, and tranquilizers may increase drowsiness

Stop use and ask a doctor if
- cough lasts more than 7 days, comes back, or occurs with fever, rash, or headache that lasts. These could be signs of a serious condition.

If pregnant or breast-feeding, ask a health professional before use.

Keep out of reach of children. In case of overdose, get medical help or contact a Poison Conrol Center right aways.

Directions:
- use dose cup or tablespoon (TBSP)
- do not exceed 4 doses per 24 huors

adults and children 12 years and over	2 TBSP (30 ml) every 6 hours
children 6 to 11 years	1 TBSP (15 ml) every 6 hours
children under 6 years	ask a doctor

Other Information:
- each tablespoon contains sodium 71 mg
- store at room temperature

Inactive Ingredients: citric acid, FD&C Red No. 40, flavor, potassium sorbate, propylene glycol, purified water, sodium citrate, sucrose

Questions? 1-800-362-1683

How Supplied: Available in 4 and 6 OZ

Shown in Product Identification Guide, page 516

PEDIATRIC VICKS® 44e® (Procter & Gamble)
Cough & Chest Congestion Relief
Cough suppressant/Expectorant

- Non-drowsy
- Alcohol-free
- Aspirin-free

Drug Facts:

Active Ingredient: Purpose:
(per 15 ml tablespoon
Dextromethorphan
    HBr 10 mg .... Cough suppressant
Guaifenesin 100mg .... Expectorant

TABLE 1
Children's Tylenol® Dosing Chart

AGE GROUP		0–3 mos	4–11 mos	12–23 mos	2–3 yrs	4–5 yrs	6–8 yrs	9–10 yrs	11 yrs	12 yrs	Maximum doses/24 hrs
WEIGHT (if possible use weight to dose; otherwise use age)		6–11 lbs	12–17 lbs	18–23 lbs	24–35 lbs	36–47 lbs	48–59 lbs	60–71 lbs	72–95 lbs	96 lbs and over	
PRODUCT FORM	**INGREDIENTS**	Dose to be administered based on weight or age†									
Infants' Drops	in each (0.8 mL)										
Concentrated Tylenol Infants' Drops	Acetaminophen 80 mg	(0.4 mL)*	(0.8 mL)*	1.2 mL (0.8 + 0.4 mL)*	1.6 mL (0.8 + 0.8 mL)	—	—	—	—	—	5 times in 24 hrs
Concentrated Tylenol Infants' Drops Plus Cold	Acetaminophen 80 mg, Phenylephrine HCl 1.25 mg	(0.4 mL)*	(0.8 mL)*	1.2 mL (0.8 + 0.4 mL)*	1.6 mL (0.8 + 0.8 mL)	—	—	—	—	—	5 times in 24 hrs
Concentrated Tylenol Infants' Drops Plus Cold & Cough	Acetaminophen 80 mg, Dextromethorphan HBr 2.5 mg, Phenylephrine HCl 1.25 mg	(0.4 mL)*	(0.8 mL)*	1.2 mL (0.8 + 0.4 mL)*	1.6 mL (0.8 + 0.8 mL)*	—	—	—	—	—	5 times in 24 hrs
Children's Liquids	Per 5 mL = 1 teaspoonful (TSP)										
Children's Tylenol Suspension Liquid	Acetaminophen 160 mg	—	½ TSP*	¾ TSP*	1 TSP	1½ TSP	2 TSP	2½ TSP	3 TSP	—	5 times in 24 hrs
Children's Tylenol with Flavor Creator	Acetaminophen 160 mg	—	—	—	1 TSP	1½ TSP	2 TSP	2½ TSP	3 TSP	—	5 times in 24 hrs
Children's Tylenol Plus Cold Suspension Liquid	Acetaminophen 160 mg, Chlorpheniramine Maleate 1 mg, Phenylephrine HCl 2.5 mg	—	½ TSP**	¾ TSP**	1 TSP**	1 TSP**	2 TSP	2 TSP	2 TSP	—	5 times in 24 hrs
Children's Tylenol Plus Multi-Symptom Cold Suspension Liquid	Acetaminophen 160 mg, Chlorpheniramine Maleate 1 mg, Dextromethorphan HBr 5 mg, Phenylephrine HCl 2.5 mg	—	½ TSP**	¾ TSP**	1 TSP**	1 TSP**	2 TSP	2 TSP	2 TSP	—	5 times in 24 hrs

Product	Active Ingredients	Dosage (youngest → oldest age/weight)	Max. doses
Children's Tylenol Plus Flu Suspension Liquid	Acetaminophen 160 mg; Chlorpheniramine Maleate 1 mg; Dextromethorphan HBr 5 mg; Phenylephrine HCl 2.5 mg	—, ½ TSP**, ¾ TSP**, 1 TSP**, 1 TSP**, 2 TSP, 2 TSP, 2 TSP, —	5 times in 24 hrs
Children's Tylenol Plus Cold & Allergy Liquid	Acetaminophen 160 mg; Diphenhydramine HCl 12.5 mg; Phenylephrine HCl 2.5 mg	—, ½ TSP**, ¾ TSP**, 1 TSP**, 1 TSP**, 2 TSP, 2 TSP, 2 TSP, —	5 times in 24 hrs
Children's Tylenol Plus Cough & Runny Nose	Acetaminophen 160 mg; Chlorpheniramine Maleate 1 mg; Dextromethorphan HBr 5 mg	—, ½ TSP**, ¾ TSP**, 1 TSP**, 1 TSP**, 2 TSP, 2 TSP, 2 TSP, —	5 times in 24 hrs
Children's Tylenol Plus Cough & Sore Throat	Acetaminophen 160 mg; Dextromethorphan HBr 5 mg	—, ½ TSP*, ¾ TSP*, 1 TSP, 1 TSP, 2 TSP, 2 TSP, 2 TSP, —	5 times in 24 hrs
Children's Tablets — *Per tablet*			
Children's Tylenol Meltaways	Acetaminophen 80 mg	—, —, 2 tablets, 3 tablets, 4 tablets, 5 tablets, 6 tablets, —	5 times in 24 hrs
Jr. Tylenol Meltaways	Acetaminophen 160 mg	—, —, —, 2 tablets, 2½ tablets, 3 tablets, 4 tablets, —	5 times in 24 hrs

†All products may be dosed every 4 hours, if needed.

*Under 2 years (under 24 lbs), consult a doctor. **Under 6 years (under 48 lbs), consult a doctor.

- Infants' Tylenol Drops are more concentrated than Children's Tylenol Liquids. The Infants' Concentrated Drops have been specifically designed for use only with enclosed dropper. Do not use any other dosing device with this product. Shake well before using; fill to prescribed level and dispense liquid slowly into child's mouth, toward inner cheek. Use original bottle cap or dropper to maintain child resistance.
- Children's Tylenol Liquids are less concentrated than Infants' Tylenol Concentrated Drops. The Children's Tylenol Liquids have been specifically designed for use with the enclosed measuring cup. Use only enclosed measuring cup to dose this product. Shake well before using.
- Children's Tylenol Meltaways Tablets are not the same concentration as Junior Strength Tylenol Meltaways Tablets; dissolve in mouth or chew before swallowing.
- Jr. Tylenol Meltaways Tablets contain twice as much medicine as Children's Tylenol Meltaways Tablets; dissolve in mouth or chew before swallowing.
- Single ingredient Infants', Children's and Junior Tylenol acetaminophen products—do not use for more than 5 days unless directed by a doctor.
- Children's Tylenol with Flavor Creator: shake the Children's Tylenol® product well before using. Use the measuring cup provided with the enclosed Children's Tylenol® in the measuring cup. Once the measuring cup contains the recommended dose, pour the entire contents of 1 flavor packet onto the Children's Tylenol® in the measuring cup. Do not stir to dissolve Flavor Crystals in the medicine. Take promptly. Reseal pouch of unopened flavor packets. Do not give for more than 5 days unless directed by a doctor.

Uses:
- temporarily relieves cough due to the common cold
- helps loosen phlegm and thin bronchial secretions to rid bronchial passageways of bothersome mucus

Warnings:

Do not use
- if you are now taking a prescription monoamine oxidase inhibitor (MAOI) (certain drugs for depression, psychiatric or emotional conditions, or Parkinson's disease), or for 2 weeks after stopping the MAOI drug. If you do not know if your prescription drug contains an MAOI, ask a doctor or pharmacist before taking this product.

Ask a doctor before use if you have:
- a sodium restricted diet
- cough that occurs with too much phlegm (mucus)
- persistent or chronic cough such as occurs with smoking, asthma, chronic bronchitis or emphysema

Stop use and ask a doctor if:
- cough lasts more than 7 days, comes back, or occurs with fever, rash, or headache that lasts. These could be signs of a serious condition.

If pregnant or breast-feeding, ask a health professional before use.

Keep out of reach of children. In case of overdose, get medical help or contact a Poison Control Center right away.

Directions:
- use tablespoon (TBSP) or dose cup
- do not exceed 6 doses per 24 hours
  Under 2 yrs. .... ask a doctor
  2–5 yrs. .... ½ TBSP (7½ ml) every 4 hours
  6–11 yrs. .... 1 TBSP (15 ml) every 4 hours
  12 yrs. & older .... 2 TBSP (30 ml) every 4 hours

Other Information:
- **each tablespoon contains** sodium 30 mg
- store at room temperature

Inactive Ingredients: Carboxymethyl-cellulose sodium, citric acid, FD&C red no. 40, flavor, high fructose corn syrup, polyethylene oxide, polyoxyl 40 stearate, propylene glycol, purified water, saccharin sodium, sodium benzoate, sodium citrate.

How Supplied: 4 FL OZ (118 ml) plastic bottles. A calibrated dose cup accompanies each bottle.

TAMPER EVIDENT: Do not use if imprinted shrinkband is missing or broken.

Questions? 1-800-342-6844

Dist. by Procter & Gamble, Cincinnati OH 45202.

US Pat 5,458,879   42434802

Shown in Product Identification Guide, page 516

**PEDIATRIC VICKS® 44m®
(Procter & Gamble)
Cough & Cold Relief
Cough Suppressant/Antihistamine**

- Alcohol-free
- Aspirin-free

Drug Facts

**Active Ingredients:
(per 15 ml tablespoon)   Purposes:**
Chlorpheniramine maleate
  2 mg .... Pain reliever/fever reducer
Dextromethorphan HBr
  15 mg .... Cough suppressant

Uses: temporarily relieves cough/cold symptoms:
- cough
- sneezing
- runny nose

Warnings:

Do not use if you are now taking a prescription monoamine oxidase inhibitor (MAOI) (certain drugs for depression, psychiatric or emotional conditions, or Parkinson's disease), or for 2 weeks after stopping the MAOI drug. If you do not know if your prescription drug contains an MAOI, ask a doctor or pharmacist before taking this product.

Ask a doctor before use if you have
- glaucoma
- a sodium-restricted diet
- a breathing problem or chronic cough that lasts or as occurs with smoking, asthma, chronic bronchitis, or emphysema
- cough that occurs with too much phlegm (mucus)
- trouble urinating due to an enlarged prostate gland

Ask a doctor or pharmacist before use if you are taking sedatives or tranquilizers.

When using this product
- **do not use more than directed**
- excitability may occur, especially in children
- drowsiness may occur
- avoid alcoholic drinks
- be careful when driving a motor vehicle or operating machinery
- alcohol, sedatives, and transquilizers may increase drowsiness

Stop use and ask a doctor if
- symptoms do not get better within 7 days or are accompanied by a fever
- cough lasts more than 7 days, comes back, or occurs with fever, rash, or headache that lasts. These could be signs of a serious condition.

If pregnant or breast-feeding, ask a health professional before use.

Keep out of reach of children. In case of overdose, get medical help or contact a Poison Control Center right away.

Directions:
- use dose cup or tablespoon (TBSP)
- do not exceed 4 doses per 24 hours

adults and children 12 yrs and over	2 TBSP (30 ml) every 6 hours
children 6 to under 12 years	1 TBSP (15 ml) every 6 hours
children under 6 years	ask a doctor

Other Information:
- each tablespoon contains sodium 30 mg
- store at room temperature

Inactive Ingredients: carboxymethylo-celluose sodium, citric acid, FD&C red no. 40, flavor, high fructose corn syrup, polyethylene oxide, polyoxyl 40 stearate, propylene glycol, purified water, saccharin sodium, sodium benzoate, sodium citrate

Questions? 1-800-342-6844

How Supplied: 4 FL OZ
Shown in Product Identification Guide, page 516

**VICKS® 44® COUGH RELIEF (Procter & Gamble)
Dextromethorphan HBr/
Cough Suppressant
Alcohol 5%**

- Maximum Strength
- Non-Drowsy
- For Adults & Children

Drug Facts:

**Active Ingredients:
(per 15 ml tablespoon)   Purpose:**
Dextromethorphan HBr
  30 mg .... Cough suppressant

Uses: Temporarily relieves cough due to minor throat and bronchial irritation associated with a cold

Warnings:

Do not use if you are now taking a prescription monoamine oxidase inhibitor (MAOI) (certain drugs for depression, psychiatric or emotional conditions, or Parkinson's disease), or for 2 weeks after stopping the MAOI drug. If you do not know if your prescription drug contains an MAOI, ask a doctor or pharmacist before taking this product.

Ask a doctor before use if you have:
- cough that occurs with too much phlegm (mucus)
- persistent or chronic cough such as occurs with smoking, asthma, or emphysema

Stop use and ask a doctor if:
- cough lasts more than 7 days, comes back, or occurs with fever, rash, or headache that lasts. These could be signs of a serious condition.

If pregnant or breast feeding, ask a health professional before use.

Keep out of reach of children. In case of overdose, get medical help or contact a Poison Control Center right away.

Directions:
- use teaspoon (tsp), tablespoon (TBSP) or dose cup

Continued on next page

Vicks 44 Cough—Cont.

- do not exceed 4 doses per 24 hours
  Under 6 yrs. .... ask a doctor
  6–11 yrs. .... 1½ tsp (7½ ml)
  every 6-8 hours
  12 yrs. & older .... 1 TBSP (15 ml)
  every 6-8 hours

Other Information:
- **each tablespoon contains** sodium 31 mg
- store at room temperature

Inactive Ingredients: Alcohol, FD&C blue no.1, FD&C red 40, carboxymethylcellulose sodium, citric acid, flavor, high fructose corn syrup, polyethylene oxide, polyoxyl 40 stearate, propylene glycol, purified water, saccharin sodium, sodium benzoate, sodium citrate.

How Supplied: Available in 4 FL OZ (118 ml) 6 FL OZ (177 ml) plastic bottle. A calibrated dose cup accompanies each bottle.
TAMPER EVIDENT: Do not use if imprinted shrinkband is missing or broken.
Questions? 1-800-342-6844
Dist. by Procter & Gamble, Cincinnati, OH 45202.
US Pat 5,458,879   42434792
Shown in Product Identification Guide, page 516

VICKS® 44D® (Procter & Gamble)
COUGH & HEAD CONGESTION RELIEF
Cough Suppressant/Nasal Decongestant
Alcohol 5%

Drug Facts
Active Ingredients:
(in each 15 ml tablespoon)   **Purposes:**
Dextromethorphan HBr
    20 mg .... Cough suppressant
Phenylephrine HCl
    10 mg .... Nasal decongestant

Uses: temporary relieves these cold symptoms:
- cough
- nasal congestion

Warnings:
Do not use if you are now taking a prescription monoamine oxidase inhibitor (MAOI) (certain drugs for depression, psychiatric or emotional conditions, or Parkinson's disease), or for 2 weeks after stopping the MAOI drug. If you do not know if your prescription drug contains an MAOI, ask a doctor or pharmacist before taking this product.
Ask a doctor before use if you have
- heart disease
- thyroid disease
- diabetes
- high blood pressure
- cough that occurs with too much phlegm (mucus)
- cough that lasts or is chronic such as occurs with smoking, asthma, or emphysema
- trouble urinating due to an enlarged prostate gland

- a sodium-restricted diet
When using this product, do not take more than directed.
Stop use and ask a doctor if
- you get nervous, dizzy or sleepless
- symptoms do not get better within 7 days or are accompanied by fever
- cough lasts more than 7 days, comes back, or occurs with fever, rash, or headache that lasts.
  These could be signs of a serious condition.
If pregnant or breast-feeding, ask a health professional before use.
Keep out of reach of children. In case of overdose, get medical help or contact a Poison Conrol Center right aways.

Directions:
- use dose cup, tablespoon (tsp), or tablespoon (TBSP)
- do not exceed 4 doses per 24 huors

adults and children 12 years and over	1 TBSP (15 ml) every 4 hours
children 6 to under 12 years	1½ tsp (7½ ml) every 4 hours
children under 6 years	ask a doctor

Other Information:
- each tablespoon contains sodium 33 mg
- store at room temperature

Inactive Ingredients: alcohol, carboxymethylcellulose sodium, citric acid, FD&C Blue No. 1, FD&C Red No. 40, flavor, glycerin, propylene glycol, purified water, saocharin sodium, sodium benzoate, sodium chloride, sorbitol, sucrose

Questions? 1-800-342-6844
How Supplied: Available in 4, 6, and 8 OZ
Shown in Product Identification Guide, page 516

VICKS® 44E® (Procter & Gamble)
Cough & Chest Congestion Relief
Cough Suppressant/Expectorant
Alcohol 5%

- Non-Drowsy
- For Adults & Children

Drug Facts:
Active Ingredients:
(per 15 ml tablespoon)   **Purpose:**
Dextromethorphan HBr
    20 mg .... Cough suppressant
Guaifenesin
    200 mg .... Expectorant

Uses:
- temporarily relieves cough due to the common cold
- helps loosen phlegm and thin bronchial secretions to rid the bronchial passageways of bothersome mucus

Warnings:
Do not use
- if you are now taking a prescription monoamine oxidase inhibitor (MAOI)

(certain drugs for depression, psychiatric or emotional conditions, or Parkinson's disease), or for 2 weeks after stopping the MAOI drug. If you do not know if your prescription drug contains an MAOI, ask a doctor or pharmacist before taking this product.
Ask a doctor before use if you have:
- a sodium restricted diet
- persistent or chronic cough such as occurs with smoking, asthma, chronic bronchitis or emphysema
- cough that occurs with too much phlegm (mucus)
Stop use and ask a doctor if:
- cough lasts more than 7 days, comes back, or occurs with fever, rash, or headache that lasts. These could be signs of a serious condition.
If pregnant or breast-feeding, ask a health professional before use.
Keep out of reach of children. In case of overdose, get medical help or contact a Poison Control Center right away.

Directions:
- use teaspoon (tsp), tablespoon (TBSP) or dose cup
- do not exceed 6 doses per 24 hours
Under 6 yrs. .... ask a doctor
6–11 yrs. .... 1½ tsp (7½ ml)
every 4 hours
12 yrs. & older. .... 1 TBSP (15 ml)
every 4 hours

Other Information:
- **each tablespoon contains** sodium 31 mg
- store at room temperature

Inactive Ingredients: Alcohol, FD&C blue 1, carboxymethylcellulose sodium, citric acid, flavor, high fructose corn syrup, polyethylene oxide, polyoxyl 40 stearate, propylene glycol, purified water, FD&C red no. 40, saccharin sodium, sodium benzoate, sodium citrate.

How Supplied: Available in 4 FL OZ (118 ml) 6 FL OZ (177 ml) and 8 FL OZ (236 ml) plastic bottles. A calibrated dose cup accompanies each bottle.
TAMPER EVIDENT: Do not use if imprinted shrinkband is missing or broken.
Questions? 1-800-342-6844
Dist. by Procter & Gamble, Cincinnati OH 45202.
US Pat 5,458,879   42434800
Shown in Product Identification Guide, page 516

VICKS® 44M® (Procter & Gamble)
COUGH, COLD & FLU RELIEF
Cough Suppressant/Antihistamine/Pain Reliever–Fever Reducer Alcohol 10%
Maximum strength cough formula

Drug Facts
Active Ingredients:
(in each 5 ml teaspoon)   **Purposes:**
Acetaminophen
    162.5 mg .... Pain reliever/
fever reducer

Chlorpheniramine maleate
 1 mg .... Antihistamine
Dextromethorphan HBr
 7.5 mg .... Cough suppressant

Uses:
temporarily relieves cough/cold/flu symptoms:
- cough due to minor throat and bronchial irritation
- sneezing
- headache
- sore throat
- fever
- runny nose

Warnings:
Alcohol warning: If you consume 3 or more alcoholic drinks every day, ask your doctor whether you should take acetaminophen or other pain relievers/fever reducers. Acetaminophen may cause liver damage.

Sore throat warning: If sore throat is severe, persists more than two days, is accompanied or followed by a fever, headache, rash, nausea or vomiting, consult a doctor promptly.
Do not use
- **with other medicines containing acetaminophen**
- if you are now taking a prescription monoamine oxidase inhibitor (MAOI) (certain drugs for depression, psychiatric or emotional conditions, or Parkinson's disease), or for 2 weeks after stopping the MAOI drug. If you do not know if your prescription drug contains an MAOI, ask a doctor or pharmacist before taking this product.

Ask a doctor before use if you have
- glaucoma
- cough that occurs with too much phlegm (mucus)
- a breathing problem or chronic cough that lasts or as occurs with smoking, asthma, chronic bronchitis or emphysema
- trouble urinating due to an enlarged prostate gland

Ask a doctor or pharmacist before use if you are taking sedatives or tranquilizers.
When using this product
- **do not use more than directed**
- excitability may occur, especially in children
- drowsiness may occur
- avoid alcoholic drinks
- be careful when driving a motor vehicle or operating machinery
- alcohol, sedatives, and tranquilizers may increase drowsiness

Stop use and ask a doctor if
- pain or cough gets worse or lasts more than 7 days
- fever gets worse or lasts more than 3 days
- redness or swelling is present
- new symptoms occur
- cough comes back or occurs with rash or headache that lasts.

These could be signs of a serious condition.
If pregnant or breast-feeding, ask a health professional before use.
Keep out of reach of children.

Overdose warning: Taking more than the recommended dose can cause serious health problems. In case of overdose, get medical help or contact a Poison Control Center right away. Quick medical attention is critical for adults as well as for children even if you do not notice any signs or symptoms.

Directions:
- take only as recommended — see Overdose warning
- use dose cup or teaspoon (tsp)
- do not exceed 4 doses per 24 hours

adults and children 12 years and over	4 tsp (20 ml) every 6 hours
children under 12 years	ask a doctor

Other Information:
- each teaspoon contains sodium 8 mg
- store at room temperature

Inactive Ingredients: alcohol, carboxymethylcellulose sodium, citric acid, FD&C Blue No. 1, FD&C Red No. 40, flavor, high fructose corn syrup, polythylene glycol, polyethylene oxide, propylene glycol, purified water, saccharin sodium, sodium citrate

Questions? 1-800-342-6844
How Supplied:
Available in 4, 6, and 8 OZ
Shown in Product Identification Guide, page 516

**VICKS® Cough Drops
(Procter & Gamble)
Menthol Cough Suppressant/
Oral Anesthetic
Menthol and Cherry Flavors**

CONSUMER INFORMATION: Vicks Cough Drops provide fast and effective relief. Each drop contains effective medicine to suppress your impulse to cough as it dissolves into a soothing syrup to relieve your sore throat.

Drug Facts:

Active Ingredient:
Menthol:

Active Ingredient: (per drop)	**Purpose:**
Menthol 3.3 mg	Cough suppressant/ oral anesthetic

Cherry:

Active Ingredient: (per drop)	**Purpose:**
Menthol 1.7 mg	Cough suppressant/ oral anesthetic

Uses: Temporarily relieves:
- sore throat
- coughs due to colds or inhaled irritants

Warnings:
Ask a doctor before use if you have:
- cough associated with excessive phlegm (mucus)
- persistent or chronic cough such as those caused by asthma, emphysema, or smoking
- a severe sore throat accompanied by difficulty in breathing or that lasts more than 2 days
- a sore throat accompanied or followed by fever, headache, rash, swelling, nausea or vomiting

Stop use and ask a doctor if:
- you need to use more than 7 days
- cough lasts more than 7 days, comes back, or occurs with fever, rash, or headache that lasts. These could be the signs of a serious condition.

If pregnant or breast-feeding, ask a health professional before use.
Keep out of reach of children.

Directions:
- under 5 yrs.: ask a doctor (menthol)
- adults & children 5 yrs & older: allow 2 drops to dissolve slowly in mouth (cherry)
- adults & children 5 yrs & older: allow 3 drops to dissolve slowly in mouth

Cough: may be repeated every hour.
Sore Throat: may be repeated every 2 hours.

Other Information:
- store at room temperature

Inactive Ingredients:
Menthol: Ascorbic acid, caramel, corn syrup, eucalyptus oil, sucrose.
Cherry: Ascorbic acid, citric acid, corn syrup, eucalyptus oil, FD&C blue 1, flavor, FD&C red 40, sucrose.

How Supplied: Vicks® Cough Drops are available in boxes of 20 triangular drops. Each red or green drop is debossed with "V."
Questions? 1-800-707-1709
Made in Mexico by Procter & Gamble Manufactura S. de R.I. de C.V. Dist. by Procter & Gamble
Cincinnati OH 45202
50144381

**VICKS® DAYQUIL® LIQUID
(Procter & Gamble)**

**VICKS® DAYQUIL® LIQUICAPS®
Multi-Symptom Cold/Flu Relief
Nasal Decongestant/Pain Reliever/
Cough Suppressant/Fever Reducer
Non-drowsy**

Drug Facts
Active Ingredients: (in each 5 ml teaspoon)	**Purposes:**
Acetaminophen 325 mg	Pain reliever/fever reducer

Continued on next page

Vicks DayQuil—Cont.

Dextromethorphan HBr
  10 mg .... Cough suppressant
Phenylephrine HCl
  5 mg .... Nasal decongestant

Uses:

temporarily relieves common cold/flu symptoms: [preferred order by most bothersome symptoms]

- nasal congestion
- cough due to minor throat and bronchial irritation
- sore throat
- headache
- minor aches and pains
- fever

Warnings:

Alcohol warning: If you consume 3 or more alcoholic drinks every day, ask your doctor whether you should take acetaminophen or other pain relievers/fever reducers. Acetaminophen may cause liver damage.

Sore throat warning: If sore throat is severe, persists for more than two days, is accompanied or followed by a fever, headache, rash, nausea, or vomiting, consult a doctor promptly.

Do not use

- **with other medicines containing acetaminophen**
- if you are now taking a prescription monoamine oxidase inhibitor (MAOI) (certain drugs for depression, psychiatric or emotional conditions, or Parkinson's disease), or for 2 weeks after stopping the MAOI drug. If you do not know if your prescription drug contains an MAOI, ask a doctor or pharmacist before taking this product.

Ask a doctor before use if you have

- heart disease
- thyroid disease
- diabetes
- high blood pressure
- trouble urinating due to enlarged prostate gland
- cough that occurs with too much phlegm (mucus)
- persistent or chronic cough as occurs with smoking, asthma, or emphysema
- a sodium-restricted diet

When using this product, do not use more than directed

Stop use and ask a doctor if

- you get nervous, dizzy or sleepless
- symptoms get worse or last more than 5 days (children) or 7 days (adults)
- fever gets worse or lasts more than 3 days
- redness or swelling is present
- new symptoms occur
- cough comes back, or occurs with rash or headache that lasts.

These could be signs of a serious condition.

If pregnant or breast-feeding, ask a health professional before use.

Keep out of reach of children.

Overdose warning: Taking more than the recommended dose can cause serious health problems. In case of overdose, get medical help or contact a Poison Conrol Center right away. Quick medical attention is critical for adults as well as for children even if you do not notice any signs or symptoms.

Directions:

- take only as recommended — see Overdose warning
- use dose cup or tablespoon (TBSP)
- do not exceed 5 doses (children) or 6 doses (adults) per 24 hours

adults and children 12 years and over	2 TBSP (30 ml) every 4 hours
children 6 to under 12 years	1 TBSP (15 ml) every 4 hours
children under 6 years	ask a doctor

- When using other DayQuil or NyQuil products, carefully read each label to Insure correct dosing

Other Information:

- each tablespoon contains sodium 71 mg
- store at room temperature

Inactive Ingredients: citric acid, FD&C yellow no. 6, flavor, glycerin, plyethylene glycol, propylene glycol, purified water, saccharin sodium citrate, sucrose

Questions? 1-800-251-3374

How Supplied:

Available in 6 and 10 OZ, twin pack and quad pack.

Drug Facts

Active Ingredients:
(in each LiquiCap)   **Purposes:**

Acetaminophen
  325 mg ..... Pain reliever/fever reducer
Dextromethorphan HBr
  10 mg .... Cough suppressant
Phenylephrine HCl
  5 mg .... Nasal decongestant

Uses:

temporary relieves common cold/flu symptoms: [preferred order by most bothersome symptoms]

- nasal congestion
- cough due to minor throat and bronchial irritation
- sore throat
- headache
- minor aches and pains
- fever

Warnings:

Alcohol warning: If you consume 3 or more alcoholic drinks every day, ask your doctor whether you should take acetaminophen or other pain relievers/fever reducers. Acetaminophen may cause liver damage.

Sore throat warning: If sore throat is severe, persists for more than two days, is

accompanied or followed by a fever, headache, rash, nausea, or vomiting, consult a doctor promptly.

Do not use

- **with other medicines containing acetaminophen**
- if you are now taking a prescription monoamine oxidase inhibitor (MAOI) (certain drugs for depression, psychiatric or emotional conditions, or Parkinson's disease), or for 2 weeks after stopping the MAOI drug. If you do not know if your prescription drug contains an MAOI, ask a doctor or pharmacist before taking this product.

Ask a doctor before use if you have

- heart disease
- thyroid disease
- diabetes
- high blood pressure
- trouble urinating due to enlarged prostate gland
- cough that occurs with too much phlegm (mucus)
- persistent or chronic cough as occurs with smoking, asthma, or emphysema

When using this product, do not use more than directed

Stop use and ask a doctor if

- you get nervous, dizzy or sleepless
- symptoms get worse or last more than 5 days (children) or 7 days (adults)
- fever gets worse or lasts more than 3 days
- redness or swelling is present
- new symptoms occur
- cough comes back, or occurs with rash or headache that lasts.

These could be signs of a serious condition.

If pregnant or breast-feeding, ask a health professional before use.

Keep out of reach of children.

Overdose warning: Taking more than the recommended dose can cause serious health problems. In case of overdose, get medical help or contact a Poison Conrol Center right away. Quick medical attention is critical for adults as well as for children even if you do not notice any signs or symptoms.

Directions:

- take only as recommended — see Overdose warning
- do not exceed 5 doses (children) or 6 doses (adults) per 24 hours

adults and children 12 years and over	2 LiquiCaps with water every 4 hours
children under 12 years	ask a doctor

- When using other DayQuil or NyQuil products, carefully read each label to Insure correct dosing

Other Information:

- store at room temperature

Inactive Ingredients: FD&C Red No. 40, FD&C yellow No. 6, gelatin, glycerin,

polyethylene glycol, povidone, propylene glycol, purified water, sorbitol special, titanium dioxide

Questions? 1-800-251-3374

How Supplied:
Available in boxes of 2, 12, 30, 24, 40, and 60.

Shown in Product Identification Guide, page 516

VICKS® NYQUIL® COUGH
(Procter & Gamble)
Antihistamine
Cough Suppressant
All Night Cough Relief
Cherry Flavor

alcohol 10%

Drug Facts:

Active Ingredients:	**Purpose:**
(per 15 ml tablespoon)	
Dextromethorphan HBr 15 mg	Cough suppressant
Doxylamine succinate 6.25 mg	Antihistamine

Uses:
Temporarily relieves cold symptoms
• cough
• runny nose and sneezing

Warnings:
Do not use if you are now taking a prescription monoamine oxidase inhibitor (MAOI) (certain drugs for depression, psychiatric or emotional conditions, or Parkinson's disease), or for 2 weeks after stopping the MAOI drug. If you do not know if your prescription drug contains an MAOI, ask a doctor or pharmacist before taking this product.
Ask a doctor before use if you have:
• asthma
• emphysema
• breathing problems
• excessive phlegm (mucus)
• glaucoma
• chronic bronchitis
• persistent or chronic cough
• cough associated with smoking
• trouble urinating due to enlarged prostate gland
Ask a doctor or pharmacist before use if you are:
taking sedatives or tranquilizers.
When using this product:
• **do not use more than directed**
• marked drowsiness may occur
• avoid alcoholic drinks
• excitability may occur, especially in children
• be careful when driving a motor vehicle or operating machinery
• alcohol, sedatives, and tranquilizers may increase drowsiness
Stop use and ask a doctor if:
• cough lasts more than 7 days, comes back, or occurs with fever, rash, or headache that lasts.

These could be signs of a serious condition.
If pregnant or breast-feeding, ask a health professional before use.
Keep out of reach of children. In case of overdose, get medical help or contact a Poison Control Center right away.

Directions: [1 oz bottle] use tablespoon (TBSP)
Use tablespoon (TBSP) or dose cup
• do not exceed 4 doses per 24 hours
Under 12 yrs. .... ask a doctor
12 yrs. and older .... 2 TBSP or 30 ml every 6 hours
[6 & 10 oz bottle, twin, quad pack]
• if taking NyQuil and DayQuil®, limit total to 4 doses per day.

Other Information:
• **each tablespoon contains** sodium 17 mg
• store at room temperature

Inactive Ingredients: Alcohol, F&C blue no. 1, citric acid, flavor, high fructose corn syrup, polyethylene glycol, propylene glycol, purified water, FD&C red no. 40, saccharin sodium, sodium citrate

How Supplied: Available in 1 FL OZ (30 ml) 6 FL OZ (177 ml), 10 FL OZ (295 ml) plastic bottles with child-resistant, tamper-evident cap and calibrated Medicine cup.
TAMPER EVIDENT: Do not use if imprinted shrinkband is missing or broken.
Questions? 1-800-362-1683
Dist. by Procter & Gamble, Cincinnati OH 45202. 42437885

Show in Product Identification Guide, page 516

VICKS® NYQUIL® LIQUICAPS®/ LIQUID MULTI-SYMPTOM COLD/ FLU RELIEF (Proctor & Gamble)

Drug Facts

Active Ingredients:	
(in each LiquiCap)	**Purpose:**
Acetaminophen 325 mg	Pain reliever/fever reducer
Dextromethorphan HBr 15 mg	Cough suppressant
Doxylamine succinate 6.25 mg	Antihistamine

Uses: temporarily relieves common cold/ flu symptoms: [preferred order by most bothersome symptoms]
• cough due to minor throat and bronchial irritation
• sore throat
• headache
• minor aches and pains
• fever
• runny nose and sneezing

Warnings:
Alcohol warning: If you consume 3 or more alcoholic drinks every day, ask your doctor whether you should take acetaminophen or other pain relievers/fever re-

ducers. Acetaminophen may cause liver damage.

Sore throat warning: If sore throat is severe, persists for more than two days, is accompanied or followed by fever, headache, rash, nausea, or vomiting, consult a doctor promptly.
Do not use
• **with other medicines containing acetaminophen**
• if you are now taking a prescription monoamine oxidase inhibitor (MAOI) (certain drugs for depression, psychiatric or emotional conditions, or Parkinson's disease), or for 2 weeks after stopping the MAOI drug. If you do not know if your prescription drug contains an MAOI, ask a doctor or pharmacist before taking this product.
Ask a doctor before use if you have
• glaucoma
• cough that occurs with too much phelgm (mucus)
• a breathing problem or chronic cough that lasts or as occurs with smoking, asthma, chronic bronchitis or emphysema
• trouble urinating due to enlarged prostate gland
Ask a doctor or pharmacist before use if you are taking sedatives or tranquilizers.
When using this product
• **do not use more than directed**
• excitability may occur, especially in children
• marked drowsiness may occur
• avoid alcoholic drinks
• be careful when driving a motor vehicle or operating machinery
• alcohol, sedatives, and tranquilizers may increase drowsiness
Stop use and ask a doctor if
• pain or cough gets worse or lasts more than 7 days
• fever gets worse or lasts more than 3 days
• redness or swelling is present
• new symptoms occur
• cough comes back or occurs with rash or headache that lasts.
These could be signs of a serious condition.
If pregnant or breast-feeding, ask a health professional before use.
Keep out of reach of children.

Overdose warning: Taking more than the recommended dose can cause serious health problems. In case of overdose, get medical help or contact a Poison Control Center right away. Quick medical attention is critical for adults as well as for children even if you do not notice any signs or symptoms.

Directions:
• take only as recommended – see Overdose warning
• do not exceed 4 doses per 24 hours

Continued on next page

Vicks NyQuil LiquiCaps—Cont.

adults and children 12 years and over	2 LiquiCaps with water every 6 hours
children under 12 years	ask a doctor

- when using other DayQuil or NyQuil products, carefully read each label to insure correct dosing

Other Information:
- store at room temperature

Inactive Ingredients: D&C Yellow No. 10, FD&C Blue No. 1, gelatin, glycerin, polyethylene glycol, povidone, propylene glycol, purified water, sorbitol special, titanium dioxide

Questions? 1–800–362–1683

Drug Facts

Active Ingredients:
(in each 15 ml tablespoon)   Purpose:

Acetaminophen
500 mg .... Pain reliever/fever reducer
Dextromethorphan HBr
15 mg .... Cough suppressant
Doxylamine succinate
6.25 mg .... Antihistamine

Uses: temporarily relieves common cold/flu symptoms: [preferred order by most bothersome symptoms]
- cough due to minor throat and bronchial irritation
- sore throat
- headache
- minor aches and pain
- fever
- runny nose and sneezing

Warnings:

Alcohol warning: If you consume 3 or more alcoholic drinks every day, ask your doctor whether you should take acetaminophen or other pain relievers/fever reducers. Acetaminophen may cause liver damage.

Sore throat warning: If sore throat is severe, persists for more than two days, is accompanied or followed by fever, headache, rash, nausea, or vomiting, consult a doctor promptly.

Do not use
- with other medicines containing acetaminophen
- if you are now taking a prescription monoamine oxidase inhibitor (MAOI) (certain drugs for depression, psychiatric or emotional conditions, or Parkinson's disease), or for 2 weeks after stopping the MAOI drug. If you do not know if your prescription drug contains an MAOI, ask a doctor or pharmacist before taking this product.

Ask a doctor before use if you have
- glaucoma
- cough that occurs with too much phlegm (mucus)

- a breathing problem or chronic cough that lasts or as occurs with smoking, asthma, chronic bronchitis or emphysema
- trouble urinating due to enlarged prostate gland

Ask a doctor or pharmacist before use if you are taking sedatives or tranquilizers.

When using this product
- do not use more than directed
- excitability may occur, especially in children
- marked drowsiness may occur
- avoid alcoholic drinks
- be careful when driving a motor vehicle or operating machinery
- alcohol, sedatives, and tranquilizers may increase drowsiness

Stop use and ask a doctor if
- pain or cough gets worse or lasts more than 7 days
- fever gets worse or lasts more than 3 days
- redness or swelling is present
- new symptoms occur
- cough comes back or occurs with rash or headache that lasts.

These could be signs of a serious condition.

If pregnant or breast-feeding, ask a health professional before use.

Keep out of reach of children.

Overdose warning: Taking more than the recommended dose can cause serious health problems. In case of overdose, get medical help or contact a Poison Control Center right away. Quick medical attention is critical for adults as well as for children even if you do not notice any signs or symptoms.

Directions:
- take only as recommended – see Overdose warning
- use dose cup or tablespoon (TBSP)
- do not exceed 4 doses per 24 hours

adults and children 12 years and over	2 TBSP (30 ml) every 6 hours
children under 12 years	ask a doctor

- when using other DayQuil and NyQuil products, carefully read each label to insure correct dosing

Other Information:
- each tablespoon contains sodium 17 mg
- store at room temperature

Inactive Ingredients: [original] alcohol, citric acid, D&C yellow no. 10, FD&C green no. 3, FD&C yellow no. 6, flavor, high fructose corn syrup, polyethylene glycol, propylene glycol, purified water, saccharin sodium, sodium citrate

[cherry] alcohol, citric acid, FD&C blue no. 1, FD&C red no. 40, flavor, high fructose corn syrup, polyethylene glycol, propylene glycol, purified water, saccharin sodium, sodium citrate

Questions? 1–800–362–1683
Shown in Product Identification Guide, page 516

VICKS® SINEX® NASAL SPRAY
(Procter & Gamble)
Ultra Fine Mist for Sinus Relief
[sĭ 'nĕx]
Phenylephrine HCl Nasal Decongestant

For full product information see page 781.

VICKS® VAPOR INHALER
(Procter & Gamble)
Levmetamfetamine/Nasal Decongestant

Drug Facts

Active Ingredient: Purpose:
(per inhaler)
Levmetamfetamine
    50mg .... Nasal decongestant

Uses: Temporarily relieves nasal congestion due to:
- a cold
- hay fever or other upper respiratory allergies
- sinusitis

Warnings:
When using this product:
- do not exceed recommended dosage
- temporary burning, stinging, sneezing, or increased nasal discharge may occur
- frequent or prolonged use may cause nasal congestion to recur or worsen
- do not use for more than 7 days
- do not use container by more than one person as it may spread infection
- use only as directed

Stop use and ask a doctor if:
- symptoms persist

If pregnant or breast-feeding, ask a health professional before use.

Keep out of reach of children. If swallowed, get medical help or contact a poison control center right away.

Directions:
The product delivers in each 800 ml air 0.04 to 0.15 mg of levmetamfetamine.
- do not use more often than every 2 hours
- under 6 yrs.: ask a doctor
- 6–11 yrs.: with adult supervision, 1 inhalation in each nostril.
- 12 yrs. & older: 2 inhalation in each nostril.

Other Information:
- store at room temperature
- keep inhaler tightly closed.

- This inhaler is effective for a minimum of 3 months after first use.

Inactive Ingredients: Bornyl acetate, camphor, lavender oil, menthol, methyl salicylate.

How Supplied: Available as a cylindrical plastic nasal inhaler.
Net weight: 0.007 OZ (204 mg).
TAMPER EVIDENT: Use only if imprinted wrap is intact.
Questions? 1-800-873-8276
Dist. by Procter & Gamble, Cincinnati OH 45202. ©2001 42438038

VICKS® VAPORUB®
(Procter & Gamble)
[vā ′pō-rub]
VICKS® VAPORUB® CREAM
(greaseless)
Cough
Suppressant/Topical Analgesic

Drug Facts

Active Ingredients:
Vicks® VapoRub®:

Active Ingredients:	**Purpose:**
Camphor 4.8%	Cough suppressant, & topical analgesic
Eucalyptus oil 1.2%	Cough suppressant
Menthol 2.6%	Cough suppressant, & topical analgesic

Vicks® VapoRub®:

Active Ingredient:	**Purpose:**
Camphor 5.2%	Cough suppressant, & topical analgesic
Eucalyptus oil 1.2%	Cough suppressant
Menthol 2.8%	Cough suppressant, & topical analgesic

Uses:
- on chest and throat, temporarily relieves cough due to the common cold
- on muscles and joints, temporarily relieves minor aches and pains

Warnings:
Failure to follow these warnings could result in serious consequences.
For external use only; avoid contact with eyes.
Do not use:
- by mouth
- with tight bandages
- in nostrils
- on wounds or damaged skin
Ask a doctor before use if you have:
- cough that occurs with too much phlegm (mucus)
- persistent or chronic cough such as occurs with smoking, asthma or emphysema
When using this product, do not:
- heat
- microwave
- add to hot water or any container where heating water. May cause splattering and result in burns.

Stop use and ask a doctor if:
- muscle aches/pains persist more than 7 days or come back
- cough lasts more than 7 days, comes back, or occurs with fever, rash, or headache that lasts.
These could be signs of a serious condition.
If pregnant or breast-feeding, ask a health professional before use.
Keep out of reach of children. If swallowed, get medical help or contact a Poison Control Center right away.

Directions:
- **See important warnings under "When using this product"**
- under 2 yrs.: ask a doctor
- adults and children 2 yrs. & older: Rub a thick layer on chest & throat or rub on sore aching muscles. If desired, cover with a warm, dry cloth. Keep clothing loose about throat/chest to help vapors reach the nose/mouth. Repeat up to three times per 24 hours or as directed by a doctor.

Other Information:
- store at room temperature

Inactive Ingredients:
Vicks® VapoRub®: Cedarleaf oil, nutmeg oil, special petrolatum, thymol, turpentine oil
Vicks® VapoRub® Cream: Carbomer 954, cedarleaf oil, cetyl alcohol, cetyl palmitate, cyclomethicone copolyol, dimethicone copolyol, dimethicone, EDTA, glycerin, imidazolidinyl urea, isopropyl palmitate, methylparaben, nutmeg oil, peg-100 stearate, propylparaben, purified water, sodium hydroxide, stearic acid, stearyl alcohol, thymol, titanium dioxide, turpentine oil

How Supplied:
Vicks® VapoRub®: Available in 1.76 oz (50 g) 3.53 oz (100 g) and 6 oz (170 g) plastic jars 0.45 oz (12 g) tin.
Vicks® VapoRub® Cream: Available in 2.99 oz (85 g) tube.
Questions? 1-800-873-8276
www.vicks.com
Vicks® VapoRub® 50142932
Vicks® VapoRub® Cream 50117758
US Pat. 5,322,689
Made in Mexico by Procter & Gamble Manufactura, S. de R.L. de C.V.
Dist. by Procter & Gamble, Cincinnati OH 45202

VICKS® VAPOSTEAM®
(Procter & Gamble)
[vā ′pō ″stēm]
Liquid Medication for Hot Steam Vaporizers.
Camphor/Cough Suppressant

Drug Facts:

Active Ingredient:	**Purpose:**
Camphor 6.2%	Cough suppressant

Uses: Temporarily relieves cough associated with a cold.

Warnings:
Failure to follow these warnings could result in serious consequences.
For external use only
Flammable Keep away from fire or flame. For steam inhalation only.
Ask a doctor before use if you have:
- a persistent or chronic cough such as occurs with smoking, emphysema or asthma
- cough that occurs with too much phlegm (mucus)
When using this product do not:
- heat
- microwave
- use near an open flame
- take by mouth
- direct steam from the vaporizer too close to the face
- add to hot water or any container where heating water except when adding to cold water only in a hot steam vaporizer. May cause splattering and result in burns.
Stop use and ask a doctor if:
- cough lasts more than 7 days, comes back, or occurs with fever, rash, or headache that lasts.
These could be signs of a serious condition.
Keep out of reach of children. In case of eye exposure (flush eyes with water); or in case of accidental ingestion; seek medical help or contact a Poison Control Center right away.

Directions:
see important warnings under "When using this product"
- under 2 yrs.: ask a doctor
- adults & children 2 yrs. & older: use 1 tablespoon of solution for each quart of water or 1½ teaspoonsful of solution for each pint of water
- add solution directly to cold water only in a hot steam vaporizer
- follow manufacturer's directions for using vaporizer. Breathe in medicated vapors. May be repeated up to 3 times a day.

Other Information:
- close container tightly and store at room temperature away from heat.

Inactive Ingredients: Alcohol 78%, cedarleaf oil, eucalyptus oil, laureth-7, menthol, nutmeg oil, poloxamer 124, silicone.

How Supplied: Available in 4 FL OZ (118 ml) and 8 FL OZ (235 ml) bottles.
Questions? 1-800-873-8276
Made in Mexico by Procter & Gamble Manufactura S. de R.L. de C.V.
Dist. by Procter & Gamble
Cincinnati OH 45202
50144018

ZICAM® Cold Remedy Nasal Gel™
[*zī-kăm*]
(Matrixx)

ZICAM® Cold Remedy Gel Swabs™

ZICAM® Cold Remedy Swabs Kids Size

ZICAM® Cold Remedy RapidMelts®

ZICAM® Cold Remedy RapidMelts® with Vitamin C

ZICAM® Cold Remedy Oral Mist™

ZICAM® Cold Remedy Chewables™

ZICAM® Cold Remedy ChewCaps

Drug Facts:
ZICAM® Cold Remedy Nasal Gel™, ZICAM® Cold Remedy Gel Swabs™, ZICAM® Cold Remedy Swabs Kids Size only:

Active Ingredient: **Purpose:**
Zincum
Gluconicum 2x .... Reduces duration
and severity of the
common cold

ZICAM® Cold Remedy RapidMelts®, ZICAM® Cold Remedy RapidMelts® with Vitamin C, ZICAM® Cold Remedy Oral Mist™, ZICAM® Cold Remedy Chewables™, ZICAM® Cold Remedy ChewCaps only:

Active Ingredient: **Purpose:**
Zincum
Aceticum 2x .... Reduces duration
and severity of the
common cold

Zincum Gluconicum 1x

Uses:
• Reduces the duration of the common cold
• Reduces severity of cold symptoms:
 • sore throat • stuffy nose • sneezing
 • coughing • congestion

Warnings:
ZICAM® Cold Remedy Nasal Gel™, ZICAM® Cold Remedy Gel Swabs™, ZICAM® Cold Remedy Swabs Kids Size only:
For nasal use only. Ask doctor before use if you have ear, nose of throat sensitivity or if you are susceptible to nose bleeds. **When using this product** avoid contact with eyes. In case of accidental contact with eyes, flush with water and immediately seek professional help. Temporary discomfort such as burning, stinging, sneezing or increased nasal discharge may result. To help avoid possible irritation, do not sniff up gel. Use of this container by more than one person may spread infection. **Stop use and ask a doctor** if symptoms persist or are accompanied by fever. ZICAM® Cold Remedy was formulated to shorten the duration of the common cold and may not be effective for flu or allergies. **If pregnant or breast**

feeding, ask a health professional before use. **Keep out of reach of children.** If swallowed, get medical help or contact a Poison Control Center right away.
ZICAM® Cold Remedy RapidMelts®, ZICAM® Cold Remedy RapidMelts® with Vitamin C, ZICAM® Cold Remedy Oral Mist™, ZICAM® Cold Remedy Chewables™, ZICAM® Cold Remedy ChewCaps only:
For oral use only. Stop use and ask a doctor if symptoms persist or are accompanied by fever. ZICAM® Cold Remedy was formulated to shorten the duration of the common cold and may not be effective for flu or allergies. **If pregnant or breast feeding,** ask a health professional before use. **Keep out of reach of children.**
ZICAM® Cold Remedy Oral Mist™ only:
When using this product avoid contact with eyes. In case of accidental contact with eyes, flush with water and immediately seek professional help.

Directions:
ZICAM® Cold Remedy Nasal Gel™:
• For best results, use at the first sign of a cold and continue to use for an additional 48 hours after symptoms subside.
• Adults and children 3 years of age and older (with adult supervision):
• Remove cap and safety clip
• Hold with thumb at the bottom of the bottle and nozzle between your fingers.
• Prior to initial use, prime pump by holding it upright and depressing several times (into a tissue) until the gel is dispensed.
• Place tip of nozzle just past nasal opening (approximately 1/8″).
• While inside nasal opening, slightly angle nozzle outward.
• Pump once into each nostril. To help avoid possible irritation, do not sniff up gel. This product helps put gel in the lower part of the nose.
• After application, press lightly on the outside of each nostril for about 5 seconds.
• Wait at least 30 seconds before blowing nose.
• Use once every 4 hours.
• Children under 3 years of age, consult doctor before use.
ZICAM® Cold Remedy Gel Swabs™:
• For best results, use at the first sign of a cold and continue to use for an additional 48 hours after symptoms subside.
• Adults and children 3 years of age and older (with adult supervison):
• Open tube (also see illustrations on side of carton & insert):
• With thumb and index finger, pinch the tube on both yellow dots.
• With other hand, gently bend base of handle back and forth until seal is broken.
• Pull out swab.
• Apply medication just inside first nostril. Press lightly on the outside of first nostril for about 5 seconds. Re-dip swab in tube. Apply medication to second nostril. Press lightly on the outside of second nostril for about 5 seconds. Do

not insert swab more than ¼″ past nasal opening.
• Discard swab after use.
• Wait at least 30 seconds before blowing nose.
• Use one tube every 4 hours.
• Children under 3 years of age: Consult a doctor before use.
ZICAM® Cold Remedy Swabs Kids Size:
• For best results, use at the first sign of a cold and continue to use for an additional 48 hours after symptoms subside.
• Adults and children 3 years of age and older (with adult supervision):
• Separate one swab from the other.
• Before opening:
 • Turn swab upside down so medication saturates swab head.
 • Return right side up and squeeze at yellow dot to move medication away from dotted tear line.
• To open:
 • Fold in half so arrow heads meet; then tear across dotted line.
 • Slide plastic sleeve halfway down swab handle to expose swab tip.
• Apply medication just inside of first nostril. During application, press lightly on the outside of nostril for about 5 seconds. Do not insert swab more than ¼″ past nasal opening.
• Re-moisten swab by pulling plastic sleeve back around swab tip. Then pull sleeve down and apply to second nostril. Discard swab after use.
• Wait at least 30 seconds before blowing nose.
• Use one tube every 4 hours.
• Children under 3 years of age, consult doctor before use.
ZICAM® Cold Remedy RapidMelts®
ZICAM® Cold Remedy RapidMelts® with Vitamin C:
• For best results, use at the first sign of a cold and continue to use for an additional 48 hours after symptoms subside.
• Adults and children 3 years of age and older (with adult supervison):
• Dissolve entire tablet in mouth. Do not chew. Do not swallow whole.
• Take one tablet at the onset of symptoms.
• Repeat every three hours until symptoms are gone.
• To avoid minor stomach upset, do not take on an empty stomach.
• Do not eat or drink for 15 minutes after use. Do not eat or drink citrus fruits or juices for 30 minutes before or after use. Otherwise, drink plenty of fluids.
• Children under 3 years of age, consult doctor before use.
ZICAM® Cold Remedy Chewables™
ZICAM® Cold Remedy ChewCaps:
• For best results, use at the first sign of a cold and continue to use for an additional 48 hours after symptoms subside.
• Adults and children 6 years of age and older (with adult supervision):
• Take one Chewable™ or ChewCap at the onset of symptoms. Chew thoroughly before swallowing.
• Repeat every three hours until symptoms are gone.

- To avoid minor stomach upset, do not take on an empty stomach.
- Do not eat or drink for 15 minutes after use. Do not eat or drink citrus fruits or juices for 30 minutes before or after use. Otherwise, drink plenty of water.
- These products are not recommended for children under the age of 6 due to the hazard of choking.

ZICAM® Cold Remedy Oral Mist™:
- For best results, use at the first sign of a cold and continue to use for an additional 48 hours after symptoms subside.
- Adults and children 3 years of age and older (with adult supervison):
- Spray four times in mouth at the onset of symptoms. Spray on inside of cheeks, roof of mouth and gums. Retain for 15 seconds. Swallow.
- Repeat every three hours until symptoms are gone.
- To avoid minor stomach upset, do not take on an empty stomach.
- Do not eat or drink for 15 minutes after use. Do not eat or drink citrus fruits or juices for 30 minutes before or after use. Otherwise, drink plenty of water.
- Children under 3 years of age, consult doctor before use.

Inactive Ingredients:

ZICAM® Cold Remedy Nasal Gel™, ZICAM® Cold Remedy Gel Swabs™, ZICAM® Cold Remedy Swabs Kids Size only: benzalkonium chloride, glycerin, hydroxyethylcellulose, purified water, sodium chloride, sodium hydroxide

ZICAM® Cold Remedy RapidMelts® only: crospovidone, magnesium stearate, mannitol, microcrystalline cellulose, natural & artificial cherry flavor, polysorbate 80, polyvinyl pyrolidone, purified talc, silicon dioxide, sodium lauryl sulphate, sodium starch glycolate, sorbitan monostearate, sucralose

ZICAM® Cold Remedy RapidMelts® with Vitamin C only: ascorbic acid, carnauba wax, crospovidone, ethylcellulose, FD&C yellow #6, magnesium stearate, mannitol, microcrystalline cellulose, mono and diglycerides, natural orange flavor, polyethylene glycol, polysorbate 80, polyvinyl pyrolidone, purified talc, silicon dioxide, sodium lauryl sulphate, sodium starch glycolate, sorbitan monostearate, sucralose.

ZICAM® Cold Remedy Chewables™ only: FD&C red #40, glycerin, HPMC, lecithin, malitol syrup, maltodextrin, mono and diglycerides, natural and artifical strawberry flavor, partially hydrogenated cotton seed and soy oil, sugar.

ZICAM® Cold Remedy ChewCaps only: acetylated mono-diglycerides, confectioner's glaze, dextrose monohydrate, FD&C red #40 and #28, FD&C yellow #6, HPMC, lecithin, magnesium stearate, maltitol syrup, maltodextrin, mono and di-glycerides, natural and artificial cinnamon flavor, opaglos red #2, partially hydrogenated cotton seed and soy oil, polyethylene glycol, purified talc, silicon dioxide, sodium carboxymethylcellulose, sucralose, sugar, titanium dioxide.

ZICAM® Cold Remedy Oral Mist™ only: benzalkonium chloride, glycerin, peppermint flavor, purified water, sucralose.

ZICAM® Cold Remedy Nasal Gel™: 0.5 FL OZ (15mL) pump bottle; ZICAM® Cold Remedy Gel Swabs™ and ZICAM® Cold Remedy Swabs Kids Size: 20 medicated swabs; ZICAM® Cold Remedy RapidMelts® and ZICAM® Cold Remedy RapidMelts® with Vitamin C: 25 quick dissolve tablets; ZICAM® Cold Remedy Chewables™: 25 chewable squares; ZICAM® Cold Remedy ChewCaps: 25 chewable caplets; ZICAM® Cold Remedy Oral Mist™: 1.0 FL OZ (30mL)

Shown in Product Identification Guide, page 507

ZICAM® Extreme Congestion Relief
[zī 'kăm]
(Matrixx)
ZICAM® Intense Sinus Relief
(Matrixx)

Drug Facts:

Active Ingredient: **Purpose:**
Oxymetazoline
HCl 0.05% .... Nasal decongestant

Uses:
- Temporarily relieves nasal congestion due to:
  *common cold *sinusitis *hay fever *upper respiratory allergies
- Helps clear nasal passages
- Shrink swollen membranes
- Temporarily relieves sinus congestion and pressure

Warnings: For nasal use only. Ask a doctor before use if you have heart disease, high blood pressure, thyroid disease, diabetes, trouble urinating due to enlarged prostrate gland. **When using this product do not use more than directed.** Do not use for more than 3 days. Use only as directed. Frequent or prolonged use may cause nasal congestion to recur or worsen. Temporary discomfort such as burning, stinging, sneezing, or an increase in nasal discharge may result. Use of this container by more than one person may spread infection. **Stop use and ask a doctor** if symptoms persist. **If pregnant or breast-feeding,** ask a health professional before use. **Keep out of reach of children. If swallowed,** get medical help or contact a Poison Control Center right away.

Directions: Adults and children 6 to under 12 years of age (with adult supervision): Pump 2 or 3 times in each nostril without tilting your head, not more often than once every 10 to 12 hours. Sniff deeply. Do not exceed 2 doses in any 24-hour period. Wipe nozzle clean after use. Children under 6 years of age: Consult a doctor.
To use pump:
Remove cap and safety clip.

Hold with thumb at bottom of bottle and nozzle between fingers.
Before using the first time, prime pump by depressing several times.
ZICAM® Extreme Congestion Relief only

Inactive Ingredients: alkoxylated diester, aloe barbadensis gel, benzalkonium chloride, benzyl alcohol, disodium EDTA, disodium phosphate, glycerin, hydroxyethylcellulose, hydroxylated lecithin, monosodium phosphate, purified water
ZICAM® Intense Sinus Relief only

Inactive Ingredients: alkoxylated diester, aloe barbadensis gel, benzalkonium chloride, benzyl alcohol, disodium EDTA, disodium phosphate, di-alpha tocopherol, eucalyptol, glycerin, hydroxyethylcellulose, hydroxylated lecithin, menthol, monosodium phosphate, polysorbate 80, purified water

How Supplied: *ZICAM®* Extreme Congestion Relief and ZICAM ® Intense Sinus Relief nasal pump: 0.5 FL OZ (15 mL) pump bottle

Shown in Product Identification Guide, page 508

ZICAM® Cough Plus D Cough Spray (Matrixx)
ZICAM® Cough Relief Cough Spray
ZICAM® Cough Max Cough Spray
ZICAM® Cough Max Nighttime Cough Spray
ZICAM® Cough Max Cough Melts

Active Ingredients:
(in each 0.25 mL spray)   **Purpose:**
Cough Plus D:
Dextromethorphan
HBr 5.0 mg .... Cough Suppressant
Phenylephrine
HCl 2.5 mg .... Nasal Decongestant

Cough Relief:
Dextromethorphan
HBr 5.0 mg .... Cough Suppressant

Cough Max:
Dextromethorphan
HBr 6.0 mg .... Cough Suppressant

Cough Max Nighttime:
Dextromethorphan
HBr 6.0 mg .... Cough Suppressant

Cough Max Cough Melts:
Dextromethorphan
HBr 30 mg .... Cough Suppressant

Uses: temporarily relieves

Cough Plus D:
- cough due to minor throat and bronchial irritation associated with a cold
- nasal congestion due to the common cold

Continued on next page

Zicam—Cont.

Cough Relief/Cough Max/Cough Max Nighttime/Cough Max Melts

Uses: temporarily relieves cough due to minor throat and bronchial irritation associated with a cold.

Warnings:

Cough Plus D/Cough Max/Cough Max Nighttime/Cough Max Cough Melts:

Do not use if you are now taking a prescription monoamine oxidase inhibitor (MAOI) (certain drugs for depression, psychiatric, or emotional conditions, or Parkinson's disease), or for 2 weeks after stopping the MAOI drug. If you do not know if your prescription drug contains an MAOI, ask a doctor or pharmacist before taking this product.

Cough Plus D:

Ask a doctor before use if you have

- heart disease
- high blood pressure
- thyroid disease
- diabetes
- trouble urinating due to an enlarged prostate gland
- cough accompanied by excessive phlegm (mucus)
- persistent or chronic cough such as occurs with smoking, asthma, or emphysema

When using this product do not use more than directed.

Stop use and ask a doctor if

- you get nervous, dizzy, or sleepless
- symptoms do not get better within 7 days or are accompanied by fever
- cough lasts more than 7 days, comes back, or occurs with fever, rash, or headache that lasts. These could be signs of a serious condition.

If pregnant or breast-feeding, ask a health professional before use.

Keep out of reach of children. In case of overdose, get medical help or contact a Poison Control Center right away.

Cough Relief/Cough Max/Cough Max Nighttime/Cough Max Melts:

Ask a doctor before use if you have

- cough accompanied by excessive phlegm (mucus).
- persistent or chronic cough such as occurs with smoking, asthma, or emphysema.

Stop use and ask a doctor if

- cough lasts more than 7 days, comes back, or occurs with fever, rash, or headache that lasts. These could be signs of a serious condition.

If pregnant or breast-feeding, ask a health professional before use.

Keep out of reach of children. In case of overdose, get medical help or contact a Poison Control Center right away.

Directions:

Cough Plus D:

- Remove safety cap.
- Prime pump by spraying into a tissue.
- Hold close to mouth and depress sprayer fully. Swallow.

12 yrs & older .... 4 sprays (20.0 mg Dextromethorphan HBr, 10.0 mg Phenylephrine HCl)

Under 12 yrs .... consult a doctor

- Repeat every 4 hours, not to exceed 6 doses per day.
- May be followed by water or liquids if desired.

Directions:

Cough Relief:

- Remove safety cap.
- Prime pump by spraying into a tissue.
- Hold close to mouth and depress sprayer fully. Swallow.

12 yrs & older .... 4 sprays (20.0 mg Dextromethorphan)

Under 12 yrs .... consult a doctor

- Repeat every 6-8 hours, not to exceed 4 doses per day.
- May be followed by water or liquids if desired.

Directions:

Cough Max/Cough Max Nighttime:

- Remove safety cap.
- Prime pump by spraying into a tissue.
- Hold close to mouth and depress sprayer fully. Swallow.

12 yrs & older .... 5 sprays (30.0 mg Dextromethorphan HBr)

Under 12 yrs .... consult a doctor

- Repeat every 6-8 hours, not to exceed 4 doses per day.
- May be followed by water or liquids if desired.

Directions:

Cough Max Melts:

- Adults and children 12 years of age and older:
  - Dissolve entire tablet in mouth. Do not swallow whole.
  - Repeat every 6-8 hours, do not exceed 4 doses per day.
  - To avoid minor stomach upset, do not take on an empty stomach.
- Under 12 years of age, consult a doctor.

Inactive Ingredients: Acetylated monodiglyceric ideides, crospovidone, dextrose monohydrate, FD&C Red #40, magnesium stearate, mannitol, microcrystalline cellulose, natural & cherry flavor, polysorbate 80, purified talc, silicon dioxide, styrene and divinyl benzene resin, sucralose

Cough Plus D:

Inactive Ingredients: acesulfame k, citric acid, flavor, glycerin, malic acid, menthol, PEG-40 hydrogenated caster oil, polyethylene glycol, potassium chloride, potassium sorbate, purified water, sodium citrate, sucralose

Cough Relief:

Inactive Ingredients: acesulfame k, citric acid, flavor, glycerin, malic acid, menthol, PEG-40 hydrogenated caster oil, polyethylene glycol, postassium chloride, potassium sorbate, purified water, sodium citrate, sucralose

Cough Max:

Inactive Ingredients: citric acid, glycerin, hydroxylated lecithin, menthol, natural flavors, polyethylene glycol, polysorbate 60, potassium sorbate, purified water, sucralose

Cough Max Nighttime:

Inactive Ingredients: alcohol, benzyl alcohol, glycerin, lecithin, menthol, natural flavors, polyethylene glycol, polysorbate 60, potassium sorbate, purified water, sucralose

Cough Max Melts:

Other Information:

Store at room temperature 15°C-29°C (59°F-84°F)

Questions?
Comments?

call 877-942-2626 toll-free or visit us on the web at www.zicam.com

Shown in Product Identification Guide, page 507

ZICAM® Maximum Strength Flu Daytime (Matrixx)

ZICAM® Maximum Strength Flu Nighttime

Drug Facts

Active Ingredients: **Purpose:**
(on each spoon)

Daytime:
Acetaminophen 1000mg .... Pain Reliever/ Fever Reducer
Chlorpheniramine maleate 4mg .... Antihistamine
Dextromethorphan HBr 30mg .... Cough Suppressant
Nighttime:
Acetaminophen 1000mg .... Pain Reliever/ Fever Reducer
Doxylamine succinate 12.5mg .... Antihistamine
Dextromethorphan HBr 30mg .... Cough Suppressant

Uses: temporarily relieves common cold and flu symptoms:

- coughs due to minor throat and bronchial irritation
- runny nose
- muscular aches
- watery eyes
- sneezing
- sore throat
- headache
- minor aches & pains
- fever

Warnings:

Alcohol Warning: If you consume 3 or more alcoholic drinks per day, ask your doctor whether you should take acetaminophen or other pain relievers/fever re-

ducers. Acetaminophen may cause liver damage.

Sore Throat Warning: If sore throat is severe, persists for more than two days, is accompanied by or followed by fever, headache, rash, nausea, or vomiting, consult a doctor promptly.

Do not use
- **with other medicines containing acetaminophen**
- if you are now taking a prescription monoamine oxidase inhibitor (MAOI) (certain drugs for depression, psychiatric or emotional conditions, or Parkinson's disease), or for 2 weeks after stopping the MAOI drug. If you do not know if your prescription drug contains an MAOI, ask a doctor or pharmacist before taking this product.

Ask a doctor before use if you have
- difficulty in urination due to enlarged prostate
- a breathing problem such as emphysema or chronic bronchitis
- cough that occurs with too much phlegm (mucus)
- persistent or chronic cough as occurs with smoking, asthma, or emphysema
- glaucoma

Ask a doctor or pharmacist before use if you are taking sedatives or tranquilizers

When using this product
- **do not use more than directed**
- may cause excitability especially in children
- alcohol, sedatives, and tranquilizers may increase drowsiness
- use caution when driving a motor vehicle or operating machinery
- may cause marked drowsiness
- avoid alcoholic beverages

Stop use and ask a doctor if
- redness or swelling is present
- fever gets worse and lasts more than 3 days
- new symptoms occur
- symptoms do not get better within 7 days or are accompanied by a fever

These could be signs of a serious condition.

If pregnant or breast feeding, ask a health professional before use. **Keep out of reach of children.**

Overdose Warning: Taking more than the recommended dose can cause serious health problems. In case of overdose, get medical help or contact a Poison Control Center right away. Quick medical attention is critical for adults as well as for children even if you do not notice any signs or symptoms.

Directions:
- Take only as directed – see overdose warning.
- Remove spoon from protective wrapper.
- Peel back lid completely from spoon.
- Stir spoon in 4 to 8 ounces of hot or cold beverage (tea, juice, soda) or take directly from spoon.
- Mix for 30 seconds or until uniform.
- Lick remaining medicine off spoon.
- Discard protective wrapper, lid and spoon.
- Take one dose [or spoon] every 6 hours as needed.
- Adults and children 12 years and over, one dose every 6 hours as needed.
- Do not exceed 4 doses every 24 hours.

Inactive Ingredients: Purified Water, Glycerin, Hydroxyethylcellulose, Sucralose, Sodium Carboxymethylcellulose, Propylene Glycol, Polyethylene Glycol 400, Polyethylene, Potassium Chloride

Shown in Product Identification Guide, page 507

Respiratory System:
Hay Fever

4-WAY® MENTHOL
(Novartis Consumer Health, Inc.)
Nasal Decongestant

For full product information see page 775.

4-WAY® Fast Acting Nasal Spray
(Novartis Consumer Health, Inc.)
Phenylephrine hydrochloride 1%,
nasal decongestant

For full product information see page 775.

ADVIL® ALLERGY SINUS
CAPLETS (Wyeth Consumer)
ADVIL® MULTI-SYMPTOM COLD
CAPLETS
Pain Reliever/Fever Reducer (NSAID)
Nasal Decongestant
Antihistamine

Active Ingredients (in each caplet):
Chlorpheniramine maleate 2 mg
Ibuprofen 200 mg (NSAID)*
Pseudoephedrine HCl 30 mg
*nonsteroidal anti-inflammatory drug

Uses:
• temporarily relieves these symptoms associated with hay fever or other upper respiratory allergies, and the common cold:
  • runny nose • sneezing • headache
  • itchy, watery eyes
  • nasal congestion • minor aches and pains • itching of the nose or throat
  • sinus pressure • fever

Warnings:
Allergy alert: Ibuprofen may cause a severe allergic reaction, especially in people allergic to aspirin. Symptoms may include:
• hives
• facial swelling
• asthma (wheezing)
• shock
• skin reddening
• rash
• blisters
If an allergic reaction occurs, stop use and seek medical help right away.
Stomach bleeding warning: This product contains a nonsteroidal anti-inflammatory drug (NSAID), which may cause stomach bleeding. The chance is higher if you:
• are age 60 or older
• have had stomach ulcers or bleeding problems
• take a blood thinning (anticoagulant) or steroid drug

• take other drugs containing an NSAID [aspirin, ibuprofen, naproxen, or others]
• have 3 or more alcoholic drinks every day while using this product
• take more or for a longer time than directed
Do not use
• if you have ever had an allergic reaction to any other pain reliever/fever reducer
• right before or after heart surgery
• if you are now taking a prescription monoamine oxidase inhibitor (MAOI) (certain drugs for depression, psychiatric, or emotional conditions, or Parkinson's disease), or for 2 weeks after stopping the MAOI drug. If you do not know if your prescription drug contains an MAOI, ask a doctor or pharmacist before taking this product.
Ask a doctor before use if you have
• a breathing problem such as emphysema or chronic bronchitis
• problems or serious side effects from taking pain relievers or fever reducers
• stomach problems that last or come back, such as heartburn, upset stomach, or stomach pain
• ulcers
• bleeding problems
• high blood pressure
• heart or kidney disease
• thyroid disease
• diabetes
• glaucoma
• trouble urinating due to an enlarged prostate gland
• taken a diuretic
• reached age 60 or older
Ask a doctor or pharmacist before use if you are
• taking any other drug containing an NSAID (prescription or nonprescription)
• taking a blood thinning (anticoagulant) or steroid drug
• under a doctor's care for any serious condition
• taking sedatives or tranquilizers
• taking any other product that contains pseudoephedrine, chlorpheniramine or any other nasal decongestant or antihistamine
• taking aspirin to prevent heart attack or stroke, because ibuprofen may decrease this benefit of aspirin
• taking any other drug
When using this product
• take with food or milk if stomach upset occurs
• long term continuous use may increase the risk of heart attack or stroke
• avoid alcoholic drinks
• be careful when driving a motor vehicle or operating machinery

• drowsiness may occur
• alcohol, sedatives, and tranquilizers may increase drowsiness
Stop use and ask a doctor if
• you feel faint, vomit blood, or have bloody or black stools. These are signs of stomach bleeding.
• pain gets worse or lasts more than 10 days
• fever gets worse or lasts more than 3 days
• nasal congestion lasts for more than 7 days
• stomach pain or upset gets worse or lasts
• redness or swelling is present in the painful area
• you get nervous, dizzy, or sleepless
• symptoms continue or get worse
• any new symptoms appear
If pregnant or breast-feeding, ask a health professional before use. It is especially important not to use this product during the last 3 months of pregnancy unless definitely directed to do so by a doctor because it may cause problems in the unborn child or complications during delivery.
Keep out of reach of children. In case of overdose, get medical help or contact a Poison Control Center right away.

Directions:
• **do not take more than directed**
• **the smallest effective dose should be used**
• do not take longer than 10 days, unless directed by a doctor (see Warnings)
• adults: take 1 caplet every 4–6 hours while symptoms persist.
• do not take more than 6 caplets in any 24-hour period, unless directed by a doctor
• children under 12 years of age: consult a doctor

Other Information:
• read all warnings and directions before use. Keep carton.
• store in a dry place 20–25°C (68–77°F)
• avoid excessive heat above 40°C (104°F)

Inactive Ingredients: carnauba wax, croscarmellose sodium, FD&C red no. 40 aluminum lake, FD&C yellow no. 6 aluminum lake, glyceryl behenate, hypromellose, iron oxide black, microcrystalline cellulose, polydextrose, polyethylene glycol, pregelatinized starch, propylene glycol, silicon dioxide, starch, titanium dioxide

How Supplied: Allergy sinus caplets in packages of 20 caplets
Multi-symptom cold caplets in packages of 10 caplets

ADVIL® COLD & SINUS
(Wyeth Consumer)
Caplets, and Liqui-Gels
Pain Reliever/Fever Reducer/(NSAID)
Nasal Decongestant

For full product information see page 723.

ALAVERT (Wyeth Consumer)
Loratadine orally disintegrating tablets
Loratadine swallow tablets
Antihistamine

Active Ingredient   (in each tablet):
Loratadine 10 mg

Uses:
- temporarily relieves these symptoms due to hay fever or other upper respiratory allergies:
  - runny nose • sneezing • itchy, watery eyes
  - itching of the nose or throat

Warnings:
Do not use if you have ever had an allergic reaction to this product or any of its ingredients
Ask a doctor before use if you have liver or kidney disease. Your doctor should determine if you need a different dose.
When using this product do not use more than directed. Taking more than recommended may cause drowsiness.
Stop use and ask a doctor if an allergic reaction to this product occurs. Seek medical help right away.
If pregnant or breast-feeding, ask a health professional before use.
Keep out of reach of children. In case of overdose, get medical help or contact a Poison Control Center right away.

Directions:
- (orally disintegrating tablet) tablet melts in mouth. Can be taken with or without water.

Age	Dose
adults and children 6 years and over	1 tablet daily; do not use more than 1 tablet in 24 hours
children under 6	ask a doctor
consumers who have liver or kidney disease	ask a doctor

Other Information:
- (orally disintegrating tablet) Phenylketonurics: Contains Phenylalanine 8.4 mg per tablet
- (orally disintegrating tablet) store at 20–25°C (68–77°F)
- (swallow tablet) store at 15–30°C (59–86°F)
- keep in a dry place

Inactive Ingredients (Loratadine orally disintegrating tablets) (original): artificial & natural flavor, aspartame, citric acid, colloidal silicon dioxide, corn syrup solids, crospovidone, magnesium stearate, mannitol, microcrystalline cellulose, modified food starch, sodium bicarbonate
(orange mint): anhydrous citric acid, aspartame, butylated hydroxyanisole, colloidal silicon dioxide, corn syrup solids, crospovidone, dextrin, ferric oxides, magnesium stearate, maltodextrin, mannitol, microcrystalline cellulose, modified food starch, natural & artificial flavors, sodium bicarbonate

Inactive Ingredients (Loratadine swallow tablets): lactose monohydrate, magnesium stearate, microcrystalline cellulose, sodium starch glycolate

How Supplied: Loratadine orally disintegrating tablets in packages of 6, 12, 24 & 48

How Supplied: Loratadine swallow tablets in packages of 15 and 30 tablets

---

ALAVERT ALLERGY & SINUS D-12 HOUR TABLETS (Wyeth Consumer)
Loratadine/Pseudoephedrine Sulfate
Extended Release Tablets
Antihistamine/Nasal Decongestant

Active Ingredients   (in each tablet):
Loratadine 5 mg
Pseudoephedrine sulfate 120 mg

Uses:
- temporarily relieves these symptoms due to hay fever or other upper respiratory allergies:
  - runny nose
  - sneezing • itchy, watery eyes
  - itching of the nose or throat
- temporarily relieves nasal congestion due to the common cold, hay fever or other respiratory allergies
- reduces swelling of nasal passages
- temporarily relieves sinus congestion and pressure
- temporarily restores freer breathing through the nose

Warnings:
Do not use
- if you have ever had an allergic reaction to this product or any of its ingredients
- if you are now taking a prescription monoamine oxidase inhibitor (MAOI) (certain drugs for depression, psychiatric, or emotional conditions, or Parkinson's disease), or for 2 weeks after stopping the MAOI drug. If you do not know if your prescription drug contains an MAOI, ask a doctor or pharmacist before taking this product.

Ask a doctor before use if you have
- heart disease • high blood pressure
- thyroid disease • diabetes
- trouble urinating due to an enlarged prostate gland
- liver or kidney disease. Your doctor should determine if you need a different dose.

When using this product do not take more than directed. Taking more than directed may cause drowsiness.
Stop use and ask a doctor if
- an allergic reaction to this product occurs. Seek medical help right away.
- symptoms do not improve within 7 days or are accompanied by a fever
- nervousness, dizziness or sleeplessness occurs

If pregnant or breast-feeding, ask a health professional before use.
Keep out of reach of children. In case of overdose, get medical help or contact a Poison Control Center right away.

Directions:
- do not divide, crush, chew or dissolve the tablet

Age	Dose
adults and children 12 years and over	1 tablet every 12 hours; not more than 2 tablets in 24 hours
children under 12 years of age	ask a doctor
consumers with liver or kidney disease	ask a doctor

Other Information:
- **each tablet contains:** calcium 30 mg
- store between 15° and 25°C (59° and 77°F)
- keep in a dry place

Inactive Ingredients: croscarmellose sodium, dibasic calcium phosphate, hypromellose, lactose monohydrate, magnesium stearate, pharmaceutical ink, povidone, titanium dioxide

How Supplied: Blister packs of 12 and 24 tablets.

CHILDREN'S CLARITIN ALLERGY
(Schering-Plough Healthcare)
loratadine oral solution, grape flavor
5mg/5mL-antihistamine

Drug Facts
Active Ingredient   Purpose:
(In each 5 ml teaspoonful):
Loratadine 5 mg .... Antihistamine

Uses: temporarily relieves these symptoms due to hay fever or other upper respiratory allergies:
- runny nose
- itchy, watery eyes
- sneezing
- itching of the nose or throat

Warnings:
Do not use if you have ever had an allergic reaction to this product or any of its ingredients

Continued on next page

Children's Claritin Allergy—Cont.

Ask a doctor before use if you have liver or kidney disease. Your doctor should determine if you need a different dose.

When using this product do not take more than directed. Taking more than directed may cause drowsiness.

Stop use and ask a doctor if an allergic reaction to this product occurs. Seek medical help right away.

If pregnant or breast-feeding, ask a health professional before use.

Keep out of reach of children. In case of overdose, get medical help or contact a Poison Control Center right away.

Directions:

adults and children 6 years and over	2 teaspoonfuls daily; do not take more than 2 teaspoonfuls in 24 hours
children 2 to under 6 years of age	1 teaspoonful daily; do not take more than 1 teaspoonful in 24 hours
consumers with liver or kidney disease	ask a doctor

Other Information:

- **each teaspoonful contains:** sodium 6 mg
- packaged with tamper-evident bottle cap. Do not use if breakable ring is separated or missing.
- store between 20° to 25° C (68° to 77° F)

Inactive Ingredients:

edetate disodium, flavor, glycerin, maltitol, phosphoric acid, polyethylene glycol, propylene glycol, sodium benzoate, sodium phosphate monobasic, sorbitol, sucralose, water

Questions or comments?

1-800-CLARITIN (1-800-252-7484) or www.claritin.com

How Supplied:

4 FL oz bottle, grape flavor

Shown in Product Identification Guide, page 517

CLARITIN 24 HOUR NON-DROWSY REDITABS

(Schering-Plough Healthcare)
loratadine 10 mg/antihistamine

CLARITIN 24 HOUR NON-DROWSY TABLETS

Loratadine 10 mg/antihistamine

FOR CLARITIN REDITABS

Drug Facts

Active Ingredient (in each tablet):   **Purpose:**

Loratadine 10 mg .... Antihistamine

Uses: temporarily relieves these symptoms due to hay fever or other upper respiratory allergies:

- runny nose
- itchy, watery eyes
- sneezing
- itching of the nose or throat

Warnings:

Do not use if you have ever had an allergic reaction to this product or any of its ingredients.

Ask a doctor before use if you have liver or kidney disease. Your doctor should determine if you need a different dose.

When using this product do not take more than directed. Taking more than directed may cause drowsiness.

Stop use and ask a doctor if an allergic reaction to this product occurs. Seek medical help right away.

If pregnant or breast-feeding, ask a health professional before use.

Keep out of reach of children. In case of overdose, get medical help or contact a Poison Control Center right away.

Directions:

- place 1 tablet on tongue: tablet disintegrates with or without water

adults and children 6 years and over	1 tablet daily: not more than 1 tablet in 24 hours
children under 6 years of age	ask a doctor
consumers with liver or kidney disease	ask a doctor

Other Information:

- safety sealed: do not use if the individual blister unit imprinted with Claritin® Reditabs® is open or torn
- store between 20° to 25° C (68° to 77° F)
- Use tablet immediately after opening individual blister

Inactive Ingredients:

anhydrous citric acid, gelatin, mannitol, mint flavor

Questions or comments?:

1-800-CLARITIN (1-800-252-7484) or www.claritin.com

How Supplied: Boxes of 4, 10, 20, and 30 count tablets.

FOR CLARITIN 24 HOUR NON-DROWSY TABLETS

Drug Facts

Active Ingredient (in each tablet):   **Purpose:**

Loratadine 10 mg .... Antihistamine

Uses: temporarily relieves these symptoms due to hay fever or other upper respiratory allergies:

- runny nose
- itchy, watery eyes
- sneezing
- itching of the nose or throat

Warnings:

Do not use if you have ever had an allergic reaction to this product or any of its ingredients.

Ask a doctor before use if you have liver or kidney disease. Your doctor should determine if you need a different dose.

When using this product do not take more than directed. Taking more than directed may cause drowsiness.

Stop use and ask a doctor if an allergic reaction to this product occurs. Seek medical help right away.

If pregnant or breast-feeding, ask a health professional before use.

Keep out of reach of children. In case of overdose, get medical help or contact a Poison Control Center right away.

Directions:

adults and children 6 years and over	1 tablet daily: not more than 1 tablet in 24 hours
children under 6 years of age	ask a doctor
consumers with liver or kidney disease	ask a doctor

Other Information:

- safety sealed: do not use if the individual blister unit imprinted with Claritin® is open or torn
- store between 20° to 25° C (68° to 77° F)
- protect from excessive moisture

Inactive Ingredients:

corn starch, lactose monohydrate, magnesium stearate

Questions or comments?:

1-800-CLARITIN (1-800-252-7484) or www.claritin.com

How Supplied: Boxes of 4, 10, 20, and 30 count tablets.

Shown in Product Identification Guide, page 517

CLARITIN-D 12 HOUR NON-DROWSY

(Schering-Plough Healthcare)
pseudoephedrine sulfate 120 mg/nasal decongestant
Loratadine 5 mg/antihistamine

CLARITIN-D NON-DROWSY 24 HOUR

pseudoephedrine sulfate 240 mg/nasal decongestant
Loratadine 10 mg/antihistamine

FOR CLARITIN-D 12 HOUR NON-DROWSY

Drug Facts

Active Ingredients (in each tablet):   **Purpose:**

Loratadine 5 mg .... Antihistamine
Pseudoephedrine sulfate 120 mg .... Nasal decongestant

Uses:
- temporarily relieves these symptoms due to hay fever or other upper respiratory allergies:
  - sneezing
  - itchy, watery eyes
  - runny nose
  - itching of the nose or throat
- temporarily relieves nasal congestion due to the common cold, hay fever or other upper respiratory allergies
- reduces swelling of nasal passages
- temporarily relieves sinus congestion and pressure
- temporarily restores freer breathing through the nose

Warnings:
Do not use
- if you have ever had an allergic reaction to this product or any of its ingredients
- if you are now taking a prescription monoamine oxidase inhibitor (MAOI) (certain drugs for depression, psychiatric, or emotional conditions, or Parkinson's disease), or for 2 weeks after stopping the MAOI drug. If you do not know if your prescription drug contains an MAOI, ask a doctor or pharmacist before taking this product.

Ask a doctor before use if you have
- heart disease
- thyroid disease
- high blood pressure
- diabetes
- trouble urinating due to an enlarged prostate gland
- liver or kidney disease. Your doctor should determine if you need a different dose.

When using this product do not take more than directed.
Taking more than directed may cause drowsiness.

Stop use and ask a doctor if
- an allergic reaction to this product occurs. Seek medical help right away.
- symptoms do not improve within 7 days or are accompanied by a fever
- nervousness, dizziness or sleeplessness occurs

If pregnant or breast-feeding, ask a health professional before use.

Keep out of reach of children. In case of overdose, get medical help or contact a Poison Control Center right away.

Directions: • do not divide, crush, chew or dissolve the tablet

adults and children 12 years and over	1 tablet every 12 hours; not more than 2 tablets in 24 hours
children under 12 years of age	ask a doctor
consumers with liver or kidney disease	ask a doctor

Other Information:
- **each tablet contains:** calcium 30 mg
- safety sealed: do not use if the individ-

ual blister unit imprinted with Claritin-D® 12 Hr. is open or torn
- store between 15° and 25° C (59° and 77°F)
- keep in a dry place

Inactive Ingredients: croscarmellose sodium, dibasic calcium phosphate, hypromellose, lactose monohydrate, magnesium stearate, pharmaceutical ink, povidone, titanium dioxide

Questions or comments?:
1-800-CLARITIN (1-800-252-7484) or www.claritin.com

How Supplied: Boxes of 10, 20, and 30 count tablets.

FOR CLARITIN-D NON-DROWSY 24 HOUR

Drug Facts

Active Ingredients
(in each tablet):   **Purpose:**

Loratadine 10 mg .... Antihistamine
Pseudoephedrine sulfate
    240 mg .... Nasal decongestant

Uses:
- temporarily relieves these symptoms due to hay fever or other upper respiratory allergies:
  - sneezing
  - itchy, watery eyes
  - runny nose
  - itching of the nose or throat
- temporarily relieves nasal congestion due to the common cold, hay fever or other upper respiratory allergies
- reduces swelling of nasal passages
- temporarily relieves sinus congestion and pressure
- temporarily restores freer breathing through the nose

Warnings:
Do not use
- if you have ever had an allergic reaction to this product or any of its ingredients
- if you are now taking a prescription monoamine oxidase inhibitor (MAOI) (certain drugs for depression, psychiatric, or emotional conditions, or Parkinson's disease) or for 2 weeks after stopping the MAOI drug. If you do not know if your prescription drug contains an MAOI, ask a doctor or pharmacist before taking this product.

Ask a doctor before use if you have
- heart disease
- thyroid disease
- high blood pressure
- diabetes
- trouble urinating due to an enlarged prostate gland
- liver or kidney disease. Your doctor should determine if you need a different dose.

When using this product do not take more than directed.
Taking more than directed may cause drowsiness.

Stop use and ask a doctor if
- an allergic reaction to this product occurs. Seek medical help right away.
- symptoms do not improve within 7 days or are accompanied by a fever
- nervousness, dizziness or sleeplessness occurs

If pregnant or breast-feeding, ask a health professional before use.

Keep out of reach of children. In case of overdose, get medical help or contact a Poison Control Center right away.

Directions:
- do not divide, crush, chew or dissolve the tablet

adults and children 12 years and over	1 tablet daily with a full glass of water; not more than 1 tablet in 24 hours
children under 12 years of age	ask a doctor
consumers with liver or kidney disease	ask a doctor

Other Information:
- **each tablet contains:** calcium 25 mg
- safety sealed: do not use if the individual blister unit imprinted with Claritin-D® 24 hour is open or torn
- store between 20° C to 25° C (68° F to 77° F)
- protect from light and store in a dry place

Inactive Ingredients: carnauba wax, dibasic calcium phosphate, ethylcellulose, hydroxypropyl cellulose, hypromellose, magnesium stearate, pharmaceutical ink, polyethylene glycol, povidone, silicon dioxide, sugar, titanium dioxide, white wax

Questions or comments?:
1-800-CLARITIN (1-800-252-7484) or www.claritin.com

How Supplied: Boxes of 5, 10, and 15 count tablets.
Shown in Product Identification Guide, page 517

CHILDREN'S DIMETAPP® COLD & ALLERGY CHEWABLE TABLETS (Wyeth Consumer)
Antihistamine/Nasal decongestant

For full product information see page 730.

CHILDREN'S DIMETAPP® Cold & Allergy Elixir (Wyeth Consumer)
Antihistamine, Nasal Decongestant

For full product information see page 730.

CHILDREN'S DIMETAPP® DM COLD & COUGH Elixir (Wyeth Consumer)
Antihistamine, Cough Suppressant, Nasal Decongestant

For full product information see page 731.

TODDLER'S DIMETAPP COLD AND COUGH DROPS (Wyeth Consumer)
Cough suppressant/Nasal decongestant

For full product information see page 732.

MUCINEX® D
(Adams Respiratory Therapeutics)
600 mg Guaifenesin and 60 mg Pseudoephedrine HCl Extended-Release Bi-Layer Tablets
Expectorant and Nasal Decongestant

For full product information see page 776.

ROBITUSSIN® Cough & Cold Nighttime (Wyeth Consumer)
ROBITUSSIN® Pediatric Cough & Cold Nighttime
ROBITUSSIN® Cough & Allergy
Nasal Decongestant, Cough Suppressant, Antihistamine

For full product information see page 736.

THERAFLU® THIN STRIPS®-MULTISYMPTOM
(Novartis Consumer Health, Inc.)
Antihistamine/Cough Suppressant
(Diphenhydramine HCl)

For full product information see page 744.

TRIAMINIC® NIGHT TIME Cold & Cough
(Novartis Consumer Health, Inc.)
Antihistamine/Cough Suppressant, Nasal Decongestant
Grape Flavor

For full product information see page 746.

TRIAMINIC® Softchews®
(Novartis Consumer Health, Inc.)
Cough & Runny Nose
Antihistamine, Cough Suppressant
Cherry Flavor

For full product information see page 748.

TRIAMINIC THIN STRIPS®
COUGH & RUNNY NOSE
(Novartis Consumer Health, Inc.)

For full product information see page 749.

TYLENOL® Severe Allergy Caplets (McNeil Consumer)

TYLENOL® Allergy Multi-Symptom Caplets with Cool Burst™ and Gelcaps

TYLENOL® Allergy Multi-Symptom Nighttime Caplets with Cool Burst™

For full product information see page 717.

VICKS® SINEX®
(Procter & Gamble)
[sī 'něx]
12-HOUR [Nasal Spray]
[Ultra Fine Mist] for Sinus Relief
Oxymetazoline HCl
Nasal Decongestant

For full product information see page 781.

VICKS® SINEX® NASAL SPRAY
(Procter & Gamble)
Ultra Fine Mist for Sinus Relief
[sī 'něx]
Phenylephrine HCl Nasal Decongestant

For full product information see page 781.

VICKS® VAPOR INHALER
(Procter & Gamble)
Levmetamfetamine/Nasal Decongestant

For full product information see page 764.

ZICAM® Allergy Relief (Matrixx)
[zī'kăm]

Drug Facts:

Active Ingredients:	Purpose:
Luffa operculata 4x, 12x, 30x	
Galphimia glauca 12x, 30x	
Histanium hydrochloricum 12x, 30x, 200x	
Sulphur 12x, 30x, 200x	Upper respiratory allergy symptom relief

Uses:
• Relieves symptoms of hay fever and

other upper respiratory allergies such as: *sinus pressure *runny nose *sneezing *itchy eyes *watery eyes *nasal congestion

Warnings: For nasal use only. Ask a doctor before use if you have ear, nose or throat sensitivity or if you are susceptible to nose bleeds. When using this product avoid contact with eyes. In case of accidental contact with eyes, flush with water and immediately seek professional help. The use of this container by more than one person may spread infection. Stop use and ask a doctor if symptoms persist. If pregnant or breast-feeding, ask a health professional before use. Keep out of reach of children. If swallowed, get medical help or contact a Poison Control Center right away.

Directions:
• Adults and children 6 years of age and older (with adult supervision):
  • Remove cap and safety clip.
  • Hold with thumb at bottom of bottle and nozzle between your fingers.
  • Before using the first time, prime pump by depressing several times.
  • Place tip of nozzle just past nasal opening (approximately 1/8").
  • While inside nasal opening, slightly angle nozzle outward.
  • Pump once into each nostril.
  • After application, press lightly on outside of each nostril for about 5 seconds.
  • Wait at least 30 seconds before blowing nose.
  • Use once every 4 hours.
  • Optimal results may not be seen for 1-2 weeks. After 1-2 weeks, may need to use only 1-2 times daily. For best results, use up to one week before contact with known causes of your allergies.
• Children under 6 years of age: Consult a doctor before use.

Inactive Ingredients: benzalkonium chloride, benzyl alcohol, edetate disodium, glycerine, hydroxyethylcellulose, potassium chloride, potassium phosphate, purified water, sodium chloride, sodium phosphate

How Supplied: *ZICAM®* Allergy Relief nasal pump: 0.5 FL OZ (15 mL) pump bottle

Shown in Product Identification Guide, page 507

ZICAM® Extreme Congestion Relief (Matrixx)
ZICAM® Intense Sinus Relief (Matrixx)
[zī 'kăm]

For full product information see page 767.

Respiratory System:
Nasal/Sinus Congestion

4-WAY® Fast Acting Nasal Spray
(Novartis Consumer Health, Inc.)
**Phenylephrine hydrochloride 1%,
nasal decongestant**

Active Ingredient:	Purpose:
Phenylephrine hydrochloride 1%	Nasal decongestant

Uses:
- temporarily relieves nasal congestion due to:
  - common cold
  - hay fever
  - upper respiratory allergies

Warnings:
Ask a doctor before use if you have
- heart disease
- high blood pressure
- thyroid disease
- diabetes
- trouble urinating due to an enlarged prostate gland

When using this product
- **do not use more than directed**
- do not use more than 3 days
- use only as directed
- frequent or prolonged use may cause nasal congestion to recur or worsen
- temporary discomfort such as burning, stinging, sneezing, or an increase in nasal discharge may occur
- infection may spread if this container is used by more than one person

Stop use and ask a doctor if symptoms persist
If pregnant or breast-feeding, ask a health professional before use.
Keep out of reach of children. If swallowed, get medical help or contact a Poison Control Center right away.

Directions:
- adults and children 12 years and older: 2 or 3 sprays in each nostril not more than every 4 hours.
- children under 12 years: ask a doctor.
Use instructions: with head in a normal, upright position, put atomizer tip into nostril. Squeeze bottle with firm, quick pressure while inhaling. Wipe nozzle clean after each use.

Other Information:
- store at room temperature
- container is filled to proper level for best spray action

Inactive Ingredients:
benzalkonium chloride, boric acid, sodium borate, water

Questions or comments?
1-800-468-7746

How Supplied:
Available in 0.5 and 1.0 oz cartons
Shown in Product Identification Guide, page 512

4-WAY® MENTHOL
(Novartis Consumer Health, Inc.)
Nasal Decongestant

Drug Facts

Active Ingredient:	Purpose:
Phenylephrine hydrochloride 1%	Nasal decongestant

Uses:
- temporarily relieves nasal congestion due to:
  - common cold • hay fever
  - upper respiratory allergies

Warnings:
Ask a doctor before use if you have
- heart disease • high blood pressure
- thyroid disease • diabetes
- trouble urinating due to an enlarged prostate gland

When using this product
- **do not use more than directed**
- do not use more than 3 days
- use only as directed
- frequent or prolonged use may cause nasal congestion to recur or worsen
- temporary discomfort such as burning, stinging, sneezing, or an increase in nasal discharge may occur
- infection may spread if this container is used by more than one person

Stop use and ask a doctor if symptoms persist
If pregnant or breast-feeding, ask a health professional before use.
Keep out of reach of children. If swallowed, get medical help or contact a Poison Control Center right away.

Directions:
- adults and children 12 years and older: 2 or 3 sprays in each nostril not more than every 4 hours.
- children under 12 years: ask a doctor.
Use instructions: with head in a normal, upright position, put atomizer tip into nostril. Squeeze bottle with firm, quick pressure while inhaling. Wipe nozzle clean after each use.

Other Information:
- store at room temperature
- container is filled to proper level for best spray action

Inactive Ingredients: benzalkonium chloride, boric acid, camphor, eucalyptol, menthol, polysorbate 80, sodium borate, water

Questions or comments?
1-800-468-7746
How Supplied:
Available in 0.5 fl oz cartons.

4-WAY® SALINE
(Novartis Consumer Health, Inc.)
Moisturizing Mist

Uses:
Helps make nasal passages feel clear and more comfortable by providing gentle, soothing, moisture to dry, irritated nasal passages due to colds, allergies, air pollution, smoke, air travel, overuse of decongestant sprays/drops and dry air (low humidity).

Directions:

Adults and children 2 years of age and over:	2 to 3 sprays in each nostril as often as needed or as directed by your doctor.
Children under 2 years of age:	Use only as directed by your doctor.

Use Instructions: With head in a normal, upright position, put atomizer tip into nostril. Squeeze bottle with firm, quick pressure while inhaling. Wipe nozzle clean after each use.

Cautions: Keep out of reach of children. The use of this dispenser by more than one person may spread infections.

Ingredients: Water, Boric Acid, Glycerin, Sodium Chloride, Sodium Borate, Eucalyptol, Menthol, Polysorbate 80, Benzalkonium Chloride

Note: Container is filled to proper level for best spray action. Store at room temperature.

Questions or comments?
1-800-468-7746

How Supplied:
Available in 1.0 fl oz cartons.

ADVIL® ALLERGY SINUS
CAPLETS (Wyeth Consumer)
ADVIL® MULTI-SYMPTOM COLD
CAPLETS
**Pain Reliever/Fever Reducer (NSAID)
Nasal Decongestant
Antihistamine**

For full product information see page 770.

ADVIL® COLD & SINUS
Caplets, and Liqui-Gels
Pain Reliever/Fever Reducer/(NSAID)
Nasal Decongestant

For full product information see page 723.

**ALAVERT ALLERGY & SINUS D-12
HOUR TABLETS (Wyeth Consumer)**
Loratadine/Pseudoephedrine Sulfate
Extended Release Tablets
Antihistamine/Nasal Decongestant

For full product information see page 771.

**ALEVE COLD & SINUS CAPLETS
(Bayer Healthcare)
(NSAID Labeling)**
[a-lēv]

For full product information see page 724.

**BC® POWDER
(GlaxoSmithKline Consumer)
ARTHRITIS STRENGTH BC®
POWDER
BC® COLD POWDER LINE**

For full product information see page 677.

**CLARITIN-D 12 HOUR
NON-DROWSY
(Schering-Plough Healthcare)**
pseudoephedrine sulfate 120 mg/nasal
decongestant
Loratadine 5 mg/antihistamine

**CLARITIN-D NON-DROWSY
24 HOUR**
pseudoephedrine sulfate 240 mg/nasal
decongestant
Loratadine 10 mg/antihistamine

For full product information see page 772.

**COMTREX®
(Novartis Consumer Health, Inc.)
MAXIMUM STRENGTH**
Pain Reliever/Fever Reducer, Cough
Suppressant, Nasal Decongestant
Acetaminophon, Dextromethorphan HBr,
Phenylephrine HCl
Non-Drowsy Cold & Cough

For full product information see page 725.

**COMTREX® Cold & Cough
Day/Night
(Novartis Consumer Health, Inc.)**
Pain Reliever/Fever Reducer

For full product information see page 726.

**CONTAC® COLD AND FLU DAY
AND NIGHT
(GlaxoSmithKline Consumer)**

For full product information see page 727.

**CONTAC COLD AND FLU NON-
DROWSY MAXIMUM STRENGTH
(GlaxoSmithKline Consumer)**

For full product information see page 728.

**CONTAC® COLD AND FLU
MAXIMUM STRENGTH
(GlaxoSmithKline Consumer)**

For full product information see page 728.

**CONTAC® Non-Drowsy
(GlaxoSmithKline Consumer)
Decongestant
12 Hour Cold Caplets**

For full product information see page 729.

**CONTAC®-D COLD NON-DROWSY
DECONGESTANT
(GlaxoSmithKline Consumer)**

For full product information see page 729.

**CHILDREN'S DIMETAPP® COLD &
ALLERGY CHEWABLE TABLETS
(Wyeth Consumer)**
Antihistamine/Nasal decongestant

For full product information see page 730.

**CHILDREN'S DIMETAPP® LONG
ACTING COUGH PLUS COLD
SYRUP (Wyeth Consumer)**
Cough suppressant/Antihistamine

For full product information see page 731.

**TODDLER'S DIMETAPP COLD AND
COUGH DROPS (Wyeth Consumer)**
Cough suppressant/Nasal decongestant

For full product information see page 732.

**EXCEDRIN® SINUS HEADACHE
(Novartis Consumer Health, Inc.)**
Acetaminophen and Phenylephrine HCl

For full product information see page 610.

**HYLAND'S COMPLETE FLU CARE 4
KIDS (Standard Homeopathic)**

For full product information see page 732.

**CHILDREN'S MOTRIN® Cold
(McNeil Consumer)**
ibuprofen/pseudoephedrine HCl
Oral Suspension

For full product information see page 733.

**MUCINEX® D
(Adams Respiratory Therapeutics)
600 mg Guaifenesin and 60 mg
Pseudoephedrine HCl Extended-
Release Bi-Layer Tablets
Expectorant and Nasal Decongestant**

Drug Facts

Active Ingredients: **Purpose:**
**(in each extended-release
bi-layer tablet)**
Guaifenesin 600 mg .... Expectorant
Pseudoephedrine HCl
60 mg .... Nasal Decongestant

Uses:
- helps loosen phlegm (mucus) and thin bronchial secretions to rid the bronchial passageways of bothersome mucus and make coughs more productive
- temporarily relieves nasal congestion due to:
  - common cold
  - hay fever
  - upper respiratory allergies
- temporarily restores freer breathing through the nose
- promotes nasal and/or sinus drainage
- temporarily relieves sinus congestion and pressure

Warnings:
Do not use if you are now taking a prescription monoamine oxidase inhibitor (MAOI) (certain drugs for depression, psychiatric or emotional conditions, or Parkinson's disease), or for 2 weeks after stopping the MAOI drug. If you do not know if your prescription drug contains a MAOI, ask a doctor or pharmacist before taking this product.

Ask a doctor before use if you have
- heart disease
- high blood pressure
- thyroid disease
- diabetes
- trouble urinating due to an enlarged prostate gland
- persistent or chronic cough such as occurs with smoking, asthma, chronic bronchitis, or emphysema
- cough accompanied by too much phlegm (mucus)

When using this product
- **do not use more than directed**

Stop use and ask a doctor if
- you get nervous, dizzy, or sleepless
- symptoms do not get better within 7 days, come back or occur with a fever, rash, or persistent headache. These could be signs of a serious illness.

If pregnant or breast-feeding, ask a health professional before use.

Keep out of reach of children. In case of overdose, get medical help or contact a Poison Control Center right away.

Directions:
- do not crush, chew, or break tablet
- take with a full glass of water
- this product can be administered without regard for timing of meals
- adults and children 12 years and older: two tablets every 12 hours; not more than 4 tablets in 24 hours
- children under 12 years of age: do not use

Other Information:
- tamper evident: do not use if printed seal on blister is broken or missing
- store at 20-25°C (68-77°F)

Inactive Ingredients: carbomer 934P, NF; FD&C yellow #6 aluminum lake; hypromellose, USP; magnesium stearate, NF; microcrystalline cellulose, NF; sodium starch glycolate, NF

How Supplied: Boxes of 18 tablets (in blisters of 6) (NDC 63824-057-18), 36 tablets (in blisters of 6) (NDC 63824-057-36). A modified oval bi-layer tablet debossed with "Adams" on the orange layer and "600" on the white layer. Each tablet provides 600 mg guaifenesin and 60 mg pseudoephedrine HCl. US Patent Nos. 6,372,252 B1 and 6,955,821 B2

Shown in Product Identification Guide, page 503

**NASAL COMFORT™ (Matrixx)
Moisture Therapy**

For full product information see page 733.

**PEDIATRIC VICKS® 44m®
(Procter & Gamble)
Cough & Cold Relief
Cough Suppressant/Antihistamine**

For full product information see page 759.

**REFENESEN™ 400 NON-DROWSY
IMMEDIATE RELEASE
EXPECTORANT CAPLETS (Reese)**
[rĕ-fĕn-ə-sĕn]

**REFENESEN™ DM NON-DROWSY
IMMEDIATE RELEASE
EXPECTORANT & COUGH
SUPPRESSANT CAPLETS**

**REFENESEN™ PE NON-DROWSY
IMMEDIATE RELEASE
EXPECTORANT & NASAL
DECONGESTANT CAPLETS**

Expectorant, nasal decongestant, cough suppressant

For full product information see page 721.

**ROBITUSSIN Cough & Cold CF
Liquid (Wyeth Consumer)
ROBITUSSIN Cough & Cold
Pediatric Drops
Cough Suppressant/Expectorant/
Nasal decongestant**

For full product information see page 735.

**ROBITUSSIN® Cough & Cold
(Wyeth Consumer)
Long-Acting
ROBITUSSIN® Pediatric Cough &
Cold Long-Acting
Cough Suppressant, Antihistamine**

For full product information see page 735.

**ROBITUSSIN COUGH, COLD & FLU
NIGHTTIME (Wyeth Consumer)
Pain Reliever/Fever Reducer, Nasal
Decongestant, Cough Suppressant,
Antihistamine**

For full product information see page 738.

**ROBITUSSIN® Head & Chest
Congestion PE Syrup
(Wyeth Consumer)
Nasal Decongestant, Expectorant**

For full product information see page 739.

**THERAFLU® Nighttime Severe Cold
(Novartis Consumer Health, Inc.)
Pain Reliever-Fever Reducer
(Acetaminophen)
Antihistamine (Pheniramine maleate)
Nasal Decongestant
(Phenylephrine HCl)**

For full product information see page 740.

**THERAFLU® Cold & Cough
(Novartis Consumer Health, Inc.)
Cough Suppressant
(Dextromethorphan HBr)
Antihistamine (Pheniramine maleate)
Nasal Decongestant
(Phenylephrine HCl)**

For full product information see page 740.

**THERAFLU® Cold & Sore Throat
(Novartis Consumer Health, Inc.)
Pain Reliever-Fever Reducer
(Acetaminophen)
Antihistamine (Pheniramine maleate)
Nasal Decongestant (Phenylephrine
HCl)**

For full product information see page 741.

**THERAFLU® Flu & Chest
Congestion
(Novartis Consumer Health, Inc.)
Pain Reliever-Fever Reducer
(Acetaminophen)
Expectorant (Guaifenesin)**

For full product information see page 741.

**THERAFLU® Flu & Sore Throat
(Novartis Consumer Health, Inc.)
Pain Reliever-Fever Reducer
(Acetaminophen)
Antihistamine (Pheniramine maleate)
Nasal Decongestant (Phenylephrine
HCl)**

For full product information see page 742.

**THERAFLU® Daytime Severe Cold
(Novartis Consumer Health, Inc.)
Pain Reliever-Fever Reducer
(Acetaminophen)
Nasal Decongestant (Phenylephrine
HCl)**

For full product information see page 742.

**THERAFLU® DAYTIME WARMING
RELIEF
(Novartis Consumer Health, Inc.)
Pain Reliever/Fever Reducer/Cough
Suppressant/Nasal Decongestant**

For full product information see page 743.

**THERAFLU® NIGHTTIME WARMING
RELIEF
(Novartis Consumer Health, Inc.)
Cough Suppressant/Antihistamine/Pain
Reliever/Fever Reducer/Nasal
Decongestant**

For full product information see page 743.

**TRIAMINIC® Day Time Cold &
Cough
(Novartis Consumer Health, Inc.)
Cough Suppressant, Nasal
Decongestant
Cherry Flavor**

For full product information see page 745.

**TRIAMINIC® NIGHT TIME Cold &
Cough
(Novartis Consumer Health, Inc.)
Antihistamine/Cough Suppressant,
Nasal Decongestant
Grape Flavor**

For full product information see page 746.

TRIAMINIC® CHEST & NASAL CONGESTION
(Novartis Consumer Health, Inc.)
Expectorant, Nasal Decongestant

For full product information see page 746.

TRIAMINIC® COLD & ALLERGY
(Novartis Consumer Health, Inc.)
Antihistamine, Nasal Decongestant
Orange Flavor

For full product information see page 746.

TRIAMINIC® COUGH & SORE THROAT
(Novartis Consumer Health, Inc.)
Pain Reliever/Fever Reducer/Cough Suppressant

For full product information see page 747.

INFANT TRIAMINIC THIN STRIPS®
(Novartis Consumer Health, Inc.)
Decongestant
Nasal Decongestant
Decongestant Plus Cough
Nasal Decongestant, Cough Suppressant

For full product information see page 747.

TRIAMINIC® Softchews®
(Novartis Consumer Health, Inc.)
Cough & Runny Nose
Antihistamine, Cough Suppressant
Cherry Flavor

For full product information see page 748.

TRIAMINIC THIN STRIPS®
Cold & Cough
(Novartis Consumer Health, Inc.)
Cough Suppressant, Nasal Decongestant

Drug Facts

Active Ingredients: **Purpose:**
(in each strip)
Dextromethorphan, 3.67 mg (equivalent to 5 mg dextromethorphan HBr) .... Cough suppressant
Phenylephrine HCl, 2.5 mg .... Nasal decongestant

Uses:
temporarily relieves
• nasal and sinus congestion due to a cold
• cough due to minor throat and bronchial irritation

Warnings:
Do not use
• in a child who is taking a prescription monoamine oxidase inhibitor (MAOI) (certain drugs for depression, psychiat-

ric, or emotional conditions, or Parkinson's disease), or for 2 weeks after stopping the MAOI drug. If you do not know if the child's prescription drug contains an MAOI, ask a doctor or pharmacist before giving this product.

Ask a doctor before use if the child has
• heart disease • high blood pressure
• thyroid disease • diabetes • glaucoma
• cough that lasts or is chronic such as occurs with asthma
• cough that occurs with too much phlegm (mucus)

When using this product
• do not exceed recommended dosage

Stop use and ask a doctor if
• nervousness, dizziness, or sleeplessness occur
• symptoms do not improve within 7 days or occur with a fever
• cough persists for more than 7 days, comes back or occurs with a fever, rash or persistent headache. These could be signs of a serious condition.

Keep out of reach of children. In case of overdose, get medical help or contact a poison control center right away.

Directions:
• take every 4 hours; not to exceed 6 doses in 24 hours or as directed by a doctor

children 6 to under 12 years of age:	allow 2 strips to dissolve on tongue
children 2 to under 6 years of age:	allow 1 strip to dissolve on tongue
children under 2 years of age:	ask a doctor

Other Information:
• contains no aspirin
• store at controlled room temperature 20-25°C (68-77°F)

Inactive Ingredients: acetone, alcohol, FD&C Blue 1, FD&C Red 40, flavors, hypromellose, microcrystalline cellulose, polacrilin, polyethylene glycol, purified water, sodium polystyrene sulfonate, sucralose, titanium dioxide

Questions? call **1-800-452-0051** 24 hours a day, 7 days a week.
Alcohol: less than 0.5%

How Supplied: 16 Wild Berry Flavored Medicated Strips in a carton.
Shown in Product Identification Guide, page 515

TRIAMINIC THIN STRIPS®
COLD
(Novartis Consumer Health, Inc.)
Nasal Decongestant

For full product information see page 748.

CHILDREN'S TYLENOL® Plus Flu
(McNeil Consumer)

For full product information see page 749.

TYLENOL® Severe Allergy Caplets
(McNeil Consumer)

TYLENOL® Allergy Multi-Symptom Caplets with Cool Burst™ and Gelcaps

TYLENOL® Allergy Multi-Symptom Nighttime Caplets with Cool Burst™

For full product information see page 717.

TYLENOL® Cold Head Congestion Daytime Caplets with Cool Burst™ and Gelcaps (McNeil Consumer)

TYLENOL® Cold Head Congestion Nighttime Caplets with Cool Burst™

TYLENOL® Cold Head Congestion Severe Caplets with Cool Burst™

For full product information see page 750.

TYLENOL® COLD
Severe Congestion Non-Drowsy Caplets with Cool Burst™ (McNeil Consumer)

For full product information see page 751.

TYLENOL® Cold Multi-Symptom Daytime Caplets with Cool Burst™ and Gelcaps (McNeil Consumer)

TYLENOL® Cold Multi-Symptom Nighttime Caplets with Cool Burst™

TYLENOL® Cold Multi-Symptom Severe Caplets with Cool Burst™

TYLENOL® Cold Multi-Symptom Daytime Liquid

TYLENOL® Cold Multi-Symptom Nighttime Liquid with Cool Burst™

TYLENOL® Cold Multi-Symptom Severe Daytime Liquid

For full product information see page 752.

TYLENOL® Sinus Congestion & Pain Daytime Caplets with Cool Burst™ and Gelcaps (McNeil Consumer)

TYLENOL® Sinus Congestion & Pain Nighttime Caplets with Cool Burst™

TYLENOL® Sinus Congestion & Pain Severe Caplets with Cool Burst™

TYLENOL® Sinus Severe Congestion Caplets with Cool Burst™
Product information for all dosage forms of TYLENOL Sinus have been combined under this heading.

Description:

Each *TYLENOL® Sinus Congestion & Pain Daytime Caplet* with Cool Burst™ *and Gelcap* contains acetaminophen 325 mg and phenylephrine HCl 5 mg. Each *TYLENOL® Sinus Congestion & Pain Nighttime Caplet with Cool Burst*™ contains acetaminophen 325 mg, chlorpheniramine maleate 2 mg and phenylephrine HCL 5 mg. Each *TYLENOL® Sinus Congestion & Pain Severe Caplet with Cool Burst*™ contains acetaminophen 325 mg, guaifenesin 200 mg and phenylephrine HCl 5 mg. Each *TYLENOL® Sinus Severe Congestion Caplet with Cool Burst*™ contains acetaminophen 325 mg, guaifenesin 200 mg, and pseudoephedrine HCl 30 mg.

Actions:

TYLENOL® Sinus Congestion & Pain Daytime Caplets with Cool Burst™ *and Gelcaps* contain a clinically proven analgesic/antipyretic and a decongestant. Acetaminophen is equal to aspirin in analgesic and antipyretic effectiveness and it is unlikely to produce many of the side effects associated with aspirin and aspirin-containing products. Acetaminophen produces analgesia by elevation of the pain threshold and antipyresis through action on the hypothalamic heat regulating center. Phenylephrine hydrochloride is a sympathomimetic amine which temporarily relieves sinus congestion and pressure. *TYLENOL® Sinus Congestion & Pain Nighttime Caplets with Cool Burst*™ contain, in addition to the above ingredients, an antihistamine which provides temporary relief of runny nose and sneezing. *TYLENOL® Sinus Congestion & Pain Severe Caplets with Cool Burst*™ contain a clinically proven analgesic-antipyretic, an expectorant, and a decongestant. Acetaminophen is equal to aspirin in analgesic and antipyretic effectiveness and it is unlikely to produce many of the side effects associated with aspirin and aspirin-containing products. Acetaminophen produces analgesia by elevation of the pain threshold and antipyresis through action on the hypothalamic heat regulating center. Guaifenesin is an expectorant which helps loosen phlegm (mucus) and thin bronchial secretions to make coughs more productive. Phenylephrine hydrochloride is a sympathomimetic amine which temporarily relieves sinus congestion and pressure. *TYLENOL® Sinus Severe Congestion Caplets with Cool Burst*™ contain a clinically proven analgesic/antipyretic and a decongestant. Maximum allowable nonprescription levels of acetaminophen, guaifenesin, and pseudoephedrine HCl provide temporary relief of sinus pain, headache, and congestion. Acetaminophen is equal to aspirin in analgesic and antipyretic effectiveness and it is unlikely to produce many of the side effects associated with aspirin and aspirin-containing products. Acetaminophen produces analgesia by elevation of the pain threshold and antipyresis through action on the hypothalamic heat regulating center.

Uses:

TYLENOL® Sinus Congestion & Pain Daytime Caplets with Cool Burst™:
• for the temporary relief of:
  • headache
  • sinus congestion and pressure
  • nasal congestion
  • minor aches and pains
• reduces swelling of nasal passages

TYLENOL® Sinus Congestion & Pain Daytime Gelcaps:
• for the temporary relief of:
  • sinus congestion and pressure
  • headache
  • minor aches and pains
  • nasal congestion
• helps decongest sinus openings and passages

TYLENOL® Sinus Congestion & Pain Nighttime Caplets with Cool Burst™:
• for the temporary relief of:
  • headache
  • sinus congestion and pressure
  • nasal congestion
  • runny nose and sneezing
  • minor aches and pains
• reduces swelling of nasal passages
• helps decongest sinus openings and passages

TYLENOL® Sinus Congestion & Pain Severe Caplets with Cool Burst™:
• for the temporary relief of:
  • sinus congestion and pressure
  • headache
  • nasal congestion
  • minor aches and pains
• helps loosen phlegm (mucus) and thin bronchial secretions to make coughs more productive
• temporarily relieves nasal congestion due to the common cold, and hay fever and other upper respiratory allergies

TYLENOL® Sinus Severe Congestion Caplets with Cool Burst™:
• temporarily relieves:
  • minor aches and pains
  • sinus headache
• temporarily relieves nasal congestion associated with sinusitis
• promotes nasal and/or sinus drainage
• helps loosen phlegm (mucus) and thin bronchial secretions to make coughs more productive

Directions:

TYLENOL® Sinus Congestion & Pain Daytime Caplets with Cool Burst™ *and Gelcaps:*
• **do not take more than directed (see overdose warning)**

adults and children 12 years and over	• take 2 caplets or gelcaps every 4 hours • swallow whole – do not crush, chew or dissolve (caplets only) • do not take more than 12 caplets or gelcaps in 24 hours
children under 12 years	• do not use this adult product in children under 12 years of age; this will provide more than the recommended dose (overdose) and may cause liver damage.

TYLENOL® Sinus Congestion & Pain Nighttime Caplets with Cool Burst™:
• **do not take more than directed (see overdose warning)**

adults and children 12 years and over	• take 2 caplets every 4 hours • swallow whole – do not crush, chew or dissolve • do not take more than 12 caplets in 24 hours
children under 12 years	• do not use this adult product in children under 12 years of age; this will provide more than the recommended dose (overdose) and may cause liver damage.

TYLENOL® Sinus Congestion & Pain Severe Caplets with Cool Burst™:
• **do not take more than directed (see overdose warning)**

adults and children 12 years and over	• take 2 caplets every 4 hours • swallow whole — do not crush, chew or dissolve • do not take more than 12 caplets in 24 hours
children under 12 years	• do not use this adult product in children under 12 years of age; this will provide more than the recommended dose (overdose) and may cause liver damage.

TYLENOL® Sinus Severe Congestion Caplets with Cool Burst™:
• **do not take more than directed (see overdose warning)**

adults and children 12 years and over	• take 2 caplets every 4 – 6 hours as needed • swallow whole — do not crush, chew or dissolve • do not take more than 8 caplets in 24 hours
children under 12 years	• do not use this adult product in children under 12 years of age; this will provide more than the recommended dose (overdose) and may cause liver damage.

Continued on next page

Tylenol Sinus—Cont.

Warnings:

Alcohol warning: If you consume 3 or more alcoholic drinks every day, ask your doctor whether you should take acetaminophen or other pain relievers or fever reducers. Acetaminophen may cause liver damage.

Do not use

- with any other product containing acetaminophen
- if you are now taking a prescription monamine oxidase inhibitor (MAOI) (certain drugs for depression, psychiatric or emotional conditions or Parkinson's disease), or for 2 weeks after stopping the MAOI drug. If you do not know if your prescription drug contains an MAOI, ask a doctor or pharmacist before taking this product.

Ask a doctor before use if you have

TYLENOL® Sinus Congestion & Pain Daytime Caplets with Cool Burst™ *and Gelcaps*

- heart disease
- high blood pressure
- thyroid disease
- diabetes
- trouble urinating due to an enlarged prostate gland

TYLENOL® Sinus Congestion & Pain Nighttime Caplets with Cool Burst™

- heart disease
- high blood pressure
- thyroid disease
- diabetes
- trouble urinating due to an enlarged prostate gland
- a breathing problem such as emphysema or chronic bronchitis
- glaucoma

TYLENOL® Sinus Congestion & Pain Severe Caplets with Cool Burst™

- heart disease
- high blood pressure
- thyroid disease
- diabetes
- trouble urinating due to an enlarged prostate gland
- cough that occurs with too much phlegm (mucus)
- persistent or chronic cough such as occurs with smoking, asthma, chronic bronchitis or emphysema

TYLENOL® Sinus Severe Congestion Caplet with Cool Burst™

- heart disease
- diabetes
- thyroid disease
- cough that occurs with too much phlegm (mucus)
- high blood pressure
- trouble urinating due to an enlarged prostate gland
- chronic cough that lasts as occurs with smoking, asthma, or emphysema

Ask a doctor or pharmacist before use if you are taking sedatives or tranquilizers (*TYLENOL® Sinus Congestion & Pain Nighttime Caplets with Cool Burst*™ only)

When using this product do not exceed recommended dosage

TYLENOL® Sinus Congestion & Pain Nighttime Caplets with Cool Burst™ *only:*

- excitability may occur, especially in children
- drowsiness may occur
- alcohol, sedatives and tranquilizers may increase the drowsiness effect
- avoid alcoholic drinks
- be careful when driving a motor vehicle or operating machinery

Stop use and ask a doctor if

TYLENOL® Sinus Congestion & Pain Daytime Caplets with Cool Burst™ *and Gelcaps, TYLENOL® Sinus Congestion & Pain Nighttime Caplets with Cool Burst*™

- nervousness, dizziness, or sleeplessness occur
- pain or nasal congestion gets worse or lasts for more than 7 days
- fever gets worse or lasts for more than 3 days
- redness or swelling is present
- new symptoms occur

These could be signs of a serious condition.

TYLENOL® Sinus Congestion & Pain Severe Caplets with Cool Burst™

- nervousness, dizziness, or sleeplessness occurs
- pain, nasal congestion or cough gets worse or lasts more than 7 days
- fever gets worse or lasts more than 3 days
- redness or swelling is present
- new symptoms occur
- cough comes back or occurs with rash or headache that lasts

These could be signs of a serious condition.

TYLENOL® Sinus Severe Congestion Caplet with Cool Burst™

- new symptoms occur
- redness or swelling is present
- pain, nasal congestion, or cough gets worse or lasts for more than 7 days
- you get nervous, dizzy or sleepless
- cough comes back or occurs with rash or headache that lasts. These could be signs of a serious condition.

If pregnant or breast feeding, ask a health professional before use.

Keep out of reach of children.

Overdose Warning: Taking more than the recommended dose (overdose) may cause liver damage. In case of overdose get medical help or contact a Poison Control Center right away (1-800-222-1222). Quick medical attention is critical for adults as well as for children even if you do not notice any signs or symptoms.

Other Information:

- each caplet contains: **sodium 3 mg** (*TYLENOL® Sinus Congestion & Pain Severe Caplets with Cool Burst*™ *and TYLENOL® Sinus Severe Congestion Caplet with Cool Burst*™)

- store between 20 – 25° C (68 – 77° F) (does not apply to *TYLENOL® Sinus Congestion & Pain Daytime Gelcaps*)
- store between 20 – 25° C (68 – 77° F). Avoid high humidity (*TYLENOL® Sinus Congestion & Pain Daytime Gelcaps*)

PROFESSIONAL INFORMATION: OVERDOSAGE INFORMATION

For overdosage information, please refer to pgs. 696–697.

Inactive Ingredients:

TYLENOL® Sinus Congestion & Pain Daytime:

Caplets: carnauba wax, cellulose, corn starch, D&C yellow #10, FD&C blue #1, FD&C red #40, flavors, hypromellose, iron oxide, polyethylene glycol, polysorbate 80, silicon dioxide, sodium starch glycolate, stearic acid, sucralose, titanium dioxide

Gelcaps: benzyl alcohol, butylparaben, castor oil, cellulose, corn starch, D&C yellow #10, edetate calcium disodium, FD&C blue #1, gelatin, hypromellose, iron oxide, methylparaben, propylparaben, silcon dioxide, sodium lauryl sulfate, sodium propionate, sodium starch glycolate, stearic acid, titanium dioxide

TYLENOL® Sinus Congestion & Pain Nighttime Caplets with Cool Burst™: black iron oxide, carnauba wax, cellulose, corn starch, flavors, hypromellose, polyethylene glycol, polysorbate 80, silicon dioxide, sodium starch glycolate, stearic acid, sucralose, titanium dioxide, yellow iron oxide

TYLENOL® Sinus Congestion & Pain Severe Caplets with Cool Burst™: carnauba wax, cellulose, corn starch, croscarmellose sodium, flavors, hydroxypropyl cellulose, hypromellose, iron oxide, mannitol, silicon dioxide, stearic acid, sucralose

TYLENOL® Sinus Severe Congestion Caplets with Cool Burst™: cellulose, corn starch, croscarmellose sodium, D&C yellow #10, FD&C blue #1 FD&C red #40, flavor, iron oxide, mannitol, polyethylene glycol, polyvinyl alcohol, povidone, silicon dioxide, stearic acid, sucralose, talc, titanium dioxide

How Supplied:

TYLENOL® Sinus Congestion & Pain Daytime:

Caplets: Light green-colored, imprinted with "TY C1080" – blister packs of 24.

Gelcaps: Green- and white-colored, imprinted with "TY C1077" – blister packs of 24.

TYLENOL® Sinus Congestion & Pain Nighttime Caplets with Cool Burst™: off-white colored, imprinted with "TY C1076" – blister packs of 24.

TYLENOL® Sinus Congestion & Pain Severe Caplets with Cool Burst™: white caplet, imprinted with "TY MS C1072" – blister packs of 24.

TYLENOL® Sinus Severe Congestion Caplet with Cool Burst™: light green-

colored caplets printed with "Tylenol Sinus SC" in black ink – blister packs of 24.

Shown in Product Identification Guide, page 512

CONCENTRATED TYLENOL®
Infants' Drops Plus Cold Nasal Decongestant, Fever Reducer & Pain Reliever (McNeil Consumer)

CONCENTRATED TYLENOL®
Infants' Drops Plus Cold & Cough Nasal Decongestant, Fever Reducer & Pain Reliever, Cough Suppressant

CHILDREN'S TYLENOL® Plus Cough & Sore Throat Suspension Liquid

CHILDREN'S TYLENOL® Plus Cough & Runny Nose Suspension Liquid

CHILDREN'S TYLENOL® Plus Multi-Symptom Cold Suspension Liquid

CHILDREN'S TYLENOL® Plus Cold Suspension Liquid

For full product information see page 754.

CHILDREN'S VICKS® NYQUIL®
(Procter & Gamble)
Antihistamine/Cough Suppressant

For full product information see page 756.

VICKS® 44D® (Procter & Gamble)
COUGH & HEAD CONGESTION RELIEF
Cough Suppressant/Nasal Decongestant
Alcohol 5%

For full product information see page 760.

VICKS® 44M® (Procter & Gamble)
COUGH, COLD & FLU RELIEF
Cough Suppressant/Antihistamine/Pain Reliever–Fever Reducer Alcohol 10%
Maximum strength cough formula

For full product information see page 760.

VICKS® DAYQUIL® LIQUID
(Procter & Gamble)

VICKS® DAYQUIL® LIQUICAPS®
Multi-Symptom Cold/Flu Relief
Nasal Decongestant/Pain Reliever/Cough Suppressant/Fever Reducer Non-drowsy

For full product information see page 761.

VICKS® NYQUIL® LIQUICAPS®/ LIQUID MULTI-SYMPTOM COLD/ FLU RELIEF (Proctor & Gamble)

For full product information see page 763.

VICKS® SINEX®
(Procter & Gamble)
[sī 'něx]
12-HOUR [Nasal Spray]
[Ultra Fine Mist] for Sinus Relief
Oxymetazoline HCl
Nasal Decongestant

Drug Facts:

Active Ingredients: (in each tablet)	**Purpose:**
Oxymetazoline HCl 0.05%	Nasal decongestant

Uses: Temporarily relieves sinus/nasal congestion due to
• colds
• hay fever
• upper respiratory allergies
• sinusitis

Warnings:
Ask a doctor before use if you have:
• heart disease
• thyroid disease
• diabetes
• high blood pressure
• trouble urinating due to enlarged prostate gland
When using this product:
• **do not exceed recommended dosage**
• temporary burning, stinging, sneezing, or increased nasal discharge may occur
• frequent or prolonged use may cause nasal congestion to recur or worsen
• use of this container by more than one person may cause infection
Stop use and ask a doctor if:
• symptoms persist for more than 3 days
If pregnant or breast-feeding, ask a health professional before use.
Keep out of reach of children. In case of accidental ingestion, get medical help or contact a poison control center right away.

Directions:
Nasal Spray:
• under 6 yrs: ask a doctor
• adults & children 6 yrs. & older (with adult supervision): 2 or 3 sprays in each nostril without tilting your head, not more often than every 10 to 12 hours. Do not exceed 2 doses in 24 hours.
Ultra Fine Mist:
Remove protective cap. Before using for the first time, prime the pump by firmly depressing its rim several times. Hold container with thumb at base and nozzle between first and second fingers. Without tilting your head, insert nozzle into nostril. Fully depress rim with a firm, even stroke and inhale deeply.
• under 6 yrs.: ask a doctor
• adults & children 6 yrs. & older (with adult supervision): 2 or 3 sprays in each nostril, not more often than every 10 to

12 hours. Do not exceed 2 doses in 24 hours.

Other Information:
• store at room temperature

Inactive Ingredients: Benzalkonium chloride, camphor, chlorhexidine gluconate, disodium EDTA, eucalyptol, menthol, potassium phosphate, purified water, sodium chloride, sodium phosphate, tyloxapol.

How Supplied: Available in ½ FL OZ (14.7 ml) plastic squeeze bottle and ½ FL OZ (14.7 ml) measured-dose Ultra Fine mist pump.
TAMPER EVIDENT: Do not use if imprinted shrinkband is missing or broken.
Questions? 1-800-873-8276
Dist. by
Procter & Gamble,
Cincinnati OH 45202

VICKS® SINEX® NASAL SPRAY
(Procter & Gamble)
Ultra Fine Mist for Sinus Relief
[sī 'něx]
Phenylephrine HCl Nasal Decongestant

Drug Facts:

Active Ingredients:	**Purpose:**
Phenylephrine HCl 0.5%	Nasal decongestant

Uses: Temporarily relieves sinus/nasal congestion due to
• colds
• hay fever
• upper respiratory allergies
• sinusitis

Warnings:
Ask a doctor before use if you have:
• heart disease
• thyroid disease
• diabetes
• high blood pressure
• trouble urinating due to enlarged prostate gland
When using this product:
• **do not exceed recommended dosage**
• use of this container by more than one person may cause infection
• temporary burning, stinging, sneezing, or increased nasal discharge may occur
• frequent or prolonged use may cause nasal congestion to recur or worsen
Stop use and ask a doctor if:
• symptoms persist for more than 3 days
If pregnant or breast-feeding, ask a health professional before use.
Keep out of reach of children. In case of accidental ingestion, get medical help or contact a poison control center right away.

Directions:
Nasal Spray:
• under 12 yrs. ask a doctor
• adults & children 12 yrs. & older: 2 or 3 sprays in each nostril without tilting

Continued on next page

Vicks Sinex—Cont.

your head, not more often than every 4 hours.

Ultra Fine Mist: Remove protective cap. Before using for the first time, prime the pump by firmly depressing its rim several times. Hold container with thumb at base and nozzle between first and second fingers. Without tilting it, insert nozzle into nostril. Fully depress rim with a firm, even stroke and inhale deeply.

- under 12 yrs.: ask a doctor
- adults & children 12 yrs. & older: 2 or 3 sprays in each nostril, not more often than every 4 hours.

Other Information:

- store at room temperature

Inactive Ingredients: Benzalkonium chloride, camphor, chlorhexidine gluconate, citric acid, disodium EDTA, eucalyptol, menthol, purified water, tyloxapol

How Supplied: Available in $\frac{1}{2}$ FL OZ (14.7 ml) plastic squeeze bottle and $\frac{1}{2}$ FL OZ (14.7 ml) measured dose Ultra Fine mist pump. Note: This container is properly filled when approximately half full. Air space equal to one half of volume is necessary to propel the fine spray.

Tamper Evident:
Do not use if imprinted shrinkband is missing or broken.

Questions? 1-800-873-8276
Nasal Spray 42436771
Ultra Fine Mist 42436765
Dist. by Procter & Gamble
Cincinnati OH 45202

VICKS® VAPOR INHALER
(Procter & Gamble)
Levmetamfetamine/Nasal
Decongestant

For full product information see page 769.

ZICAM® Allergy Relief (Matrixx)
[zī'kăm]

For full product information see page 774.

ZICAM® Cold Remedy Nasal Gel™ (Matrixx)
[zī-kăm]

ZICAM® Cold Remedy Gel Swabs™

ZICAM® Cold Remedy Swabs Kids Size

ZICAM® Cold Remedy RapidMelts®

ZICAM® Cold Remedy RapidMelts® with Vitamin C

ZICAM® Cold Remedy Oral Mist™

ZICAM® Cold Remedy Chewables™

ZICAM® Cold Remedy ChewCaps

For full product information see page 766.

ZICAM® Extreme Congestion Relief (Matrixx)
ZICAM® Intense Sinus Relief (Matrixx)
[zī 'kăm]

For full product information see page 767.

Respiratory System:
Runny Nose

ADVIL® ALLERGY SINUS
CAPLETS (Wyeth Consumer)
ADVIL® MULTI-SYMPTOM COLD
CAPLETS
Pain Reliever/Fever Reducer (NSAID)
Nasal Decongestant
Antihistamine

For full product information see page 770.

ALAVERT (Wyeth Consumer)
Loratadine orally disintegrating tablets
Loratadine swallow tablets
Antihistamine

For full product information see page 771.

ALAVERT ALLERGY & SINUS D-12
HOUR TABLETS (Wyeth Consumer)
Loratadine/Pseudoephedrine Sulfate
Extended Release Tablets
Antihistamine/Nasal Decongestant

For full product information see page 771.

BC® POWDER
(GlaxoSmithKline Consumer)
ARTHRITIS STRENGTH BC®
POWDER
BC® COLD POWDER LINE

For full product information see page 677.

CLARITIN 24 HOUR NON-DROWSY
REDITABS
(Schering-Plough Healthcare)
loratadine 10 mg/antihistamine

CLARITIN 24 HOUR NON-DROWSY
TABLETS
Loratadine 10 mg/antihistamine

For full product information see page 772.

CLARITIN-D 12 HOUR
NON-DROWSY
(Schering-Plough Healthcare)
pseudoephedrine sulfate 120 mg/nasal
decongestant
Loratadine 5 mg/antihistamine

CLARITIN-D NON-DROWSY
24 HOUR
pseudoephedrine sulfate 240 mg/nasal
decongestant
Loratadine 10 mg/antihistamine

For full product information see page 772.

COMTREX®
(Novartis Consumer Health, Inc.)
MAXIMUM STRENGTH
Day/Night Severe Cold & Sinus
Pain Reliever/Fever Reducer – Nasal
Decongestant – Antihistamine*
Acetaminophen, Phenylephrine HCl,
Chlorpheniramine Maleate*

For full product information see page 725.

COMTREX® Cold & Cough
Day/Night
(Novartis Consumer Health, Inc.)
Pain Reliever/Fever Reducer

For full product information see page 726.

CONTAC® COLD AND FLU DAY
AND NIGHT
(GlaxoSmithKline Consumer)

For full product information see page 727.

CONTAC® COLD AND FLU
MAXIMUM STRENGTH
(GlaxoSmithKline Consumer)

For full product information see page 728.

CHILDREN'S DIMETAPP® COLD &
ALLERGY CHEWABLE TABLETS
(Wyeth Consumer)
Antihistamine/Nasal decongestant

For full product information see page 730.

CHILDREN'S DIMETAPP® Cold &
Allergy Elixir (Wyeth Consumer)
Antihistamine, Nasal Decongestant

For full product information see page 730.

CHILDREN'S DIMETAPP® DM
COLD & COUGH Elixir
(Wyeth Consumer)
Antihistamine, Cough Suppressant,
Nasal Decongestant

For full product information see page 731.

ROBITUSSIN® Cough & Cold
Nighttime (Wyeth Consumer)
ROBITUSSIN® Pediatric Cough &
Cold Nighttime
ROBITUSSIN® Cough & Allergy
Nasal Decongestant, Cough
Suppressant, Antihistamine

For full product information see page 736.

THERAFLU® NIGHTTIME WARMING
RELIEF
(Novartis Consumer Health, Inc.)
Cough Suppressant/Antihistamine/Pain
Reliever/Fever Reducer/Nasal
Decongestant

For full product information see page 743.

THERAFLU® THIN
STRIPS®-MULTISYMPTOM
(Novartis Consumer Health, Inc.)
Antihistamine/Cough Suppressant
(Diphenhydramine HCl)

For full product information see page 744.

TRIAMINIC® NIGHT TIME Cold &
Cough
(Novartis Consumer Health, Inc.)
Antihistamine/Cough Suppressant,
Nasal Decongestant
Grape Flavor

For full product information see page 746.

TRIAMINIC® COLD & ALLERGY
(Novartis Consumer Health, Inc.)
Antihistamine, Nasal Decongestant
Orange Flavor

For full product information see page 746.

TRIAMINIC® Softchews®
(Novartis Consumer Health, Inc.)
Cough & Runny Nose
Antihistamine, Cough Suppressant
Cherry Flavor

For full product information see page 748.

TRIAMINIC THIN STRIPS®
COUGH & RUNNY NOSE
(Novartis Consumer Health, Inc.)

For full product information see page 749.

CHILDREN'S TYLENOL® Plus Cold
& Allergy (McNeil Consumer)

For full product information see page 716.

CHILDREN'S TYLENOL® Plus Flu
(McNeil Consumer)

For full product information see page 749.

TYLENOL® Severe Allergy Caplets (McNeil Consumer)

TYLENOL® Allergy Multi-Symptom Caplets with Cool Burst™ and Gelcaps

TYLENOL® Allergy Multi-Symptom Nighttime Caplets with Cool Burst™

For full product information see page 717.

TYLENOL® Cold Head Congestion Daytime Caplets with Cool Burst™ and Gelcaps (McNeil Consumer)

TYLENOL® Cold Head Congestion Nighttime Caplets with Cool Burst™

TYLENOL® Cold Head Congestion Severe Caplets with Cool Burst™

For full product information see page 750.

TYLENOL® Cold Multi-Symptom Daytime Caplets with Cool Burst™ and Gelcaps (McNeil Consumer)

TYLENOL® Cold Multi-Symptom Nighttime Caplets with Cool Burst™

TYLENOL® Cold Multi-Symptom Severe Caplets with Cool Burst™

TYLENOL® Cold Multi-Symptom Daytime Liquid

TYLENOL® Cold Multi-Symptom Nighttime Liquid with Cool Burst™

TYLENOL® Cold Multi-Symptom Severe Daytime Liquid

For full product information see page 751.

TYLENOL® Sinus Congestion & Pain Daytime Caplets with Cool Burst™ and Gelcaps (McNeil Consumer)

TYLENOL® Sinus Congestion & Pain Nighttime Caplets with Cool Burst™

TYLENOL® Sinus Congestion & Pain Severe Caplets with Cool Burst™

TYLENOL® Sinus Severe Congestion Caplets with Cool Burst™
Product information for all dosage forms of TYLENOL Sinus have been combined under this heading.

For full product information see page 752.

TYLENOL® Sore Throat Daytime Liquid with Cool Burst™ (McNeil Consumer)

TYLENOL® Sore Throat Nighttime Liquid with Cool Burst™

TYLENOL® Cough & Sore Throat Daytime Liquid with Cool Burst™

TYLENOL® Cough & Sore Throat Nighttime Liquid with Cool Burst™

For full product information see page 790.

CONCENTRATED TYLENOL® Infants' Drops Plus Cold Nasal Decongestant, Fever Reducer & Pain Reliever (McNeil Consumer)

CONCENTRATED TYLENOL® Infants' Drops Plus Cold & Cough Nasal Decongestant, Fever Reducer & Pain Reliever, Cough Suppressant

CHILDREN'S TYLENOL® Plus Cough & Sore Throat Suspension Liquid

CHILDREN'S TYLENOL® Plus Cough & Runny Nose Suspension Liquid

CHILDREN'S TYLENOL® Plus Multi-Symptom Cold Suspension Liquid

CHILDREN'S TYLENOL® Plus Cold Suspension Liquid

For full product information see page 754.

CHILDREN'S VICKS® NYQUIL® (Procter & Gamble)
Antihistamine/Cough Suppressant

For full product information see page 756.

PEDIATRIC VICKS® 44m® (Procter & Gamble)
Cough & Cold Relief
Cough Suppressant/Antihistamine

For full product information see page 759.

VICKS® 44M® (Procter & Gamble)
COUGH, COLD & FLU RELIEF
Cough Suppressant/Antihistamine/Pain Reliever–Fever Reducer Alcohol 10%
Maximum strength cough formula

For full product information see page 760.

VICKS® NYQUIL® LIQUICAPS®/ LIQUID MULTI-SYMPTOM COLD/ FLU RELIEF (Proctor & Gamble)

For full product information see page 763.

ZICAM® Allergy Relief (Matrixx)
[zī′kăm]

For full product information see page 774.

ZICAM® Flu Daytime (Matrixx)

ZICAM® Nighttime

For full product information see page 768.

Respiratory System:
Sinus Pressure/Pain

ADVIL® ALLERGY SINUS CAPLETS (Wyeth Consumer)
ADVIL® MULTI-SYMPTOM COLD CAPLETS
Pain Reliever/Fever Reducer (NSAID)
Nasal Decongestant
Antihistamine

For full product information see page 770.

ALAVERT ALLERGY & SINUS D-12 HOUR TABLETS (Wyeth Consumer)
Loratadine/Pseudoephedrine Sulfate
Extended Release Tablets
Antihistamine/Nasal Decongestant

For full product information see page 771.

ALEVE COLD & SINUS CAPLETS (Bayer Healthcare)
(NSAID Labeling)
[a-lēv]

For full product information see page 771.

CLARITIN-D 12 HOUR NON-DROWSY
(Schering-Plough Healthcare)
pseudoephedrine sulfate 120 mg/nasal decongestant
Loratadine 5 mg/antihistamine

CLARITIN-D NON-DROWSY 24 HOUR
pseudoephedrine sulfate 240 mg/nasal decongestant
Loratadine 10 mg/antihistamine

For full product information see page 772.

CONTAC® COLD AND FLU DAY AND NIGHT
(GlaxoSmithKline Consumer)

For full product information see page 727.

CONTAC COLD AND FLU NON-DROWSY MAXIMUM STRENGTH
(GlaxoSmithKline Consumer)

For full product information see page 728.

CONTAC®-D COLD NON-DROWSY DECONGESTANT
(GlaxoSmithKline Consumer)

For full product information see page 729.

EXCEDRIN® SINUS HEADACHE
(Novartis Consumer Health, Inc.)
Acetaminophen and Phenylephrine HCl

For full product information see page 610.

MUCINEX® D
(Adams Respiratory Therapeutics)
600 mg Guaifenesin and 60 mg Pseudoephedrine HCl Extended-Release Bi-Layer Tablets
Expectorant and Nasal Decongestant

For full product information see page 776.

TYLENOL® Severe Allergy Caplets (McNeil Consumer)

TYLENOL® Allergy Multi-Symptom Caplets with Cool Burst™ and Gelcaps

TYLENOL® Allergy Multi-Symptom Nighttime Caplets with Cool Burst™

For full product information see page 717.

TYLENOL® Cold Head Congestion Daytime Caplets with Cool Burst™ and Gelcaps (McNeil Consumer)

TYLENOL® Cold Head Congestion Nighttime Caplets with Cool Burst™

TYLENOL® Cold Head Congestion Severe Caplets with Cool Burst™

For full product information see page 750.

TYLENOL® Cold Multi-Symptom Daytime Caplets with Cool Burst™ and Gelcaps (McNeil Consumer)

TYLENOL® Cold Multi-Symptom Nighttime Caplets with Cool Burst™

TYLENOL® Cold Multi-Symptom Severe Caplets with Cool Burst™

TYLENOL® Cold Multi-Symptom Daytime Liquid

TYLENOL® Cold Multi-Symptom Nighttime Liquid with Cool Burst™

TYLENOL® Cold Multi-Symptom Severe Daytime Liquid

For full product information see page 751.

TYLENOL® Sinus Congestion & Pain Daytime Caplets with Cool Burst™ and Gelcaps (McNeil Consumer)

TYLENOL® Sinus Congestion & Pain Nighttime Caplets with Cool Burst™

TYLENOL® Sinus Congestion & Pain Severe Caplets with Cool Burst™

TYLENOL® Sinus Severe Congestion Caplets with Cool Burst™
Product information for all dosage forms of TYLENOL Sinus have been combined under this heading.

For full product information see page 752.

ZICAM® Allergy Relief (Matrixx)
[zī'kăm]

For full product information see page 774.

Respiratory System:
Sinusitis

ADVIL® COLD & SINUS
(Wyeth Consumer)
Caplets, and Liqui-Gels
Pain Reliever/Fever Reducer/(NSAID)
Nasal Decongestant

For full product information see page 723.

CONTAC® Non-Drowsy
(GlaxoSmithKline Consumer)
Decongestant
12 Hour Cold Caplets

For full product information see page 729.

CHILDREN'S DIMETAPP® Cold &
Allergy Elixir (Wyeth Consumer)
Antihistamine, Nasal Decongestant

For full product information see page 730.

CHILDREN'S DIMETAPP® DM
COLD & COUGH Elixir
(Wyeth Consumer)
Antihistamine, Cough Suppressant,
Nasal Decongestant

For full product information see page 731.

TODDLER'S DIMETAPP COLD AND
COUGH DROPS (Wyeth Consumer)
Cough suppressant/Nasal decongestant

For full product information see page 732.

EXCEDRIN® EXTRA STRENGTH
(Novartis Consumer Health, Inc.)
PAIN RELIEVER

For full product information see page 684.

THERAFLU® Nighttime Severe Cold
(Novartis Consumer Health, Inc.)
Pain Reliever-Fever Reducer
(Acetaminophen)
Antihistamine (Pheniramine maleate)
Nasal Decongestant
(Phenylephrine HCl)

For full product information see page 740.

THERAFLU® Cold & Cough
(Novartis Consumer Health, Inc.)
Cough Suppressant
(Dextromethorphan HBr)
Antihistamine (Pheniramine maleate)
Nasal Decongestant
(Phenylephrine HCl)

For full product information see page 740.

THERAFLU® Cold & Sore Throat
(Novartis Consumer Health, Inc.)
Pain Reliever-Fever Reducer
(Acetaminophen)
Antihistamine (Pheniramine maleate)
Nasal Decongestant (Phenylephrine
HCl)

For full product information see page 741.

THERAFLU® Flu & Chest
Congestion
(Novartis Consumer Health, Inc.)
Pain Reliever-Fever Reducer
(Acetaminophen)
Expectorant (Guaifenesin)

For full product information see page 741.

THERAFLU® Flu & Sore Throat
(Novartis Consumer Health, Inc.)
Pain Reliever-Fever Reducer
(Acetaminophen)
Antihistamine (Pheniramine maleate)
Nasal Decongestant (Phenylephrine
HCl)

For full product information see page 742.

THERAFLU® Daytime Severe Cold
(Novartis Consumer Health, Inc.)
Pain Reliever-Fever Reducer
(Acetaminophen)
Nasal Decongestant (Phenylephrine
HCl)

For full product information see page 742.

TRIAMINIC® CHEST & NASAL
CONGESTION
(Novartis Consumer Health, Inc.)
Expectorant, Nasal Decongestant

For full product information see page 746.

TRIAMINIC® COUGH & SORE
THROAT
(Novartis Consumer Health, Inc.)
Pain Reliever/Fever Reducer/Cough
Suppressant

For full product information see page 747.

VICKS® SINEX®
(Procter & Gamble)
[sĭ 'nĕx]
12-HOUR [Nasal Spray]
[Ultra Fine Mist] for Sinus Relief
Oxymetazoline HCl
Nasal Decongestant

For full product information see page 781.

VICKS® SINEX® NASAL SPRAY
(Procter & Gamble)
Ultra Fine Mist for Sinus Relief
[sĭ 'nĕx]
Phenylephrine HCl Nasal
Decongestant

For full product information see page 781.

VICKS® VAPOR INHALER
(Procter & Gamble)
Levmetamfetamine/Nasal
Decongestant

For full product information see page 764.

ZICAM® Extreme Congestion Relief
(Matrixx)
ZICAM® Intense Sinus Relief
[zĭ 'kăm]

For full product information see page 767.

Respiratory System:
Sneezing

ADVIL® ALLERGY SINUS CAPLETS (Wyeth Consumer)
ADVIL® MULTI-SYMPTOM COLD CAPLETS
Pain Reliever/Fever Reducer (NSAID)
Nasal Decongestant
Antihistamine

For full product information see page 770.

ALAVERT (Wyeth Consumer)
Loratadine orally disintegrating tablets
Loratadine swallow tablets
Antihistamine

For full product information see page 771.

ALAVERT ALLERGY & SINUS D-12 HOUR TABLETS (Wyeth Consumer)
Loratadine/Pseudoephedrine Sulfate
Extended Release Tablets
Antihistamine/Nasal Decongestant

For full product information see page 771.

BC® POWDER
(GlaxoSmithKline Consumer)
ARTHRITIS STRENGTH BC® POWDER
BC® COLD POWDER LINE

For full product information see page 677.

CHILDREN'S CLARITIN ALLERGY
(Schering-Plough Healthcare)
loratadine oral solution, grape flavor
5mg/5mL-antihistamine

For full product information see page 771.

CLARITIN 24 HOUR NON-DROWSY REDITABS
(Schering-Plough Healthcare)
loratadine 10 mg/antihistamine

CLARITIN 24 HOUR NON-DROWSY TABLETS
Loratadine 10 mg/antihistamine

For full product information see page 772.

CLARITIN-D 12 HOUR NON-DROWSY
(Schering-Plough Healthcare)
pseudoephedrine sulfate 120 mg/nasal
decongestant
Loratadine 5 mg/antihistamine

CLARITIN-D NON-DROWSY 24 HOUR
pseudoephedrine sulfate 240 mg/nasal
decongestant
Loratadine 10 mg/antihistamine

For full product information see page 772.

COMTREX®
(Novartis Consumer Health, Inc.)
MAXIMUM STRENGTH
Day/Night Severe Cold & Sinus
Pain Reliever/Fever Reducer – Nasal
Decongestant – Antihistamine*
Acetaminophen, Phenylephrine HCl,
Chlorpheniramine Maleate*

For full product information see page 725.

COMTREX® Cold & Cough Day/Night
(Novartis Consumer Health, Inc.)
Pain Reliever/Fever Reducer

For full product information see page 726.

CONTAC® COLD AND FLU DAY AND NIGHT
(GlaxoSmithKline Consumer)

For full product information see page 727.

CONTAC® COLD AND FLU MAXIMUM STRENGTH
(GlaxoSmithKline Consumer)

For full product information see page 728.

CHILDREN'S DIMETAPP® COLD & ALLERGY CHEWABLE TABLETS
(Wyeth Consumer)
Antihistamine/Nasal decongestant

For full product information see page 730.

CHILDREN'S DIMETAPP® Cold & Allergy Elixir (Wyeth Consumer)
Antihistamine, Nasal Decongestant

For full product information see page 730.

CHILDREN'S DIMETAPP® DM COLD & COUGH Elixir
(Wyeth Consumer)
Antihistamine, Cough Suppressant,
Nasal Decongestant

For full product information see page 731.

ROBITUSSIN® Cough & Cold Nighttime (Wyeth Consumer)
ROBITUSSIN® Pediatric Cough & Cold Nighttime
ROBITUSSIN® Cough & Allergy
Nasal Decongestant, Cough
Suppressant, Antihistamine

For full product information see page 736.

THERAFLU® NIGHTTIME WARMING RELIEF
(Novartis Consumer Health, Inc.)
Cough Suppressant/Antihistamine/Pain
Reliever/Fever Reducer/Nasal
Decongestant

For full product information see page 743.

THERAFLU® THIN STRIPS®-MULTISYMPTOM
(Novartis Consumer Health, Inc.)
Antihistamine/Cough Suppressant
(Diphenhydramine HCl)

For full product information see page 744.

TRIAMINIC® NIGHT TIME Cold & Cough
(Novartis Consumer Health, Inc.)
Antihistamine/Cough Suppressant,
Nasal Decongestant
Grape Flavor

For full product information see page 746.

TRIAMINIC® COLD & ALLERGY
(Novartis Consumer Health, Inc.)
Antihistamine, Nasal Decongestant
Orange Flavor

For full product information see page 746.

TRIAMINIC® Softchews®
(Novartis Consumer Health, Inc.)
Cough & Runny Nose
Antihistamine, Cough Suppressant
Cherry Flavor

For full product information see page 748.

**TRIAMINIC THIN STRIPS®
COUGH & RUNNY NOSE
(Novartis Consumer Health, Inc.)**

For full product information see page 749.

**CHILDREN'S TYLENOL® Plus Cold
& Allergy (McNeil Consumer)**

For full product information see page 716.

**CHILDREN'S TYLENOL® Plus Flu
(McNeil Consumer)**

For full product information see page 749.

**TYLENOL® Severe Allergy Caplets
(McNeil Consumer)**

**TYLENOL® Allergy Multi-Symptom
Caplets with Cool Burst™ and
Gelcaps**

**TYLENOL® Allergy Multi-Symptom
Nighttime Caplets with Cool
Burst™**

For full product information see page 717.

**TYLENOL® Cold Head Congestion
Daytime Caplets with Cool Burst™
and Gelcaps (McNeil Consumer)**

**TYLENOL® Cold Head Congestion
Nighttime Caplets with Cool
Burst™**

**TYLENOL® Cold Head Congestion
Severe Caplets with Cool Burst™**

For full product information see page 750.

**TYLENOL® Cold Multi-Symptom
Daytime Caplets with Cool Burst™
and Gelcaps (McNeil Consumer)**

**TYLENOL® Cold Multi-Symptom
Nighttime Caplets with Cool
Burst™**

**TYLENOL® Cold Multi-Symptom
Severe Caplets with Cool Burst™**

**TYLENOL® Cold Multi-Symptom
Daytime Liquid**

**TYLENOL® Cold Multi-Symptom
Nighttime Liquid with Cool Burst™**

**TYLENOL® Cold Multi-Symptom
Severe Daytime Liquid**

For full product information see page 751.

**TYLENOL® Sinus Congestion &
Pain Daytime Caplets with Cool
Burst™ and Gelcaps
(McNeil Consumer)**

**TYLENOL® Sinus Congestion &
Pain Nighttime Caplets with Cool
Burst™**

**TYLENOL® Sinus Congestion &
Pain Severe Caplets with Cool
Burst™**

**TYLENOL® Sinus Severe
Congestion Caplets with Cool
Burst™**
Product information for all dosage
forms of TYLENOL Sinus have been
combined under this heading.

For full product information see page 752.

**TYLENOL® Sore Throat Daytime
Liquid with Cool Burst™
(McNeil Consumer)**

**TYLENOL® Sore Throat Nighttime
Liquid with Cool Burst™**

**TYLENOL® Cough & Sore Throat
Daytime Liquid with Cool Burst™**

**TYLENOL® Cough & Sore Throat
Nighttime Liquid with Cool Burst™**

For full product information see page 790.

**CONCENTRATED TYLENOL®
Infants' Drops Plus Cold Nasal
Decongestant, Fever Reducer &
Pain Reliever (McNeil Consumer)**

**CONCENTRATED TYLENOL®
Infants' Drops Plus Cold & Cough
Nasal Decongestant, Fever Reducer
& Pain Reliever, Cough
Suppressant**

**CHILDREN'S TYLENOL® Plus
Cough & Sore Throat Suspension
Liquid**

**CHILDREN'S TYLENOL® Plus
Cough & Runny Nose Suspension
Liquid**

**CHILDREN'S TYLENOL® Plus Multi-
Symptom Cold Suspension Liquid**

**CHILDREN'S TYLENOL® Plus
Cold Suspension Liquid**

For full product information see page 754.

**CHILDREN'S VICKS® NYQUIL®
(Procter & Gamble)**
Antihistamine/Cough Suppressant

For full product information see page 756.

**PEDIATRIC VICKS® 44m®
(Procter & Gamble)**
Cough & Cold Relief
Cough Suppressant/Antihistamine

For full product information see page 759.

VICKS® 44M® (Procter & Gamble)
COUGH, COLD & FLU RELIEF
Cough Suppressant/Antihistamine/Pain
Reliever–Fever Reducer Alcohol 10%
Maximum strength cough formula

For full product information see page 760.

**VICKS® NYQUIL® LIQUICAPS®/
LIQUID MULTI-SYMPTOM COLD/
FLU RELIEF (Proctor & Gamble)**

For full product information see page 763.

ZICAM® Allergy Relief (Matrixx)
[zī'kăm]

For full product information see page 774.

ZICAM® Flu Daytime (Matrixx)

ZICAM® Nighttime

For full product information see page 768.

Respiratory System:
Sore Throat

CHILDREN'S ADVIL CHEWABLE TABLETS (Wyeth Consumer)
Fever Reducer/Pain Reliever (NSAID)

For full product information see page 603.

CHILDREN'S ADVIL SUSPENSION (Wyeth Consumer)
Fever Reducer/Pain Reliever (NSAID)

For full product information see page 603.

JUNIOR STRENGTH ADVIL® SWALLOW TABLETS (Wyeth Consumer)
Fever Reducer/Pain Reliever (NSAID)

For full product information see page 605.

COMTREX®
(Novartis Consumer Health, Inc.)
MAXIMUM STRENGTH
Pain Reliever/Fever Reducer, Cough Suppressant, Nasal Decongestant
Acetaminophon, Dextromethorphan HBr, Phenylephrine HCl
Non-Drowsy Cold & Cough

For full product information see page 725.

COMTREX® Cold & Cough Day/Night
(Novartis Consumer Health, Inc.)
Pain Reliever/Fever Reducer

For full product information see page 726.

CONTAC® COLD AND FLU DAY AND NIGHT
(GlaxoSmithKline Consumer)

For full product information see page 727.

CONTAC COLD AND FLU NON-DROWSY MAXIMUM STRENGTH
(GlaxoSmithKline Consumer)

For full product information see page 728.

CONTAC® COLD AND FLU MAXIMUM STRENGTH
(GlaxoSmithKline Consumer)

For full product information see page 728.

HURRICAINE® Topical Anesthetic
20% Benzocaine Oral Anesthetic
(Beutlich LP)

For full product information see page 712.

CHILDREN'S MOTRIN® Cold (McNeil Consumer)
ibuprofen/pseudoephedrine HCl
Oral Suspension

For full product information see page 733.

INFANTS' MOTRIN® ibuprofen Concentrated Drops (McNeil Consumer)

CHILDREN'S MOTRIN® ibuprofen Oral Suspension

JUNIOR STRENGTH MOTRIN® ibuprofen Caplets and Chewable Tablets
Product information for all dosages of Children's MOTRIN have been combined under this heading

For full product information see page 685.

ROBITUSSIN® COUGH DROPS (Wyeth Consumer)
Menthol Eucalyptus, Cherry and Honey-Lemon Flavors

ROBITUSSIN® HONEY COUGH DROPS
Honey-Lemon Tea, Natural Honey Center

ROBITUSSIN® SUGAR FREE Throat Drops
Natural Citrus

For full product information see page 737.

THERAFLU® Nighttime Severe Cold
(Novartis Consumer Health, Inc.)
Pain Reliever-Fever Reducer (Acetaminophen)
Antihistamine (Pheniramine maleate)
Nasal Decongestant (Phenylephrine HCl)

For full product information see page 740.

THERAFLU® Cold & Cough
(Novartis Consumer Health, Inc.)
Cough Suppressant (Dextromethorphan HBr)
Antihistamine (Pheniramine maleate)
Nasal Decongestant (Phenylephrine HCl)

For full product information see page 740.

THERAFLU® Cold & Sore Throat
(Novartis Consumer Health, Inc.)
Pain Reliever-Fever Reducer (Acetaminophen)
Antihistamine (Pheniramine maleate)
Nasal Decongestant (Phenylephrine HCl)

For full product information see page 741.

THERAFLU® Flu & Chest Congestion
(Novartis Consumer Health, Inc.)
Pain Reliever-Fever Reducer (Acetaminophen)
Expectorant (Guaifenesin)

For full product information see page 741.

THERAFLU® Flu & Sore Throat
(Novartis Consumer Health, Inc.)
Pain Reliever-Fever Reducer (Acetaminophen)
Antihistamine (Pheniramine maleate)
Nasal Decongestant (Phenylephrine HCl)

For full product information see page 742

THERAFLU® Daytime Severe Cold
(Novartis Consumer Health, Inc.)
Pain Reliever-Fever Reducer (Acetaminophen)
Nasal Decongestant (Phenylephrine HCl)

For full product information see page 742.

THERAFLU® DAYTIME WARMING RELIEF
(Novartis Consumer Health, Inc.)
Pain Reliever/Fever Reducer/Cough Suppressant/Nasal Decongestant

For full product information see page 743.

THERAFLU® NIGHTTIME WARMING RELIEF
(Novartis Consumer Health, Inc.)
Cough Suppressant/Antihistamine/Pain Reliever/Fever Reducer/Nasal Decongestant

For full product information see page 743.

TRIAMINIC® COUGH & SORE THROAT
(Novartis Consumer Health, Inc.)
Pain Reliever/Fever Reducer/Cough Suppressant

For full product information see page 747.

CHILDREN'S TYLENOL® Plus Cold & Allergy (McNeil Consumer)

For full product information see page 716.

CHILDREN'S TYLENOL® Plus Flu (McNeil Consumer)

For full product information see page 749.

TYLENOL® Cold Head Congestion Daytime Caplets with Cool Burst™ and Gelcaps (McNeil Consumer)

TYLENOL® Cold Head Congestion Nighttime Caplets with Cool Burst™

TYLENOL® Cold Head Congestion Severe Caplets with Cool Burst™

For full product information see page 750.

TYLENOL® COLD
Severe Congestion Non-Drowsy Caplets with Cool Burst™ (McNeil Consumer)

For full product information see page 751.

TYLENOL® Cold Multi-Symptom Daytime Caplets with Cool Burst™ and Gelcaps (McNeil Consumer)

TYLENOL® Cold Multi-Symptom Nighttime Caplets with Cool Burst™

TYLENOL® Cold Multi-Symptom Severe Caplets with Cool Burst™

TYLENOL® Cold Multi-Symptom Daytime Liquid

TYLENOL® Cold Multi-Symptom Nighttime Liquid with Cool Burst™

TYLENOL® Cold Multi-Symptom Severe Daytime Liquid

For full product information see page 752.

TYLENOL® Sore Throat Daytime Liquid with Cool Burst™ (McNeil Consumer)

TYLENOL® Sore Throat Nighttime Liquid with Cool Burst™

TYLENOL® Cough & Sore Throat Daytime Liquid with Cool Burst™

TYLENOL® Cough & Sore Throat Nighttime Liquid with Cool Burst™

Description:
TYLENOL® Sore Throat Daytime Liquid with Cool Burst™ contains acetaminophen 500 mg in each 15 mL (1 tablespoon).
TYLENOL® Sore Throat Nighttime Liquid with Cool Burst™ contains acetaminophen 500 mg and diphenhydramine HCl 25 mg in each 15 mL (1 tablespoon).
TYLENOL® Cough & Sore Throat Daytime Liquid with Cool Burst™ contains acetaminophen 500 mg and dextromethorphan HBr 15 mg in each 15 mL (1 tablespoon).
TYLENOL® Cough & Sore Throat Nighttime Liquid with Cool Burst™ contains acetaminophen 500 mg, dextromethorphan HBr 15 mg and doxylamine succinate 6.25 mg in each 15 mL (1 tablespoon).

Actions:
Acetaminophen is a clinically proven analgesic/antipyretic. Acetaminophen produces analgesia by elevation of the pain threshold and antipyresis through action on the hypothalamic heat regulating center. Acetaminophen is equal to aspirin in analgesic and antipyretic effectiveness and it is unlikely to produce many of the side effects associated with aspirin and aspirin-containing products. *TYLENOL® Cough & Sore Throat Daytime Liquid with Cool Burst™*, in addition to acetaminophen, contains the cough suppressant dextromethorphan hydrobromide. *TYLENOL® Cough & Sore Throat Nighttime Liquid with Cool Burst™*, in addition to acetaminophen and dextromethorphan hydrobromide, contains the antihistamine doxylamine succinate. *TYLENOL® Sore Throat Nighttime Liquid with Cool Burst™*, in addition to acetaminophen, contains the antihistamine diphenhydramine HCl.

Uses:
TYLENOL® Sore Throat Daytime Liquid with Cool Burst™
• temporarily relieves minor aches and pains due to:
  • the common cold
  • headache
  • sore throat
  • muscular aches
• temporarily reduces fever
TYLENOL® Sore Throat Nighttime Liquid with Cool Burst™
• temporarily relief of:
  • sore throat
  • headache

• minor aches and pains
• sneezing
• runny nose
• temporarily reduces fever
TYLENOL® Cough & Sore Throat Daytime Liquid with Cool Burst™
• temporarily relieves:
  • minor aches and pains
  • headache
  • sore throat
  • cough due to a cold
TYLENOL® Cough & Sore Throat Nighttime Liquid with Cool Burst™
• temporarily relieves the following cold/flu symptoms:
  • minor aches and pains
  • headache
  • sore throat
  • runny nose and sneezing
  • cough

Directions:
TYLENOL® Sore Throat Daytime and Nighttime Liquid with Cool Burst™
• **do not take more than directed (see overdose warning)**
• do not take for more than 10 days unless directed by a doctor. (daytime only)

adults and children 12 years and over	• take 2 tablespoons (tbsp) or 30 mL in dosing cup provided every 4 to 6 hours while symptoms last (daytime) • take 2 tablespoons (tbsp) or 30 mL in dosing cup provided every 4 to 6 hours or as directed by a doctor (nighttime) • do not take more than 8 tablespoons in 24 hours
children under 12 years	• do not use this adult product in children under 12 years of age; this will provide more than the recommended dose (overdose) and may cause liver damage

TYLENOL® Cough & Sore Throat Daytime and Nighttime Liquid with Cool Burst™
• **do not take more than directed (see overdose warning)**

adults and children 12 years and over	• take 2 tablespoons (tbsp) or 30 mL in dosing cup provided every 6 hours as needed (daytime) • take 2 tablespoons (tbsp) or 30 mL in dosing cup provided every 6 hours while symptoms last (nighttime) • do not take more than 8 tablespoons in 24 hours

children under 12 years	• do not use this adult product in children under 12 years of age; this will provide more than the recommended dose (overdose) and may cause liver damage

Warnings:

Alcohol warning: If you consume 3 or more alcoholic drinks every day, ask your doctor whether you should take acetaminophen or other pain relievers or fever reducers.
Acetaminophen may cause liver damage.

Sore throat warning: If sore throat is severe, persists for more than 2 days, is accompanied or followed by fever, headache, rash, nausea or vomiting, consult a doctor promptly.

Do not use
• with any other product containing acetaminophen
• with any other product containing diphenhydramine, even one used on skin. (for *TYLENOL® Sore Throat Nighttime Liquid with Cool Burst*™ only)
• if you are now taking a prescription monoamine oxidase inhibitor (MAOI) (certain drugs for depression, psychiatric or emotional conditions, or Parkinson's disease), or for 2 weeks after stopping the MAOI drug. If you do not know if your prescription drug contains an MAOI, ask a doctor or pharmacist before taking this product. (for *TYLENOL® Cough & Sore Throat Daytime and Nighttime Liquid with Cool Burst*™ only)

Ask a doctor before use if you have
(for *TYLENOL® Sore Throat Nighttime Liquid with Cool Burst*™ and *TYLENOL® Cough & Sore Throat Nighttime Liquid with Cool Burst*™)
• a breathing problem such as emphysema or chronic bronchitis
• trouble urinating due to an enlarged prostate gland
• glaucoma
(for *TYLENOL® Cough & Sore Throat Daytime Liquid with Cool Burst*™ and *TYLENOL® Cough & Sore Throat Nighttime Liquid with Cool Burst*™)
• cough that occurs with too much phlegm (mucus)
• persistent or chronic cough such as occurs with smoking, asthma, or emphysema

Ask a doctor or pharmacist before use if you are taking sedatives or tranquilizers (for *TYLENOL® Sore Throat Nighttime Liquid with Cool Burst*™ and *TYLENOL® Cough & Sore Throat Nighttime Liquid with Cool Burst*™)

When using this product
(for *TYLENOL® Sore Throat Nighttime Liquid with Cool Burst*™ and *TYLENOL® Cough & Sore Throat Nighttime Liquid with Cool Burst*™)

• excitability may occur, especially in children
• marked drowsiness may occur
• alcohol, sedatives and tranquilizers may increase the drowsiness effect
• avoid alcoholic drinks
• be careful when driving a motor vehicle or operating machinery (*TYLENOL® Cough & Sore Throat Nighttime Liquid with Cool Burst*™ only)
• do not drive a motor vehicle or operate machinery (*TYLENOL® Sore Throat Nighttime Liquid with Cool Burst*™ only)

Stop use and ask a doctor if
• pain gets worse or lasts for more than 10 days
• pain or cough gets worse or lasts for more than 7 days (*TYLENOL® Cough & Sore Throat Daytime & Nighttime Liquid with Cool Burst*™ only)
• fever gets worse or lasts for more than 3 days
• redness or swelling is present
• new symptoms occur
• cough comes back or occurs with rash or headache that lasts (*TYLENOL® Cough & Sore Throat Daytime & Nighttime Liquid with Cool Burst*™ only)

These could be signs of a serious condition.

If pregnant or breast-feeding, ask a health professional before use.

Keep out of the reach of children.

Overdose warning: Taking more than the recommended dose (overdose) may cause liver damage. In case of overdose, get medical help or contact a Poison Control Center (1-800-222-1222) right away. Quick medical attention is critical for adults as well as for children even if you do not notice any signs or symptoms.

Other Information:
• each tablespoon contains: **sodium 11 mg**
• store between 20-25C° (68-77°F)
• see label for lot number and expiration date

PROFESSIONAL INFORMATION: OVERDOSAGE INFORMATION

For overdosage information, please refer to pgs. 696–697.

Inactive Ingredients:
TYLENOL® Sore Throat Daytime Liquid with Cool Burst™: citric acid, FD&C blue #1, flavors, polyethylene glycol, propylene glycol, purified water, sodium benzoate, sodium carboxymethylcellulose, sorbitol, sucralose, sucrose
TYLENOL® Sore Throat Nighttime Liquid with Cool Burst™: citric acid, FD&C blue #1, flavors, polyethylene glycol, propylene glycol, purified water, sodium benzoate, sodium carboxymethylcellulose, sorbitol, sucralose, sucrose
TYLENOL® Cough & Sore Throat Daytime Liquid with Cool Burst™: citric acid, FD&C blue #1, flavors, polyethylene glycol, propylene glycol, purified water,

sodium benzoate, sodium carboxymethylcellulose, sorbitol, sucralose, sucrose
TYLENOL® Cough & Sore Throat Nighttime Liquid with Cool Burst™: citric acid, FD&C blue #1, flavors, polyethylene glycol, propylene glycol, purified water, sodium benzoate, sodium carboxymethylcellulose, sorbitol, sucralose, sucrose

How Supplied:
TYLENOL® Sore Throat Daytime and Nighttime Liquid with Cool Burst™ blue in color, in child-resistant tamper-evident bottles of 8 fl. oz.
TYLENOL® Cough & Sore Throat Daytime and Nighttime Liquid with Cool Burst™ blue in color, in child-resistant tamper-evident bottles of 8 fl. oz.
Shown in Product Identification Guide, page 512

CONCENTRATED TYLENOL® Infants' Drops Plus Cold Nasal Decongestant, Fever Reducer & Pain Reliever (McNeil Consumer)

CONCENTRATED TYLENOL® Infants' Drops Plus Cold & Cough Nasal Decongestant, Fever Reducer & Pain Reliever, Cough Suppressant

CHILDREN'S TYLENOL® Plus Cough & Sore Throat Suspension Liquid

CHILDREN'S TYLENOL® Plus Cough & Runny Nose Suspension Liquid

CHILDREN'S TYLENOL® Plus Multi-Symptom Cold Suspension Liquid

CHILDREN'S TYLENOL® Plus Cold Suspension Liquid

For full product information see page 754.

VICKS® 44M® (Procter & Gamble) COUGH, COLD & FLU RELIEF Cough Suppressant/Antihistamine/Pain Reliever–Fever Reducer Alcohol 10% Maximum strength cough formula

For full product information see page 760.

VICKS® Cough Drops (Procter & Gamble) Menthol Cough Suppressant/ Oral Anesthetic Menthol and Cherry Flavors

For full product information see page 761.

VICKS® DAYQUIL® LIQUID
(Procter & Gamble)

VICKS® DAYQUIL® LIQUICAPS®
Multi-Symptom Cold/Flu Relief
Nasal Decongestant/Pain Reliever/
Cough Suppressant/Fever Reducer
Non-drowsy

For full product information see page 761.

VICKS® NYQUIL® LIQUICAPS®/
LIQUID MULTI-SYMPTOM COLD/
FLU RELIEF (Proctor & Gamble)

For full product information see page 763.

ZICAM® Cold Remedy Nasal Gel™
(Matrixx)
[zĭ-kăm]

ZICAM® Cold Remedy Gel Swabs™

ZICAM® Cold Remedy Swabs Kids
Size

ZICAM® Cold Remedy RapidMelts®

ZICAM® Cold Remedy RapidMelts®
with Vitamin C

ZICAM® Cold Remedy Oral Mist™

ZICAM® Cold Remedy Chewables™

ZICAM® Cold Remedy ChewCaps

For full product information see page 766.

ZICAM® Flu Daytime (Matrixx)

ZICAM® Nighttime

For full product information see page 768.

Respiratory System:
Throat and Nose Itching

TRIAMINIC® NIGHT TIME Cold & Cough
(Novartis Consumer Health, Inc.)
Antihistamine/Cough Suppressant,
Nasal Decongestant
Grape Flavor

For full product information see page 746.

TRIAMINIC® COLD & ALLERGY
(Novartis Consumer Health, Inc.)
Antihistamine, Nasal Decongestant
Orange Flavor

For full product information see page 746.

Vascular System:

Angina Pectoris (unstable/chronic stable) Risk Reduction

BAYER® ASPIRIN
(Bayer Healthcare)
Comprehensive Prescribing
Information

For full product information see page 796.

Vascular System:
Ischemic Stroke Risk Reduction

BAYER® ASPIRIN
(Bayer Healthcare)
Comprehensive Prescribing
Information

For full product information see page 796.

Vascular System:
Myocardial Infarction Risk Reduction

BAYER® ASPIRIN
(Bayer Healthcare)
Comprehensive Prescribing Information

Description:
Aspirin for Oral Administration
Regular Strength 325 mg and Low Strength 81 mg Tablets
Antiplatelet, Antiarthritic

Aspirin

$C_9H_8O_4$
Mol. Wt.: 180.16
C 60.00 %; H 4.48 %; O 35.52%

Aspirin is an odorless white, needle-like crystalline or powdery substance. When exposed to moisture, aspirin hydrolyzes into salicylic and acetic acids, and gives off a vinegary-odor. It is highly lipid soluble and slightly soluble in water.

Clinical Pharmacology:
Mechanism of Action

Aspirin is a more potent inhibitor of both prostaglandin synthesis and platelet aggregation than other salicylic acid derivatives. The differences in activity between aspirin and salicylic acid are thought to be due to the acetyl group on the aspirin molecule. This acetyl group is responsible for the inactivation of cyclooxygenase via acetylation.

Pharmacokinetics

Absorption: In general, immediate release aspirin is well and completely absorbed from the gastrointestinal (GI) tract. Following absorption, aspirin is hydrolyzed to salicylic acid with peak plasma levels of salicylic acid occurring within 1-2 hours of dosing (see **Pharmacokinetics—Metabolism**). **The rate of absorption from the GI tract is dependent upon the dosage form, the presence or absence of food, gastric pH (the presence or absence of GI antacids or buffering agents), and other physiologic factors. Enteric coated aspirin products are erratically absorbed from the GI tract.**

Distribution: Salicylic acid is widely distributed to all tissues and fluids in the body including the central nervous system (CNS), breast milk, and fetal tissues. The highest concentrations are found in the plasma, liver, renal cortex, heart, and lungs. The protein binding of salicylate is concentration-dependent, i.e.,

non-linear. At low concentrations (< 100 micrograms/milliliter (mcg/mL)), approximately 90 percent of plasma salicylate is bound to albumin while at higher concentrations (>400 mcg/mL), only about 75 percent is bound. The early signs of salicylic overdose (salicylism), including tinnitus (ringing in the ears), occur at plasma concentrations approximating 200 mcg/mL. Severe toxic effects are associated with levels >400 mcg/mL. (See **ADVERSE REACTIONS** and **OVERDOSAGE**.)

Metabolism: Aspirin is rapidly hydrolyzed in the plasma to salicylic acid such that plasma levels of aspirin are essentially undetectable 1–2 hours after dosing. Salicylic acid is primarily conjugated in the liver to form salicyluric acid, a phenolic glucuronide, an acyl glucuronide, and a number of minor metabolites. Salicylic acid has a plasma half-life of approximately 6 hours. Salicylate metabolism is saturable and total body clearance decreases at higher serum concentrations due to the limited ability of the liver to form both salicyluric acid and phenolic glucuronide. Following toxic doses (10–20 grams (g)), the plasma half-life may be increased to over 20 hours.

Elimination: The elimination of salicylic acid follows zero order pharmacokinetics; (i.e., the rate of drug elimination is constant in relation to plasma concentration). Renal excretion of unchanged drug depends upon urine pH. As urinary pH rises above 6.5, the renal clearance of free salicylate increases from < 5 percent to >80 percent. Alkalinization of the urine is a key concept in the management of salicylate overdose. (See **OVERDOSAGE**.) Following therapeutic doses, approximately 10 percent is found excreted in the urine as salicylic acid, 75 percent as salicyluric acid, 10 percent phenolic and 5 percent acyl glucuronides of salicylic acid.

Pharmacodynamics

Aspirin affects platelet aggregation by irreversibly inhibiting prostaglandin cyclooxygenase. This effect lasts for the life of the platelet and prevents the formation of the platelet aggregating factor thromboxane A2. Non-acetylated salicylates do not inhibit this enzyme and have no effect on platelet aggregation. At somewhat higher doses, aspirin reversibly inhibits the formation of prostaglandin I2 (prostacyclin), which is an arterial vasodilator and inhibits platelet aggregation. At higher doses aspirin is an effective anti-inflammatory agent, partially due to inhibition of inflammatory mediators via cyclooxygenase inhibition in peripheral tis-

sues. In vitro studies suggest that other mediators of inflammation may also be suppressed by aspirin administration, although the precise mechanism of action has not been elucidated. It is this nonspecific suppression of cyclo-oxygenase activity in peripheral tissues following large doses that leads to its primary side effect of gastric irritation. (See **ADVERSE REACTIONS**.)

Clinical Studies:
Ischemic Stroke and Transient Ischemic Attack (TIA): In clinical trials of subjects with TIA's due to fibrin platelet emboli or ischemic stroke, aspirin has been shown to significantly reduce the risk of the combined endpoint of stroke or death and the combined endpoint of TIA, stroke, or death by about 13–18 percent.

Suspected Acute Myocardial Infarction(MI): In a large, multi-center study of aspirin, streptokinase, and the combination of aspirin and streptokinase in 17,187 patients with suspected acute MI, aspirin treatment produced a 23-percent reduction in the risk of vascular mortality. Aspirin was also shown to have an additional benefit in patients given a thrombolytic agent.

Prevention of Recurrent MI and Unstable Angina Pectoris: These indications are supported by the results of six large, randomized, multi-center, placebo-controlled trials of predominantly male post-MI subjects and one randomized placebo-controlled study of men with unstable angina pectoris. Aspirin therapy in MI subjects was associated with a significant reduction (about 20 percent) in the risk of the combined endpoint of subsequent death and/or nonfatal reinfarction in these patients. In aspirin-treated unstable angina patients the event rate was reduced to 5 percent from the 10 percent rate in the placebo group.

Chronic Stable Angina Pectoris: In a randomized, multi-center, double-blind trial designed to assess the role of aspirin for prevention of MI in patients with chronic stable angina pectoris, aspirin significantly reduced the primary combined endpoint of nonfatal MI, fatal MI, and sudden death by 34 percent. The secondary endpoint for vascular events (first occurrence of MI, stroke, or vascular death) was also significantly reduced (32 percent).

Revascularization Procedures: Most patients who undergo coronary artery revascularization procedures have already had symptomatic coronary artery disease for which aspirin is indicated. Similarly, patients with lesions of the carotid bifur-

cation sufficient to require carotid endarterectomy are likely to have had a precedent event. Aspirin is recommended for patients who undergo revascularization procedures if there is a preexisting condition for which aspirin is already indicated.

Rheumatologic Diseases: In clinical studies in patients with rheumatoid arthritis, juvenile rheumatoid arthritis, ankylosing spondylitis and osteoarthritis, aspirin has been shown to be effective in controlling various indices of clinical disease activity.

Animal Toxicology:

The acute oral 50 percent lethal dose in rats is about 1.5 g/kilogram (kg) and in mice 1.1 g/kg. Renal papillary necrosis and decreased urinary concentrating ability occur in rodents chronically administered high doses. Dose-dependent gastric mucosal injury occurs in rats and humans. Mammals may develop aspirin toxicosis associated with GI symptoms, circulatory effects, and central nervous system depression. (See **OVERDOSAGE**.)

Indications and Usage:

Vascular Indications (Ischemic Stoke, TIA, Acute MI, Prevention of Recurrent MI, Unstable Angina Pectoris, Chronic Stable Angina Pectoris): Aspirin is indicated to: (1) Reduce the combined risk of death and nonfatal stroke in patients who have had ischemic stroke or transient ischemia of the brain due to fibrin platelet emboli, (2) reduce the risk of vascular mortality in patients with a suspected acute MI, (3) reduce the combined risk of death and nonfatal MI in patients with a previous MI or unstable angina pectoris, (4) reduce the combined risk of MI and sudden death in patients with chronic stable angina pectoris.

Revascularization Procedures (Coronary Artery Bypass Graft (CABG), Percutaneous Transluminal Coronary Angioplasty (PTCA), and Carotid Endarterectomy): Aspirin is indicated in patients who have undergone revascularization procedures (i.e., CABG, PTCA, or carotid endarterectomy) when there is a preexisting condition for which aspirin is already indicated.

Rheumatologic Disease Indications (Rheumatoid Arthritis, Juvenile Rheumatoid Arthritis, Spondyloarthropathies, Osteoarthritis, and the Arthritis and Pleurisy of Systemic Lupus Erythematosus (SLE)): Aspirin is indicated for the relief of the signs and symptoms of rheumatoid arthritis, juvenile rheumatoid arthritis, osteoarthritis, spondyloarthropathies, and arthritis and pleurisy associated with SLE.

Contraindications:

Allergy: Aspirin is contraindicated in patients with known allergy to nonsteroidal anti- inflammatory drug products and in patients with the syndrome of asthma, rhinitis, and nasal polyps. Aspirin may cause severe urticaria, angioedema, or bronchospasm (asthma).

Reye's Syndrome: Aspirin should not be used in children or teenagers for viral infections, with or without fever, because of the risk of Reye's syndrome with concomitant use of aspirin in certain viral illnesses.

Warnings:

Alcohol Warning: Patients who consume three or more alcoholic drinks every day should be counseled about the bleeding risks involved with chronic, heavy alcohol use while taking aspirin.

Coagulation Abnormalities: Even low doses of aspirin can inhibit platelet function leading to an increase in bleeding time. This can adversely affect patients with inherited (hemophilia) or acquired (liver disease or vitamin K deficiency) bleeding disorders.

GI Side Effects: GI side effects include stomach pain, heartburn, nausea, vomiting, and gross GI bleeding. Although minor upper GI symptoms, such as dyspepsia, are common and can occur anytime during therapy, physicians should remain alert for signs of ulceration and bleeding, even in the absence of previous GI symptoms. Physicians should inform patients about the signs and symptoms of GI side effects and what steps to take if they occur.

Peptic Ulcer Disease: Patients with a history of active peptic ulcer disease should avoid using aspirin, which can cause gastric mucosal irritation and bleeding.

Precautions:
General

Renal Failure: Avoid aspirin in patients with severe renal failure (glomerular filtration rate less than 10 mL/minute).

Hepatic Insufficiency: Avoid aspirin in patients with severe hepatic insufficiency.

Sodium Restricted Diets: Patients with sodium-retaining states, such as congestive heart failure or renal failure, should avoid sodium-containing buffered aspirin preparations because of their high sodium content.

Laboratory Tests

Aspirin has been associated with elevated hepatic enzymes, blood urea nitrogen and serum creatinine, hyperkalemia, proteinuria, and prolonged bleeding time.

Drug Interactions

Angiotensin Converting Enzyme (ACE) Inhibitors: The hyponatremic and hypotensive effects of ACE inhibitors may be diminished by the concomitant administration of aspirin due to its indirect effect on the renin-angiotensin conversion pathway.

Acetazolamide: Concurrent use of aspirin and acetazolamide can lead to high serum concentrations of acetazolamide (and toxicity) due to competition at the renal tubule for secretion.

Anticoagulant Therapy (Heparin and Warfarin): Patients on anticoagulation therapy are at increased risk for bleeding because of drug-drug interactions and the effect on platelets. Aspirin can displace warfarin from protein binding sites, leading to prolongation of both the prothrombin time and the bleeding time. Aspirin can increase the anticoagulant activity of heparin, increasing bleeding risk.

Anticonvulsants: Salicylate can displace protein-bound phenytoin and valproic acid, leading to a decrease in the total concentration of phenytoin and an increase in serum valproic acid levels.

Beta Blockers: The hypotensive effects of beta blockers may be diminished by the concomitant administration of aspirin due to inhibition of renal prostaglandins, leading to decreased renal blood flow, and salt and fluid retention.

Diuretics: The effectiveness of diuretics in patients with underlying renal or cardiovascular disease may be diminished by the concomitant administration of aspirin due to inhibition of renal prostaglandins, leading to decreased renal blood flow, and salt and fluid retention.

Methotrexate: Salicylate can inhibit renal clearance of methotrexate, leading to bone marrow toxicity, especially in the elderly or renal impaired.

Nonsteroidal Anti-inflammatory Drugs (NSAID's): The concurrent use of aspirin with other NSAID's should be avoided because this may increase bleeding or lead to decreased renal function.

Oral Hypoglycemics: Moderate doses of aspirin may increase the effectiveness of oral hypoglycemic drugs, leading to hypoglycemia.

Uricosuric Agents (Probenecid and Sulfinpyrazone): Salicylates antagonize the uricosuric action of uricosuric agents.

Carcinogenesis, Mutagenesis, Impairment of Fertility

Administration of aspirin for 68 weeks at 0.5 percent in the feed of rats was not carcinogenic. In the Ames Salmonella assay, aspirin was not mutagenic; however, aspirin did induce chromosome aberrations in cultured human fibroblasts. Aspirin inhibits ovulation in rats. (See **Pregnancy**).

Pregnancy

Pregnant women should only take aspirin if clearly needed. Because of the known effects of NSAIDs on the fetal cardiovascular system (closure of the third trimester of pregnancy should be avoided. Salicylate products have also been associated with alterations in maternal and neonatal hemostasis mechanisms, decreased birth weight, and with perinatal mortality.

Labor and Delivery

Aspirin should be avoided 1 week prior to and during labor and delivery because it

Continued on next page

Bayer Aspirin—Cont.

can result in excessive blood loss at delivery. Prolonged gestation and prolonged labor due to prostaglandin inhibition have been reported.

Nursing Mothers

Nursing mothers should avoid using aspirin because salicylate is excreted in breast milk. Use of high doses may lead to rashes, platelet abnormalities, and bleeding in nursing infants.

Pediatric Use

Pediatric dosing recommendations for juvenile rheumatoid arthritis are based on well-controlled clinical studies. An initial dose of 90–130 mg/kg/day in divided doses, with an increase as needed for anti-inflammatory efficacy (target plasma salicylate levels of 150–300 mcg/mL) are effective. At high doses (i.e., plasma levels of greater than 200 mcg/mL), the incidence of toxicity increases.

Adverse Reactions:

Many adverse reactions due to aspirin ingestion are dose-related. The following is a list of adverse reactions that have been reported in the literature. (See **WARNINGS**.)

Body as a Whole: Fever, hypothermia, thirst.

Cardiovascular: Dysrhythmias, hypotension, tachycardia.

Central Nervous System: Agitation, cerebral edema, coma, confusion, dizziness, headache, subdural or intracranial hemorrhage, lethargy, seizures.

Fluid and Electrolyte: Dehydration, hyperkalemia, metabolic acidosis, respiratory alkalosis.

Gastrointestinal: Dyspepsia, GI bleeding, ulceration and perforation, nausea, vomiting, transient elevations of hepatic enzymes, hepatitis, Reye's syndrome, pancreatitis.

Hematologic: Prolongation of the prothrombin time, disseminated intravascular coagulation, coagulopathy, thrombocytopenia.

Hypersensitivity: Acute anaphylaxis, angioedema, asthma, bronchospasm, laryngeal edema, urticaria.

Musculoskeletal: Rhabdomyolysis.

Metabolism: Hypoglycemia (in children), hyperglycemia.

Reproductive: Prolonged pregnancy and labor, stillbirths, lower birth weight infants, antepartum and postpartum bleeding.

Respiratory: Hyperpnea, pulmonary edema, tachypnea.

Special Senses: Hearing loss, tinnitus. Patients with high frequency hearing loss may have difficulty perceiving tinnitus. In these patients, tinnitus cannot be used as a clinical indicator of salicylism.

Urogenital: Interstitial nephritis, papillary necrosis, proteinuria, renal insufficiency and failure.

Drug Abuse and Dependence:

Aspirin is nonnarcotic. There is no known potential for addiction associated with the use of aspirin.

Overdosage:

Salicylate toxicity may result from acute ingestion (overdose) or chronic intoxication. The early signs of salicylic overdose (salicylism), including tinnitus (ringing in the ears), occur at plasma concentrations approaching 200 mcg/mL. Plasma concentrations of aspirin above 300 mcg/mL are clearly toxic. Severe toxic effects are associated with levels above 400 mcg/mL. (See **CLINICAL PHARMACOLOGY**). A single lethal dose of aspirin in adults in not known with certainty but death may be expected at 30 g. For real or suspected overdose, a Poison Control Center should be contacted immediately. Careful medical management is essential.

Signs and Symptoms: In acute overdose, severe acid-base and electrolyte disturbances may occur and are complicated by hyperthermia and dehydration. Respiratory alkalosis occurs early while hyperventilation is present, but is quickly followed by metabolic acidosis.

Treatment: Treatment consists primarily of supporting vital functions, increasing salicylate elimination, and correcting the acid-base disturbance. Gastric emptying and/or lavage is recommended as soon as possible after ingestion, even if the patient has vomited spontaneously. After lavage and/or emesis, administration of activated charcoal, as a slurry, is beneficial, if less than 3 hours have passed since ingestion. Charcoal adsorption should not be employed prior to emesis and lavage. Severity of aspirin intoxication is determined by measuring the blood salicylate level. Acid-base status should be closely followed with serial blood gas and serum pH measurements. Fluid and electrolyte balance should also be maintained.

In severe cases, hyperthermia and hypovolemia are the major immediate threats to life. Children should be sponged with tepid water. Replacement fluid should be administered intravenously and augmented with correction of acidosis. Plasma electrolytes and pH should be monitored to promote alkaline diuresis of salicylate if renal function is normal. Infusion of glucose may be required to control hypoglycemia.

Hemodialysis and peritoneal dialysis can be performed to reduce the body drug content. In patients with renal insufficiency or in cases of life-threatening intoxication, dialysis is usually required. Exchange transfusion may be indicated in infants and young children.

Dosage and Administration:

Each dose of aspirin should be taken with a full glass of water unless patient is fluid restricted. Anti-inflammatory and analgesic dosages should be individualized. When aspirin is used in high doses, the development of tinnitus may be used as a clinical sign of elevated plasma salicylate levels except in patients with high frequency hearing loss.

Ischemic Stroke and TIA:
50–325 mg once a day. Continue therapy indefinitely.

Suspected Acute MI:
The initial dose of 160–162.5 mg is administered as soon as an MI is suspected. The maintenance dose of 160–162.5 mg a day is continued for 30 days post-infarction. After 30 days, consider further therapy based on dosage and administration for prevention of recurrent MI.

Prevention of Recurrent MI:
75–325 mg once a day. Continue therapy indefinitely.

Unstable Angina Pectoris:
75–325 mg once a day. Continue therapy indefinitely.

Chronic Stable Angina Pectoris:
75–325 mg once a day. Continue therapy indefinitely.

CABG:
325 mg daily starting 6 hours post-procedure. Continue therapy for one year post-procedure.

PTCA:
The initial dose of 325 mg should be given 2 hours pre-surgery. Maintenance dose is 160–325 mg daily. Continue therapy indefinitely.

Carotid Endarterectomy:
Doses of 80 mg once daily to 650 mg twice daily, started pre-surgery, are recommended. Continue therapy indefinitely.

Rheumatoid Arthritis:
The initial dose is 3 g a day in divided doses. Increase as needed for anti-inflammatory efficacy with target plasma salicylate levels of 150–300 mcg/mL. At high doses (i.e., plasma levels of greater than 200 mcg/mL), the incidence of toxicity increases.

Juvenile Rheumatoid Arthritis:
Initial dose is 90–130 mg/kg/day in divided doses. Increase as needed for anti-inflammatory efficacy with target plasma salicylate levels of 150–300 mcg/mL. At high doses (i.e., plasma levels of greater than 200 mcg/mL), the incidence of toxicity increases.

Spondyloarthropathies:
Up to 4 g per day in divided doses.

Osteoarthritis:
Up to 3 g per day in divided doses.

Arthritis and Pleurisy of SLE:
The initial dose is 3 g a day in divided doses. Increase as needed for anti-inflammatory efficacy with target plasma salicylate levels of 150–300 mcg/mL. At high doses (i.e., plasma levels of greater than 200 mcg/mL), the incidence of toxicity increases.

Storage Conditions

Store at room temperature.
Bayer HealthCare LLC
Consumer Care Division
36 Columbia Road
PO Box 1910
Morristown, NJ 07962-1910
Shown in Product Identification Guide, page 504

Vascular System:
Revascularization Procedures

BAYER® ASPIRIN
(Bayer Healthcare)
Comprehensive Prescribing
Information

For full product information see page 796.

Vascular System:
Transient Ischemic Attack Risk Reduction

BAYER® ASPIRIN
(Bayer Healthcare)
Comprehensive Prescribing
Information

For full product information see page 796.

Women's Health:
Feminine Hygiene

MASSENGILL®
(GlaxoSmithKline Consumer)
[*mas 'sen-gil*]
Baby Powder Scent Soft Cloth Towelette

Ingredients: Purified Water, Octoxynol-9, Lactic Acid, Disodium Edta, Fragrance, Potassium Sorbate, Cetylpyridinium Chloride, and Sodium Bicarbonate.

Indications: For cleansing and refreshing the external vaginal area.

Actions: Massengill Baby Powder Scent Soft Cloth Towelette safely cleanse the external vaginal area. The towelette delivery system makes the application soft and gentle.

Directions: Remove towelette from foil packet, unfold, and gently wipe from front to back. After towelette has been used once, return towelette to foil packet and throw it away. Safe to use daily as often as needed. For external use only.

How Supplied: 50 individually sealed soft cloth towelettes per carton.
Comments, questions or for information about STD's and vaginal health, call toll free 1-800-245-1040 weekdays.

MASSENGILL Feminine Cleansing Wash, Floral
(GlaxoSmithKline Consumer)
[*mas 'sen-gil*]

Ingredients: Purified Water, sodium laureth sulfate, magnesium laureth sulfate, sodium laureth-8 sulfate, magnesium laureth-8 sulfate, sodium oleth sulfate, magnesium oleth sulfate, lauramidopropyl betaine, myristamine oxide, lactic acid, PEG-120 methyl glucose dioleate, fragrance, sodium methylparaben, sodium ethylparaben, sodium propylparaben, methylchloroisothiazolinone, methylisothiazolinone, D&C Red #33.

Indications: For cleansing and refreshing of external vaginal area.

Actions: Massengill feminine cleansing wash safely and gently cleanses the external vaginal area.

Directions: Pour small amount into palm of hand or wash cloth and lather into wet skin. Rinse clean. Safe to use daily. For external use only.

How Supplied: 8 fl. oz plastic flip-top bottle.

Women's Health:
Menstrual Cramps/Pain

ADVIL® (Wyeth Consumer)
Ibuprofen Tablets, USP
Ibuprofen Caplets (Oval-Shaped Tablets)
Ibuprofen Gel Caplets (Oval-Shaped Gelatin Coated Tablets)
Ibuprofen Liqui-Gel Capsules
Pain reliever/Fever Reducer (NSAID)
For full product information see page 674.

———————————

ALEVE CAPLETS (Bayer Healthcare)
(NSAID Labeling)
[a-lēv]
For full product information see page 675.

———————————

ALEVE GELCAPS
(Bayer Healthcare)
(NSAID Labeling)
[a-lēv]
For full product information see page 675.

———————————

ALEVE TABLETS (Bayer Healthcare)
(NSAID Labeling)
[a-lēv]
For full product information see page 676.

———————————

BC® POWDER
(GlaxoSmithKline Consumer)
ARTHRITIS STRENGTH BC®
POWDER
BC® COLD POWDER LINE
For full product information see page 677.

BUFFERIN®
(Novartis Consumer Health, Inc.)
Regular/Extra Strength
Pain Reliever/Fever Reducer
For full product information see page 678.

———————————

EXCEDRIN® EXTRA STRENGTH
(Novartis Consumer Health, Inc.)
PAIN RELIEVER
For full product information see page 684.

———————————

GOODY'S®
(GlaxoSmithKline Consumer)
Extra Strength Pain Relief Tablets
For full product information see page 685.

———————————

MOTRIN® IB (Ibuprofen)
Pain Reliever/Fever Reducer
Tablets and Caplets
(McNeil Consumer)
For full product information see page 687.

———————————

THERMA-CARE HEAT ACTIVATED
WRAPS (Procter & Gamble)
Therapeutic heat wraps
For full product information see page 692.

REGULAR STRENGTH TYLENOL®
acetaminophen Tablets
(McNeil Consumer)
EXTRA STRENGTH TYLENOL®
acetaminophen Geltabs, Caplets,
Cool Caplets, and EZ Tabs
EXTRA STRENGTH TYLENOL®
acetaminophen Rapid Release Gels
EXTRA STRENGTH TYLENOL®
acetaminophen Adult Liquid Pain
Reliever
TYLENOL® Arthritis Pain
Acetaminophen Extended Release
Geltabs/Caplets
TYLENOL® 8 Hour Acetaminophen
Extended Release Caplets

Product information for all dosage forms of Adult TYLENOL acetaminophen have been combined under this heading.

For full product information see page 695.

———————————

WOMEN'S TYLENOL®
(McNeil Consumer)
Menstrual Relief Pain Reliever/
Diuretic Caplets
For full product information see page 803.

Women's Health:
Premenstrual Syndrome

BUFFERIN®
(Novartis Consumer Health, Inc.)
Regular/Extra Strength
Pain Reliever/Fever Reducer

For full product information see page 678.

EXCEDRIN® EXTRA STRENGTH
(Novartis Consumer Health, Inc.)
PAIN RELIEVER

For full product information see page 684.

WOMEN'S TYLENOL®
(McNeil Consumer)
Menstrual Relief Pain Reliever/
Diuretic Caplets

Description:
Each *Women's Tylenol® Menstrual Relief Caplet* contains acetaminophen 500 mg and pamabrom 25 mg.

Actions:
Women's TYLENOL® Menstrual Relief Caplets contain a clinically proven analgesic-antipyretic and a diuretic. Maximum allowable non-prescription levels of acetaminophen and pamabrom provide temporary relief of minor aches and pains due to cramps, headache, and backache and water retention, weight gain, bloating, swelling and full feeling associated with the premenstrual and menstrual periods. Acetaminophen is equal to aspirin in analgesic and antipyretic effectiveness and it is unlikely to produce many of the side effects associated with aspirin containing products. Acetaminophen produces analgesia by elevation of the pain threshold. Pamabrom is a diuretic which relieves water retention.

Uses:
• temporarily relieves minor aches and pains due to:
  • cramps • headache • backache
  • premenstrual and menstrual cramps
• temporarily relieves water-weight gain, bloating, swelling and/or full feeling associated with the premenstrual and menstrual periods

Directions:
• **do not take more than directed** (see overdose warning)

adults and children 12 years and over	• take 2 caplets every 4 to 6 hours • do not take more than 8 caplets in 24 hours
children under 12 years	• do not use this adult product in children under 12 years of age; this will provide more than the recommended dose (overdose) and may cause liver damage

Warnings
Alcohol warning: If you consume 3 or more alcoholic drinks every day, ask your doctor whether you should take acetaminophen or other pain relievers/fever reducers. Acetaminophen may cause liver damage.
Do not use
• with any other product containing acetaminophen
Stop use and ask a doctor if
• new symptoms occur
• redness or swelling is present
• pain gets worse or lasts for more than 10 days
If pregnant or breast-feeding, ask a health professional before use.
Keep out of reach of children.

Overdose Warning: Taking more than the recommended dose (overdose) may cause liver damage. In case of overdose, get medical help or contact a Poison Control Center (1-800-222-1222) right away. Quick medical attention is critical for adults as well as for children even if you do not notice any signs or symptoms.

Other Information:
• store between 20–25°C (68–77°F)

Professional Information:
Overdosage Information
For overdosage information, please refer to pgs. 696–697.

Inactive Ingredients:
cellulose, corn starch, hypromellose, magnesium stearate, polydextrose, polyethylene glycol, sodium starch glycolate, titanium dioxide, triacetin

How Supplied:
White capsule shaped caplets with TYME printed on one side in tamper-evident bottles of 24.

Shown in Product Identification Guide, page 512

Women's Health:

Vaginal Candidiasis

VAGISTAT®-1
Vaginal antifungal
(Novartis Consumer Health, Inc.)

Drug Facts

Active Ingredient: **Purpose:**
(in each applicator)
Tioconazole 300 mg (6.5%) .... Vaginal antifungal

Use:
• treats vaginal yeast infections

Warnings:

For vaginal use only

Do not use if you have never had a vaginal yeast infection diagnosed by a doctor

Ask a doctor before use if you have
• **vaginal itching and discomfort for the first time**
• **lower abdominal, back or shoulder pain, fever, chills, nausea, vomiting, or foul-smelling vaginal discharge. You may have a more serious condition.**
• vaginal yeast infections often (such as once a month or 3 in 6 months). You could be pregnant or have a serious underlying medical cause for your symptoms, including diabetes or a weakened immune system.

• been exposed to the human immuno-deficiency virus (HIV) that causes AIDS

When using this product
• do not use tampons, douches, spermicides, or other vaginal products. Condoms and diaphragms may be damaged and fail to prevent pregnancy or sexually transmitted disease (STDs).
• do not have vaginal intercourse
• mild increase in vaginal burning, itching, or irritation may occur

Stop use and ask a doctor if
• **symptoms do not get better after 3 days**
• **symptoms last more than 7 days**
• **you get a rash or hives, abdominal pain, fever, chills, nausea, vomiting, or foul-smelling vaginal discharge**

If pregnant or breast-feeding, ask a health professional before use.

Keep out of reach of children. If swallowed, get medical help or contact a Poison Control Center right away.

Directions:
• before using this product read the enclosed brochure and instructions on foil packet for complete directions and information
• adults and children 12 years of age and over:
  • open the foil packet just before use and remove blue cap

• insert entire contents of applicator into the vagina at bedtime. Throw applicator away after use.
• children under 12 years of age: ask a doctor

Other Information:
• this product is a 1-dose treatment, most women do not experience complete relief of their symptoms in just one day. Most women experience some relief within one day and complete relief of symptoms within 7 days.
• if you have questions about vaginal yeast infections, consult your doctor
• store at 15°-30°C (59°-86°F)
• see end flap of carton for lot number and expiration date

Inactive Ingredients: butylated hydroxyanisole, magnesium aluminum silicate, white petrolatum
Questions or comments?
1-888-824-4782

How Supplied: VAGISTAT-1 is supplied in a ready-to-use prefilled single close vaginal applicator. Each applicatorful will deliver approximately 4.6 grams of VAGISTAT-1 containing 6.5% of tioconazole per gram of ointment.

Shown in Product Identification Guide, page 515

SECTION 8

DIETARY SUPPLEMENT INFORMATION

This section presents information on natural remedies and nutritional supplements marketed under the Dietary Supplement Health and Education Act of 1994. It is made possible through the courtesy of the manufacturers whose products appear on the following pages. The information concerning each product has been prepared, edited, and approved by the manufacturer's professional staff.

The descriptions of products appearing in this section are designed to provide all information necessary for informed use, including, when applicable, active ingredients, inactive ingredients, actions, warnings, cautions, interactions, symptoms and treatment of oral overdosage, dosage and directions for use, and how supplied. Descriptions in this section must be in full compliance with the Dietary Supplement Health and Education Act, which permits claims regarding a product's effect on the structure or functioning of the body, but forbids claims regarding a product's ability to treat, diagnose, cure, or prevent any specific disease. Descriptions of products marketed under the act do not receive formal evaluation or approval from the Food and Drug Administration.

In compiling this section, the publisher has emphasized the necessity of describing products comprehensively. The descriptions seen here include all information made available by the manufacturer. The publisher does not warrant or guarantee any product described here, and does not perform any independent analysis of the information provided. Inclusion of a product in this book does not represent an endorsement, and the publisher does not necessarily advocate the use of any product listed.

Dietary Supplements

BAUSCH & LOMB OCUVITE®
Adult 50+ Formula
Eye Vitamin and Mineral Supplement
(Bausch & Lomb)

For full product information see page .

BAUSCH & LOMB PRESERVISION®
AREDS
High Potency Eye Vitamin and Mineral Supplement Original, 4 per day tablets
(Bausch & Lomb)

Description: see supplement facts (table A)
[See first table below]

Other Ingredients: Lactose Monohydrate, Microcrystalline Cellulose, Crospovidone, Stearic Acid, Magnesium Stearate, Silicon Dioxide, Polysorbate 80, Triethyl Citrate, FD&C Yellow #6, FD&C Red #40. Contains Soy.
- Age-related macular degeneration is the leading cause of vision loss and blindness in people over 55. The National Institutes of Health (NIH) Age Related Eye Disease Study (AREDS) proved that a unique high-potency vitamin and mineral supplement was effective in helping to preserve the sight of certain people most at risk.*
- Bausch & Lomb **Ocuvite PreserVision** was the only eye vitamin and mineral supplement clinically proven effective in the NIH AREDS Study.
- Bausch & Lomb **Ocuvite PreserVision** is a high-potency antioxidant supplement with the antioxidant vitamins A, C, E and select minerals at levels that are well above those in ordinary multivitamins and generally cannot be attained through diet alone.

For a FREE 16-page brochure on Age-Related Macular Degeneration call toll-free 1-866-467-3263 (1-866-HOPE-AMD)

Recommended Intake: To get the same levels proven in the NIH AREDS Study it is important to take 4 tablets per day – 2 in the morning, 2 in the evening taken with meals.
Current and Former Smokers: Consult your eye care professional about the risks associated with smoking and using Beta-Carotene.
Bausch & Lomb Ocuvite PreserVision is the #1 recommended eye vitamin and mineral supplement brand among Retinal Specialists.[1]

---

*This statement has not been evaluated by the Food and Drug Administration. This product is not intended to diagnose, treat, cure or prevent any disease.

How Supplied: NDC 24208-432 Orange, eye shaped film coated tablet, engraved BL 01 on one side, scored on the other side. Available in bottles of 120 or 240 count tablets
DO NOT USE IF SEAL UNDER CLOSURE IS BROKEN.
Keep this product out of the reach of children.
STORE AT ROOM TEMPERATURE.
Made in USA
Marketed by
Bausch & Lomb
Rochester, NY 14609

References: 1. Data on file, Bausch & Lomb, Inc.
© Bausch & Lomb Incorporated. All Rights Reserved.
Bausch & Lomb, Ocuvite and PreserVision are registered trademarks of Bausch & Lomb Incorporated or its affiliates. Other brand names are trademarks of their respective owners.

Shown in Product Identification Guide, page 503

BAUSCH & LOMB PRESERVISION®
AREDS
Eye Vitamin and Mineral Supplement AREDS: The ONLY clinically proven effective formula.
(Bausch & Lomb)
Easy to swallow 2 per day Soft Gels

Description: see supplement facts (table A)
[See second table below]

Other Ingredients: Gelatin, Glycerin, Soybean Oil, Unbleached Lecithin (soy), Yellow Wax, Annatto Oil, Titanium Dioxide
- Age-related macular degeneration (AMD) is the leading cause of vision loss and blindness in people over 55. The landmark National Institutes of Health AREDS trial proved that a high potency antioxidant vitamin and mineral supplement was effective in helping to preserve the sight of certain people most at risk.*
- The patented Bausch & Lomb PreserVision® is the ONLY eye vitamin and mineral supplement clinically proven effective in the 10 year National Institutes of Health (NIH) Age Related Eye Disease Study (AREDS). US Patent 6,660,297.
- Bausch & Lomb PreserVision® is a high potency antioxidant and mineral supplement with the antioxidant vitamins A, C, E, and selected minerals in amounts above those in ordinary multivitamins and generally cannot be obtained through diet alone.
- **Recommended Intake:** Instead of taking 4 tablets per day to get the high levels proven effective in the National Institutes of Health (NIH) Age Related Eye Disease Study (AREDS), you only need to take: 2 softgels per day – 1 in the morning. 1 in the evening taken with meals.

Bausch & Lomb PreserVision® is the #1 recommended eye vitamin and mineral supplement among vitreoretinal eye doctors.*

Table A

Supplement Facts
Serving Size: 4 tablets daily; 2 in the morning, 2 in the evening taken with meals.

Contents	Two tablets		Daily Dosage (4 tablets)	
	Amount	% of Daily Value	Amount	% of Daily Value
Vitamin A (10% as beta-carotene)	14,320 IU	286%	28,640 IU	573%
Vitamin C (ascorbic acid)	226 mg	376%	452 mg	753%
Vitamin E (dl-alpha tocopheryl acetate)	200 IU	666%	400 IU	1333%
Zinc (zinc oxide)	34.8 mg	232%	69.6 mg	464%
Cooper (cupric oxide)	0.8 mg	40%	1.6 mg	80%

Table A

Supplement Facts
Serving Size: 2 Soft Gels; 2 in the morning, 1 in the evening taken with meals.

Contents	Daily Dosage (2 Soft Gels)	
	Amount	% of Daily Value
Vitamin A (beta-carotene)	28,640 IU	573%
Vitamin C (ascorbic acid)	452 mg	753%
Vitamin E (dl-alpha tocopheryl acetate)	400 IU	1333%
Zinc (zinc oxide)	69.6 mg	464%
Copper (cupric oxide)	1.6 mg	80%

CURRENT AND FORMER SMOKERS:
Consult your eye doctor or eye care professional about the risks associated with smoking and Beta-Carotene.

> * This statement has not been evaluated by the Food and Drug Administration. This product is not intended to diagnose, treat, cure or prevent any disease.

---

* Data on file, Bausch & Lomb Incorporated.

How Supplied: NDC 24208-532-10 60 ct. NDC 24208-532-30 120 ct. Available in bottles of 60 count and 120 count soft gels. Orange, oval shaped soft gelatin capsule imprinted with BL-PV on one side.
DO NOT USE IF SEAL UNDER CLOSURE IS BROKEN
Keep this product out of the reach of children.
STORE AT ROOM TEMPERATURE
Made in the USA
Marketed by:
Bausch & Lomb Incorporated, Rochester NY 14609
Bausch & Lomb and Preservision are registered trademarks of Bausch & Lomb Incorporated.
© Bausch & Lomb Incorporated. All rights reserved.

Shown in Product Identification Guide, page 503

BAUSCH & LOMB PRESERVISION®
LUTEIN
Eye Vitamin and Mineral Supplement
Beta-carotene free formulation.
(Bausch & Lomb)
Easy to swallow 2 per day Soft Gels

Description: see supplement facts (table A)
[See table below]

Other Ingredients: Gelatin, Glycerin, Soybean Oil, Unbleached Lecithin, Yellow Wax, Annatto Oil, Titanium Dioxide
This product is Vitamin A (beta-carotene) Free.
• The Bausch & Lomb PreserVision® Lutein patented formula is based on the Bausch & Lomb PreserVision® AREDS formula*, with the beta-carotene substituted with 10 mg of FloraGlo® Lutein.

• Lutein is a carotenoid found in dark leafy green vegetables such as spinach. Carotenoids are concentrated in the macula, the part of the eye responsible for central vision. Studies suggest that lutein plays an essential role in maintaining healthy central vision by protecting against free radical damage and filtering blue light.**
• Lutein levels in your eye are related to the amount in your diet. Bausch & Lomb PreserVision® Lutein contains 5 mg of lutein per soft gel, which gives you 10 mg of lutein per day. The leading multivitamin contains only a fraction of the amount of lutein used in clinical studies.

*Bausch & Lomb Ocuvite® PreserVision® AREDS formula was the only antioxidant vitamin and mineral supplement proven effective in the 10-year National Institutes of Health (NIH) Age-Related Eye Disease Study (AREDS). AREDS was a 10-year, independent study conducted by the National Eye Institute (NEI) of the National Institutes of Health (NIH).

Recommended Intake: 2 soft gels per day – 1 in the morning, 1 in the evening taken with meals.

> **This statement has not been evaluated by the Food and Drug Administration. This product is not intended to diagnose, treat, cure or prevent any disease.

How Supplied: NDC 24208-632-10. Available in bottles of 50 count soft gels. Orange, oval shaped soft gelatin capsule, imprinted with BL-LPV on one side.
DO NOT USE IF SEAL UNDER CLOSURE IS BROKEN
Keep out of reach of children.
STORE AT ROOM TEMPERATURE
®FloraGLO is a registered trademark of Kemin Industries, Inc.
Made in the USA
Marketed by:
Bausch & Lomb Incorporated, Rochester NY 14609
© Bausch & Lomb Incorporated. All rights reserved.
Bausch & Lomb and Preservision are registered trademarks of Bausch & Lomb or its affiliates.

Shown in Product Identification Guide, page 503

BEELITH TABLETS (Beach)
magnesium supplement with pyridoxine HCl

Description: Each tablet contains magnesium oxide 600 mg and pyridoxine hydrochloride (Vitamin B_6) 25 mg equivalent to Vitamin B_6 20 mg.

Supplement Facts
Serving Size: 1 Tablet

	Amount Per Tablet	% Daily Value
Vitamin B_6 (pyridoxine HCl)	20 mg	1000%
Magnesium (from magnesium oxide)	362 mg	90%

Inactive Ingredients: FD&C Yellow No. 6, hydroxypropyl methylcellulose, magnesium stearate, microcrystalline cellulose, polyethylene glycol, sodium starch glycolate, titanium dioxide.
May also contain D&C Yellow No. 10, FD&C Yellow No. 5 (Tartrazine), hydroxypropyl cellulose, polydextrose, stearic acid and/or triacetin.

Indications: As a dietary supplement for patients with magnesium and/or Vitamin B_6 deficiencies resulting from malnutrition, alcoholism, magnesium depleting drugs, chemotherapy, and inadequate nutritional intake or absorption. Also, increases urinary magnesium levels.

Dosage: One tablet daily or as directed by a physician.

Warnings: Do not take this product if you are presently taking a prescription drug without consulting your physician or other health professional. If you have kidney disease, take only under the supervision of a physician. Excessive dosage may cause laxation. If pregnant or breast-feeding, ask a health professional before use.
KEEP OUT OF THE REACH OF CHILDREN.

How Supplied: Golden yellow, film-coated tablet with the letters **BP** and the number **132** imprinted on each tablet. Packaged in bottles of 100 (Item No. 0486-1132-01) tablets.

BENEFIBER®
(Novartis Consumer Health, Inc.)
Fiber Supplement

Description:
Doctors agree that fiber is an important part of a healthy diet. However most people only get half the daily recommended amount of fiber.[1] Now it's easier than ever to add fiber to your diet with Benefiber®, a 100% natural fiber that you can mix with almost anything. It's

---

Table A

Supplement Facts
Serving size: 2 soft gels daily; 1 in the morning, 1 in the evening taken with meals

Contents	Daily Dosage (2 Soft Gels) Amount	% Daily Value
Vitamin C (ascorbic acid)	452 mg	753%
Vitamin E (dl-alpha tocopheryl acetate)	400 IU	1333%
Zinc (zinc oxide)	69.6 mg	464%
Copper (cupric oxide)	1.6 mg	80%
Lutein	10 mg	†

†Daily value not established

Continued on next page

Benefiber—Cont.

• Taste-free • Grit-free • Non-thickening so it won't alter the taste or texture of your foods or beverages.

Be creative with Benefiber®. Try it in your coffee, juice, yogurt, your baked goods, favorite recipes or whatever you desire. You won't even know it's there!

Supplement Facts
Serving Size: 2 tsp (3.5g)

Amount Per Serving	%DV*
Calories 15	
Sodium 0mg	0%*
Total Carbohydrate 4g	1%*
Dietary Fiber 3g	12%*
Soluble Fiber 3g	†
Sugars 0g	†

* Percent Daily Values (DV) are based on a 2,000 calorie diet.
† Daily Value not established.

Ingredients: Wheat dextrin
Gluten Free (less than 10 ppm gluten)

Directions for Use:

Stir 2 teaspoons of Benefiber into 4-8 oz. of any beverage or soft food (hot or cold). Stir well until dissolved.
Not recommended for carbonated beverages.

AGE	DOSAGE	
12 yrs. to adult	2 tsp	3 times daily
7 to 11 yrs.	1 tsp	3 times daily
Under 6 yrs.	Ask your doctor	

tsp = teaspoon
[1] The American Dietetic recommends a healthy diet include 25-35 grams of fiber a day.

Other Information:
Store at controlled room temperature 20-25°C (68-77°F). Protect from moisture. Use within 6 months of opening.

Warning:
Keep out of reach of children.
If you are pregnant or nursing a baby, ask a health professional before use.

Tamper Evident Feature: Do not use if printed inner seal is broken or missing.

Questions? Call 1-800-452-0051
24 hours a day, 7 days a week or visit us at www.Benefiber.com for recipe ideas and additional information.

How Supplied: Available in 2.8 oz, 5.4 oz, 8.6 oz, 12.3 oz, and 16.7 oz powder bottles.

Shown in Product Identification Guide, page 512

BENEFIBER®
(Novartis Consumer Health, Inc.)
Fiber Supplement
Chewable Tablets
Orange Creme Flavor

Benefiber Chewable Tablets are an easy way to add fiber to your diet. These great tasting tablets provide as much fiber per dose as the leading bulk fiber, but because there's no need for water or mixing, you can take them virtually anywhere, anytime.

Supplement Facts:
Serving Size: 3 Tablets

Amount Per Serving	%DV*
Calories 35	
Total Carbohydrate 8g	3%*
Dietary Fiber 3g	12%*
Soluble Fiber 3g	†
Sugars 4g	
Sodium 10mg	<1%

*Percent Daily Values (DV) are based on a 2,000 calorie diet.
†Daily Value (DV) not established.

Ingredients: partially hydrolyzed guar gum, sorbitol, maltodextrin, confectioner's sugar, dextrates, citric acid, magnesium stearate, sucralose, sucrose, natural and artificial flavors, modified food starch, acacia, FD&C yellow 6 aluminum lake, silicon dioxide, lecithin, tocopherols, soybean oil

Directions for use: Adults: Chew 1 to 3 tablets up to 5 times daily to supplement the fiber content of your diet. Do not take more than 15 tablets in a 24 hour period.

Age	Dosage
12 yrs. to adult	1–3 tablets up to 5 times daily[1]
7 to 11 yrs.	1/2–1 1/2 tablets up to 5 times daily[2]
Under 6 yrs.	ask your doctor

[1] Not to exceed 15 tablets per day.
[2] Not to exceed 7 1/2 tablets per day.

Other Information: Store at controlled room temperature 20–25°C (68–77°F). Protect from excessive heat and moisture. **Keep out of reach of children.**
If you are pregnant or nursing a baby, ask a health professional before use.
Tamper Evident Feature: Notice! Protective printed inner seal beneath cap. If missing or damaged, do not use contents.
Product may contain dark specks due to the processing of natural ingredients.
Benefiber guarantees your satisfaction or your money back.

Questions? call **1-800-452-0051** 24 hours a day, 7 days a week or visit us at

www.benefiber.com for additional information.

How Supplied: Available in bottles of 36 ct. and 100 ct. tablets.
Shown in Product Identification Guide, page 513

BENEFIBER® CAPLETS
(Novartis Consumer Health, Inc.)
Fiber supplement

Supplement Facts
Serving Size: 3 Caplets

Amount Per Serving	%DV*
Calories 15	
Sodium 0mg	0%*
Total Carbohydrate 4g	1%*
Dietary Fiber 3g	12%*
Soluble Fiber 3g	†
Sugars 0g	†

* Percent Daily Values (DV) are based on a 2,000 calorie diet.
† Daily Value not established.

Ingredients: Wheat dextrin, microcrystalline cellulose, magnesium stearate, colloidal silicon dioxide
Gluten Free (less than 10 ppm gluten)

Directions for use:

Adults: Take 3 caplets up to 3 times daily to supplement the fiber content of your diet. Swallow with liquid. Do not exceed 9 caplets per day.
Keep out of reach of children.
If you are pregnant or nursing a baby, ask a health professional before use.

Tamper Evident Feature:

Protective printed inner seal "sealed for your protection" beneath cap. If missing or damaged, do not use contents.
Benefiber® guarantees your satisfaction or your money back.

Questions? Call 1-800-452-0051
24 hours a day, 7 days a week or visit us at www.benefiber.com for additional information.

Other Information:
Store at controlled room temperature 20-25°C (68-77°F). Protect from excessive heat and moisture.

How Supplied:
Available in 72 ct. and 114 ct. bottles.

BIOLEAN® PROXTREME™
(Wellness International)
Multi-Protein Dietary Supplement

Description: BioLean® ProXtreme™ is a multi-protein formula containing a scientific blend of ion-exchange whey pro-

tein isolates, cross flow ultra filtration isolates, whey protein concentrates, hydrolyzed whey peptides, glutamine peptides and egg albumen. This combination of various protein sources provides 25 grams of protein per serving while only having 2 grams of carbohydrates. BioLean® ProXtreme™ provides an ideal ratio of essential and non-essential amino acids in their most easily assimilated forms, while also providing high levels of the branched chain amino acids (BCAAs). To increase absorption and digestibility, the proteins in BioLean® ProXtreme™ are enzymatically predigested. These proteins are further processed with whey protein to minimize protein cross-linking.

Uses: BioLean® ProXtreme™ may:
• Enhance weight loss and aid weight maintenance
• Increase metabolic rate via increased lean body mass and thermic effect of protein metabolism
• Increase ratio of lean muscle mass to total body mass
• Combat catabolic muscle breakdown
• Reduce fatigue and post-exercise recovery time

Directions: As a dietary supplement, add 1 packet BioLean® ProXtreme™ to 1 cup water, milk, or juice. Stir, shake, or blend thoroughly.

Warnings: Not for use by young children. If you are pregnant or nursing, consult a health professional before using this product. Accidental overdose of iron-containing products is a leading cause of fatal poisoning in children under 6. Keep this product out of reach of children. In case of accidental overdose, call a doctor or poison control center immediately.

Ingredients: Sugar 1 g, Potassium 240 mg, Carbohydrate 2 g, Cholesterol 13 mg, Sodium 80 mg, Protein 25 g, Vitamin A 1,125 IU, Vitamin C 27 mg, Vitamin D 90 IU, Vitamin E 14 IU, Riboflavin 450 mcg, Niacin 5 mg, Vitamin B6 450 mcg, Folic Acid 63 mcg, Vitamin B12 1.4 mcg, Biotin 68 mcg, Pantothenic Acid 2 mg, Calcium 185 mg, Chromium 55 mcg, Proprietary Amino Acid Blend 1 g (Glutamine Peptides, L-Leucine, L-Isoleucine, L-Valine, Zytrix®* 100 mg), Protein Complex (Whey Protein Isolate, Whey Protein Concentrate, Egg Albumen, Whey Peptides, Glutamine Peptides), Cocoa, Natural and Artificial Flavor, Lecithin, Vitamin/Mineral Blend (Ascorbic Acid, Chromium GTF Polynicotinate, d-alpha Tocopheryl Succinate [Natural Vitamin E], Calcium Phosphate Dibasic, Biotin, Vitamin A Palmitate, Niacinamide, d-Calcium Pantothenate, Cholecalciferol, Folic Acid, Pyridoxine Hydrochloride, Riboflavin, Cyanocobalamin), Xanthan Gum, Acesulfame Potassium, Salt, Sucralose.

*Zytrix® is a registered trademark of Custom Nutriceutical Laboratories.

How Supplied: One box contains 14 single serving packets.

Additional Information: For additional information on ingredients or uses, please visit www.winltd.com.

These statements have not been evaluated by the Food & Drug Administration. This product is not intended to diagnose, treat, cure or prevent any disease.

CALTRATE® 600 + D
(Wyeth Consumer)

Supplement Facts
Serving Size 1 Tablet

Amount Per Serving	% DV
Vitamin D 400 IU	100%
Calcium 600 mg	60%

Ingredients: Calcium Carbonate, Starch. Contains < 2% of: Acacia, Cholecalciferol (Vit.D₃), Croscarmellose Sodium, dl-Alpha Tocopherol, FD&C Yellow 6 Aluminum Lake, Magnesium Stearate, Medium-Chain Triglycerides, Polyethylene Glycol, Polyvinyl Alcohol, Sucrose, Talc, Titanium Dioxide, Tricalcium Phosphate.
As with any supplement, if you are pregnant, nursing, or taking medication, consult your doctor before use.
Keep out of reach of children.

Suggested Use: Take one tablet twice daily with food or as directed by your physician. Not formulated for use in children.
Storage:
Store at room temperature. Keep bottle tightly closed. Bottle sealed with printed foil under cap. Do Not Use if foil is torn.

How Supplied:
Bottles of 60, 120 tablets

CALTRATE® 600 PLUS™ Tablets
(Wyeth Consumer)
CALTRATE® 600 PLUS™
Chewables
Calcium Carbonate
Calcium Supplement With Vitamin D & Minerals

Supplement Facts
Serving Size 1 Tablet

Amount Per Serving	%DV
Vitamin D 400 IU	100%
Calcium 600 mg	60%
Magnesium 50 mg	13%
Zinc 7.5 mg	50%
Copper 1 mg	50%
Manganese 1.8 mg	90%
Boron 250 mcg	*

* Daily Value (%DV) not established.

Ingredients: Calcium Carbonate, Starch, Magnesium Oxide. Contains <2% of: Acacia, Cholecalciferol (Vit. D₃), Cros-

carmellose Sodium, Cupric Sulfate, dl-Alpha Tocopherol, FD&C Blue 1 Aluminum Lake, FD&C Red 40 Aluminum Lake, FD&C Yellow 6 Aluminum Lake, Hypromellose, Magnesium Stearate, Manganese Sulfate, Medium-Chain Triglycerides, Microcrystalline Cellulose, Polysorbate 80, Sodium Borate, Sucrose, Titanium Dioxide, Triacetin, Tricalcium Phosphate, Zinc Oxide.

Chewables

Supplement Facts
Serving Size 1 Tablet

Amount Per Serving	% DV
Calories 10	
Total Carbohydrate 2 g	<1%+
Sugars 2 g	*
Vitamin D 400 IU	100%
Calcium 600 mg	60%
Magnesium 40 mg	10%
Zinc 7.5 mg	50%
Copper 1 mg	50%
Manganese 1.8 mg	90%
Boron 250 mcg	*

* Daily Value (%DV) not established.
+ Percent Daily Value based on a 2,000 calorie diet

Ingredients: Dextrose, Calcium Carbonate, Maltodextrin. Contains <2% of: Adipic Acid, BHT, Cholecalciferol (Vit. D₃), Corn Starch, Crospovidone, Cupric Oxide, dl-Alpha Tocopherol, FD&C Blue 2 Aluminum Lake, FD&C Red 40 Aluminum Lake, FD&C Yellow 6 Aluminum Lake, Gelatin, Hypromellose, Magnesium Oxide, Magnesium Stearate, Manganese Sulfate, Mineral Oil, Modified Starch, Natural and Artificial Flavor, Partially Hydrogenated Soybean Oil, Powdered Cellulose, Sodium Borate, Stearic Acid, Sucrose, Zinc Oxide.

Suggested Use: Take one tablet twice daily with food or as directed by your physician. Not formulated for use in children.

As with any supplement, if you are pregnant, nursing, or taking medication, consult your doctor before use.
Keep out of reach of children.
Store at room temperature. Keep bottle tightly closed.
Bottle sealed with printed foil under cap. Do Not Use if foil is torn.

How Supplied: Tablets; Bottles of 60 & 120
Chewables, Bottles of 60 & 90.
(Orange, cherry and fruit flavors)

CENTRUM® (Wyeth Consumer)
High Potency
Multivitamin/Multimineral Supplement
From A to Zinc®

Supplement Facts
Serving Size 1 Tablet

Continued on next page

Centrum—Cont.

Each Tablet Contains	% DV
Vitamin A 3500 IU	70%
(29% as Beta Carotene)	
Vitamin C 60 mg	100%
Vitamin D 400 IU	100%
Vitamin E 30 IU	100%
Vitamin K 25 mcg	31%
Thiamin 1.5 mg	100%
Riboflavin 1.7 mg	100%
Niacin 20 mg	100%
Vitamin B_6 2 mg	100%
Folic Acid 400 mcg	100%
Vitamin B_{12} 6 mcg	100%
Biotin 30 mcg	10%
Pantothenic Acid 10 mg	100%
Calcium 162 mg	16%
Iron 18 mg	100%
Phosphorus 109 mg	11%
Iodine 150 mcg	100%
Magnesium 100 mg	25%
Zinc 15 mg	100%
Selenium 20 mcg	29%
Copper 2 mg	100%
Manganese 2 mg	100%
Chromium 120 mcg	100%
Molybdenum 75 mcg	100%
Chloride 72 mg	2%
Potassium 80 mg	2%
Boron 150 mcg	*
Nickel 5 mcg	*
Silicon 2 mg	*
Tin 10 mcg	*
Vanadium 10 mcg	*
Lutein 250 mcg	*
Lycopene 300 mcg	*

*Daily Value (%DV) not established.

Ingredients: Dibasic Calcium Phosphate, Magnesium Oxide, Potassium Chloride, Microcrystalline Cellulose, Ascorbic Acid (Vit. C), Ferrous Fumarate, Calcium Carbonate, dl-Alpha Tocopheryl Acetate (Vit. E), Starch. Contains < 2% of: Acacia, Ascorbyl Palmitate, Beta Carotene, Biotin, BHT, Calcium Pantothenate, Calcium Stearate, Chromic Chloride, Citric Acid, Crospovidone, Cupric Oxide, Cyanocobalamin (Vit. B_{12}), dl-Alpha Tocopherol, Ergocalciferol (Vit. D), FD&C Yellow 6 Aluminum Lake, Folic Acid, Gelatin, Hypromellose, Lutein, Lycopene, Magnesium Borate, Magnesium Stearate, Manganese Sulfate, Niacinamide, Nickelous Sulfate, Phytonadione (Vit. K), Potassium Iodide, Pyridoxine Hydrochloride (Vit. B_6), Riboflavin (Vit. B_2), Silicon Dioxide, Sodium Aluminum Silicate, Sodium Ascorbate, Sodium Benzoate, Sodium Borate, Sodium Citrate, Sodium Metavanadate, Sodium Molybdate, Sodium Selenate, Sorbic Acid, Stannous Chloride, Sucrose, Thiamine Mononitrate (Vit. B_1), Titanium Dioxide, Tribasic Calcium Phosphate, Vitamin A Acetate (Vit. A), Zinc Oxide. May also contain <2%: Lactose (milk).

Suggested Use:

Adults – One tablet daily with food. Not formulated for use in children.

As with any supplement, if you are pregnant, nursing, or taking medication, consult your doctor before use.

Warning: Accidental overdose of iron-containing products is a leading cause of fatal poisoning in children under 6. Keep this product out of reach of children. In case of accidental overdose, call a doctor or poison control center immediately.

IMPORTANT INFORMATION: Long-term intake of high levels of vitamin A (excluding that sourced from beta-carotene) may increase the risk of osteoporosis in adults. Do not take this product if taking other vitamin A supplements.

How Supplied: Bottles of 15, 50, 130, 180, 250 tablets
Storage: Store at room temperature. Keep bottle tightly closed.
Bottle sealed with printed foil under cap. Do not use if foil is torn.

CENTRUM KIDS COMPLETE
(Wyeth Consumer)
DORA the EXPLORER, RUGRATS, SPONGEBOB SQUAREPANTS, & NICKTOONS
Multivitamin/Multimineral Supplement
(Orange, Cherry, Fruit Punch)++

Supplement Facts:
[See table below]

++Combined Ingredients List for 3 flavors

Ingredients: Sucrose, Dibasic Calcium Phosphate, Mannitol (wheat), Calcium Carbonate, Stearic Acid (soybean), Magnesium Oxide, Ascorbic Acid (Vit. C), Pregelatinized Starch, Microcrystalline Cellulose, dl-Alpha Tocopheryl Acetate (Vit. E). Contains < 2% of: Acacia, Aspartame,** Beta Carotene, Biotin, BHT, Calcium Pantothenate, Carbonyl Iron, Carrageenan, Chromic Chloride, Citric Acid, Cupric Oxide, Cyanocobalamin (Vit. B_{12}), Dextrose, Ergocalciferol (Vit. D), FD&C Blue 2 Aluminum Lake, FD&C Red 40 Aluminum Lake (sulfite), FD&C Yellow 6 Aluminum Lake, Folic Acid, Gelatin, Glucose, Guar Gum, Lactose (milk), Magnesium Stearate, Malic Acid, Maltodextrin, Manganese Sulfate, Mono- and Di-glycerides, Natural and Artificial Flavors, Niacinamide, Phytonadione (Vit. K), Potassium Iodide, Potassium Sorbate, Purified Water, Pyridoxine Hydrochloride (Vit. B_6), Riboflavin (Vit. B_2), Silicon Dioxide, Sodium Ascorbate, Sodium Benzoate, Sodium Citrate, Sodium Molybdate, Sodium Silicoaluminate, Sorbic Acid, Starch, Thiamine Mononitrate (Vit. B_1), Tocopherol, Tribasic Calcium Phosphate, Vanillin, Vitamin A Acetate (Vit. A), Zinc Oxide.

Suggested Use: Children 2 and 3 years of age, chew approximately ½ tablet daily with food. Children 4 years of age and older, chew 1 tablet daily with food. Not formulated for use in children less than 2 years of age.

Warning: Accidental overdose of iron-containing products is a leading cause of

Serving Size:		½ Tablet	1 Tablet
Amount Per Tablet:		% DV for Children 2 and 3 Years (1/2 Tablet)	% DV for Children 4 Years and Older (1 Tablet)
Calories 5			
Total Carbohydrate <1g		*	<1%+
Vitamin A 3500 IU		70%	70%
(29% as Beta Carotene)			
Vitamin C 60 mg		75%	100%
Vitamin D 400 IU		50%	100%
Vitamin E 30 IU		150%	100%
Vitamin K 10 mcg		*	13%
Thiamin 1.5 mg		107%	100%
Riboflavin 1.7 mg		106%	100%
Niacin 20 mg		111%	100%
Vitamin B_6 2 mg		143%	100%
Folic Acid 400 mcg		100%	100%
Vitamin B_{12} 6 mcg		100%	100%
Biotin 45 mcg		15%	15%
Pantothenic Acid 10 mg		100%	100%
Calcium 108 mg		7%	11%
Iron 18 mg		90%	100%
Phosphorus 50 mg		3%	5%
Iodine 150 mcg		107%	100%
Magnesium 40 mg		10%	10%
Zinc 15 mg		94%	100%
Copper 2 mg		100%	100%
Manganese 1 mg		*	50%
Chromium 20 mcg		*	17%
Molybdenum 20 mcg		*	27%

*Daily Value (%DV) not established.
+Percent Daily Values based on a 2,000 calorie diet.

fatal poisoning in children under 6. Keep this product out of reach of children. In case of accidental overdose, call a doctor or poison control center immediately.

CONTAINS ASPARTAME.

** PHENYLKETONURICS: CONTAINS PHENYLALANINE.

Storage: Store at room temperature. Keep bottle tightly closed.
Bottle sealed with printed foil under cap. Do not use if foil is torn.

How Supplied: Assorted Flavors—Uncoated Tablet—Bottles of 60, 100 tablets
Marketed by: Wyeth Consumer Healthcare, Madison, NJ 07940

CENTRUM® PERFORMANCE
Multivitamin/Multimineral Supplement (Wyeth Consumer)

Supplement Facts
Serving Size 1 Tablet

Each Tablet Contains	% DV
Vitamin A 3500 IU	70%
(29% as Beta Carotene)	
Vitamin C 120 mg	200%
Vitamin D 400 IU	100%
Vitamin E 60 IU	200%
Vitamin K 25 mcg	31%
Thiamin 4.5 mg	300%
Riboflavin 5.1 mg	300%
Niacin 40 mg	200%
Vitamin B$_6$ 6 mg	300%
Folic Acid 400 mcg	100%
Vitamin B$_{12}$ 18 mcg	300%
Biotin 40 mcg	13%
Pantothenic Acid 10 mg	100%
Calcium 100 mg	10%
Iron 18 mg	100%
Phosphorus 48 mg	5%
Iodine 150 mcg	100%
Magnesium 40 mg	10%
Zinc 15 mg	100%
Selenium 70 mcg	100%
Copper 2 mg	100%
Manganese 4 mg	200%
Chromium 120 mcg	100%
Molybdenum 75 mcg	100%
Chloride 72 mg	2%
Potassium 80 mg	2%
Ginseng Root (*Panax ginseng*) 50 mg Standardized Extract	*
Ginkgo Biloba Leaf (*Ginkgo biloba*) 60 mg Standardized Extract	*
Boron 60 mcg	*
Nickel 5 mcg	*
Silicon 4 mg	*
Tin 10 mcg	*
Vanadium 10 mcg	*

*Daily Value (%DV) not established.

Ingredients: Dibasic Calcium Phosphate, Potassium Chloride, Ascorbic Acid (Vit. C), Microcrystalline Cellulose, Calcium Carbonate, dl-Alpha Tocopheryl Acetate (Vit. E), Magnesium Oxide, Ginkgo Biloba Leaf (*Ginkgo biloba*) Standardized Extract, Gelatin, Ginseng Root (*Panax ginseng*) Standardized Extract, Ferrous Fumarate, Niacinamide, Crospovidone, Starch. Contains <2% of: Acacia Gum, Ascorbyl Palmitate, Beta Carotene, Biotin, BHT, Calcium Pantothenate, Chromic Chloride, Citric Acid, Cupric Oxide, Cyanocobalamin (Vit. B$_{12}$), Ergocalciferol (Vit. D), FD&C Red 40 Aluminum Lake, FD&C Yellow 6 Aluminum Lake, Folic Acid, Glucose, Hypromellose, Lactose (milk), Magnesium Borate, Magnesium Stearate, Manganese Sulfate, Nickelous Sulfate, Phytonadione (Vit. K), Polyethylene Glycol, Polysorbate 80, Potassium Iodide, Potassium Sorbate, Purified Water, Pyridoxine Hydrochloride (Vit. B$_6$), Riboflavin (Vit. B$_2$), Silicon Dioxide, Sodium Ascorbate, Sodium Benzoate, Sodium Borate, Sodium Citrate, Sodium Metavanadate, Sodium Molybdate, Sodium Selenate, Sodium Silicoaluminate, Sorbic Acid, Stannous Chloride, Sucrose, Thiamin Mononitrate (Vit. B$_1$), Titanium Dioxide, Tocopherol, Tribasic Calcium Phosphate, Vitamin A Acetate (Vit. A), Zinc Oxide. May also contain <2%: Maltodextrin.

Suggested Use: Adults—One tablet daily with food. Not formulated for use in children.

Warning: Accidental overdose of iron-containing products is a leading cause of fatal poisoning in children under 6. Keep this product out of reach of children. In case of accidental overdose, call a doctor or poison control center immediately.

Precaution: As with any supplement, if you are pregnant, nursing, or taking medication, contact your doctor before use.

IMPORTANT INFORMATION: Long-term intake of high levels of vitamin A (excluding that sourced from beta-carotene) may increase the risk of osteoporosis in adults. Do not take this product if taking other vitamin A supplements.

Store at Room Temperature. Keep bottle tightly closed. Bottle is sealed with printed foil under cap. Do not use if foil is torn.

How Supplied: Bottles of 45, 75 and 120 Tablets.

CENTRUM® SILVER®
(Wyeth Consumer)
Multivitamin/Multimineral Supplement Specially Formulated for Adults 50+ From A to Zinc®

Supplement Facts
Serving Size 1 Tablet

Each Tablet Contains	% DV
Vitamin A 3500 IU	70%
(29% as Beta Carotene)	
Vitamin C 60 mg	100%
Vitamin D 400 IU	100%
Vitamin E 45 IU	150%
Vitamin K 10 mcg	13%
Thiamin 1.5 mg	100%
Riboflavin 1.7 mg	100%
Niacin 20 mg	100%
Vitamin B$_6$ 3 mg	150%
Folic Acid 400 mcg	100%
Vitamin B$_{12}$ 25 mcg	417%
Biotin 30 mcg	10%
Pantothenic Acid 10 mg	100%
Calcium 200 mg	20%
Phosphorus 48 mg	5%
Iodine 150 mcg	100%
Magnesium 100 mg	25%
Zinc 15 mg	100%
Selenium 20 mcg	29%
Copper 2 mg	100%
Manganese 2 mg	100%
Chromium 150 mcg	125%
Molybdenum 75 mcg	100%
Chloride 72 mg	2%
Potassium 80 mg	2%
Boron 150 mcg	*
Nickel 5 mcg	*
Silicon 2 mg	*
Vanadium 10 mcg	*
Lutein 250 mcg	*
Lycopene 300 mcg	*

*Daily Value (%DV) not established.

Ingredients: Calcium Carbonate, Dibasic Calcium Phosphate, Magnesium Oxide, Potassium Chloride, Microcrystalline Cellulose, Starch, Ascorbic Acid (Vit. C), dl-Alpha Tocopheryl Acetate (Vit. E), Crospovidone. Contains < 2% of: Acacia, Ascorbyl Palmitate, Beta Carotene, Biotin, BHT, Calcium Pantothenate, Calcium Stearate, Chromic Chloride, Citric Acid, Cupric Oxide, Cyanocobalamin (Vit. B$_{12}$), dl-Alpha Tocopherol, Ergocalciferol (Vit. D), FD&C Blue 2 Aluminum Lake, FD&C Red 40 Aluminum Lake, FD&C Yellow 6 Aluminum Lake, Folic Acid, Gelatin, Lutein, Lycopene, Magnesium Borate, Magnesium Stearate, Manganese Sulfate, Niacinamide, Nickelous Sulfate, Phytonadione (Vit. K), Polyethylene Glycol, Polyvinyl Alcohol, Potassium Iodide, Pyridoxine Hydrochloride (Vit. B$_6$), Riboflavin (Vit. B$_2$), Silicon Dioxide, Sodium Aluminum Silicate, Sodium Ascorbate, Sodium Benzoate, Sodium Borate, Sodium Citrate, Sodium Metavanadate, Sodium Molybdate, Sodium Selenate, Sorbic Acid, Sucrose, Talc, Thiamine Mononitrate (Vit. B$_1$), Titanium Dioxide, Tribasic Calcium Phosphate, Vitamin A Acetate (Vit. A), Zinc Oxide. May also contain < 2%: Lactose (milk).

Suggested Use:
Adults – One tablet daily with food. Not formulated for use in children.

Warnings: As with any supplement, if you are pregnant, nursing, or taking medication, contact your doctor before use.

IMPORTANT INFORMATION: Long-term intake of high levels of vitamin A

Continued on next page

Centrum Silver—Cont.

(excluding that sourced from beta-carotene) may increase the risk of osteoporosis in adults. Do not take this product if taking other vitamin A supplements.

How Supplied: Bottles of 60, 100, 150 tablets

Storage:
Store at Room Temperature. Keep bottle tightly closed. Bottle is sealed with printed foil under cap. Do not use if foil is torn.

CITRACAL® CAPLETS
ULTRADENSE® Calcium Citrate
with Vitamin D Dietary
Supplement
(Mission Pharmacal)

For full product information see page 703.

D-CAL™ (A & Z Pharmaceutical)
Calcium Supplement with Vitamin D
Chewable Caplets

Ingredients: Calcium Carbonate, Vitamin D, Sorbitol, Flavor, D&C Red #27 Lake, Magnesium Stearate. No sugar, No salt, No lactose, No preservative.

Supplement Facts

Serving Size One Caplet

Each Caplet Contains		% Daily Value
Calcium (as calcium carbonate)	300 mg	30%
Vitamin D	100 IU	25%

Recommended Intake: Take two caplets daily for adult and one caplet for child, or as directed by your physician.

Warnings: KEEP OUT OF REACH OF CHILDREN. Do not accept if safety seal under cap is broken or missing.

Actions: D-Cal™ provides a concentrated form of calcium to help build healthy bones. It contains Vitamin D to help the body absorb calcium. D-Cal™ can also help prevent osteoporosis. It is helpful to pregnant and nursing women, children's growth, and calcium deficiency at all ages.

How Supplied: Bottles of 30 and 60 caplets

DDS®-ACIDOPHILUS (UAS Labs)
Capsule, Tablet & Powder free of
dairy products, corn, soy, and
preservatives

Description: DDS®-Acidophilus is the source of a special strain of Lactobacillus acidophilus free of dairy products, corn, soy and preservatives. Each capsule or tablet contains one billion viable DDS®-1 L.acidophilus at the time of manufacturing. One gram of powder contains two billion viable DDS®-1 L.acidophilus.

Indications and Usages: An aid in implanting the gut with beneficial Lactobacillus acidophilus under conditions of digestive disorders, acne, yeast infections, and following antibiotic therapy.

Administration: One to two capsules or tablets twice daily before meals. One-fourth teaspoon powder can be substituted for two capsules or tablets.

How Supplied: Bottles of 100 capsules or tablets. 12 bottles per case. Powder is available in 2 oz. bottle; 12 bottles per case.

Storage: Keep refrigerated under 40°F.

FEOSOL® Caplets
(GlaxoSmithKline Consumer)
Hematinic
Iron Supplement

Description: FEOSOL Caplets contain pure iron micro particles called carbonyl iron. Replacing FEOSOL Capsules, this advanced formula is specially designed to be well absorbed, gentle on the stomach and offers enhanced safety in the event of an accidental overdose. Each FEOSOL carbonyl iron caplet delivers 45 mg of pure elemental iron, the same amount of elemental iron contained in the 225 mg ferrous sulfate capsule. At equivalent doses, carbonyl iron and ferrous sulfate were shown to be equally efficacious in correcting hemoglobin, hematocrit and serum iron levels in iron-deficient patients[1].

Safety: According to the American Association of Poison Control Centers, iron containing supplements are the leading cause of pediatric poisoning deaths for children under six in the United States[2]. Widely used as a food additive, carbonyl iron must be gastrically solubilized before it can be absorbed, giving it lower toxicity and enhancing its safety versus any of the ferrous salts[3]. As a result, carbonyl iron presents less chance of harm from accidental overdose. In addition, at equivalent doses, carbonyl iron side effects are no greater than those experienced with ferrous sulfate[4].

Warnings: Do not exceed recommended dosage. The treatment of any anemic condition should be under the advice and supervision of a physician. Since oral iron products interfere with absorption of oral tetracycline antibiotics, these products should not be taken within two hours of each other. Occasional gastrointestinal discomfort (such as nausea) may be minimized by taking with meals. Iron containing medication may occasionally cause constipation or diarrhea. If you are pregnant or nursing a baby, seek the advice of a health professional before using this product.

WARNING: Accidental overdose of iron-containing products is a leading cause of fatal poisoning in children under 6. Keep this product out of reach of children. In case of accidental overdose, call a doctor or poison control center immediately.

SUPPLEMENT FACTS
Serving Size: 1 Tablet

Amount per Caplet	% Daily Value
Iron 45 mg	250%

Ingredients: Lactose, Sorbitol, Carbonyl Iron, Hypromellose. Contains 1% or less of the following ingredients: Carnauba Wax, Crospovidone, FD&C Blue #2 Al Lake, FD&C Red #40 Al Lake, FD&C Yellow #6 Al Lake, Magnesium Stearate, Polydextrose, Polyethylene Glycol, Polyethylene Glycol 8000 (Powder), Stearic Acid, Titanium Dioxide, Triacetin.

Directions: Adults—one caplet daily or as directed by a physician. Children under 12 years: Consult a physician.

Tamper-Evident Feature: Each caplet is encased in a plastic cell with a foil back; do not use if cell or foil is broken.

References: [1]Devasthali SD, Gordeuk VR, Brittenham GM, et al, "Bioavailability of Carbonyl Iron: A randomized, double-blind study." Eur J Haematology, 1991; 46:272–278.
[2]FDA Consumer; March 1996:7
[3]Heubers, JA, Brittenham GM, Csiba E and Finch CA. "Absorption of carbonyl iron." J Lab Clin Med 1986; 108:473–78.
[4]Devasthali SD, Gordeuk VR, Brittenham GM, et al, "Bioavailability of a Carbonyl Iron: A randomized, double-blind study." Eur J Haematology, 1991; 46:272–278.
Store at room temperature, avoid excessive heat (greater than 100°F) or humidity.

How Supplied: Boxes of 30 and 60 caplets in blisters. Also available in single unit packages of 100 caplets intended for institutional use
Also available: Feosol Tablets.
Comments or Questions? Call Toll-Free 1-800-245-1040 Weekdays.
GlaxoSmithKline Consumer Healthcare, L.P.
Moon Township, PA 15108

Made in USA
Shown in Product Identification Guide, page 505

FEOSOL® TABLETS
(GlaxoSmithKline Consumer)
Hematinic
Iron Supplement

Description: Feosol tablets provide the body with ferrous sulfate—an iron supplement for iron deficiency and iron deficiency anemia when the need for such

therapy has been determined by a physician.

SUPPLEMENT FACTS
Serving Size: 1 Tablet

Amount per Tablet	% Daily Value
Iron 65 mg	360%

Ingredients: Dried ferrous sulfate 200 mg (65 mg of elemental iron) equivalent to 325 mg of ferrous sulfate per tablet. Lactose, Sorbitol, Crospovidone, Magnesium Stearate, Carnauba Wax. Contains 2% or less of the following ingredients: FD&C Blue #1, FD&C Yellow #6, Hypromellose, Polydextrose, Polyethylene Glycol, Titanium Dioxide, Triacetin.

Directions: Adults and children 12 years and over—One tablet daily or as directed by a physician. Children under 12 years—Consult a physician.

Tamper-Evident Feature: Each tablet is encased in a plastic cell with a foil back; do not use if cell or foil is broken.

Warnings: Do not exceed recommended dosage. The treatment of any anemic condition should be under the advice and supervision of a physician. Since oral iron products interfere with absorption of oral tetracycline antibiotics, these products should not be taken within two hours of each other. Occasional gastrointestinal discomfort (such as nausea) may be minimized by taking with meals. Iron containing medication may occassionally cause constipation or diarrhea.

If you are pregnant or nursing a baby, seek the advice of a health professional before using this product.

WARNING: Accidental overdose of iron-contraining products is a leading cause of fatal poisoning in children under 6. Keep this product out of reach of children. In case of accidental overdose, call a doctor, or poison control center immediately.

Store at room temperature (59–86°F). Not USP for dissolution.

How Supplied: Cartons of 100 tablets in child-resistant blisters.
Previously packaged in bottles.
Also available: Feosol caplets.

Comments or Questions?
Call toll-free 1-800-245-1040 weekdays.
GlaxoSmithKline Consumer Healthcare, L.P.
Moon Township, PA 15108

Made in USA
Shown in Product Identification Guide, page 505

FLINTSTONES® COMPLETE with Choline
(Bayer Healthcare)

Supplement Facts
Serving Size: ½ tablet (2 & 3 years of age); 1 tablet (4 years of age and older)

Servings Per Container: *(number of tablets × 2); (number of tablets)*

Amount Per Tablet	% Daily Value for Children 2 & 3 Years of Age (½ Tablet)	%Daily Value for Adults and Children 4 Years of Age and older (1 Tablet)
Total Carbohydrate <1 g	**	<1%*
Vitamin A 3000 IU (33% as beta-carotene)	60%	60%
Vitamin C 60 mg	75%	100%
Vitamin D 400 IU	50%	100%
Vitamin E 30 IU	150%	100%
Thiamin (B₁) 1.5 mg	107%	100%
Riboflavin (B₂) 1.7 mg	106%	100%
Niacin 15 mg	83%	75%
Vitamin B₆ 2 mg	143%	100%
Folic Acid 400 mcg	100%	100%
Vitamin B₁₂ 6 mcg	100%	100%
Biotin 40 mcg	13%	13%
Pantothenic Acid 10 mg	100%	100%
Calcium (elemental) 100 mg	6%	10%
Iron 18 mg	90%	100%
Phosphorus 100 mg	6%	10%
Iodine 150 mcg	107%	100%
Magnesium 20 mg	5%	5%
Zinc 12 mg	75%	80%
Copper 2 mg	100%	100%
Sodium 10 mg	**	<1%
Choline 38 mg	**	**

* Percent Daily Values are based on a 2,000 calorie diet.
** Daily value not established.

Ingredients: Sorbitol, Dicalcium Phosphate, Magnesium Phosphate, Choline Bitartrate, Sodium Ascorbate, Ferrous Fumarate, Gelatin, Natural & Artificial Flavors (including fruit acids), Pregelatinized Starch, Vitamin E Acetate, Stearic Acid, Carrageenan, Hydrogenated Vegetable Oil, Magnesium Stearate, Zinc Oxide, Niacinamide, D-Calcium Pantothenate, FD&C Red #40 Aluminum Lake, FD&C Yellow #6 Aluminum Lake, Xylitol, Aspartame†, FD&C Blue #2 Lake, Cupric Oxide, Pyridoxine Hydrochloride, Sucrose, Riboflavin, Thiamine Mononitrate, Vitamin A Acetate, Beta-Carotene, Monoammonium Glycyrrhizinate, Folic Acid, Soybean Oil, Potassium Iodide, Butylated Hydroxytoluene, Biotin, Vitamin D, Magnesium Oxide, Vitamin B₁₂.

†**PHENYLKETONURICS: CONTAINS PHENYLALANINE**
KEEP OUT OF REACH OF CHILDREN

WARNING: Accidental overdose of iron-containing products is a leading cause of fatal poisoning in children under 6. Keep this product out of reach of children. In case of accidental overdose, call a doctor or Poison Control Center immediately.

Directions: 2 & 3 years of age – **Chew** one-half tablet daily. Adults and children 4 years of age and older – **Chew** one tablet daily.
Store in a cool, dry place. Tightly reseal after each use.

CHILD RESISTANT CAP
Do not use this product if printed safety seal bearing "Bayer HealthCare" under cap is torn or missing.

How Supplied: Available in 60 and 150 tablets
Made in USA
Bayer HealthCare LLC
Consumer Care Division
P.O. Box 1910
Morristown, NJ 07962-1910 USA

Shown in Product Identification Guide, page 504

FLINTSTONES® Gummies
(Bayer Healthcare)

Supplement Facts
Serving Size: 1 Gummy (2 & 3 years of age); 2 gummies (4 years of age and older)
Servings Per Container: *(number of gummies); (number of gummies/2)*

Amount Per 2 Gummies	% Daily Value for Children 2 & 3 Years of Age (1 Gummy)	% Daily Value for Adults and Children 4 Years of Age and older (2 Gummies)
Calories 15		
Total Carbohydrate 3g	**	1%*

Continued on next page

Flintstones Gummies—Cont.

Sugars 3 g	**	**
Vitamin A 2000 IU	40%	40%
Vitamin C 30 mg	38%	50%
Vitamin D 200 IU	25%	50%
Vitamin E 20 IU	100%	67%
Vitamin (B$_6$) 1 mg	71%	50%
Folic Acid 200 mcg	50%	50%
Vitamin B$_{12}$ 5 mcg	83%	83%
Biotin 75 mcg	25%	25%
Pantothenic Acid 5 mg	50%	50%
Iodine 40 mcg	29%	27%
Zinc 2.5 mg	16%	17%
Choline 30 mcg	**	**
Inositol 20 mcg	**	**

* Percent Daily Values are based on a 2,000 calorie diet.
** Daily value not established.

Ingredients: Glucose Syrup, Sucrose, Gelatin, Water, Citric Acid, Ascorbic Acid, Vitamin E Acetate, Modified Starch, D-Calcium Pantothenate, Maltodextrin, Zinc Sulfate, Vegetable Oil, Artificial Flavors, Corn Starch, Acacia Gum, Pyridoxine Hydrochloride, Vitamin A Acetate, Silicon Dioxide, Carnauba Wax, Folic Acid, Vitamin D3 (cholecalciferol), Bees Wax, FD&C Red #40, dl-Alpha-Tocopherol, D-Biotin, Choline Bitartrate, Potassium Iodide, FD&C Yellow #6, Inositol, Vitamin B$_{12}$, FD&C Blue #1.

KEEP OUT OF REACH OF CHILDREN
Not for children under 2 years of age due to risk of choking.

Directions: Children 2 to 3 years of age: **Chew** one gummy daily. Adults and children 4 years of age and older: **Chew** two gummies daily.

CHILD RESISTANT CAP
Do not use this product if safety seal bearing "SEALED for YOUR PROTECTION" under cap is torn or missing.
Made in Germany

How Supplied: Available in 60 ct.
Bayer HealthCare LLC
Consumer Care Division
P.O. Box 1910
Morristown, NJ 07962-1910 USA

Shown in Product Identification Guide, page 504

MY FIRST FLINTSTONES®
(Bayer Healthcare)

Directions: Children 2 & 3 years of age — **Chew** one tablet daily. Tablet should be fully chewed or crushed for children who cannot chew.

Supplement Facts
Serving Size: One tablet

	Amount Per Tablet	% Daily Value for Children 2 & 3 Years of Age
Total Carbohydrate	< 1 g	< 1%*
Sugars	< 1 g	**
Vitamin A (25% as beta carotene)	1998 IU	80%
Vitamin C	69 mg	150%
Vitamin D	400 IU	100%
Vitamin E	15 IU	150%
Thiamin (B$_1$)	1.05 mg	150%
Riboflavin (B$_2$)	1.2 mg	150%
Niacin	10 mg	111%
Vitamin B$_6$	1.05 mg	150%
Folic Acid	300 mcg	150%
Vitamin B$_{12}$	4.5 mcg	150%
Sodium	10 mg	**

* Percent Daily Values are based on a 2,000 calorie diet.
** Daily value not established.

Ingredients: Sucrose (a natural sweetener), Sodium Ascorbate, Invert Sugar, Artificial Flavors (including fruit acids), Stearic Acid, Gelatin, Vitamin E Acetate, Niacinamide, FD&C Red #40 Lake, FD&C Yellow #6 Lake, FD&C Blue #2 Lake, Pyridoxine Hydrochloride, Riboflavin, Thiamine Mononitrate, Vitamin A Acetate, Folic Acid, Soybean Oil, Beta-Carotene, Butylated Hydroxytoluene, Vitamin D, Vitamin B$_{12}$.

KEEP OUT OF REACH OF CHILDREN
CHILD RESISTANT CAP
Do not use this product if printed safety seal bearing "Bayer HealthCare" under cap is torn or missing.

How Supplied: bottles of 60 Chewable Tablets
Made in USA
Bayer HealthCare LLC
Consumer Care Division
P.O. Box 1910
Morristown, NJ 07962-1910 USA

Shown in Product Identification Guide, page 504

FOOD FOR THOUGHT™
(Wellness International)
Choline-Enriched Supplement

Description: Food For Thought™, ideal anytime peak mental performance is needed, contains a proprietary blend of amino acids and choline along with powerful antioxidants and B vitamins that are essential in the production of the acetylcholine, the most abundant neurotransmitter in the body. Adequate acetylcholine is vital because of its role in neuromuscular control and cognitive functioning. Low levels of acetylcholine can contribute to a lack of concentration and forgetfulness, and may interfere with sleep patterns. Food For Thought™ further enhances its effectiveness through the utilization of essential vitamins and minerals required for promoting the synthesis of the brain neurotransmitter serotonin, which is crucial for sleep regulation.

Uses: Food For Thought™ may:
- Increase mental performance and acuity
- Improve neuromuscular control
- Augment physical performance

Directions: As a dietary supplement, add 3/4 cup of chilled water or fruit juice to one packet of mix. Stir briskly. Consume 1–2 times per day. Keep in a cool, dry place. For maximum results, combine this product with one serving of Winrgy®.

Warnings: Not for use by children under the age of 18, pregnant or lactating women. Persons taking medications should seek medical advice before taking this product. Persons with ulcers or a history of ulcers should consult their physician before using a choline supplement. Do not consume more than four servings per day. Avoid the use of antacids containing aluminum with this product.

Ingredients: Carbohydrates 6g, Sugars 6g, Vitamin C 72mg (as Ascorbic Acid), Vitamin E 30 IU (as DL-Alpha Tocopheryl Acetate), Thiamin 2.9mg (as Thiamin Mononitrate), Riboflavin 2.8, Niacin 73mg (as Niacinamide Niacin), Vitamin B6 4.7mg (as Pyridoxine HCL), Vitamin B12 100mg (as Cyanocobalamin), Pantothenic Acid 380mg (as Calcium Pantothenate), Calcium 34mg (as calcium pantothenate), Zinc 2.9mg (as Zinc Gluconate), Copper 0.4mg (as Copper Gluconate), Chromium 250mcg (as Chromium Aspartate), Choline 770mg (as Choline Bitartrate), Glycine 130mg, Lysine 35mg (as L-Lysine HCL), Fructose, Natural Flavors, Silicon Dioxide and Magnesium Gluconate.

How Supplied: One box contains 28 single serving packets.

Additional Information: For additional information on ingredients or uses, please visit www.winltd.com.

These statements have not been evaluated by the Food & Drug Administration. This product is not intended to diagnose, treat, cure or prevent any disease.

IMMUNE²⁶® (Legacy for Life)

Description: immune²⁶ ("hyperimmune" egg) is derived from both the white and the yolk of eggs of hens stimulated with over 26 inactivated pathogens. The polyvalent preparation is primarily bacteria of enteric human origin.

Clinical Background: Upon oral administration, a wide range of immune components, of both a specific and non-specific nature, are passively transferred to the recipient. Although the Igs stay within the lumen, the other components appear to help the body support immune function, modulate autoimmune responses, support and balance cardiovascular function, help maintain healthy cholesterol levels, a vital circulatory system, a functional digestive tract, flexible and healthy joints, and energy levels. immune²⁶ appears to help the body "balance" immune function, rather than "boost" immune function. It may be used concomitantly with prescription medications.

Precautions: Those with known allergies to eggs should consult with a health practitioner before consuming this product.
Note: immune²⁶ is not intended to diagnose, treat, cure, or prevent any disease. These statements have not been evaluated by the Food and Drug Administration.

How Supplied: One serving (4.5g) of immune²⁶ is available as: pure hyperimmune (HIE) egg powder, capsules (9/serving), and as chewable tablets (3/serving). immune²⁶ COMPLETE Support®, with 4.5g of HIE egg, is enriched with essential vitamins, minerals, and protein. immune²⁶ is available for children as Legacy Power Chews, a chewable tablet fortified with vitamins and minerals. immune²⁶, at 4.5g, is the essential ingredient in the high protein, low carbohydrate BALANCE Shake, utilized for weight management and athletic performance. COMPANION for Life pet chewables feature immune²⁶, as well as glucosamine and taurine for optimal pet health. And LEGACY Skincare contains immune²⁶ for healthy, balanced skin.

LACTAID® ORIGINAL STRENGTH CAPLETS (McNeil Consumer)
(lactase enzyme)

LACTAID® FAST ACT CAPLETS AND CHEWABLE TABLETS
(lactase enzyme)

For full product information see page 668.

METAMUCIL® DIETARY FIBER SUPPLEMENT (Procter & Gamble)
[met uh-mū sil]
(psyllium husk)

For full product information see page 650.

BAUSCH & LOMB OCUVITE®
Adult Formula
Eye Vitamin and Mineral Supplement
(Bausch & Lomb)

For full product information see page 706.

BAUSCH & LOMB OCUVITE® LUTEIN
[lu 'teen]
Vitamin and Mineral Supplement
(Bausch & Lomb)

For full product information see page 707.

ONE-A-DAY® Cholesterol Plus
(Bayer Healthcare)
Dietary Supplement

Supplement Facts
Serving Size: One tablet

	Amount Per Serving	% Daily Value
Vitamin A (30% as beta-carotene)	2500 IU	50%
Vitamin C	60 mg	100%
Vitamin D	400 IU	100%
Vitamin E	30 IU	100%
Thiamin (B₁)	1.5 mg	100%
Riboflavin (B₂)	1.7 mg	100%
Niacin	20 mg	100%
Vitamin B₆	2 mg	100%
Folic Acid	400 mcg	100%
Vitamin B₁₂	6 mcg	100%
Biotin	50 mcg	17%
Pantothenic Acid	10 mg	100%
Calcium (elemental)	100 mg	10%
Iodine	150 mcg	100%
Magnesium	100 mg	25%
Zinc	15 mg	100%
Selenium	70 mcg	100%
Copper	2 mg	100%
Manganese	2 mg	100%
Chromium	120 mcg	100%
Molybdenum	75 mcg	100%
Potassium	99 mg	3%
Boron	150 mcg	*
Policosanol (Saccharum officinarum, L.)	10 mg	*

* Daily Value not established.

Ingredients: Calcium Carbonate, Cellulose, Potassium Chloride, Magnesium Oxide, Ascorbic Acid, Gelatin, Dicalcium Phosphate, dl-Alpha-Tocopheryl Acetate, Croscarmellose Sodium, Stearic Acid, Niacinamide, Zinc Oxide, D-Calcium Pantothenate, Acacia, Silicon Dioxide, Crospovidone, Magnesium Stearate, Talc, Corn Starch, Policosanol, Manganese Sulfate, Boron Citrate, Povidone, Cupric Oxide, Pyridoxine Hydrochloride, Polyethylene Glycol, Hypromellose, Thiamine Mononitrate, Riboflavin, Vitamin A Acetate, Chromium Chloride, Folic Acid, Beta-Carotene, Potassium Iodide, Sodium Molybdate, Sodium Selenate, Biotin, Ergocalciferol, Cyanocobalamin.

If pregnant or breast-feeding, ask a health professional before use.
Before using this product, consult a health professional if you are taking medication for anticoagulation (blood thinning), including daily aspirin.
KEEP OUT OF REACH OF CHILDREN

Directions: Adults: One tablet daily, with food.
CHILD RESISTANT CAP
Do not use this product if safety seal bearing "SEALED FOR YOUR PROTECTION" under cap is torn or missing.

How Supplied: Available in 3 sizes:
50 count bottle
100 count bottle
125 count bottle
Distributed by:
Bayer HealthCare LLC
Consumer Care Division
P.O. Box 1910
Morristown, NJ 07962-1910 USA

Shown in Product Identification Guide, page 504

ONE-A-DAY® Men's Health Formula
(Bayer Healthcare)

Directions: Adults: One tablet daily, with food.

Supplement Facts
Serving Size: One tablet

	Amount Per Serving	% Daily Value
Vitamin A (14% as beta-carotene)	3500 IU	70%
Vitamin C	90 mg	150%
Vitamin D	400 IU	100%
Vitamin E	45 IU	150%
Vitamin K	20 mcg	25%
Thiamin (B₁)	1.2 mg	80%
Riboflavin (B₂)	1.7 mg	100%
Niacin	16 mg	80%

Continued on next page

One-A-Day Men's Health—Cont.

Vitamin B_6	3 mg	150%
Folic Acid	400 mcg	100%
Vitamin B_{12}	18 mcg	300%
Biotin	30 mcg	10%
Pantothenic Acid	5 mg	50%
Calcium (elemental)	210 mg	21%
Magnesium	120 mg	30%
Zinc	15 mg	100%
Selenium	105 mcg	150%
Copper	2 mg	100%
Manganese	2 mg	100%
Chromium	120 mcg	100%
Potassium	100 mg	3%
Lycopene	600 mcg	*

* Daily Value not established.

Ingredients: Calcium Carbonate, Magnesium Oxide, Potassium Chloride, Cellulose, Ascorbic Acid, dl-Alpha-Tocopheryl Acetate, Gelatin, Croscarmellose Sodium, Acacia, Dicalcium Phosphate, Zinc Oxide, Niacinamide, Stearic Acid, Silicon Dioxide, Dextrin, Magnesium Stearate, Corn Starch, D-Calcium Pantothenate, Manganese Sulfate, Calcium Silicate, Pyridoxine Hydrochloride, Sucrose, Hypromellose, Cupric Oxide, Resin, Glucose, Riboflavin, Thiamine Mononitrate, Vitamin A Acetate, Dextrose, Lecithin, Chromium Chloride, Lycopene, Sodium Carboxymethylcellulose, Folic Acid, Ascorbyl Palmitate, Beta-Carotene, Sodium Selenate, Sodium Ascorbate, Sodium Citrate, dl-Alpha-Tocopherol, Biotin, Phytonadione, Cyanocobalamin, Tricalcium Phosphate, Ergocalciferol.

Contains: Fish (cod, pollock, haddock, hake, cusk, redfish) and soy.

KEEP OUT OF REACH OF CHILDREN

CHILD RESISTANT CAP

Do not use this product if safety seal bearing "SEALED FOR YOUR PROTECTION" under cap is torn or missing.

How Supplied: Available in 4 sizes:
60 count bottle
100 count bottle
200 count bottle
250 count bottle
Made in USA
Distributed by:
Bayer HealthCare LLC
Consumer Care Division
P.O. Box 1910
Morristown, NJ 07962-1910 USA

Shown in Product Identification Guide, page 504

ONE-A-DAY® WEIGHT SMART
(Bayer Healthcare)
Dietary Supplement

Supplement Facts
Serving Size: One tablet

	Amount Per Serving	% Daily Value
Vitamin A (100% as beta-carotene)	2500 IU	50%
Vitamin C	60 mg	100%
Vitamin D	400 IU	100%
Vitamin E	30 IU	100%
Vitamin K	80 mcg	100%
Thiamin (B_1)	1.9 mg	127%
Riboflavin (B_2)	2.125 mg	125%
Niacin	25 mg	125%
Vitamin B_6	2.5 mg	125%
Folic Acid	400 mcg	100%
Vitamin B_{12}	7.5 mcg	125%
Pantothenic Acid	12.5 mg	125%
Calcium (elemental)	300 mg	30%
Iron	18 mg	100%
Magnesium	50 mg	12%
Zinc	15 mg	100%
Selenium	70 mcg	100%
Copper	2 mg	100%
Manganese	2 mg	100%
Chromium	200 mcg	167%
EGCG (from Green Tea Extract, *camellia sinensis* leaf)	32 mg	*

* Daily Value not established.

Ingredients: Calcium Carbonate, Cellulose, Green Tea Extract (leaf), Magnesium Oxide, Ascorbic Acid, Ferrous Fumarate, Acacia, Sodium Starch Glycolate, dl-Alpha-Tocopheryl Acetate, Niacinamide, Croscarmellose Sodium, Zinc Oxide, Dicalcium Phosphate, Dextrin, D-Calcium Pantothenate, Caffeine Powder, Silicon Dioxide, Hypromellose, Magnesium Stearate, Titanium Dioxide, Gelatin, Corn Starch, Glucose, Crospovidone, Calcium Silicate, Manganese Sulfate, Cupric Sulfate, Polyethylene Glycol, Pyridoxine Hydrochloride, Riboflavin, Dextrose, Thiamine Mononitrate, Lecithin, Beta-Carotene, Chromium Chloride, Resin, Folic Acid, FD&C Blue #1 Lake, Sodium Selenate, Phytonadione, Tricalcium Phosphate, Cholecalciferol, Cyanocobalamin.

Contains: fish (cod, pollock, haddock, hake, cusk, redfish) and soy

> **Warning:** Accidental overdose of iron-containing products is a leading cause of fatal poisoning in children under 6. Keep this product out of reach of children. In case of accidental overdose, call a doctor or Poison Control Center immediately.

If pregnant or breast-feeding, ask a health professional before use.
KEEP OUT OF REACH OF CHILDREN

Directions: Adults: One tablet daily, with food.
CHILD RESISTANT CAP
Do not use this product if safety seal bearing "SEALED for YOUR PROTECTION" under cap is torn or missing.

How Supplied: Available in 4 sizes:
50 count bottle
100 count bottle
125 count bottle
175 count bottle
Made in U.S.A.
Distributed by:
Bayer HealthCare LLC
Consumer Care Division
P.O. Box 1910
Morristown, NJ 07962-1910 USA

Shown in Product Identification Guide, page 504

ONE-A-DAY® Women's
(Bayer Healthcare)

Directions: Adults: One tablet daily, with food.

Supplement Facts
Serving Size: One tablet

	Amount Per Serving	% Daily Value
Vitamin A (20% as beta carotene)	2500 IU	50%
Vitamin C	60 mg	100%
Vitamin D	400 IU	100%
Vitamin E	30 IU	100%
Vitamin K	25 mcg	31%
Thiamin (B_1)	1.5 mg	100%
Riboflavin (B_2)	1.7 mg	100%
Niacin	10 mg	50%
Vitamin B_6	2 mg	100%
Folic Acid	400 mcg	100%
Vitamin B_{12}	6 mcg	100%
Biotin	30 mcg	10%
Pantothenic Acid	5 mg	50%

Calcium (elemental)	450 mg	45%
Iron	18 mg	100%
Magnesium	50 mg	13%
Zinc	15 mg	100%
Selenium	20 mcg	29%
Copper	2 mg	100%
Manganese	2 mg	100%
Chromium	120 mcg	100%

Ingredients: Calcium Carbonate, Cellulose, Magnesium Oxide, Ascorbic Acid, Ferrous Fumarate, Corn Starch, Maltodextrin, dl-Alpha-Tocopheryl Acetate, Acacia, Croscarmellose Sodium, Zinc Oxide, Titanium Dioxide, Dextrin, Hypromellose, Magnesium Stearate, Dicalcium Phosphate, Niacinamide, Silicon Dioxide, D-Calcium Pantothenate, Manganese Sulfate, Gelatin, Polyethylene Glycol, Cupric Sulfate, Dextrose, Pyridoxine Hydrochloride, Glucose, Lecithin, Riboflavin, Thiamine Mononitrate, Vitamin A Acetate, Chromium Chloride, Folic Acid, Beta-Carotene, FD&C Yellow #5 (tartrazine) Lake, FD&C Yellow #6 Lake, Sodium Selenate, Biotin, Phytonadione, FD&C Blue #2 Lake, Tricalcium Phosphate, Cholecalciferol, Cyanocobalamin.

Contains: Fish (cod, pollock, haddock, hake, cusk, redfish) and soy.

WARNING: Accidental overdose of iron-containing products is a leading cause of fatal poisoning in children under 6. Keep this product out of reach of children. In case of accidental overdose, call a doctor or Poison Control Center immediately.

CHILD RESISTANT CAP
Do not use this product if safety seal bearing "SEALED FOR YOUR PROTECTION" under cap is torn or missing.

How Supplied: Available in 4 sizes:
60 count bottle
100 count bottle
200 count bottle
250 count bottle
Made in U.S.A.
Distributed by:
Bayer HealthCare LLC
Consumer Care Division
P.O. Box 1910
Morristown, NJ 07962-1910 USA

Shown in Product Identification Guide, page 504

OS-CAL® 250 + D
(GlaxoSmithKline Consumer)
Calcium with Vitamin D Supplement

Description: Calcium supplement to help reduce the risk of osteoporosis (see below*). Also contains Vitamin D.

Amount Per Tablet	% Daily Value for Pregnant or Lactating Women	% Daily Value for Adults and Children 4 or More Years of Age
Vitamin D 125 IU	31%	31%
Calcium 250 mg	19%	25%

Amount Per Tablet	% Daily Value for Pregnant or Lactating Women	% Daily Value for Adults and children 4 or more years of age
Calcium 500 mg	38%	50%

Supplement Facts
Serving Size 1 Tablet

Amount Per Tablet	% Daily Value for Pregnant or Lactating Women	% Daily Value for Adults and Children 4 or more years of age
Vitamin D 200 IU	50%	50%
Calcium 500 mg	38%	50%

Supplement Facts   Serving Size 1 Tablet
[See first table above]

Ingredients: Oyster shell powder, corn syrup solids, talc, corn starch, hypromellose. Contains less than 1% of calcium stearate, polysorbate 80, titanium dioxide, polyethylene glycol, Vitamin D, propylparaben and methylparaben (preservative), simethicone, yellow 5 lake, blue 1 lake, carnauba wax, edetate sodium.

Directions: One tablet three times a day with meals, or as recommended by your physician.

How Supplied: Bottle of 100 and 240 tablets
Store at room temperature.
Keep out of reach of children.

*Osteoporosis affects middle-aged and older persons, especially Caucasian and Asian women, and those whose families tend to have fragile bones in later years. A lifetime of regular exercise and eating a healthful diet that includes enough calcium, especially during teen and early adult years, builds and maintains good bone health and may reduce the risk of osteoporosis in later life. Adequate calcium intake is important, but daily intakes above 2000 mg are not likely to provide any additional benefit.

Shown in Product Identification Guide, page 506

OS-CAL® 500
(GlaxoSmithKline Consumer)
Calcium Supplement

Description: Calcium supplement to help reduce the risk of osteoporosis. Osteoporosis affects middle-aged and older persons, especially Caucasian and Asian women, and those whose families tend to have fragile bones in later years. A lifetime of regular exercise and eating a healthful diet that includes enough calcium, especially during teen and early adult years, builds and maintains good bone health and may reduce the risk of osteoporosis in later life. Adequate calcium intake is important, but daily intakes above 2000 mg are not likely to provide any additional benefit.

Supplement Facts
Serving Size 1 Tablet
[See second table above]

Ingredients: Oyster shell powder, corn syrup solids, talc, corn starch. Contains less than 1% of sodium starch glycolate, calcium stearate, polysorbate 80, hypromellose, polydextrose, titanium dioxide, propylparaben and methylparaben (preservative), triacetin, yellow 5 lake, blue 1 lake, polyethylene glycol, carnauba wax.

Directions: One tablet two to three times a day with meals, or as recommended by your physician.

How Supplied: Bottles of 75 and 160 tablets
Store at room temperature.
Keep out of reach of children.

Shown in Product Identification Guide, page 506

OS-CAL® 500 + D
(GlaxoSmithKline Consumer)
Calcium with Vitamin D Supplement

Description: Calcium supplement to help reduce the risk of osteoporosis (see below*). Also contains Vitamin D.

[See third table above]

Ingredients: Oyster shell powder, corn syrup solids, talc, corn starch. Contains less than 1% of sodium starch glycolate, calcium stearate, polysorbate 80, hypromellose, polydextrose, titanium dioxide,

Continued on next page

Os-Cal 500 + D—Cont.

Vitamin D, propylparaben and methylparaben (preservative), triacetin, yellow 5 lake, blue 1 lake, polyethylene glycol, carnauba wax.

Directions: One tablet two to three times a day with meals, or as recommended by your physician.

How Supplied: Bottle of 75 and 160 tablets
Store at room temperature.
Keep out of reach of children.
*Osteoporosis affects middle-aged and older persons, especially Caucasian and Asian women, and those whose families tend to have fragile bones in later years. A lifetime of regular exercise and eating a healthful diet that includes enough calcium, especially during teen and early adult years, builds and maintains good bone health and may reduce the risk of osteoporosis in later life.
Adequate calcium intake is important, but daily intakes above 2000 mg are not likely to provide any additional benefit.

Shown in Product Identification Guide, page 506

OS-CAL® CHEWABLE
(GlaxoSmithKline Consumer)
Calcium Supplement

Description: Calcium supplement to help reduce the risk of osteoporosis. Osteoporosis affects middle-aged and older persons, especially Caucasian and Asian women, and those whose families tend to have fragile bones in later years. A lifetime of regular exercise and eating a healthful diet that includes enough calcium, especially during teen and early adult years, builds and maintains good bone health and may reduce the risk of osteoporosis in later life.
Adequate calcium intake is important, but daily intakes above 2000 mg are not likely to provide any additional benefit.
[See table below]

Ingredients: Calcium carbonate, dextrose monohydrate, maltodextrin, microcrystalline cellulose, magnesium stearate, artificial flavors, sodium chloride.
Each tablet provides 500 mg of elemental calcium

Directions: One tablet two to three times a day with meals, or as recommended by your physician.

How Supplied: Bottle of 60 tablets
Store at room temperature.

Keep out of reach of children.
Shown in Product Identification Guide, page 506

PERIDIN-C®
Vitamin C Supplement
(Beutlich LP)

Dietary supplement helps alleviate hot flashes by improving capillary strength and maintaining vascular integrity, reducing the physiologic potential for flushing.[*]
Suggested Use for Hot Flashes[*] - 2 tablets, 3 times per day after meals. Reduce servings gradually after one month until effective daily intake is determined.

Ingredients:
Vitamin C (as ascorbic acid) – 200 mg.
Natural Citrus Bioflavonoids Complex (as Hesperidin Complex standardized to contain 45% total bioflavonoids) – 150 mg.
Natural Citrus Bioflavonoid (as Hesperidin Methyl Chalcone) – 50 mg.

Other Ingredients: hypromellose, microcrystalline cellulose, crospovidone, stearic acid, polydextrose, titanium dioxide, yellow 6 lake, polyethylene glycol, magnesium stearate, silicon dioxide, triacetin, carnauba wax and polysorbate 80.

How Supplied:
Bottles of 100 tablets – Product # 0283–0597–01

---

*This statement has not been evaluated by the Food and Drug Administration. This product is not intended to diagnose, treat, cure or prevent any disease.

PREMCAL
(Dannmarie)

Description: PremCal is a combination calcium and vitamin D nutritional supplement that offers three different strengths of vitamin D3 per tablet- 500 IU, 1000 IU, and 2000 IU with 500 mg of elemental calcium as the carbonate. PremCal is indicated in those requiring higher than the currently recommended doses of vitamin D such as vitamin D deficiency, premenstrual syndrome, osteoporosis, osteomalacia or malabsorption.

Ingredients: PremCal tablets are supplied in 3 different strengths of vitamin D3 (Light- 500 IU; Regular- 1000 IU; Extra

strength -2000 IU) with a constant amount of calcium 500 mg as calcium carbonate and 15 mg of magnesium oxide. Each tablet also contains hypromellose, croscarmellose sodium, malto dextrin, povidone, stearic acid, magnesium stearate, triacetin, polyethylene glycol, silicon dioxide. Free of sugar, soy, wheat, gluten, corn, shellfish, and artificial colors.

Directions: One tablet two times a day with meals or as recommended by your physician.

Warnings: Do not take more than two tablets per day unless directed by your physician. Do not use with prolonged or intense exposure to sunlight unless directed by your physician. Do not use if you have a calcium disorder such as primary hyperparathyroidism, hypercalciuria, elevated calcium levels, kidney stones or kidney disease without consulting your physician.

How Supplied: PremCal Light, Regular and Extra strength are supplied in bottles of 180 tablets. UPC#8-80569-00013-6 (PremCal-Light):UPC#8-80569-00010-5 (PremCal-Regular): UPC#8-80569-00016-7 (PremCal-Extra strength).

PURETRIM™ MEDITERRANEAN WELLNESS SHAKE
(Awareness Corporation)

Description: Vegetarian Natural Wholefood High Protein Low Carb Energy Shake. No Dairy, No Soy

Ingredients: Vegetable Pea & Brown Rice Protein, Antioxidants, Prebiotics, Essential Fatty Acids & Enzyme Active Greens

Directions: Mix contents in 10 oz. of cold water.

Warnings: Not for use by pregnant or lactating women. Must be 18 years or older to use.

How Supplied: 10 Packets (Net Wt 500 g)
Shown in Product Identification Guide, page 503

SLOW FE®
(Novartis Consumer Health, Inc.)
Slow Release Iron Tablets

Supplement Facts

Serving Size	1 Tablet
Amount Per Tablet	**%Daily Value**
160 mg dried ferrous sulfate, USP (equivalent to 47.5 mg elemental iron)	264%

Description:
SLOW FE® with its unique controlled delivery system gives you the high potency iron you need with the gentleness you want.

Supplement Facts
Serving Size 1 Tablet

Amount Per Serving	% Daily Value for Pregnant or Lactating Women	% Daily Value for Adults and Children 4 or more years of age
Calories 5		
Calcium 500 mg	38%	50%

- *Gentle to Your System*–clinically shown to reduce the side effects (constipation and abdominal discomfort) common to iron use.
- *Doctor Recommended Ingredient*– SLOW FE contains ferrous sulfate, the ingredient most recommended by doctors.
- *Small Tablet*–once a day dosage easy-to-swallow SLOW FE provides the high dose of iron your body needs.

Other Ingredients: lactose, hypromellose, talc, magnesium stearate, cetostearyl alcohol, polysorbate 80, titanium dioxide, yellow iron oxide, FD&C blue #2 aluminum lake.

> **WARNING:** Accidental overdose of iron-containing products is a leading cause of fatal poisoning in children under 6. **Keep this product out of reach of children.** In case of accidental overdose, call a doctor or poison control center immediately.

If pregnant or breast-feeding, ask a health care professional before use.
The treatment of any anemic condition should be under the advice and supervision of a doctor. As oral iron products interfere with absorption of oral tetracycline antibiotics, these products should not be taken within two (2) hours of each other.

Iron-containing supplements may occasionally cause bowel effects such as constipation.

Dosage: ADULTS – One or two tablets daily or as recommended by a physician. CHILDREN UNDER 12 – Consult a doctor. Tablets must be swallowed whole.

Blister packaged for your protection. Do not use if individual seals are broken.

Store at controlled room temperature 20°-25°C (68°-77°F). Protect from moisture.

Tablets non-USP (disintegration, content uniformity)
Tablets made in Great Britain

Questions? call **1-800-452-0051** 24 hours a day, 7 days a week.

How Supplied: Available in 30 ct., 60 ct., and 90 ct. cartons.

SLOWFE® WITH FOLIC ACID
(Novartis Consumer Health, Inc.)
Slow Release Iron, Folic Acid Dietary Supplement

Description:
Neural tube defects have many causes. Research has shown that by maintaining an adequate intake of folic acid, a woman in her childbearing years may reduce the risk of conceiving a baby with the birth defects spina bifida or anencephaly. These birth defects that, while not widespread, are extremely significant and may occur in the unborn baby before a woman realizes that she is pregnant. That's why the U.S. Public Health Service is recommend-

ing a daily intake of at least 400 mcg of folic acid for all women capable of becoming pregnant, regardless of when they plan to do so. And while sources of folate include fruits, vegetables, whole grain products, fortified cereals, and dietary supplements, women who do not eat a well-balanced diet or who may be concerned about their diets may choose to obtain folate or folic acid from SlowFe® with Folic Acid. Folic acid consumption should be limited to 1000 mcg per day from all sources.

Supplement Facts

Serving Size	1 Tablet
Servings Per Container	20

Amount Per Tablet		% Daily Value
Folate	350 mcg	87%
Iron (ferrous sulfate 160 mg)	47.5 mg	264%

Other Ingredients: lactose, hydroxypropyl methylcellulose, talc, magnesium stearate, cetostearyl alcohol, polysorbate 80, titanium dioxide, yellow iron oxide.

Dosage: ADULTS – One or two tablets once a day or as recommended by a physician. A maximum of two tablets daily may be taken. CHILDREN UNDER 12 – Consult a physician. Tablets must be swallowed whole.

Warning: The treatment of any anemic condition should be under the advice and supervision of a physician. As oral iron products interfere with absorption of oral tetracycline antibiotics, these products should not be taken within two hours of each other. Intake of folic acid from all sources should be limited to 1000 mcg per day to prevent the masking of Vitamin B12 deficiencies. Should you become pregnant while using this product, consult a physician as soon as possible about good prenatal care and the continued use of this product. If you are already pregnant or nursing a baby, seek the advice of a health care professional before using this product.

> **Warning:** Accidental overdose of iron-containing products is a leading cause of fatal poisoning in children under 6. Keep this product out of reach of children. In case of accidental overdose, call a doctor or poison control center immediately.

> **Child Resistant**
> Blister packaged for your protection. Do not use if individual seals are broken.

Questions? call **1-800-452-0051** 24 hours a day, 7 days a week.

Other Information:
Store at controlled room temperature 20°-25°C (68°-77°F). Protect from moisture.

How Supplied:
Available in 20ct. cartons.
Shown in Product Identification Guide, page 515

STEPHAN™ CLARITY®
(Wellness International)
Nutritional Supplement

Description: StePHan™ Clarity®, contains specific vitamins, minerals, amino acids and nutrients important for memory and concentration. Key ingredients such as lecithin, glutamic acid and ginkgo biloba promote increased brain functioning. These nutrients provide fuel for the brain as well as increased blood flow to the entire central nervous system. These ingredients and their effects ensure that StePHan™ Clarity® is a natural and effective way to better one's health.

Uses: StePHan™ Clarity® may:
- Improve memory and concentration
- Enhance metabolism of carbohydrates and fats
- Detoxify

Directions: As a dietary supplement, take one or more capsules daily as needed.

Warnings: CAUTION PHENYLKE-TONURICS: Contains 9.2 mg phenylalanine per serving.

Ingredients: Proprietary blend (Lecithin, Bee Pollen, L-Glutamic Acid, Ribonucleic Acid Yeast, L-Aspartic Acid, L-Arginine HCL, L-Leucine, L-Lysine HCL, L Phenylalanine, L-Serine, L-Proline, L Valine, L Isoleucine, L-Alanine, L-Glycine, L Threonine, L-Tyrosine, L-Histidine, L Cysteine HCL, L-Methionine, Adenosine Triphosphate, Ginkgo Biloba 50:1 Extract), Hydroxypropylmethylcellulose, DL-Alpha Tocopheryl Acetate, Ascorbic Acid, Niacinamide, Stearic Acid, Ethylcellulose, Vitamin A Acetate, D-Calcium Pantothenate, Thiamine HCL, Silicon Dioxide, Dicalcium Phosphate, Pyridoxine HCL, Riboflavin, Folic Acid, Cholecalciferol, Biotin, Cyancobalamin.

How Supplied: One bottle contains 60 easy-to-swallow capsules.

Additional Information: For additional information on ingredients or uses, please visit www.winltd.com.

These statements have not been evaluated by the Food & Drug Administration. This product is not intended to diagnose, treat, cure or prevent any disease.

STEPHAN™ ELASTICITY®
(Wellness International)
Nutritional Supplement

Description: StePHan™ Elasticity® contains a scientifically balanced mixture

Continued on next page

StePHan Elasticity—Cont.

of specific amino acids and nutrients established as important for skin tone and texture. Vitamin A and selenium, two key ingredients known for their antioxidant properties, help protect the skin from premature aging and provide a protective effect against sun damage that can later lead to skin cancer.

Uses: StePHan™ Elasticity® may:
• Improve skin tone and texture
• Reduce premature skin aging
• Reduce risk of certain types of skin cancers

Directions: As a dietary supplement, take one or more capsules daily as needed.

Warnings: Accidental overdose of iron-containing products is a leading cause of fatal poisoning in children under 6. Keep this product out of reach of children. In case of accidental overdose, call a doctor or poison control center immediately.

Ingredients: Proprietary Blend (Shavegrass Herb, L-Glutamic Acid, Bladderwrack Extract, Ribonucleic Acid Yeast, L-Aspartic Acid, L-Arginine HCL, L-Leucine, L-Lysine HCL, L-Phenylalanine, L-Serine, L-Proline, L-Valine, L-Isoleucine, L-Alanine, L-Glycine, L-Threonine, L-Tyrosine, L-Histidine, L-Cysteine HCL, L-Methionine, Adenosine Triphosphate), Hydroxypropylmethylcellulose, DL-Alpha Tocopheryl Acetate, Ascorbic Acid, Ethylcellulose, Stearic Acid, Silicon Dioxide, Calcium Amino Acid Chelate, Manganese Amino Acid Chelate, Iron Amino Acid Chelate, Magnesium Amino Acid Chelate, Zinc Amino Acid Chelate, Vitamin A Acetate, Selenium Amino Acid Chelate, Chromium Amino Acid Chelate.

How Supplied: One bottle contains 60 easy-to-swallow capsules.

Additional Information: For additional information on ingredients or uses, please visit www.winltd.com.

These statements have not been evaluated by the Food & Drug Administration. This product is not intended to diagnose, treat, cure or prevent any disease.

STEPHAN™ ESSENTIAL®
(Wellness International)
Nutritional Supplement

Description: StePHan™ Essential® contains specific vitamins, minerals, herbs and amino acids that are proactive to cardiovascular and circulatory management. Two primary ingredients, L-carnitine and vitamin E, provide increased energy utilization in the heart and skeletal muscles as well as protective antioxidant effects, thereby reducing certain types of cellular cardiovascular damage. Another key ingredient, linoleic acid, also provides protection against coronary heart disease by lowering serum cholesterol levels and decreasing platelet stickiness.

Uses: StePHan™ Essential® may:
• Protect against cardiovascular disease
• Lower serum cholesterol
• Decrease platelet aggregation and stickiness
• Increase immune system integrity
• Aid in therapy for certain neurologic disorders

Directions: As a dietary supplement, take one or more capsules daily as needed.

Warnings: CAUTION PHENYLKETONURICS: Contains 6.9 mg phenylalanine per serving.

Ingredients: Proprietary Blend (Isolated Soy Protein, L-Carnitine Bitartrate, Bee Pollen, Marine Lipid Concentrate, Ribonucleic Acid Yeast, Adenosine Triphosphate), Hydroxypropylmethylcellulose, Magnesium Amino Acid Chelate, Starch, D-Alpha Tocopheryl Succinate, Selenium Amino Acid Chelate, Silicon Dioxide.

How Supplied: One bottle contains 60 easy-to-swallow capsules.

Additional Information: For additional information on ingredients or uses, please visit www.winltd.com.

These statements have not been evaluated by the Food & Drug Administration. This product is not intended to diagnose, treat, cure or prevent any disease.

STEPHAN™ FLEXIBILITY®
(Wellness International)
Nutritional Supplement

Description: StePHan™ Flexibility® is rich in vitamins, minerals and amino acids recognized as beneficial to the health of joints and soft tissues. Two important amino acids utilized in StePHan™ Flexibility® include glycine and histidine. These amino acids are known to improve neuromuscular control as well as provide relief from symptoms associated with rheumatoid arthritis. Boron, another key ingredient, is vital in protecting joints from mineral losses and vitamin E is added to reduce muscular cramps and spasms.

Uses: StePHan™ Flexibility® may:
• Increase integrity of joints and their soft tissues
• Minimize bone loss by reducing excretion of calcium and magnesium
• Decrease symptoms associated with rheumatoid arthritis
• Relieve muscular cramps and spasms

Directions: As a dietary supplement, take one or more capsules daily as needed.

Warnings: CAUTION PHENYLKETONURICS: Contains 9.2 mg phenylalanine per serving.

Ingredients: Proprietary Blend (Boron Gluconate, L-Glutamic Acid, Ribonucleic Acid Yeast, L-Aspartic Acid, L-Arginine HCL, L-Leucine, L-Lysine HCL, Bee Pollen, L-Phenylalanine, L-Serine, L-Proline, L-Valine, L-Isoleucine, L-Alanine, L-Glycine, L-Threonine, L-Tyrosine, L-Histidine, L-Cysteine HCL, L-Methionine, Adenosine Triphosphate), Hydroxypropylmethylcellulose, Zinc Amino Acid Chelate, Calcium Amino Acid Chelate, Stearic Acid, Ascorbic Acid, Whey, D-Alpha Tocopheryl Succinate, Magnesium Stearate, Niacinamide, Silicon Dioxide, Cellulose, Vitamin A Palmitate, D-Calcium Pantothenate, Thiamine HCL, Dicalcium Phosphate, Pyridoxine HCL, Riboflavin, Folic Acid, Selenomethionine, Cholecalciferol, Biotin, Cyanocobalamin.

How Supplied: One bottle contains 60 easy-to-swallow capsules.

Additional Information: For additional information on ingredients or uses, please visit www.winltd.com.

These statements have not been evaluated by the Food & Drug Administration. This product is not intended to diagnose, treat, cure, or prevent and disease.

STEPHAN™ LOVPIL™
(Wellness International)
Nutritional Supplement

Description: StePHan™ Lovpil™ is a nutritional supplement formulated with vitamins, minerals, herbs and amino acids recognized as important for general health and sexual vitality. Damiana, typically thought of as an aphrodisiac by those who are familiar with its effects, is an important ingredient utilized in StePHan™ Lovpil™ and is known for its stimulating properties on male virility and libido. Two other key ingredients, arginine and vitamin C, are essential in maintaining healthy sperm counts and protecting sperm from oxidative DNA damage.

Uses: StePHan™ Lovpil™ may:
• Increase overall health and well-being
• Improve sexual vitality and libido

Directions: As a dietary supplement, take one or more capsules daily as needed.

Ingredients: Proprietary Blend (Damiana Leaf, Isolated Soy Protein, Ribonucleic Acid Yeast, Adenosine Triphosphate), Calcium Carbonate, Hydroxypropylmethylcellulose, Ascorbic Acid, Stearic Acid, Zinc Amino Acid Chelate, Magnesium Stearate, Manganese Amino Acid Chelate, Silicon Dioxide, Vitamin A Acetate, Dicalcium Phosphate, Cholecalciferol, Folic acid, Selenomethionine, Cyanocobalamin.

How Supplied: One bottle contains 60 easy-to-swallow capsules.

Additional Information: For additional information on ingredients or uses, please visit www.winltd.com.

These statements have not been evaluated by the Food & Drug Administration. This product

is not intended to diagnose, treat, cure or prevent any disease.

STEPHAN™ MASCULINE®
(Wellness International)
Nutritional Supplement

Description: StePHan™ Masculine® contains a special blend of nutrients with vitamins, minerals, herbs and amino acids shown to be essential for healthy male reproductive systems. Zinc, a key ingredient in StePHan™ Masculine®, is important in maintaining healthy testosterone levels. A deficiency in this mineral often results in regression of the male sex glands, decreased sexual interest, mental lethargy, emotional problems and even poor appetite. In males with only a mild zinc deficiency, zinc supplementation was accompanied by increased sperm count and plasma testosterone.

Uses: StePHan™ Masculine® may:
- Ensure overall health of the male reproductive system
- Enhance libido
- Decrease mental lethargy and emotional problems
- Increase sperm count and plasma testosterone

Directions: As a dietary supplement, take one or more capsules daily as needed.

Ingredients: Proprietary Blend (L-Histidine, Bee Pollen, Parsley Leaf, Ribonucleic Acid, Adenosine Triphosphate), Calcium Carbonate, Zinc Amino Acid Chelate, Hydroxypropylmethylcellulose, Magnesium Amino Acid Chelate, Stearic Acid, Magnesium Stearate.

How Supplied: One bottle contains 60 easy-to-swallow capsules.

Additional Information: For additional information on ingredients or uses, please visit www.winltd.com.

These statements have not been evaluated by the Food & Drug Administration. This product is not intended to diagnose, treat, cure or prevent any disease.

STEPHAN™ PROTECTOR®
(Wellness International)
Nutritional Supplement

Description: StePHan™ Protector® is a nutritional supplement that combines specific vitamins, minerals and amino acids recognized as important for the health of areas associated with the human immune system. Astragalus is a key ingredient known for improving immune system integrity by relieving stress-induced immune system suppression. Additionally, research indicates that kelp supplies dozens of important nutrients for improved cardiovascular health and function.

Uses: StePHan™ Protector® may:
- Strengthen the immune and digestive systems
- Function as an adaptogen to reduce stress-induced immune system suppression
- Improve cardiovascular health

Directions: As a dietary supplement, take one or more capsules daily as needed.

Warnings: CAUTION PHENYLKETONURICS: Contains 9.2 mg phenylalanine per serving.

Ingredients: Proprietary Blend (Isolated Soy Protein, Astragalus Root, Bee Pollen, Kelp, Ribonucleic Acid Yeast, Adenosine Triphosphate), Hydroxypropylmethylcellulose, Cellulose, Stearic acid, Magnesium Stearate, Silicon Dioxide.

How Supplied: One bottle contains 60 easy-to-swallow capsules.

Additional Information: For additional information on ingredients or uses, please visit www.winltd.com.

These statements have not been evaluated by the Food & Drug Administration. This product is not intended to diagnose, treat, cure or prevent any disease.

STEPHAN™ RELIEF®
(Wellness International)
Nutritional Supplement

Description: StePHan™ Relief® is formulated with a special combination of nutrients, vitamins, minerals, amino acids and herbs recognized as important to the digestive and excretory systems. Parsley, a key ingredient in StePHan™ Relief®, aids digestion with its carminative effects. Also included is psyllium, a gel-forming fiber that promotes both bowel regularity and healthy cholesterol levels.

Uses: StePHan™ Relief® may:
- Aid digestion
- Help maintain bowel regularity
- Prevent flatulence
- Promote healthy cholesterol levels

Directions: As a dietary supplement, take one or more capsules daily as needed.

Ingredients: Proprietary Blend (Psyllium Seed Powder, L-Isoleucine, L-Leucine, L-Valine, Bee Pollen, Bladderwrack Herb 5:1 Extract, Parsley Leaf 4:1 Extract, Ribonucleic Acid Yeast, Adenosine Triphosphate), Hydroxypropylmethylcellulose, Starch, D-Calcium Pantothenate, Silicon Dioxide.

How Supplied: One bottle contains 60 easy-to-swallow capsules.

Additional Information: For additional information on ingredients or uses, please visit www.winltd.com.

These statements have not been evaluated by the Food & Drug Administration. This product is not intended to diagnose, treat, cure or prevent any disease.

STEPHAN™ TRANQUILITY™
(Wellness International)
Nutritional Supplement

Description: StePHan™ Tranquility™ is a nutritional supplement which contains a blend of vitamins, minerals and amino acids recognized as important to areas involved in stress management. Two primary ingredients are myo-inositol and valerian root, both of which exert beneficial effects on insomnia and anxiety. Additionally, myo-inositol has been shown to lower serum triglyceride and cholesterol levels.

Uses: StePHan™ Tranquility™ may:
- Lower serum triglycerides and cholesterol
- Reduce periods of insomnia and anxiety
- Produce a mild sedative effect

Directions: As a dietary supplement, take one or more capsules daily as needed.

Warnings: CAUTION PHENYLKETONURICS: Contains 9.2 mg phenylalanine per serving.

Ingredients: Proprietary Blend (Isolated Soy Protein, Choline Bitartrate, Inositol, Lecithin, Ribonucelic Acid Yeast, Valerian Root Extract, Adenosine Triphosphate), Hydroxypropylmethylcellulose, DL-Alpha Tocopheryl Acetate, Calcium Aspartate, Silicon Dioxide, Ascorbic Acid, Stearic Acid, Niacinamide, Magnesium Amino Acid Chelate, Vitamin A Palmitate, Hydroxypropylcellulose, D-Calcium Pantothenate, Thiamine HCL, Dicalcium Phosphate, Pyridoxine HCL, Riboflavin, Folic Acid, Cholecalciferol, Biotin, Cyanocobalamin.

How Supplied: One bottle contains 60 easy-to-swallow capsules.

Additional Information: For additional information on ingredients or uses, please visit www.winltd.com.

These statements have not been evaluated by the Food & Drug Administration. This product is not intended to diagnose, treat, cure or prevent any disease.

SURE2ENDURE™
(Wellness International)
Herbal, Vitamin and Mineral Workout Supplement

Description: Sure2Endure™ is formulated to enhance the body's endurance, stamina, and ability to recover through an innovative blend of herbs, vitamins and minerals. Among these specially selected ingredients is ciwujia, known to alleviate fatigue and boost the immune system. This herb has been shown to improve overall performance in aerobic exercise, endurance activities and weight lifting without any stimulant side effects. Ciwujia increases fat metabolism during

Continued on next page

Sure2Endure—Cont.

exercise by shifting toward the use of fat as an energy source instead of carbohydrates. Additionally, this herb improves endurance by reducing lactic acid production thereby delaying fatigue that can often lead to muscle pain and cramps. Sure2Endure™ also provides antioxidant coverage and enzyme cofactors to meet the high demands that exercise places on the body. These antioxidants and cofactors scavenge free radicals formed during exercise as well as enhance carbohydrate metabolism, further leading to increased physical performance. Since tissue stress and damage are often the result of strenuous exercise, it is important to maintain proper integrity and recovery of connective tissue. To protect joints from exercise and ensure healthy connective tissue, Glucosamine is a key ingredient in Sure2Endure™. In addition to promoting healthy connective tissue, natural anti-inflammatory compounds bromelain and boswellia are included to further prove beneficial to the health of joint and soft tissues.

Uses: Sure2Endure™ may:

• Increase physical endurance and stamina
• Decrease post-exercise recovery time
• Reduce fatigue
• Alleviate muscle pain and cramps
• Improve joint integrity
• Reduce free-radical formation (antioxidant)
• Enhance carbohydrate metabolism

Directions: As a dietary supplement, take three tablets one hour prior to exercise. For optimum performance, use in conjunction with BioLean II® or BioLean Free® one hour before exercise. Phyto-Vite® may be taken with this product to maximize the antioxidant effect necessary with exercise. Mass Appeal™ may also be consumed for maximum effectiveness. Needs may vary with each individual.

Warnings: Not for use by children under the age of 18, pregnant or lactating women. Consult your physician before using this product if you have any medical conditions. Discontinue immediately if allergic symptoms develop. Keep out of reach of children.

Ingredients: Vitamin C 500 mg (as Ascorbic Acid), Vitamin E 100 IU (as D-Alpha Tocopheryl Succinate), Thiamin 10 mg (as Thiamin Mononitrate), Riboflavin 12 mg, Vitamin B6 15 mg (as Pyridoxine HCL), Vitamin B12 20 mcg (as Cyanocobalamin), Chromium 200 mcg (as patented Chelavite® Chromium Dinicotinate Glycinate), Eleuthero, Magnesium L-aspartate, Potassium L-aspartate, Indian Frankincense, Bromelain (600 GDU/g), Glucosamine HCL, Dicalcium Phosphate, Microcrystalline Cellulose, Croscarmellose Sodium, Stearic Acid, Silica, Magnesium Stearate and Sugar Coat (calcium sulfate, sucrose,

kaolin, talc, gelatin, shellac, titanium dioxide, wintergreen oil, FD&C yellow #5, FD&C blue #1, beeswax and carnauba wax).

How Supplied: One box contains 28 packets, three tablets per packet.

Additional Information: For additional information on ingredients or uses, please visit www.winltd.com.

These statements have not been evaluated by the Food & Drug Administration. This product is not intended to diagnose, treat, cure or prevent any disease.

VIBE® (Eniva)

[vīb]

Liquid Multi-Nutrient Supplement

Key Facts: Leading medical researchers and clinicians recommend that individuals ingest a multi-nutrient dietary supplement on a daily basis. The Eniva VIBE liquid nutraceutical not only meets medical recommendations in terms of nutrient content, but has been specifically formulated to allow for enhanced absorption and bioavailability due to the predigested nature of its pharmaceutical grade liquid contents.

Major Uses: Due to the predigested nature of the vitamins and minerals in the VIBE nutraceutical, nutrient absorption and cellular bio-availability of nutrients appear to be enhanced. This results in the support of healthy body structure and function. Through mechanisms not fully elucidated, the anti-oxidant capacity of VIBE appears to have a significant impact on free radicals generated through cellular replication and metabolism, as well as during health challenge processes.

Supplement Facts

| Serving size: | 1 Fluid Ounce |
| Serving Per Container: | 32 |

	Amount Per Serving	% Daily Value
Calories	24	
Total Carbohydrate	5 g	2%*
Sugars	3 g	†
Vitamin A	3,000 IU	60%
Vitamin C	120 mg	200%
Vitamin D	500 IU	125%
Vitamin E	30 IU	100%
Thiamin (Vitamin B1)	1.5 mg	100%
Riboflavin (Vitamin B2)	1.7 mg	100%
Niacin	20 mg	100%
Vitamin B6	2 mg	100%
Folic Acid	400 mcg	100%
Vitamin B12	12 mcg	200%
Biotin	300 mcg	100%
Pantothenic Acid	10 mg	100%
Calcium	100 mg	10%
Phosphorus	20 mg	2%
Iodine	150 mcg	100%
Magnesium	200 mg	50%
Zinc	5 mg	33%
Selenium	25 mcg	36%
Copper	.5 mg	25%
Manganese	1.5 mg	75%
Chromium	120 mcg	100%
Potassium	175 mg	5%
Boron	1 mg	†
Germanium	25 mcg	†
Strontium	500 mcg	†
Sulfur	35 mg	†
Vanadium	5 mcg	†
AntiOX2® Proprietary Blend	6,500 mg	†

Natural Extracts: Acai, Cranberry, Raspberry, Blueberry, Blackberry, Strawberry, Cherry, Carrot, Elderberry, Hibiscus (flower), Lemon, Lime, Apple, Blackcurrant, Oregano, Chokeberry, Grape, Pumpkin, Tomato, Pomegranate, Wolfberry, Stevia (leaf), Citrus Bioflavonoids, Grape Seed, Mixed Tocopherols

HeartPRO™ Proprietary Blend	280 mg	†

D-Ribose, CoQ10, L-Carnitine, Malic Acid, Lecithin

CollaMAX® Proprietary Blend	3,300 mg	†

Green Tea Leaf Extract, L-Lysine, L-Proline, Aloe Vera Gel, Glucosamine HCl (vegetable), Glycine, Alanine, Valine, Isoleucine, Leucine

* Percent Daily Values are based on a 2,000 calorie diet.

† Daily Value not established.

Ingredients: Purified water, natural extracts and flavors (acai, cranberry, raspberry, blueberry, blackberry, strawberry, cherry, carrot, elderberry, hibiscus, lemon, lime, apple, blackcurrant, oregano, chokeberry, grape, pumpkin, tomato, pomegranate, wolfberry, stevia), natural beet sugar, magnesium (from magnesium malate, magnesium citrate, magnesium glycerophosphate, magnesium sulfate, magnesium chloride), citric acid, malic acid, potassium (from potassium citrate, potassium chloride), green tea leaf extract, calcium (from calcium citrate, calcium malate, calcium chloride), ascorbic acid, l-proline, l-lysine, d-ribose, d-alpha-tocopherol acetate with mixed tocopherols, aloe vera gel, guar gum, niacin, niacinamide, vitamin A palmitate, zinc (from zinc sulfate), l-carnitine fumarate, potassium sorbate and sodium benzoate (naturally protect freshness), d-calcium pantothenate, boron (from sodium borate), manganese (from manganese chloride), folic acid, riboflavin-5-phosphate, pyridoxine HCl, glucosamine HCl, copper (from copper sulfate), strontium (from strontium chloride), thiamin HCl, cholecalciferol, chromium (from chromium chloride), biotin, lecithin, CoQ10 (ubidecarenone), selenium (from sodium selenate,

selenium chloride), germanium (from germanium sesquioxide), vanadium (from vanadyl sulfate), cyanocobalamin, n-methyl-cobalamin.

Dosing: Ingest 1-2 ounces per day. Do not exceed 3 ounces per day. For best results, ingest half dose in the a.m. hours and the other half in p.m. hours, unless otherwise directed by a physician.

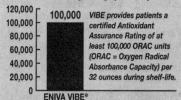

Antioxidant Capacity (ORAC) Score

VIBE provides patients a certified Antioxidant Assurance Rating of at least 100,000 ORAC units (ORAC = Oxygen Radical Absorbance Capacity) per 32 ounces during shelf-life.

ORAC Score Per 32 Ounces, 2006

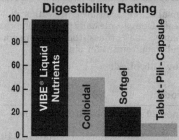

Digestibility Rating

Based upon US Pharmacopeia digestibility studies and standards

Certified Safety Assurance Testing
- *Heavy Metals*
- *Pesticides / Herbicides*
- *Full Microbiologic, Including Mold & Yeast*
- *Fungal Toxin Screen (mycotoxin)*
- *Allergen & Food Additive Screening*
- *GMO Testing*

Data on file, Eniva Nutraceutics, 2006.

Quality Testing
- *Ingredient Potency Testing & Verification*
- *Antioxidant ORAC Analysis*
- *Shelf-Life Stability*
- *Biomass Assays*
- *Particle Size Analysis*

Data on file, Eniva Nutraceutics, 2006.

Effectiveness Studies
- *Several in vivo and in vitro studies performed demonstrating efficacy.*

Data on file, Eniva Nutraceutics, 2006.

Safety Information: As with all dietary supplements, contact your doctor before use, especially if you are pregnant or lactating. Although VIBE is manufactured from natural and safe pharmaceutical grade ingredients, rare sensitivity may develop; should this occur, discontinue use. Keep this and all dietary supplements out of the reach of children. Eniva VIBE is not habit forming and is safe to be taken over time. Long-term high intake of Vitamin A (excluding that sourced form beta-carotene) may lead to health challenges. It is recommended that individuals be aware of all sources of

Vitamin A (excluding beta-carotene) in their diet.
- Scientific evidence suggests that consumption of ANTIOXIDANT VITAMINS may reduce the risk of certain forms of cancer. However, FDA has determined that this evidence is limited and not conclusive.
- As part of a well-balanced diet that is low in saturated fat and cholesterol, Folic Acid, Vitamin B6 and B12 may reduce the risk of vascular disease. However, the FDA has determined that this evidence is limited and not conclusive.

[See figure at left]

Shown in Product Identification Guide, page 504

WINRGY® (Wellness International)
Nutritional Supplement with Vitamin C

Description: Utilizing key ingredients such as riboflavin, vitamin B12, vitamin C, niacin and a proprietary blend of amino acids and caffeine, Winrgy® provides individuals with the necessary alertness and energy required for an active lifestyle. Winrgy® incorporates a unique blend of vitamins and minerals that are important in the creation of noradrenaline, a powerful neurotransmitter responsible for regulating alertness and the sleep-wakefulness cycle as well as being essential for memory and the learning process. Additionally, essential ingredients in Winrgy® help the body convert energy from carbohydrates, protein, and fat, as well as combat physical and mental fatigue. Unlike caffeine alone, Winrgy® offers the raw materials necessary to continue the production of noradrenaline and is ideal for anytime performance is required.

Uses: Winrgy® may:
- Increase energy and alertness
- Improve mental acuity
- Enhance conversion of macronutrients to energy
- Augment physical performance

Directions: As a dietary supplement, add 3/4 cup of chilled water or fruit juice to one packet of mix. Stir briskly. Consume 1–2 times per day. Keep in a cool, dry place. For maximum results, combine this product with one serving size of Food For Thought™.

Warnings: CAUTION PHENYLKETONURICS: Contains phenylalanine. Not for use by children under the age of 18, pregnant or lactating women. Persons taking medications should seek medical advice before taking this product. Do not consume more than four servings per day. Avoid the use of antacids containing aluminum with this product.

Ingredients: Carbohydrates 11 g, Sugars 10 g, Vitamin C 150 mg (as Ascorbic Acid), Vitamin E 30 IU (as DL-Alpha Tocopheryl Acetate), Thiamin 1.5 mg (as Thiamin Mononitrate), Riboflavin 3 mg, Niacin

73 mg (as Niacinamide), Vitamin B6 13 mg (as Pyridoxine HCL), Folate 180 mcg (as Folic Acid), Vitamin B12 19 mcg (as Cyanocobalamin), Pantothenic Acid 48 mg (as Calcium Pantothenate), Zinc 4.5 mg (as Zinc Gluconate), Copper 0.62 mg (as Copper Gluconate), Manganese 2.6 mg (as Manganese Aspartate), Chromium 260 mcg (as Chromium Aspartate), Potassium 25 mg (as Potassium Aspartate), Phenylalanine 570 mg (as L-phenylalanine), Taurine 180 mg, Glycine 135 mg, Caffeine 80 mg, Fructose, Natural Flavor, Citric Acid and Silicon Dioxide.

How Supplied: One box contains 28 single serving packets.

Additional Information: For additional information on ingredients or uses, please visit www.winltd.com.

These statements have not been evaluated by the Food & Drug Administration. This product is not intended to diagnose, treat, cure or prevent any disease.

ZAVITA—WE'VE BOTTLED THE RAINFOREST© (Zavita)
Liquid Herbal supplement

Uses:

Zavita™ is an exclusive liquid herbal supplement containing the legendary formula of rare botanicals used for centuries by the indigenous people and tribal healers of the Amazon Rainforest. The powerful combination of these natural botanical wonders, often referred to as "Elixa de Vida" (the Elixir of Life), promotes whole body wellness, vitality, internal cleansing, mental clarity, energy and longevity.*
The botanicals in Zavita are "wild-harvested" and processed using our state-of-the-art extraction method called "PureExtraction." Every phytoceutical factor is drawn out — while retaining the full authenticity, potency and efficacy of the original plants, making Zavita the only product of its kind in the world. (patent pending).

Actions and Uses:

Over 50 clinical studies, ethnomedical reports, and research on the biological activities on the botanical extracts in Zavita support using Zavita for the following: immune system enhancement, antimicrobial effects, neuroprotection, cardiovascular support, cell mutation protection, anti-inflammation, respiratory system support, weight control, GI protection, digestive aid, cognitive enhancement, adaptogenic stress defense, dermatological correction, sexual system support, nervous system control, free radical quenching, detoxification and ergogenics, (references available upon request, please contact Zavita at 1-888-492-8482).

Continued on next page

Zavita—Cont.

SUPPLEMENT FACTS

Serving size: 1 fl. oz. (30 ml)
Servings Per Container: 25

Amount per serving		% DV
Calories	14	
Total Carbohydrate	4g	2%*
Sugars	3g	†
Proprietary Rainforest Plant Blend	30 ml	†

Cat's claw (Uncaria tomentosa) inner bark extract, Tayuya (Cayaponia tayuya) root extract, Iporuru (Alchomea castanefolia) leaf extract, Chuchuhuasi (Maytenus krukovii) bark extract, Samambaia (Polypodium decumanum) bark extract, Catuaba (Erythroxylum catuaba) bark extract, Cha de bugre (Cordia ecalyculata) whole plant extract, Acai (Euterpe oleracea) fruit pulp concentrate, Stevia (Stevia rebaudiana) leaf extract

* Percent Daily Values (DV) are based on a 2,000 calorie diet.
† Daily Value not established.

Other Ingredients: Purified Water, Raspberry, Pineapple, Orange and other juices from Concentrate, Glycerin, Fructose, Natural Flavor, Xanthum Gum, Sodium Benzoate (to preserve freshness), and Potassium Sorbate (to preserve freshness).

Suggested Use:
Drink 1 fl oz 1–3 times daily / 30 – 90 ml daily.
Shake well before each use. Serve chilled.
Refrigerate after opening.
Best to use within 30 days after opening.
Do not use if safety seal is broken.

How Supplied:
Available in 25.35 FL OZ
Manufactured Exclusively for Zavita™
1430 Bradley Lane, Suite 196
Carrollton, TX 75007
Visit our website: www.zavita.com
© Zavita™ 2006
R6/2006

---

* These statements have not been evaluated by the Food and Drug Administration. This product is not intended to diagnose, treat, cure or prevent any disease.

Shown in Product Identification Guide, page 517

ZINC-220® CAPSULES (Alto)
[zĭnk]
(zinc sulfate 220 mg.)

Composition: Each opaque blue and pink capsule contains zinc sulfate 220 mg. delivering 78.5 mg. of elemental zinc. Zinc-220 Capsules do not contain dextrose or glucose. Inactive Ingredients dicalcium phosphate, cellulose, magnesium stearate, magnesium trisilicate and gelatin (capsule shell).

Action and Uses: Zinc-220 Capsules are indicated as a dietary supplement. Normal growth and tissue repair are directly dependent upon an adequate supply of zinc in the diet. Zinc functions as an integral part of a number of enzymes important to protein and carbohydrate metabolism. Zinc-220 Capsules are recommended for deficiencies or the prevention of deficiencies of zinc.

Warnings: Zinc-220 if administered in stat dosages of 2 grams (9 capsules) will cause an emetic effect. This product should not be used by pregnant or lactating women.

Precaution: It is recommended that Zinc-220 Capsules be taken with meals or milk to avoid gastric distress.

Dosage: One capsule daily with milk or meals. One capsule daily provides approximately 523% times the recommended adult requirement for zinc.

How Supplied:

Product	NDC	SIZE
Zinc-220® Capsules	0731-0401-06	Unit Dose Boxes... 100 (10 × 10)
Zinc-220® Capsules	0731-0401-01	Bottles 100

ALTO® Pharmaceuticals, Inc.

HERBAL MEDICINE INFORMATION

This section presents information on herbal remedies marketed under the Dietary Supplement Health and Education Act of 1994. It is made possible through the courtesy of the manufacturers whose products appear on the following pages. The information concerning each product has been prepared, edited, and approved by the manufacturer's professional staff.

The descriptions of products appearing in this section are designed to provide all information necessary for informed use, including, when applicable, active ingredients, inactive ingredients, actions, warnings, cautions, interactions, symptoms and treatment of oral overdosage, dosage and directions for use, and how supplied. Descriptions in this section must be in full compliance with the Dietary Supplement Health and Education Act, which permits claims regarding a productcs effect on the structure or functioning of the body, but forbids claims regarding a product's ability to treat, diagnose, cure, or prevent any specific disease. Descriptions of products marketed under the act do not receive formal evaluation or approval from the Food and Drug Administration.

In compiling this section, the publisher has emphasized the necessity of describing products comprehensively. The descriptions seen here include all information made available by the manufacturer. The publisher does not warrant or guarantee any product described here, and does not perform any independent analysis of the information provided. Inclusion of a product in this book does not represent an endorsement, and the publisher does not necessarily advocate the use of any product listed.

Herbal Medicine

AMBROTOSE® (Mannatech)
A Glyconutritional Dietary Supplement

Supplement Facts:
Ambrotose® powder:
Serving Size 0.44 g (approx. ¼ teaspoon)
Powder canister: 100g or 50g

Amount Per Serving	% Daily Value
0.44g	*

*Daily Value not established.

Ambrotose® capsules:
Serving Size: one capsule (2 times daily)
Capsules per container: 60

Amount Per Serving	% Daily Value
1 capsule	*

*Daily Value not established.

Ambrotose® with Lecithin capsules:
Ambrotose® with Lecithin
Supplement Facts:
Serving Size: one capsule (2 times daily)
Capsules per container: 60

Amount Per Serving	% Daily Value
1 capsule	*

*Daily Value not established.

Ingredients:
Ambrotose® Powder
Ambrotose® complex
(Internationally patented)
Arabinogalactan (Larix *decidua*) (gum), rice starch, Manapol® aloe vera gel extract (inner leaf gel), gum ghatti, Glucosamine HCl, and gum tragacanth.
Ambrotose® capsules
Ambrotose® complex
(Internationally patented)
Arabinogalactan (Larix *decidua*) (gum), Manapol® aloe vera gel extract (inner leaf gel), gum ghatti and gum tragacanth.
Other ingredients: Brown rice flour, silicon dioxide, stearic acid, gelatin.
Ambrotose® with Lecithin capsules
Ambrotose® complex
(Internationally patented)
Arabinogalactan (Larix *decidua*) (gum), Manapol® aloe vera gel extract (inner leaf gel), gum ghatti and gum tragacanth. Lecithin powder.
Other ingredients: Calcium carbonate, dibasic calcium phosphate, gelatin, brown rice flour, cellulose, silicon dioxide, magnesium stearate.
For additional information on ingredients, visit www.glycoscience.com
Use: Ambrotose® complex is a proprietary formula designed to help provide sac-

charides used in glycoconjugate synthesis to promote cellular communication and immune support.** Consumers who are healthy may notice improved concentration, more energy, better sleep, improved athletic performance, and a greater sense of well-being.

Directions: The recommended intake of Ambrotose® powder is ¼ teaspoon two times a day; the recommended intake of Ambrotose® capsules or Ambrotose® with Lecithin is one capsule two times daily. If desired, you may begin by taking less than the recommended intake. If well tolerated, you may gradually increase to the recommended intake. Children between the ages of 12 and 48 months with growth/nutritional problems (failure to thrive) have been given 1 tablespoon a day of Ambrotose powder for 3 months with no adverse effects. The amount needed by each individual may vary with time, age, genetic makeup, metabolic rate, and activities, stress level, current dietary intake, and health challenges of the moment. A health care professional experienced with use of Ambrotose complex may be helpful.

Warning: Anyone who is taking medication may wish to advise his/her physician. One teaspoon of Ambrotose® powder (equivalent to approximately 12 Ambrotose® capsules) contains the amount of glucose equivalent to 1/25 teaspoon of sucrose (table sugar)
KEEP BOTTLE TIGHTLY CLOSED.
STORE IN A COOL, DRY PLACE.

How Supplied: Bottle of 3.50 oz (100g) powder. Bottle of 1.75 oz (50g) powder. Bottle of 60 (150mg) capsules.

** This statement has not been evaluated by the Food and Drug Administration. This product is not intended to diagnose, treat, cure or prevent any disease.

Mannatech Inc.
600 S. Royal Lane, Suite 200
Coppell, Texas 75019
www.mannatech.com
Shown in Product Identification Guide, page 507

AMBROTOSE AO™ (Mannatech)
[*ăm-brō-tōs*]
Glyco-Antioxidant Supplement

[See table below]
For additional information on ingredients, Visit www.glycoscience.org

Use: Ambrotose AO™ capsules helps protect both water and fat soluble portions of cells from free radical attacks while supporting your immune system.** Defend your health by supporting overall immune function through the natural glyconutrients in Ambrotose™ phytoformula.** Protect against the daily onslaught of toxins, poor food, stress and the environment, all of which contribute to the increase in free radicals, that can accelerate the aging process. ** Help restore cellular damage and the overall balance your body may have lost due to the harmful effect of free radical damage that results from pollutants in the air we breathe, the water we drink and the lives we live.**
** This statement has not been evaluated by the Food and Drug Administra-

Supplement Facts:
Serving Size - 1 Capsule

	Amount Per Serving	% Daily Value
Vitamin E (as mixed d-alpha-, d-beta, d-delta and d-gamma tocopherols)	18 IU	60%
Mtech AO Blend™	113mg	
Quercetin dihydrate		*
Grape pomace extract (fruit)		*
Green tea extract (leaves)		*
Australian Bush Plum (Terminalia ferdinandiana) (fruit)		*
Ambrotose® Phyto Formula	333mg	
Gum Arabic		*
Xanthan Gum		*
Gum Tragacanth		*
Gum Ghatti		*
Aloe vera gel extract (inner leaf gel)- Manapol® powder		*
Phyt•Aloe complex (broccoli, Brussels sprout, cabbage, carrot, cauliflower, garlic, kale, onion, tomato, turnip, papaya, pineapple)		*

Other Ingredients: Vegetable-based cellulose capsules

*Daily value not established.

tion. This product is not intended to diagnose, treat, cure or prevent any disease.

Directions: The recommended intake of Ambrotose AO™ capsules is one capsule two times daily.

Oxygen Radical Absorption Capacity (ORAC) can be used to assess the antioxidant status of human blood and serum. One recent study reported that increasing fruit and vegetable consumption from the usual five to an experimental ten servings per day over two weeks can increase serum ORAC values by roughly 13%.[1] In an open-label pilot study of 12 healthy human volunteers, the antioxidant effects of increasing amounts of supplementation with Ambrotose AO™ were evaluated. A battery of tests was selected in order to assess both oxidative damage and protection. Independent companies were contracted to conduct blood and urine chemistry tests and statistical data analyses. An increase in ORAC$_{\beta\text{-PE}}$, a measure of oxidative protection, was found at all three doses: 19.1% at 500 mg per day, 37.4% at 1.0 g per day, and 14.3% at 1.5 g per day. A trend of decreased urinary lipid hydroperoxides/creatinine, a marker of oxidative damage, was observed as well. No significant trends were found in regard to urinary alkenal or 8-OHdG levels.[2] Thus, over the same time period, 1.0 g per day of Ambrotose AO™ provided over twice the antioxidant protection (37.4%) provided by 5 servings of fruits and vegetables (13%).

1. Cao G; Booth SL; Sadowski JA; Prior RL;. Increases in human plasma antioxidant capacity after consumption of controlled diets high in fruit and vegetables. *Am J Clin Nutr.* 1998 Nov; 68: 1081-1087.
2. Boyd S, Gary K, Koepke CM, et al. An open-label pilot study of the antioxidant activity in humans of Ambrotose AO™: Results. *GlycoScience & Nutrition (Official Publication of GlycoScience com: The Nutrition Science Site).* 2003;4(6).

Shown in Product Identification Guide, page 507

ATHENA 7 MINUTELIFT™ Cream
(Greek Island Labs)

Description: A Natural Clinically Proven Cream that reduces the appearance of sagging skin, lines, and wrinkles. No dangerous muscle relaxers & No Harsh chemicals.

Ingredients: Proprietary Greek Blend of 12 essential Botanical Oils

Directions: External skin application

Warnings: Keep out of reach of children.

How Supplied: .5 fl oz Jar

AWARENESS CLEAR™
(Awareness Corporation)

Description: May help with general digestion.*

Ingredients: Proprietary blend of Oregano Leaf, Clove Flowers, Black Walnut Seed Husk, Peppermint Leaf, Nigella, Grapefruit, Winter Melon Seed, Gentian, Hyssop Leaf, Crampbark, Thyme Leaf, Fennel.

Directions: Take 2 capsules a day each morning on an empty stomach, 1–2 hours before eating with 1 glass of water

Warnings: Do not use if Pregnant or Breastfeeding. Keep out of reach of children.

How Supplied: 90 Vegetarian Capsules per Bottle

*These statements have not been evaluated by the Food and Drug Administration. These products are not intended to diagnose, treat, cure, or prevent any disease.

Shown in Product Identification Guide, page 503

BIOLEAN® ACCELERATOR™
(Wellness International)
Herbal & Amino Acid Formulation

For full product information see page 631.

BIOLEAN FREE®
(Wellness International)
Herbal & Amino Acid Dietary Supplement

For full product information see page 631.

BIOLEAN® LIPOTRIM™
(Wellness International)
All-Natural Dietary Supplement

For full product information see page 631.

DAILY COMPLETE®
(Awareness Corporation)

Description: Liquid Supplement. 100% vegetarian ingredients delivers 211 vitamins, minerals, antioxidants, enzymes, fruits and vegetables, amino acids and herbs, in one ounce liquid a day (great orange taste) Helps to Provide Energy & Reduce Stress Levels*.

Ingredients: Rich in Vitamins & Minerals, Ionic Plant Minerals, Botanical Antioxidants with Phenalgin™, 32 Fruit & Vegetable Whole Juice Complex, Whole Superfood Green complex, 34 Mediterranean Herbs, Essential Fatty Acid Complex, Special Ocean Vegetable Blend

Directions: Take 1 ounce (30 ml) per day, during or immediately after a meal

Warnings: Do not use if pregnant or breast-feeding. Keep out of reach of children.

How Supplied: 30 ounces per Bottle, Clinically Tested Ingredients.

Shown in Product Identification Guide, page 503

DHEA PLUS™
(Wellness International)
Pharmaceutical-Grade Formulation

Description: DHEA Plus™ uniquely combines dihydroxyepiandrosterone (DHEA), Bioperine® and ginkgo biloba leaf to safely and effectively aid the body in age management. DHEA, the primary ingredient, is used by the body to manufacture the sex hormones estrogen and testosterone. As DHEA levels decline with age, women produce less estrogen and have an increased risk of heart disease. Additionally, men lose the metabolic boost that testosterone provides and are at increased risk for fat accumulation. Supplemental DHEA can therefore slow down this hormonal decline. In fact, scientific research has indicated that adequate levels of DHEA in the body can actually slow the aging process. A second key ingredient is Bioperine®, which enhances thermogenic activity and can lead to increases in fat mobilization and utilization. To further ward off the affects of aging, ginkgo biloba has been added to DHEA Plus™ to augment blood flow to the peripheral arteries and the brain. Some improvement in cognitive abilities has been noted as well as inhibition of lipid peroxidation, thereby stabilizing the cell wall against free-radical attack.

Uses: DHEA Plus™ may:
• Combat the effects of aging
• Increase thermogenesis and reduce body fat
• Reduce free-radical formation (antioxidant)
• Increase blood flow to the brain and peripheral arteries

Directions: As a dietary supplement, take one tablet daily with food.

Warnings: Not for use by children under the age of 18, pregnant or lactating women. Consult your physician before using this product if you are taking prescription medications. Persons with a history of prostate cancer should seek medical advice before using this product.

Ingredients: Dihydroxyepiandrosterone 50mg (DHEA), Ginkgo Biloba Leaf 25mg, Bioperine* 5mg (Piper Nigrum L.), Calcium Phosphate Dibasic, Partially Hydrogenated Vegetable Oil, Starch, Magnesium Stearate, Silicon Dioxide and Croscarmellose Sodium.

* Bioperine is a registered trademark of Sabinsa Corporation.

How Supplied: One bottle contains 60 enteric-coated tablets.

Additional Information: For additional information on ingredients or uses, please visit www.winltd.com.

These statements have not been evaluated by the Food & Drug Administration. This product is not intended to diagnose, treat, cure or prevent any disease.

Continued on next page

EXPERIENCE®
(Awareness Corporation)

Description: Promotes Regularity & Cleanses the Colon*

Ingredients: Proprietary Blend of Senna, Blonde Psyllium Seed Husk, Fennel Seed, Cornsilk, Solomon's seal, Rhubarb Root, Kelp

Directions: Take 1 to 2 Capsules before bedtime with a full glass of water.

Warnings: Do not use if pregnant or breast-feeding or if you have colitis. Keep out of reach of children

How Supplied: 90 Capsules per bottle, Clinically tested

Shown in Product Identification Guide, page 503

HYLAND'S BACKACHE WITH ARNICA (Standard Homeopathic)

Active Ingredients: Benzoicum Acidum 3X HPUS, Colchicum Autumnale 3X HPUS, Sulphur 3X HPUS, Arnica Montana 6X HPUS, RHUS Toxicodendron 6X HPUS.

Inactive Ingredients: Lactose, N.F.

Indications: A homeopathic medicine for the temporary relief of symptoms of low back pain due to strain or overexertion.

Directions: Adults and children over 12 years of age: Take 1–2 caplets with water every 4 hours or as needed.

Warnings: Do not use if imprinted cap band is broken or missing. If symptoms persist for more than seven days or worsen, contact a licensed health care professional. As with any drug, if you are pregnant or nursing a baby, seek the advice of a licensed health care professional before using this product. Keep this and all medications out of the reach of children. In case of accidental overdose, contact a poison control center immediately. In case of emergency, the manufacturer may be reached 24 hours a day, 7 days a week at 800/624-9659.

How Supplied: Bottles of 40 5.5 grain caplets (NDC 54973-2965-2). Store at room temperature.

HYLAND'S CALMS FORTÉ™
(Standard Homeopathic)

Active Ingredients: *Passiflora* (Passion Flower) 1X triple strength HPUS, *Avena Sativa* (Oat) 1X double strength HPUS, *Humulus Lupulus* (Hops) 1X double strength HPUS, *Chamomilla* (Chamomile) 2X HPUS, *Calcarea Phosphorica* (Calcium Phosphate) 3X HPUS, *Ferrum Phosphorica* (Iron Phosphate) 3X HPUS, *Kali Phosphoricum* (Potassium Phosphate) 3X HPUS, *Natrum Phosphoricum* (Sodium Phosphate) 3X HPUS, *Magnesia Phosphoricum* (Magnesium Phosphate) 3X HPUS.

Inactive Ingredients: Lactose, N.F., Calcium Sulfate, Starch (Corn and Tapiocal), Magnesium Stearate.

Indications: Temporary symptomatic relief of simple nervous tension and sleeplessness.

Directions: Adults: As a relaxant: Swallow 1–2 tablets with water as needed, three times daily, preferably before meals. For insomnia: 1 to 3 tablets ½ to 1 hour before retiring. Repeat as needed without danger of side effects. Children: As a relaxant: Swallow 1 tablet with water as needed, three times daily, preferably before meals. For insomnia: 1 to 2 tablets ½ to 1 hour before retiring. Repeat as needed without danger of side effects.

Warning: Do not use if imprinted cap band is broken or missing. If symptoms persist for more than seven days or worsen, consult a licensed health care professional. As with any drug, if you are pregnant or nursing a baby, seek the advice of a licensed health care professional before using this product. Keep this and all medications out of the reach of children. In case of accidental overdose, contact a Poison Control Center immediately. In case of emergency, the manufacturer may be reached 24 hours a day, 7 days a week by calling 800/624-9659.

How Supplied: Bottles of 100 4-grain tablets (NDC 54973-1121-02), 50 4-grain tablets (NDC 54973-1121-01) and 32 5.5-grain caplets (NDC 54973-1121-48). Store at room temperature.

HYLAND'S CALMS FORTE' 4 KIDS
(Standard Homeopathic)

Active Ingredients: ACONITUM NAP. 6X HPUS, CALC. PHOS. 12X HPUS, CHAMOMILLA 6X HPUS, CINA 6X HPUS, LYCOPODIUM 6X HPUS, NAT. MUR. 6X HPUS, PULSATILLA 6X HPUS, SULPHUR 6X HPUS

Inactive Ingredients: Lactose, N.F.

Indications: Temporarily relieves the symptoms restlessness, sleeplessness, night terrors, growing pains, causeless crying, occasional sleeplessness due to travel and lack of focus in children.

Directions: Children ages 2-5: dissolve 2 tablets under tongue every 15 minutes for up to 8 doses until relieved; Then every 4 hours as required.
Children ages 6-11: Dissolve 3 tablets under tongue Every 15 minutes for up to 8 doses until relieved; Then every 4 hours as required.
Children 12 years and over: Dissolve 4 tablets under tongue every 15 minutes for up to 8 does until relieved; then every 4 hours as are required or as recommended by a health care professional

Warnings: Ask a doctor before use if: pregnant or nursing, child is taking any prescription medications. If symptoms don't improve within 7 days, discontinue use and seek the advice of a licensed medical practitioner.
Keep this and all medications out of reach of children. Do not use if imprinted tamper band is broken or missing. In case of accidental overdose, contact a poison control center immediately. In case of emergency, the manufacturer may be contacted 24 hours a day, 7 days a week at 800/624-9659.

How Supplied: Bottles of 125 1 grain tablets (NDC 54973-7518-03). Store at room temperature.

HYLAND'S COMPLETE FLU CARE TABLETS (Standard Homeopathic)

Active Ingredients: Eupatorium Perfoliatum 3X, HPUS; Bryonia Alba 3X, HPUS; Gelsemium Sempervirens 3X, HPUS; Euphrasia Officinalis 3X, HPUS; Kali Iodatum 3X, HPUS; Anas Barbariae Hepatis Et Cordis Extractum 200C HPUS.

Inactive Ingredients: Lactose N.F.

Indications: Temporarily relieves the symptoms of fever, chills, body aches, headache, cough and congestion from the flu or common cold.

Directions: Adults: Take 2–3 Quick Dissolving Tablets under tongue every 4 hours or as needed.
Children 6–12 years old: ½ adult dose.

Warnings: Ask a doctor before use if you are pregnant or nursing a baby. Stop use and ask a doctor if symptoms persist for more than 7 days or worsen. Keep out of the reach of children. Do not use if imprinted tamper band is broken or missing. In case of accidental overdoes, contact a poison control center immediately. In case of emergency, the manufacturer may be contacted 24 hours a day, 7 days a week at 800/624-9659.

How Supplied: 2 Bottles of 60 Tablets (NDC 54973-3015-02)

HYLAND'S EARACHE DROPS
(Standard Homeopathic)

Active Ingredients:
Pulsatilla 30C HPUS, Chamomilla 30C HPUS, Sulphur 30C HPUS, Calc Carb 30C HPUS, Belladonna 30C HPUS, Lycopodium 30C HPUS.

Inactive Ingredients:
Citric Acid USP, Purified Water, Sodium Benzoate USP, Vegetable Glycerin USP.

Indications:
Temporarily relieves the symptoms of fever, pain, irritability and sleeplessness associated with earaches after diagnosis by a physician. Relieves common pain and itching of "swimmer's ear." If symptoms persist for more than 48 hours, or if there is a discharge from the ear, discontinue use and contact your physician.

Directions:
Adults and children of all ages: Tilt head sideways and apply 3–4 drops into involved ear 4 times daily or as needed. Tilt ear upward for at least 2 minutes after application or gently place cotton in ear to keep drops in.

Warnings:
Keep away from eyes. Do not take by mouth. Earache drops are only to be used in the ears. Tip of applicator should not enter ear canal. Ask a doctor before use if pregnant or nursing. Consult a physician if symptoms persist for more than 48 hours or if there is discharge from the ear. Keep this and all medications out of reach of children. Do not use if imprinted tamper band is broken or missing. In case of accidental overdose, contact a poison control center immediately. In case of emergency, the manufacturer may be contacted 24 hours a day, 7 days a week at 800/624-9659.

How Supplied: Bottle of .33 ounce (NDC 54973-7516-1)

HYLAND'S EARACHE TABLETS (Standard Homeopathic)

Active Ingredients: Pulsatilla (Wind Flower) 30C, HPUS; Chamomilla (Chamomile) 30C, HPUS; Sulphur 30C, HPUS; Calcarea Carbonica (Carbonate of Lime) 30C, HPUS; Belladonna 30C, HPUS; $(3 \times 10^{-60}$ % Alkaloids) and Lycopodium (Club Moss) 30C, HPUS.

Inactive Ingredients: Lactose NF

Indications: For the relief of symptoms of fever, pain, irritability and sleeplessness associated with earaches in children after diagnosis by a physician. If symptoms persist for more than 48 hours or if there is a discharge from the ear, discontinue use and contact your health care professional.

Directions: Dissolve 4 tablets under the tongue 3 times per day for 48 hours or until symptoms subside. If you prefer, tablets may be dissolved in a teaspoon of water and then given to the child. Earache Tablets are very soft and dissolve almost instantly under the tongue.

Warnings: Do not use if imprinted blisters are broken or damaged. If symptoms persist for more than 48 hours, or if there is a discharge from the ear, discontinue use and consult a licensed health care professional. As with any drug, if you are pregnant or nursing a baby, seek the ad-

vice of a licensed health care professional before using this product. Keep this and all medications out of the reach of children. In case of accidental overdose, contact a poison control center immediately. In cases of emergency, the manufacturer may be contacted 24 hours a day, 7 days a week at 800/624-9659.

How Supplied: Blister pack of 40 tablets (NDC 54973-7507-1). Store at room temperature.

HYLAND'S LEG CRAMPS WITH QUININE (Standard Homeopathic)

Active Ingredients: Cinchona Officinalis 3X, HPUS (Quinine), Viscum Album 3X, HPUS; Gnaphalium Polycephalum 3X, HPUS; Rhus Toxicodendron 6X, HPUS; Aconitum Napellus 6X, HPUS; Ledum Palustre 6X, HPUS; Magnesia Phosphorica 6X, HPUS.

Inactive Ingredients: Lactose, N.F.

Indications: Hyland's Leg Cramps is a traditional homeopathic formula for the relief of symptoms of cramps and pains in lower back and legs often made worse by damp weather. Working without contraindications or side effects, Hyland's Leg Cramps stimulates your body's natural healing response to relieve symptoms. Hyland's Leg Cramps is safe for adults and can be used in conjuction with other medications.

Directions: Adults: Dissolve 2–3 tablets under tongue every 4 hours as needed.

Warnings: Do not use if imprinted cap band is missing or broken. If symptoms persist for more than seven days or worsen, contact a licensed health care professional. As with any drug, if you are pregnant or nursing a baby, seek the advice of a licensed health care professional before using this product. Do not use if pregnant, sensitive to quinine or under 12 years of age. Keep this and all medications out of the reach of children. In case of accidental overdose, contact a poison control center immediately. In case of emergency, the manufacturer may be reached 24 hours a day, 7 days a week at 800-624-9659.

How Supplied: Bottles of 100 three-grain sublingual tablets (NDC 54973-2956-02), Bottles of 50 three-grain sublingual tablets (NDC 54973-2956-01), Bottles of 40 5.5 grain caplets (NDC 54973-2956-68). Store at room temperature.

HYLAND'S NERVE TONIC (Standard Homeopathic)

Active Ingredients: Calcarea Phosphorica (Calcium Phosphate) 3X HPUS; Ferrum Phosphorica (Iron Phosphate) 3X HPUS; Kali Phosphoricum (Potassium

Phosphate) 3X HPUS; Natrum Phosphoricum (Sodium Phosphate) 3X HPUS; Magnesia Phosphoricum (Magnesium Phosphate) 3X HPUS.

Inactive Ingredients: Lactose, N.F.

Indications: Temporary symptomatic relief of simple nervous tension and stress.

Directions: Adults take 2–6 tablets before each meal and at bedtime. Children: 2 tablets. In severe cases take 3 tablets every 2 hours.

Warnings: Do not use if imprinted cap band is broken or missing. If symptoms persist for more than seven days or worsen, contact a licensed health care professional. As with any drug, if you are pregnant or nursing a baby, seek the advice of a licensed health care professional before using this product. Keep this and all medications out of the reach of children. In case of accidental overdose, contact a poison control center immediately. In cases of emergency, the manufacturer may be contacted 24 hours a day, 7 days a week at 800/624-9659.

How Supplied: Bottles of 32 caplets (NDC 54973-1129-68), Bottles of 500 tablets (NDC 54973-1129-1), Bottles of 1000 tablets (NDC 54973-1129-2), Bottles of 100 tablets (NDC 54973-3014-02)

HYLAND'S RESTFUL LEGS (Standard Homeopathic)

Active Ingredients: ARSENICUM ALBUM 12X HPUS, LYCOPODIUM 6X HPUS, PULSATILLA 6X HPUS, RHUS TOXICODENDRON 6X HPUS, SULPHUR 6X HPUS, ZINC METALLICUM 12X HPUS.

Inactive Ingredients: Lactose, N.F.

Indications: Temporarily relieves the symptoms of the compelling urge to move legs to relieve sensations of itching, tingling, crawling, and restlessness of legs. Symptoms may occur while sitting or lying down, and improve with activity.

Directions: Adults dissolve 2–3 quick dissolving tablets under tongue every 4 hours or as needed. Children ages 6–12 ½ adult dose.

Warnings: Ask a doctor before use if pregnant or nursing a baby. Consult a physician if symptoms persist for more than 7 days. Keep this and all medications out of reach of children. Do not use if imprinted tamper band is broken or missing. In case of accidental overdose, contact a poison control center immediately. In case of emergency, the manufacturer may be contacted 24 hours a day, 7 days a week at 800/624-9659.

How Supplied: Bottles of 50 3 grain tablets (NDC 54973-2966-1). Store at room temperature.

HYLAND'S TEETHING GEL
(Standard Homeopathic)

Active Ingredients: Calcarea Phosphorica (Calcium Phosphate) 12X, HPUS; Chamomilla (Chamomile) 6X, HPUS; Coffea Cruda (Coffee) 6X, HPUS; and Belladonna 6X, HPUS (Alkaloids 0.0000003%)

Inactive Ingredients: Deionized water, Vegetable Glycerin, Hydroxyethyl Cellulose, Methyl Paraben and Propyl Paraben.

Indications: A homeopathic combination for the temporary relief of symptoms of simple restlessness and wakeful irritability due to cutting teeth.

Directions: Apply to gums as necessary. If symptoms persist for more than seven days or worsen, discontinue use and contact your health care professional. Please note, if your baby has been crying or has been very upset, your baby may fall asleep after using this product because the pain has been relieved and your child can rest.

Warnings: Do not use if tube tip is broken or missing. If symptoms persist for more than seven days or if irritation persists, inflammation develops or fever or infection develop, discontinue use and consult a licensed health care professional. As with any drug, if you are pregnant or nursing a baby, seek the advice of a licensed health care professional before using this product. Keep this and all medications out of the reach of children. In case of accidental overdose, contact a poison control center immediately. In case of emergency, the manufacturer may be contacted 24 hours a day, 7 days a week at 800/624-9659.

How Supplied: Tubes of 1/3 OZ. (NDC 54973-7504-3). Store at room temperature.

HYLAND'S TEETHING TABLETS
(Standard Homeopathic)

Active Ingredients: *Calcarea Phosphorica* (Calcium Phosphate) 3X HPUS, *Chamomilla* (Chamomile) 3X HPUS, *Coffea Cruda* (Coffee) 3X HPUS, *Belladonna* 3X HPUS (Alkaloids 0.0003%).

Inactive Ingredients: Lactose N.F.

Indications: A homeopathic combination for the temporary relief of symptoms of simple restlessness and wakeful irritability due to cutting teeth.

Directions: Dissolve 2 to 3 tablets under the tongue 4 times per day. If you prefer, tablets may first be dissolved in a teaspoon of water and then given to the child. If the child is restless or wakeful, 2 tablets every hour for 6 doses or as recommended by a licensed health care professional. Teething Tablets are very soft and dissolve almost instantly under the tongue. Please note, if your baby has been crying or has been very upset, your baby may fall asleep after using this product because the pain has been relieved and your child can rest.

Warning: Do Not use if imprinted cap band is broken or missing. If symptoms persist for more than seven days, or if irritation persist, inflammation develops or fever or infection develop, discontinue use and consult a licensed health care professional. As with any drug, if you are pregnant or nursing a baby, seek the advice of a health care professional before using this product. Keep this and all medications out of the reach of children. In case of accidental overdose, contact a poison control center immediately. In case of emergency, the manufacturer may be contacted 24 hours a day, 7 days a week at 800/624-9659.

How Supplied: Bottles of 125—one grain sublingual tablets (NDC 54973-7504-01). Store at room temperature.

INTELECTOL® MEMORY ENHANCER (Memory Secret)
VINPOCETINE TABLETS MEMORY SECRET

Description: INTELECTOL® is the purest form of Vinpocetine available. Vinpocetine is a derivative of Vincamine, which is extracted from the Periwinkle plant (*Vinca Minor, Vinca Pervinca*). Research suggests that Vinpocetine helps to maintain healthy blood circulation in the brain and supports certain neurotransmitters in the memory process.* Vinpocetine supports and protects brain blood vessel health and aids mental function.*

Directions: As a dietary supplement, take 2 tablets twice daily with meals. Vinpocetine should be taken as part of an on-going regimen with exercise, a healthy diet and keeping active the mind. Do not use if tamper-evident seal is broken.

Cautions: Take product with food to avoid stomach upset. Not recommended for use by pregnant women, nursing mothers or anyone under 18 years old. Consult a doctor or health care professional before use if you have any medical condition or if taking any medication. Not recommended for use by anyone with hemophilia, heart problems or low blood pressure. **Keep out of reach of children.**
Store in a cool, dry place.

Supplement Facts
Serving Size 2 tablets
Servings Per Container: 25

	Amount Per Serving	% DV
Vinpocetine (from Periwinkle seed extract)	10 mg	*

*Daily Value not established.
Other Ingredients: Lactose, hydroxypropylcellulose, magnesium stearate and talc.

Distributed by: The Memory Secret, Inc.
1221 Brickell Ave., Suite 1540, Miami, FL 33131/USA
memorysecret™
www.memorysecret.net
Shown in Product Identification Guide, page 512

MASS APPEAL™
(Wellness International)
Amino Acid & Mineral Workout Supplement

Description: Utilizing natural compounds which mimic the beneficial effects of anabolic steroids, Mass Appeal™ is specifically formulated to enhance athletic performance without the harmful side effects of steroids. Creatine, the primary ingredient in Mass Appeal™, works as a storage molecule for high-energy phosphate bonds, providing greater energy during exercise requiring short periods of intense activity, such as weight lifting, sprinting, and jumping. Creatine causes a "cell volumizing" effect within the muscle by forcing additional water into the muscle cells, promoting an increase in protein synthesis within the muscle which facilitates growth while slowing down the destructive breakdown of muscle cells during exercise. Mass Appeal™ also contains the branched chain amino acids (BCAAs) L- leucine, L-valine and L-isoleucine, which also increase protein synthesis and are oxidized inside muscle cells leading to a protein-sparing effect which indirectly increases anabolism by reducing the muscle's need to burn its own proteins during strenuous exercise. Other key ingredients used to protect against muscle catabolism include alpha-ketoglutaric acid and L-glutamine. Inosine and vanadyl sulfate, two important compounds known for increasing oxygen utilization within red blood cells and the flow of these cells into the muscles, are also found in Mass Appeal™. Vanadyl sulfate not only augments blood flow into muscle tissue, it increases the transport of glucose into these muscles, thusly increasing glycogen storage and exhibiting an additional muscle-sparing effect. Through supplementation, the catabolic breakdown of muscle can be minimized and the muscle tissue preserved.

Uses: Mass Appeal™ may:
• Enhance athletic performance
• Augment muscle size and strength
• Combat catabolic muscle breakdown
• Reduce fatigue and post-exercise recovery time

Directions: Adults (18 years and older) may take a loading dose of three packets in the morning and two packets in the late

afternoon for one week. This dose may be repeated every three months. Following one week of the loading dose, begin the maintenance dose of 1 packet daily two hours after exercise. Needs may vary with each individual. For individuals desiring enhanced effects, increase the loading dose to three to four packets, three times per day (morning, afternoon and evening). Following one week of this enhanced loading dose, begin the enhanced maintenance dose of two packets in the morning and two packets in the late afternoon. It is recommended that one maintain a low-fat, high-protein diet; drink at least eight glasses of water per day; and engage in 30 to 60 minutes of aerobic and anaerobic exercise three to four times per week. For optimal effects, take in conjunction with Phyto-Vite® and Sure2Endure™.

Warnings: Not for use by children under the age of 18, pregnant or lactating women. Consult your physician before using this product if you have any medical conditions. Do not take if you have kidney disease, muscle disease or are on a protein restricted diet. Discontinue immediately if allergic symptoms develop.

Ingredients: Proprietary Supplement Blend 3255 mg: Creatine Monohydrate, Inosine (phosphatebonded), L-Leucine, L-Valine, L-Isoleucine, Alpha-Ketoglutaric Acid, KIC (Calcium Keto-Isocaproate), L-Glutamine, Vanadyl Sulfate; Dicalcium Phosphate, Microcrystalline Cellulose, Stearic Acid, Croscarmellose Sodium, Silica, Magnesium Stearate and film coating (Hydroxypropyl Methylcellulose, Hydroxypropyl Cellulose, Polyethylene Glycol, Titanium Dioxide and Propylene Glycol).

How Supplied: One box contains 28 packets, four tablets per packet.

Additional Information: For additional information on ingredients or uses, please visit www.winltd.com.

These statements have not been evaluated by the Food & Drug Administration. This product is not intended to diagnose, treat, cure or prevent any disease.

NATURALJOINT™
dietary supplement (Greek Island Labs)

Description: Natural Dietary Supplement that Promotes Healthy Joints Supports Flexibility & Mobility*

Ingredients: Proprietary Greek Blend of 37 Natural Ingredients

Directions: 1 Capsules daily with meal

Warnings: Keep out of reach of children. Consult your doctor prior to using this product if you are taking any prescription medication

How Supplied: 30 Capsules (Vegetarian) Per Box

*The statements have not been reviewed or approved by the Food & Drug Administration. This product is not intended to diagnose, treat, cure or prevent any disease

PHYTO-VITE®
(Wellness International)
Advanced Antioxidant, Vitamin and Mineral Supplement

Description: Phyto-Vite® is a state-of-the-art nutritional supplement providing chelated minerals, vitamins and a diverse group of antioxidants. The antioxidant coverage provided by Phyto-Vite® is both comprehensive and diverse. First, it includes optimal amounts of vitamins A, C, and E as well as the provitamins alpha and beta carotene. The inclusion of these powerful antioxidants provides protection against the oxidative damage caused by free-radicals. Improved immune function, increased protein and steroid hormone synthesis, improved wound healing, increased soft tissue integrity and decreased platelet aggregation are just a few of the many effects of these antioxidants. Esterified vitamin C is used in Phyto-Vite® to ensure quicker uptake and a decreased rate of excretion. Ginkgo biloba helps increase vasodilation of blood vessels leading to the brain and peripheral tissues as well as to inhibit lipid peroxidation. A phytonutrient blend obtained from entire plant sources has been incorporated into Phyto-Vite® to further enhance its antioxidant effects. Key phytonutrients included are lutein, lycopene, soy isoflavones, and allicin. To ensure optimum absorption and maximum antioxidant effects, Phyto-Vite® includes the minerals copper, zinc, manganese and selenium in a chelated form. Phyto-Vite® has several unique features such as the inclusion of canola oil to ensure proper absorption of fat-soluble vitamins even on an empty stomach, an extended-release formulation to allow flexibility in dosing and a Betacoat™ casing. This is a beta carotene coating that is designed to provide antioxidant coverage to the tablet itself. This helps protect the integrity and activity of the product.

Uses: Phyto-Vite® may:
• Reduce free-radical formation (antioxidant)
• Increase immune system integrity
• Increase blood flow to brain and peripheral arteries
• Decrease platelet aggregation and stickiness
• Improve cognitive functioning

Directions: As a dietary supplement, take six tablets per day with eight ounces of liquid. Tablets may be taken all at once or staggered throughout the day.

Warnings: If pregnant or lactating, consult physician before using. Accidental overdose of iron-containing products is a leading cause of fatal poisoning in children under 6. Keep this product out of reach of children. In case of accidental overdose, call a doctor or poison control center immediately.

Ingredients: Vitamin A (25,000 IU), Vitamin C 500 mg, Vitamin D 200 IU, Vitamin E 400 IU, Vitamin K 70 mcg, Thiamin 15 mg, Riboflavin 17 mg, Niacin 100 mg, Vitamin B6 20 mg, Folate 400 mcg, Vitamin B12 60 mcg, Biotin 300 mcg, Pantothenic Acid 75 mg, Calcium 500 mg, Iron 4 mg, Phosphorus 250 mg, Iodine 150 mcg, Magnesium 400 mg, Zinc 15mg, Selenium 200 mcg, Copper 2 mg, Manganese 5 mg, Chromium 200 mcg, Potassium 70 mg, Phytonutrient Blend 800mg (alfalfa leaf, aged garlic bulb concentrate, Pur-Gar® A-10,000 [garlic bulb], soy protein isolate, broccoli floret, cabbage leaf, cayenne pepper fruit, green onion bulb, parsley leaf, tomato, spirulina), canola oil concentrate 100 mg, citrus bioflavonoid complex 50 mg, rutin 26 mg, quercetin dihydrate 24 mg, choline 50 mg, Inositol 50 mg, PABA 25 mg, ginkgo biloba leaf standardized extract 20 mg, bilberry fruit standardized extract 10 mg, catalase enzymes 10 mg, grape seed proanthocyanidins 5 mg, red grape skin extract 5 mg, boron 1 mg, dicalcium phosphate, magnesium oxide, calcium carbonate, calcium ascorbate, microcrystalline cellulose, d-alpha-tocopheryl succinate, croscarmellose sodium, stearic acid, potassium citrate, choline bitartrate, beta-carotene, niacinamide, silica, d-calcium pantothenate, magnesium stearate, copper Chelazome® glycinate, zinc Chelazome® glycinate, calcium citrate, calcium lactate, magnesium amino acid chelate, inositol, L-selenomethionine, kelp, manganese Chelazome® glycinate, biotin, pyridoxine HCl, Ferrochel® iron bisglycinate, boron chelate, riboflavin, magnesium citrate, thiamin mononitrate, retinyl palmitate, chromium Chelavite® glycinate, phylloquinone, cyanocobalamin, vanillin, cholecalciferol, folic acid.

How Supplied: One bottle contains 180 hypoallergenic Betacoat™ tablets. This hypoallergenic formula is free of dairy, yeast, wheat, sugar, starch, animal products, dyes, preservatives, artificial flavors and pesticide residues.

Additional Information: For additional information on ingredients or uses, please visit www.winltd.com.

These statements have not been evaluated by the Food & Drug Administration. This product is not intended to diagnose, treat, cure or prevent any disease.

PLUS WITH AMBROTOSE®
Complex (Mannatech)
Herbal-Amino Acid Dietary Supplement

Supplement Facts:
Serving Size - 1 Caplet (3 times daily)

	Amount Per Serving	% Daily Value
Iron	1mg	5
Wild Yam (root) Standardized for 25mg Phytosterols	200mg	*

Continued on next page

Plus with Ambrotose—Cont.

L-Glutamic acid	200mg	*
L-Glycine	200mg	*
L-Lysine	200mg	*
L-Arginine	100mg	*
Beta Sitosterol	25mg	*
Ambrotose® Complex (patent pending)	2.5mg	*

Arabinogalactan (Larix decidua) (gum), Aloe vera (inner leaf gel powder), gum ghatti and gum tragacanth.

Other Ingredients: Microcrystalline cellulose, stearic acid, croscarmellose sodium, silicon dioxide, magnesium stearate, titanium dioxide coating.

*Daily value not established.

For additional information on ingredients, visit www.glycoscience.com

Use: PLUS caplets provide nutrients to help support the endocrine system's natural production and balance of hormones.** A well-functioning endocrine system works in harmony with the body's immune system, helps support the efficient metabolism of fat, and supports natural recovery from physical or emotional stress.** The nutritional components of PLUS caplets are wild yam extract, amino acids, and beta sitosterol. PLUS caplets contain no hormones.

Directions: The recommended intake of PLUS caplets is one caplet three times daily.
KEEP BOTTLE TIGHTLY CLOSED. STORE IN A COOL, DRY PLACE.

How Supplied: Bottle of 90 caplets.

** This statement has not been evaluated by the Food and Drug Administration. This product is not intended to diagnose, treat, cure or prevent any disease.

Shown in Product Identification Guide, page 507

PURE GARDENS CREAM®
(Awareness Corporation)

Description: Natural botanical cream may help to improve appearance of dry skin, fine lines and helps to tone the skin.

Ingredients: Apple oil, vitamin C, vitamin E, Aloe Vera Leaf, Almond Oil, Cold Press Virgin Olive Oil, Sesame Oil, Chamomile Flowers Oil, Calendula Officinalis Oil, Beeswax, Jojoba Oil, Linseed Oil.

Directions: Application for both face and body. External use only

How Supplied: 2 ounce jar, Clinically tested

SATIETE® (Wellness International)
Herbal and Amino Acid Supplement

Description: Satiete® has a synergistic blend of herbs and amino acids that help regulate the neurotransmitter serotonin, decrease cravings for sweets and normalize blood sugar levels. Satiete's® key ingredient, 5-HTP, derived from griffonia seed extract, is a precursor to serotonin, which normalizes mood, sleep, appetite and energy levels. Also included is gymnema sylvestre, an important ingredient which has an effect on the oral cavity that reduces appetite for sweets as well as an ability to reduce metabolism of simple carbohydrates in the gastrointestinal system, thus leading to more manageable blood sugar levels. Vanadyl sulfate is also included to help normalize blood sugar levels. Additional ingredients included to improve energy levels and combat fatigue are St. John's Wort extract, malic acid, and magnesium. The combination of these ingredients provides a positive impact on serotonin function.

Uses: Satiete® may:
• Regulate mood
• Curb appetite and reduce carbohydrate cravings
• Improve sleep
• Increase energy levels

Directions: As a dietary supplement, begin dosage by taking one tablet three times per day 30 to 60 minutes before meals. If needed after two weeks of use, increase the dosage to two tablets three times per day. Do not exceed nine tablets daily without medical supervision.

Warnings: If you are taking MAO inhibitors, tricyclic antidepressants, SSRI antidepressants (Prozac®, Paxil™, Zoloft®) or prescription diet drugs, do not take this product without medical supervision. If you suffer from liver or kidney diseases, serious gastrointestinal disorders or carcinoid syndrome, do not take this product without medical supervision. If gastrointestinal upset develops and persists, reduce dosage, take only with large meals or discontinue use.

Ingredients: Griffonia Seed Extract (Supplying 95% min. naturally occurring L-5HTP), Gymnema 33 mg, Vanadyl Sulfate 7 mg, Vitamin B-2 6.5 mg, Niacinamide 6.5 mg, Magnesium 55mg (Oxide), Vitamin B-1 6.5 mg, Vitamin B-6 6.5 mg, Malic Acid 100 mg, St. John's Wort Extract 50 mg, Ginkgo Biloba Extract 20 mg, Vitamin B-12 100 mcg, Folic Acid 33 mcg, Microcrystalline Cellulose, Stearic Acid, Croscarmelose Sodium, Magnesium Stearate, Silicon Dioxide, Ethylcellulose and Hydroxypropylcellulose.

How Supplied: One bottle contains 84 hypoallergenic enteric-coated tablets.

Additional Information: For additional information on ingredients or uses, please visit www.winltd.com.

These statements have not been evaluated by the Food & Drug Administration. This product is not intended to diagnose, treat, cure or prevent any disease.

SLEEP-TITE™
(Wellness International)
Herbal Sleep Aid

Description: Sleep-Tite™ is a non-addicting herbal sleep aid formulated to promote a deeper, more restorative sleep without the use of pharmaceutically synthesized hormones. This powerful tool's primary function is to rejuvenate and restore by assisting the body in initiating and maintaining sleep. Sleep-Tite™ is a blend of 10 all-natural herbs, including California poppy, passion flower, valerian, and skullcap. These herbs help prevent insomnia because of their calming effects and ability to relieve muscle tension. Additional ingredients, including hops, celery seed and chamomile all provide a generalized calming effect and are especially helpful for indigestion, gastrointestinal and smooth muscle relaxation. In addition to these calming herbs, Sleep-Tite™ also contains feverfew, an herb that reduces the body's production of prostaglandin and serotonin, which can lead to inflammation, fever and the vasoactive response that triggers migraine headaches. By utilizing this unique blend of herbs to aid in the effective initiation and maintenance of sleep patterns, Sleep-Tite™ can be consumed by adults, thereby promoting physical and emotional well-being in a safe, active manner.

Uses: Sleep-Tite™ may:
• Promote restorative sleep and healthy sleep patterns
• Reduce muscle tension and joint inflammation
• Diminish occurrences of migraine headaches
• Improve physical and emotional well-being

Directions: As a dietary supplement, take two Sleep-Tite™ caplets approximately 30 to 60 minutes prior to bedtime. Some persons may require less than two caplets to achieve optimum results. Do not exceed recommended nightly amounts. Needs may vary with each individual.

Warnings: Not for use by children under the age of 18, pregnant or lactating women. Consult your physician before using this product if you have any medical condition or are taking antidepressants, sedatives or hypnotic medications. Do not take this product if using Monoamine Oxidase Inhibitors (MAOI). This product may cause drowsiness and should not be taken with alcohol or while operating a vehicle or other machinery. If allergic symptoms develop, discontinue use. Keep out of reach of children.

Ingredients: European Valerian Root 4:1 extract, Celery Seed 4:1 extract, Hops Strobile 4:1 extract, Passion Flower 4:1 extract (whole plant), California Poppy 5:1 extract (aerial parts), Chamomile Flower 5:1 extract, Chinese Fu Ling 5:1 extract (Poria Cocos), Jujube Seed 5:1 extract, Feverfew 5:1 extract (aerial parts), Skullcap (aerial parts), Dicalcium Phosphate, Microcrystalline Cellulose, Croscarmellose Sodium, Stearic Acid, Silica, Magnesium Stearate and Sugar Coat (calcium sulfate, sucrose, kaolin, talc, gelatin, shellac, titanium dioxide, anise oil, beeswax and carnauba wax).

How Supplied: One box contains 28 packets, two caplets per packet.

Additional Information: For additional information on ingredients or uses, please visit www.winltd.com.

These statements have not been evaluated by the Food & Drug Administration. This product is not intended to diagnose, treat, cure or prevent any disease.

SMILE'S PRID®
(Standard Homeopathic)

Contains: Acidum Carbolicum 2X HPUS, Ichthammol 2X HPUS, Arnica Montana 3X HPUS, Calendula Off 3X HPUS, Echinacea Ang 3X HPUS, Sulphur 12X HPUS, Hepar Sulph 12X HPUS, Silicea 12X HPUS, Rosin, Beeswax, Petrolatum, Stearyl Alcohol, Methyl & Propyl Paraben.

Indications: Temporary topical relief of pain symptoms associated with boils, minor skin eruptions, redness and irritation. Also aids in relieving the discomfort of superficial cuts, scratches and wounds.

Directions: Wash affected parts with hot water, dry and apply PRID® twice daily on clean bandage or gauze. Do not squeeze or pressure irritated skin area. After irritation subsides, repeat application once a day for several days. Children under two years: consult a physician. CAUTION: If symptoms persist for more than seven days or worsen, or if fever occurs, contact a licensed health care professional. Do not use on broken skin. Keep out of reach of children. In case of accidental ingestion, seek professional assistance or contact a poison control center. For external use only. Avoid contact with eyes.

How Supplied: 18GM tin (NDC 0619-4202-54). Keep in a cool dry place.

STEPHAN™ FEMININE®
(Wellness International)
Nutritional Supplement

Description: StePHan™ Feminine® contains selected vitamins, minerals and amino acids regarded as important to the ever-changing female body. This is achieved through such scientifically researched ingredients as magnesium and boron. Magnesium is important for regulating the flow of calcium between cells and is essential for adequate calcium uptake, which can lead to fewer PMS symptoms such as irritability, depression, headaches, backaches and menstrual cramps. Boron is vital at reducing excretion of both calcium and magnesium. This in turn leads to a healthy defense against diseases such as osteoporosis.

Uses: StePHan™ Feminine® may:
- Reduce estrogen and testosterone fluctuations that can lead to PMS symptoms
- Lessen PMS symptoms such as irritability, depression, headaches, backaches and menstrual cramps
- Increase calcium intake and reduce urinary excretion of calcium and magnesium
- Slow progression of bone loss contributed to osteoporosis

Directions: As a dietary supplement, take one or more capsules daily as needed.

Warnings: CAUTION PHENYLKETONURICS: Contains 9.2 mg phenylalanine per serving.

Ingredients: Proprietary blend (Isolated Soy Protein, Magnesium Oxide, Boron Aspartate, Ribonucelic Acid Yeast, Adenosine Triphosphate), Hydroxypropylmethylcellulose, DL-Alpha Tocopheryl Acetate, Starch, Silicon Dioxide, Selenium Amino Acid Chelate.

How Supplied: One bottle contains 60 easy-to-swallow capsules.

Additional Information: For additional information on ingredients or uses, please visit www.winltd.com.

These statements have not been evaluated by the Food & Drug Administration. This product is not intended to diagnose, treat, cure or prevent any disease.

SYNERGYDEFENSE® CAPSULES
(Awareness Corporation)

Description: Improves Digestion, Boosts the Immune System, & strengthens the body's natural defenses*.

Ingredients: Proprietary Blend of Enzymes, Probiotics, Antioxidants, Prebiotics

Directions: Take 1 capsule with a glass of water during or before your largest meal of the day. Take once or twice a daily.

Warnings: Do not use if pregnant or lactating. If under 18, consult a physician before use.

How Supplied: 30 Vegetarian Capsules individually sealed

*These statements have not been evaluated by the Food and Drug Administra-

---

tion. These products are not intended to diagnose, treat, cure, or prevent any disease.

Shown in Product Identification Guide, page 503

TAHITIAN NONI® Leaf Serum
(Tahitian Noni Int'l)
TAHITIAN NONI® Leaf Serum Soothing Gel

Description: In an exclusive process known only to Tahitian Noni International, we've extracted the juice of the long-treasured noni leaf and made it into a soothing balm. Especially for skin that's been exposed to the elements, this serum will condition and revitalize irritated, wind-chaffed, or sunburned skin with lasting relief.

Ingredients: TAHITIAN NONI® Exclusive Noni Leaf Formula [Purified Water, *Morinda citrifolia* (Noni) Leaf Juice, *Morinda citrifolia* (Noni) Leaf Extract, *Vanilla tahitensis* (Tahitian Vanilla) Fruit Extract], Pentylene Glycol, Propylene Glycol, SD Alcohol 40-B, PEG-400 Laurate and Laureth-4, Sodium Dehydroacetate, Disodium EDTA, Phenoxyethanol, Fragrance, Acrylates/C10-30 Alkyl Acrylate Crosspolymer, Potassium Hydroxide.

Suggested Use: Smooth over irritated skin as needed.

Storage: Keep tightly closed in a dry place; do not expose to excessive heat.

How Supplied:
Packaged for Tahitian Noni International, a subsidiary of Morinda, Inc. Provo, UT 84604. USA.

References:
Su C, Palu 'AK et al., TNI Patent Pending. A Noni leaf extract demonstrated significant wound healing effects in the mouse cutaneous assay by doubling the wound closure rate.
Su C, Palu 'AK et al., TNI Patent Pending Noni leaf extracts and Noni leaf juice inhibited the proliferation of a human epidermoid carcinoma cell line, A431, with an IC_{50} 76 ug/ml and 0.2% respectively.
Mannetje L. Morinda citrifolia L. in: Plant-Resources of South-East Asia (Edit.: E. Westphal, P. and C. M. Jansen). **Pudoc Wageningen 1989, p. 185-187.** A Noni leaf preparation is used as a tonic and antiseptic. Leaves are placed directly on wounds and the leaf juice produces pain-killing effects.
Saludes JP et al., Antitubercular constituents from the hexane fraction of Morinda citrifolia Linn. (Rubiaceae). Phytother. Res. 2002. (16): 683-685 Ethanol and hexane fractions from Morinda citrifolia leaf showed antitubercular activity by killing 89% of the bacteria *in vitro*, comparable to 97% kill by the anti-TB drug rifampicin at the same concentration.

Continued on next page

Tahitian Noni—Cont.

Zin ZM et al., Antioxidant activities of chromatographic fractions obtained from roots, fruit and leave of Mengkudu (Morinda citrifolia L.). Food Chemistry 2006. 94: 169-178.
Methanol fractions from defatted Noni leaf juice showed strong antioxidant activities comparable to that of alpha-tocopherol.

---

* This statement has not been evaluated by the Food and Drug Administration. This product is not intended to diagnose, treat, cure or prevent any disease

---

Shown in Product Identification Guide, page 517

TAHITIAN NONI® LIQUID DIETARY SUPPLEMENT (Tahitian Noni Int'l)

Description: TAHITIAN NONI® Juice has a heritage, a pedigree that distinguishes it from every other product on the market. This pedigree extends back 2,000 years to the people who used the noni fruit for its benefits. The countless benefits of this unique fruit can only be enjoyed if the fruit is revealed in its most pure form. Our proprietary formulation captures this precisely. It's no wonder that TAHITIAN NONI Juice touches the lives of millions worldwide. You'll find 2,000 years of goodness in every bottle of TAHITIAN NONI Juice! Always look for the TAHITIAN NONI Juice Footprint: Your only assurance of quality, purity, and authenticity.

Supplement Facts

Serving Size: 1 fluid ounce (30 ml)
Servings Per Container 33

Amount Per Serving	%Daily Value*
Calories 13	
Total Carbohydrate 3g	1%
Surgars 2g	†

*Percent Daily Values are based on a 2,000 calorie diet.
†Daily Value not established.

Ingredients: Reconstituted *Morinda citrifolia* fruit juice from pure juice puree from French Polynesia, natural grape juice concentrate, natural blueberry juice concentrate, and natural flavors. Not made from dried or powdered *Morinda citrifolia*.

How Supplied: 1 FL. OZ./30 mL daily. Preferably before meals
Shake well before using and refrigerate after opening
Do not use if seal around cap is broken
Packaged by Tahitian Noni International, a subsidiary of Morinda, Inc. Provo, UT 84604. USA.

References:
Mugglestone C, Davies S, et al., A single centre, double-blind, three dose level, parallel group, and placebo controlled safety study with TAHITIAN NONI® Juice in healthy subjects. BIBRA International LtD, Clinical Studies Department. Woodmansterne Road, Carshalton UK. 2003
Drinking 750 ml TAHITIAN NONI® Juice (TNJ) per day found to be safe in a human clinical safety study involving 96 subjects.
Wang MY et al., Noni Juice May Lower Cholesterol and Triglycerides in Adult Smokers. American Heart Association 46th Annual Conference on Cardiovascular Disease Epidemiology and Prevention Meeting Report. Phoenix, Ariz., March 2 2006.
A placebo control clinical trial involving smokers drinking 4 ounces of TAHITIAN NONI® Juice daily for 4 weeks, showed an average decrease in total cholesterol levels from 235.2/dL to 190.2 mg/dL and an average triglyceride decrease from 242.5 mg/dL to 193.5 mg/dL.
TAHITIAN NONI® Juice Does Not Contain Athletic Banned Substances. http://www.consumerlab.com/bannedsub.asp
Analysis of TNJ revealed the absence of steroids, illegal drugs, or other performance-enhancing substances, such as growth hormones, EPO, high levels of caffeine and chemical stimulants.
Jensen et al., Noni Juice Protects the Liver. Eur J Gastroenterol Hepatol. 2006 May; 18(5):575–7.
Isolated cases of hepatotoxicity were reported from Noni juice. However, other factors were likely responsible. Published safety data show that noni juice is not toxic to the liver. In fact, it demonstrates TNJ actually protects the liver.
Wang MY et al., Morinda citrifolia (Noni): A Literature Review and Recent Advances in Noni Research. Acta Pharmacol Sin. 2002 Dec; 23 (12): 1127–41.
Noni fruit juice, *Morinda citrifolia* L., has been used in folk remedies by Polynesians for over 2000 years; with reports of antiviral, antibacterial, anti-inflammatory, antifungal, antitumor, antihelminth, hypotensive, analgesic, and immune-modulating effects.
Furusawa E, Hirazumi A, Story SP, Jensen CJ. Antitumor Potential of a Polysaccharide-rich Substance from the Fruit Juice of *Morinda citrifolia* (Noni) on Sarcoma 180 Ascites Tumor in Mice. Phytother Res. 2003, 17(1158–1164)
A Polysaccharide-rich precipitate (noni-ppt) from the fruit juice of *Morinda citrifolia* and from TNJ inhibited the spread of Sarcoma 180 tumors in mice, with a cure rate of 25%–45%. Noni-ppt also showed synergistic benefits when combined with a broad spectrum of chemotherapeutic drugs.
Gerson S. Green L. Preliminary Evaluation of the Antimicrobial Activity of Extracts of *Morinda citrifolia* L. 2002 General Meeting of American Society for Microbiology.
Morinda citrifolia was shown to have antimicrobial and antifungal properties against *A. niger, C. albicans, E. coli, S. aureus* and *T. mentagrophytes.*
Opinion of the Scientific Committee on Foods on Tahitian Noni® Juice. European Commission. SCF/CS/NF/DOS/18 ADD 2 Final. 11, December 2002.
The EU's Scientific Committee on Foods found the consumption of TAHITIAN NONI® Juice to be safe, following a review of acute and subchronic oral toxicity studies, genotoxicity tests, chemical analyses, and allergenicity studies. The No-Observable-Adverse-Effect-Level (NOAEL) was 80 ml/kg, equivalent to >8% body weight.
TAHITIAN NONI® Juice Not a Significant Source of Potassium.
A case report stated that the potassium content of noni juice was 56.3 mEq/L, or 65 mg/ounce, and may be a "surreptitious" source of potassium for patients with renal disease. (Mueller et al. Am J. Kidney Dis. 2000 Feb; 35(2): 330–2.) Mueller (USA Today, March 28, 2000) clarified his research, stating he did not analyze TAHITIAN NONI® Juice, but rather a different brand of noni juice and that the amount of potassium was only "as much as you'd get in 2 inches of banana."
Tolson CB, Vest RG, West BJ. Quantitative ICP Mineral Analysis of TAHITIAN NONI® Juice. Tahitian Noni International Research Center. American Fork, Utah. USA 84003. Internal Data.
Potassium content of TAHITIAN NONI® Juice is 40 mg per 1 ounce serving. Compared to Grape juice * 42 mg per 1 ounce serving, Banana* 102 mg per 1 ounce serving and Yogurt* 66 mg per 1 ounce.
Not All Liquid Dietary Supplements Are Created Equal. Palu 'AK, West BJ, Jensen JC. Am J. Hematology 79: 79–82.
TAHITIAN NONI® Juice does not contain any significant quantity of vitamin K. A case of coumadin resistance was reported in a patient drinking juice from the "Noni Juice 4 Everything" brand, which is fortified with vitamin K (Carr ME, Koltz J, Bergeron M. Coumadin Resistance and the Vitamin Supplement "Noni." 2004 Am J. Hematology 77:103–104). This case of coumadin resistance is due to vitamin K and does not apply to the TAHITIAN NONI® Juice Brand.

---

* Source: USDA Nutrient Database for Standard Reference.
This statement has not been evaluated by the Food and Drug Administration. This product is not intended to diagnose, treat, cure or prevent any disease

Shown in Product Identification Guide, page 517

TAHITIAN NONI® Seed Oil (Tahitian Noni Int'l)

Product Information

This exclusive oil delivers intense moisture and relief to dry or distressed

skin. It is designed to help improve skin health issues that come from within.

The first and only essential oil derived from noni seeds. High in linoleic acid, a powerful ally in skin hydration and cellular health.

This world exclusive light oil delivers intense healing moisture and relief to rough, distressed skin. It takes over 50,000 seeds to make just one ounce of this rare and precious oil. Absorbs easily into skin.

Product Benefits

- Hydrates and softens skin to hasten the healing process of distressed skin
- Protects with valuable antioxidants
- An essential building block for healthy looking skin
- High in linoleic acid which helps relieve dry, flaky, or rough skin and helps maintain smooth, moist skin
- Won't clog pores

Featured Ingredients

Pure Noni Seed Oil

Hydrates and softens while protecting skin with valuable antioxidants

Recommended Use

Gently apply a small amount of Noni Seed Oil to distressed skin anywhere healing moisture can be beneficial.

How Supplied:

33 FL oz (10 ml) bottle
Packaged for Tahitian Noni International, a subsidiary of Morinda, Inc. Provo, UT 84604. USA.

References:

West BJ, Palu 'AK, Jensen CJ. Noni Seed Oil Analysis. TNI Patent Pending. Noni seed oil analysis reveal that it has natural phytosterols, vitamin E and a significant source of omega-6 fatty acid, an essential fatty acid.
Palu 'AK, Zhou BN, West BJ et al. TNI Patent Pending. Noni seed oil can reduce pain and inflammation due to its significant and selective inhibition of COX-2 enzymes.
Douglas M. Rope, M.D. Midwest Clinical Trials. A study to Asses the Comedogenicity of a Test Product When Applied Topically to the Skin of Healthy Human Subjects. May 19, 2004. Noni seed oil significantly reduced the number of closed comedones (white heads) on the skin of 26 teenage volunteers during a clinical trial.

* Source: USDA Nutrient Database for Standard Reference.

Shown in Product Identification Guide, page 517

**4LIFE® TRANSFER FACTOR PLUS®
Advanced Formula
(4Life Research, LLC)**

Description: Transfer factors are small peptides of approximately 44 amino acids that "transfer" or have the ability to express cell-mediated immunity from immune donors to non-immune recipients. 4Life Transfer Factor® products are derived from egg yolk and cow colostrum extracts. Combined, these compounds comprise the Transfer Factor E-XF™ blend, which provides the broadest spectrum transfer factor available. The extraction of 4Life Transfer Factor E-XF is protected by US patents 6,468,534; 6,866,868; with other patents pending.
Transfer factors educate the immune system to recognize self from non-self, thus supporting healthy immune system function. Because they instruct the immune system to act appropriately, transfer factors are effective in supporting normal inflammation response in the body, a key to healthy body system function.
4Life Transfer Factor Plus Advanced Formula combines Transfer Factor E-XF with a proprietary formulation of innate and adaptive immune system enhancers such as Inositol Hexaphosphate, Cordyceps, Beta Glucans, Maitake and Shiitake Mushrooms. These ingredients work together to trigger and enhance the various immune protective mechanisms of the body. Clinical studies show that 4Life Transfer Factor Plus Advanced Formula can increase Natural Killer cell activity up to 437 percent above baseline.*

---

* Blind Independent study conducted by Dr. Anatoli Vorobiev, head of Immunology, at the Russian Academy of Medical Science.

Summary of Research: In 1949 transfer factors were discovered by Dr. H. Sherwood Lawrence. Since that time hundreds of studies have been completed involving transfer factors effect on various diseases. Due to new studies conducted in Russia, the Russian Health Ministry has approved 4Life Transfer Factor and 4Life Transfer Factor Plus to be the first supplements used by doctors and hospitals in Russia. Recent studies on transfer factor include:
Rak, AV et al. Effectiveness of Transfer Factor (TF) in the Treatment of Osteomyelitis Patients. *International Symposium in* Moscow 2002, Nov 5–7, 62–63.
Granitov, VM et al. Usage of Transfer Factor Plus in Treatment of HIV - Infected Patients. *Russian Journal of HIV, AIDS and Related Problems* 2002, 1, 79–80.
Karbuisheva NV, Tatarintsev PB, Granitov BM, Karbishev IA, McCausland CW, Oganova E, *Use of Transfer Factor in Treatment of Chronic Viral Hepatitides B and C,* Siberian J. of Gastroenterology and Hepatology. 2003, (16), p. 147.
Rak AV, Dadali VA, Stolpnik ES, McCausland CW, Oganova E, Gaykovaya LB, *Immunological Test Results from Chronic Osteomyelitis Patients under going Complex Treatment with Transfer Factor,* St. Petersburg State Medical Academy R.F. Annals of Sci. Conf., I-RIID. Barnaul, 2003 p. 55.

Recommended Dose:

600mg Transfer Factor E-XF daily. If used in combination with other immune ingredients, such as 4Life Transfer Factor Plus Advanced Formula, less may be taken. No toxicity level of Transfer Factor E-XF has been established.
See www.transferfactorinstitute.com for more information on transfer factor.

4Life Transfer Factor™ Products Include:

4Life Transfer Factor Advanced Formula
4Life Transfer Factor Plus Advanced Formula
4Life Transfer Factor RioVida

Targeted Transfer Factor® Products:

4Life Transfer Factor MalePro®
4Life Transfer Factor Cardio™
4Life Transfer Factor ReCall®
4Life Transfer Factor GluCoach™
4Life Transfer Factor Belle Vie™

Other Transfer Factor Delivery:

4Life Transfer Factor Go Stix™
4Life Transfer Factor Chewable
4Life Transfer Factor Immune Spray™
4Life Transfer Factor RenewAll™
4Life Transfer Factor Kids
4Life Transfer Factor Toothpaste
4Life tf Age-Defying Effects™

**VEMMA NUTRITION PROGRAM™
(Vemma)**

Description: The Vemma Nutrition Program provides two powerful liquid formulas that make it easy to get the vitamins, minerals and antioxidants you need to form a solid nutritional foundation. The first half of the program is Mangosteen Plus™, a powerful multivitamin formulation that contains 12 full-spectrum vitamins in a base of antioxidant-rich mangosteen fruit and mangosteen pericarp (rind) extract, whole leaf aloe vera and decaffeinated green tea. This amazing formula provides powerful benefits:

Mangosteen Powered Antioxidants. Mangosteen provides powerful plant-based antioxidant protection and features a full array of phytonutrients including naturally-occurring xanthones.* Xanthones are effective antioxidants and provide the body with important nutritional benefits.* Current lab tests reveal that Vemma provides more total mangostin xanthones than the competition with 94.11 milligrams per ounce.**

Vitamin Powered Antioxidants. Contains critical antioxidant vitamins A (as beta carotene), C and E to help fight free radical damage and prevent oxidative stress to the body.* This product has an ORAC value totaling 114,163 units per liter.** Some scientific evidence suggests that consumption of antioxidant vitamins may reduce the risk of certain forms of cancer. However, the FDA has determined that this evidence is limited and not conclusive.

Continued on next page

Vemma Nutrition—Cont.

Whole Leaf Aloe Vera. This wonderful leaf succulent contains an impressive selection of minerals, amino acids and nutritional sugars such as polysaccharides, enzymes, lignins, saponins and anthraquinones that are known to provide the body with many beneficial effects for health and wellness.*

Beneficial Levels of Selenium. Some scientific evidence suggests that consumption of selenium may produce anticarcinogenic effects in the body. However, the FDA has determined that this evidence is limited and not conclusive.

Powerful B Vitamins. Supplies additional B vitamins at heart-healthy levels for added energy and provides a good source of folate.* Healthful diets with adequate folate may reduce a woman's risk of having a child with a brain and spinal cord defect.

The second half of the program is Essential Minerals®. Minerals support the health of organs, bones and the immune system.* The body does not inherently produce the minerals it needs, this is why supplementation and diet are important. In fact, our physical well-being is more directly dependent upon the minerals we take into our bodies than almost any other factor.* Vemma's Essential Minerals is a completely balanced, 100% natural mineral supplement that contains a combination of 65 major, trace and ultra-trace minerals. Essential Minerals is offered in a bioavailable (body-ready) liquid form that consists of pristine plant-sourced minerals totally dissolved in an ionic state.

The Vemma Nutrition Program's bioavailable (body-ready) formulas are easy to take and easy for the body to use. They are ideal supplements for patients who have trouble swallowing pills or tablets.

---

* These statements have not been approved by the Food and Drug Administration. This product is not intended to diagnose, treat, cure, or prevent any disease.

** Based on independent lab tests conducted in April 2006 (Lot #01B614).

Supplement Facts:

Mangosteen Plus™

[See first table above]

Essential Minerals®

[See second table above]

Directions: Shake well and serve cold. Take one fluid ounce (2 tablespoons) of Mangosteen Plus and one fluid ounce (2 tablespoons) of Essential Minerals daily. For best results, take both products together. For children ages two to twelve, take ½ dosages daily. Children under two, seek the advice of a healthcare professional.

Warnings: Keep out of reach of children. As with any nutritional supplement, always consult your healthcare professional if you are pregnant, lactating or if you have any other health condition. Discontinue if allergic reaction occurs.

Note: Store in a cool, dry place. Refrigerate after opening. Avoid exposure to direct sunlight.

Mangosteen Plus™

Supplement Facts
Serving Size 2 Tbsp (30 mL/1 fl oz)
Servings Per Container 32

	Amount Per Serving	%Daily Value
Calories	20	
Total Carbohydrate	5 g	2%*
Sugars	5 g	†
Vitamin A (100% as beta carotene)	5000 IU	100%
Vitamin C (as ascorbic acid)	300 mg	500%
Vitamin D3 (as cholecalciferol)	1000 IU	250%
Vitamin E (as d-alpha tocopheryl acetate)	60 IU	200%
Thiamin (as thiamine hydrochloride)	1.5 mg	100%
Riboflavin (as riboflavin U.S.P.)	1.7 mg	100%
Niacin (as niacinamide)	20 mg	100%
Vitamin B6 (as pyridoxine hydrochloride)	5 mg	250%
Folate (as folic acid)	800 mcg	200%
Vitamin B12 (as cyanocobalamin)	15 mcg	250%
Biotin (as d-Biotin)	300 mcg	100%
Pantothenic Acid (as calcium d-pantothenate)	10 mg	100%
Selenium (as amino acid chelate)	140 mcg	200%
Proprietary Mangosteen, Whole Leaf Aloe Vera and Green Tea Blend	25.2 g	†

Reconstituted Mangosteen (*Garcinia mangostana L.*) (fruit), Aloe Vera Leaf, Green Tea (Leaf) (decaffeinated), Mangosteen Extract (pericarp) (standardized for 10% xanthones).

Other ingredients: fructose, natural flavors, potassium sorbate, sodium benzoate, malic acid and xanthan gum.

* Percent Daily Values are based on a 2,000 calorie diet.
† Daily Value not established.

Essential Minerals®

Supplement Facts
Serving Size 2 Tbsp (30 mL/1 fl oz)
Servings Per Container 32

	Amount Per Serving	%Daily Value
Calories	15	
Total Carbohydrate	3 g	1%*
Sugars	3 g	†
Proprietary Mineral Blend	956 mg	†

Carbon (Organic), Calcium, Sodium, Sulfur, Magnesium, Chloride, Bromide, Fluoride, Iodine, Potassium, Niobium, Aluminum, Iron, Phosphorus, Silica, Manganese, Boron, Strontium, Titanium, Tungsten, Copper, Zinc, Tin, Zirconium, Molybdenum, Vanadium, Chromium, Selenium, Nickel, Cobalt, Lithium, Gallium, Barium, Yttrium, Neodymium, Hafnium, Cadmium, Thorium, Antimony, Cerium, Tellurium, Beryllium, Samarium, Dysprosium, Erbium, Bismuth, Gadolinium, Cesium, Lanthanum, Praseodymium, Europium, Lutetium, Terbium, Ytterbium, Holmium, Thallium, Thulium, Tantalum, Germanium, Gold, Platinum, Rhodium, Rubidium, Ruthenium, Scandium, Silver, Indium.

Other ingredients: purified water, fructose, plant mineral extract, natural kiwi flavor, natural strawberry flavor, citric acid, xanthan gum and carmine color.

* Percent Daily Values are based on a 2,000 calorie diet.
† Daily Value not established.

How Supplied: 32 oz. bottle of Mangosteen Plus and 32 oz. bottle of Essential Minerals. Additionally, pre-mixed 2 oz. versions are also available.

Shown in Product Identification Guide, page 517

VIBE® (Eniva)
[*vīb*]
Liquid Multi-Nutrient Supplement

For full product information see page 822.

POPULAR HERBS

Reliable information on herbal remedies is still hard to come by, yet Americans spend more than $4 billion each year on herbal products. Even more surprising are the findings from a recent *Prevention* magazine survey: Nearly 23 million consumers use herbal remedies *instead* of taking prescription medicine, and about 20 million take botanicals along with either OTC or prescription drugs.

To prepare you for those times when patients ask about the latest herbal "discovery"—as they surely will—we've compiled a quick reference of the most commonly used herbs. The information is based on the findings of the German Regulatory Authority's "Commission E"—currently the most authoritative source of information on botanical medicines. For a more thorough discussion of over 700 herbs, consult the second edition of the *PDR® for Herbal Medicines™*.

Aloe (Aloe vera). The gel from the Aloe plant is an ancient remedy used externally for its antibacterial, antiviral, anti-inflammatory, and pain-relieving effects. It is used topically in skin moisturizers and to treat burns, wounds, psoriasis, and frostbite. While the internal use of Aloe is suggested as a treatment for several conditions including constipation, there is no evidence of its efficacy. In fact, internal use is not recommended because of the risk of serious adverse effects.

Warning: Aloe should not be used by pregnant or breast-feeding women, or by people with severe intestinal disorders. Aloe should not be taken with certain drugs associated with potassium loss—such as diuretics, corticosteroids, and antiarrhythmics and other heart medications—or with the herb Licorice.

Arnica (Arnica montana). The Arnica plant is used externally for pain and inflammation due to injury, and as an anti-infectious agent. Arnica should be discontinued immediately in the event of an allergic reaction to external application. The herb should not be used on open skin wounds.

Warning: Although Europeans take Arnica internally to treat respiratory infections, internal use is not recommended due to the risk of serious cardiac adverse effects.

Astragalus (Astragalus species). Astragalus, or Huang-Qi, is used to improve immune function and strengthen the cardiovascular system. Compounds in Astragalus may also have beneficial antiviral, antioxidant, memory-enhancing, and liver-protecting effects, although the nature of those effects on specific diseases has not been established.

Warning: The use of Astragalus must be carefully monitored by a physician due to its potentially dangerous adverse effects, particularly in people with immune disorders or those taking blood-thinning medications.

Barberry (Berberis vulgaris). Both the fruit and root bark of the Barberry plant are used in folk medicine. The berry is a source of vitamin C, which stimulates the immune system, improves iron absorption, and protects against scurvy. The fruit's acid content has a mild diuretic effect that is thought to aid in urinary tract infections. Barberry root bark may reduce blood pressure, relieve constipation, and have some antibiotic effects.

Warning: Pregnant and nursing women should not use Barberry.

Bilberry (Vaccinium myrtillus). The astringent effects of Bilberry fruit are used to treat inflammation of the mouth and throat, and both the fruit and leaves are used for diarrhea. Reports citing Bilberry as a treatment for diabetic retinopathy need further confirmation.

Warning: The herb should not be used with blood-thinning drugs, including aspirin.

Black Cohosh (Cimicifuga racemosa). The hormone-modulating effects of Black Cohosh make it useful for women with menopausal symptoms and premenstrual syndrome.

Warning: Due to a risk of spontaneous abortion, Black Cohosh should not be used during pregnancy. The herb should not be taken with drugs that lower blood pressure.

Butcher's Broom (Ruscus aculeatus). This herb, native to the Mediterranean regions of Europe, Africa, and western Asia, is used medicinally as a diuretic, anti-inflammatory, and for its beneficial effects on circulation. Butcher's Broom is used to relieve the discomforts of hemorrhoids, such as itching and burning, and the leg heaviness, pain, cramping, and swelling of chronic venous insufficiency.

Cat's Claw (Uncaria tomentosa). The root of the South American Cat's Claw contains compounds that have immune-stimulating, anti-inflammatory, and anticancer effects. Although human studies have yet to be conducted, Cat's Claw is often used to treat cancer; arthritis and rheumatic disorders; and AIDS and other viral diseases.

Warning: Cat's Claw should not be used by pregnant or breastfeeding women, or by people with autoimmune disorders, multiple sclerosis, tuberculosis, transplant recipients, and children under 2 years of age.

Cayenne (Capsicum annuum). Externally, Cayenne is used to relieve the pain of muscle tension and spasm, diabetic neuropathy, and rheumatism. Cayenne is sometimes taken internally to relieve gastrointestinal disorders, although human studies have yet to confirm such uses.

Warning: Topical Cayenne preparations should not be used for more than two consecutive days, with a two-week break between applications. It should never be used on broken skin or near the eyes. When used internally, Cayenne preparations should not be taken with aspirin or antifungal drugs.

Chamomile (Matricaria recutita). Chamomile tea—which has anti-inflammatory, antispasmodic, and muscle-relaxing effects—is used to treat gastrointestinal disorders such as indigestion and gas.

Warning: Chamomile should not be used by pregnant women.

Comfrey (Symphytum officinale). This herb is applied topically as an anti-inflammatory; it is used for bruises and sprains and to promote bone healing.

Warning: Because of possible toxic adverse effects, Comfrey should not be taken internally. The herb is contraindicated in pregnant and breastfeeding women.

Dandelion (Taraxacum officinale). Dandelion, commonly used as an addition to the salad bowl, is recommended as an effective remedy for digestive and liver complaints, urinary tract infection, and as an appetite stimulant.

Warning: Although the herb is sometimes used for gallbladder complaints, this should only be done under a doctor's supervision. People with bile duct obstruction or stomach ulcer should not use Dandelion.

Dong Quai (Angelica sinensis). Dong Quai root is used in China as a women's health tonic. It is particularly used as a remedy for fibrocystic breast disease, premenstrual syndrome, painful periods, and menopausal symptoms. Dong Quai is also used in cardiovascular disease to treat high blood pressure and improve poor circulation.

Warning: Dong Quai should not be used by pregnant or breastfeeding women. The herb can also cause photosensitivity.

Echinacea (Echinacea purpurea). This species of Echinacea is a well-established immune-system stimulator; it is used to treat flu, coughs and colds, bronchitis, urinary tract infections, wounds and burns, and inflammation of the mouth and pharynx.

Warning: It should not be used in patients who have autoimmune disorders such as multiple sclerosis, collagen disease, AIDS, or tuberculosis. The herb is also contraindicated in patients who have diabetes and in pregnant or breastfeeding women. Echinacea should not be used with the following: anticancer agents, anti-organ rejection drugs, corticosteroids, or immunosuppressants.

Evening Primrose (Oenothera biennis). The anti-inflammatory compounds in Evening Primrose oil have been extensively studied, but no definitive indication has been accepted. Some herbalists consider the oil useful for treating breast pain, premenstrual syndrome, and menopausal symptoms. Capsules containing at least 500 milligrams of the oil are approved in Germany as a remedy for eczema.

Warning: People with seizure disorder or schizophrenia should not take Evening Primrose oil.

Feverfew (Tanacetum parthenium). Feverfew is used to treat migraine headaches, allergies, and arthritic and rheumatic diseases.

Warning: Feverfew should not be used during pregnancy or breastfeeding. It is also contraindicated in people with bleeding disorders, and in those who are taking anticoagulants, including aspirin.

Flax (Linum usitatissimum). Ground Flax (also known as Linseed) is used internally to relieve constipation. It is also used externally as a compress to relieve skin inflammation.

Warning: Flax should not be used internally in the cases of bowel or esophageal obstruction; or in the presence of gastrointestinal or esophageal inflammation.

Fo-Ti (Polygonum multiflorum). The Asian herb Fo-Ti is used for constipation, atherosclerosis, high cholesterol, and as an immune enhancer.

Warning: Because of its laxative action, the herb may cause diarrhea. Taking the unprocessed root may cause skin rash; and overdosage may cause numbness in the extremities.

Garlic (Allium sativum). Garlic is used as a treatment for hardening of the arteries, high blood pressure, and to reduce cholesterol levels. It may also have antibacterial and antiviral effects.

Warning: Garlic can cause allergic skin and respiratory reactions. It should not be used by people with bleeding disorders, or by those taking blood thinners (including aspirin) or NSAID therapy. Nursing women should also not use Garlic.

Ginger (Zingiber officinale). Ginger root is a treatment for motion sickness and loss of appetite. It is also indicated for nausea and vomiting associated with chemotherapy, and to help control nausea and vomiting in postoperative patients.

Warning: Ginger should not be used for morning sickness associated with pregnancy, or by nursing mothers. People who have gallstones or bleeding disorders

should not take Ginger. The herb is also contraindicated in those taking blood thinners (including aspirin) or NSAID therapy.

Ginkgo (Gingko biloba). Ginkgo has proven useful for dementia, Alzheimer's disease, peripheral arterial occlusive disease, vertigo, and tinnitus of vascular origin.

Warning: Ginkgo should not be used by people who have bleeding disorders, or who are taking blood thinners (including aspirin) or NSAID therapy.

Ginseng (Panax ginseng). The Ginseng root is used for fatigue and to improve concentration and stamina. Ginseng may also have antiviral, antioxidant, and anticancer effects.

Warning: Caution with Ginseng is urged in people with cardiovascular disease or diabetes. People who are taking diabetes drugs, diuretics, blood thinners (including aspirin), MAO inhibitors, or NSAIDs should not take Ginseng. It should not be used during pregnancy or breastfeeding, or by those with bleeding disorders. Taking large amounts can result in Ginseng abuse syndrome, which is characterized by high blood pressure, insomnia, water retention, and muscle tension.

Goldenseal (Hydrastis canadensis). Goldenseal contains the compound berberine, which is used for gastritis, gastric ulcer, gallbladder disease, and acute diarrhea. It can be useful as an adjunct therapy in cancer treatment, and is also used to treat chronic eye infection.

Warning: Goldenseal should not be used by pregnant or breastfeeding women, or by people who have bleeding disorders; it should also not be combined with blood thinners (including aspirin) or NSAIDs. Use of Goldenseal for extended periods can result in digestive disorders, constipation, excitement, hallucination or delirium, and decreased vitamin B absorption. **Overdosage can result in convulsion, difficulty breathing, and paralysis.**

Gotu Kola (Centella asiatica). Gotu Kola is used internally for chronic venous insufficiency and venous hypertension. In animal and lab studies, Gotu Kola was also effective for ulcers and varicose veins. The herb is used externally to treat wounds; if a rash develops, discontinue topical use.

Great Burnet (Sanguisorba officinalis). Great Burnet may be used both externally and internally for its astringent, decongestant, and diuretic properties. Internal uses include menopausal symptoms, intestinal bladder problems, and venous disorders. It is also prepared for external use as a plaster for wounds and ulcers.

Green Tea (Camellia sinensis). Green Tea, which is rich in catechins and flavonoids, is used to help prevent cancer. The antibacterial effects of Green Tea mouthwash are useful in the prevention of dental cavities. Keep in mind that Green Tea contains caffeine and should be used sparingly by pregnant and breastfeeding women, and by those who are caffeine-sensitive.

Hawthorn (Crataegus laevigata). Hawthorn contains several compounds that are considered beneficial to the heart. It is used for cardiac insufficiency, angina, congestive heart failure, and irregular heartbeat.

Warning: Hawthorn should not be used in children under 12, or in the first trimester of pregnancy. People taking Hawthorn must be carefully monitored by a physician, especially in cases where it is combined with cardiac glycosides, beta-blockers, or calcium channel blockers. Hawthorn should not be taken with cisapride. Overuse can lead to low blood pressure, irregular heartbeat, and excessive sleepiness.

Horse Chestnut (Aesculus hippocastanum). Both the seed and leaf of Horse Chestnut are used medicinally. The seed is indicated for the symptoms of chronic venous insufficiency, including pain, cramping, swelling, sensations of heaviness, and night cramping. Horse Chestnut leaf is used for venous disorders such as varicose veins, hemorrhoids, and phlebitis.

Warning: People taking blood thinners (including aspirin) should not use Horse Chestnut.

Kava-kava (Piper methysticum). The active compounds in Kava are lactones, which have antispasmodic, muscle-relaxing, and anticonvulsive effects; Kava can also thin the blood. The herb is used for nervousness, insomnia, tension, stress, and agitation.

Warning: People who are depressed should not take Kava. The herb is also contraindicated in pregnant or nursing women and in those with liver disorders. Overuse of Kava can result in skin rash or weight loss. Kava use for more than three months should be supervised by a physician. The herb should not be combined with alcohol, anti-anxiety or mood-altering drugs (including barbiturates), or levodopa.

Licorice (Glycyrrhiza glabra). The sweet root of the Licorice plant has a long history of use in traditional medicine. It contains various compounds with anti-inflammatory and other soothing effects that make it helpful as a treatment for ulcers and digestive disorders such as gastritis. It also acts as an expectorant for cough and bronchitis.

Warning: Licorice should not be taken with digoxin, diuretics, or medications that lower blood pressure. Licorice should also not be used in people with hepatitis and other liver disorders, kidney disease, diabetes, arrhythmias, high blood pressure, muscle cramping, low potassium levels, and pregnancy

Ma-Huang (Ephedra sinica). Ma-Huang contains compounds that alleviate bronchial constriction and is used in folk remedies as a treatment for coughs and bronchitis.

Warning: The adverse effects of Ma-Huang outweigh any possible benefits. The herb should not be taken by pregnant or breastfeeding women, or by people with the following: anxiety, high blood pressure, glaucoma, brain tumors, prostate disorders, adrenal tumors, cardiac arrhythmia, or thyroid disease. Ma-Huang should not be combined with caffeine, decongestants, stimulants, glaucoma medication, MAO inhibitors, anesthetics, or labor-inducing drugs. **Overdosage can result in death.**

Milk Thistle *(Silybum marianum).* The compounds in Milk Thistle seed have protective and regenerative effects on the liver. It is used as a treatment for liver and gallbladder disorders such as jaundice, toxic liver damage, cirrhosis of the liver, and gallbladder pain.

Warning: The herb should not be used with antipsychotic drugs, yohimbine, or male hormones.

Pumpkin Seed *(Cucurbita pepo).* Pumpkin Seed has anti-inflammatory and antioxidant properties. It is used to treat irritable bladder and symptoms of benign prostatic hyperplasia (eg, obstructed urinary flow). It does not, however, appear to relieve an enlarged prostate.

Pygeum *(Pygeum africanum).* Pygeum bark contains compounds that inhibit the inflammation and swelling associated with benign prostatic hyperplasia.

Warning: The herb should not be used by pregnant or breastfeeding women. People with stomach disorders should check with their physician before using Pygeum.

Saw Palmetto *(Serenoa repens).* The anti-inflammatory and testosterone-moderating effects of Saw Palmetto make it useful for treating benign prostatic hyperplalsia; the herb is used for treating irritable bladder as well.

Warning: Saw Palmetto should not be used by pregnant or breastfeeding women. The herb should be avoided by those who have hormone-driven cancers or a family history of such cancers. People with stomach disorders and those who are taking hormones or hormone-like drugs should check with their physician before taking it.

St. John's Wort *(Hypericum perforatum).* St. John's Wort is one of the better studied herbs. Various compounds in St. John's Wort have antidepressant, anti-inflammatory, and antibacterial effects. It is used internally for depression and anxiety, and externally for wounds, burns, skin inflammation, and blunt injuries.

Warning: St. John's Wort can cause photosensitivity if taken for too long or at high doses. It can also cause gastrointestinal discomfort and headache. Combining St. John's Wort with other antidepressant medications such as MAO inhibitors, selective serotonin reuptake inhibitors (including fluoxetine, paroxetine, sertraline, fluvoxamine, or citalopram), or nefazodone could cause "serotonin syndrome"—a condition characterized by sweating, tremor, confusion, and agitation. The herb should also not be combined with the following: antibiotics that have photosensitizing effects, cyclosporine, indinavir, combination oral contraceptives, reserpine, barbiturates, theophylline, or digoxin.

Stinging Nettle *(Urtica dioica).* Both the flowers and root of the Stinging Nettle plant contain beneficial compounds used in various conditions. The flower is used internally and externally for rheumatism; it is used internally for urinary tract infections and kidney and bladder stones. The root is used for irritable bladder and to help relieve symptoms of benign prostatic hyperplasia (eg, obstructed urinary flow), although it does not reduce prostate enlargement.

Warning: Stinging Nettle should not be used by people who suffer from fluid retention due to impaired cardiac or kidney function.

Uva-Ursi *(Arctostaphylos uva-ursi).* Uva-ursi is used in the treatment of urinary tract infections because of its astringent and antibacterial effects.

Warning: The herb should not be used by pregnant or breastfeeding women; it should also not be used in children under 12 years of age, as it could cause liver damage. Uva-ursi should not be combined with diuretics, NSAIDs, or with substances (food or medication) that promote acidity in the urine.

Valerian *(Valeriana officinalis).* Valerian root contains sedative compounds that are useful in nervousness and insomnia. It is recommended for many other unproven uses such as headache, anxiety disorders, premenstrual syndrome, and menopausal symptoms.

Warning: Patients should avoid operating motor vehicles for several hours after taking Valerian. The herb should not be used by pregnant or breastfeeding women. Valerian extract or bath oils should not be used by people suffering from skin disorders, fever, infectious disease, heart disease, or muscle tension. Valerian should not be taken with barbituates or benzodiazepenes.

Vitex *(Vitex agnus-castus).* Vitex (also known as Chaste Tree) is used as a treatment for premenstrual syndrome and menopausal symptoms.

Warning: Because of its hormonal effects, Vitex should not be used by pregnant or breastfeeding women. Occasionally, rash can occur. The herb should not be used with drugs that affect dopamine levels.

Wild Yam *(Dioscorea villosa).* Popular reports have led to the belief that Wild Yam is a "natural" source of the hormone progesterone. While Wild Yam is used as a constituent of artificial progesterone pharmaceutically, the body cannot complete the conversion process by itself. The herb can also be useful in treating high cholesterol.

Warning: Because of possible hormonal effects, pregnant and nursing women should not use Wild Yam. The herb should not be taken with estrogen-containing drugs or indomethacin.

Yohimbe *(Pausinystalia yohimbe).* Yohimbe is pre-

pared pharmaceutically under the brand name Yocon and is used to treat erectile dysfunction. Compounds in Yohimbe stimulate norepinephrine, which improves blood flow to the penis. The risks, however, of unregulated ingestion of the herb are thought to outweigh the benefits. Therefore, it is recommended that Yohimbe be taken only under strict medical supervision.

Warning: Yohimbe should not be used by women, especially pregnant or breastfeeding women. It is also contraindicated in patients with liver or kidney disease, post-traumatic stress disorder, high blood pressure, panic disorder, or Parkinson's disease. The herb should not be taken with naltrexone, blood pressure medication, alcohol, or morphine. Patients should check with their doctor before taking Yohimbe with any OTC product.

POISON CONTROL CENTERS

The American Association of Poison Control Centers (AAPCC) uses a single, nationwide emergency number to automatically link callers with their regional poison center. This toll-free number, 800-222-1222, also works for teletype lines (TTY) for the hearing-impaired and telecommunication devices (TTD) for individuals who are deaf. However, a few local poison centers and the ASPCA/Animal Poison Control Center are not part of this nationwide system and continue to use separate numbers.

Most of the centers listed below are certified by the AAPCC. Certified centers are marked by an asterisk after the name. Each has to meet certain criteria. It must, for example, serve a large geographic area; it must be open 24 hours a day and provide direct-dial or toll-free access; it must be supervised by a medical director; and it must have registered pharmacists or nurses available to answer questions from the public.

Within each state, centers are listed alphabetically by city. Some state poison centers also list their original emergency numbers (including TTY/TDD) that only work within that state. For these listings, callers may use either the state number or the nationwide 800 number.

ALABAMA

BIRMINGHAM

Regional Poison Control Center, The Children's Hospital of Alabama (*)

1600 7th Ave. South
Birmingham, AL 35233-1711
Business: 205-939-9201
Emergency: 800-222-1222
               800-292-6678 (AL)
www.chsys.org

TUSCALOOSA

Alabama Poison Center (*)

2503 Phoenix Dr.
Tuscaloosa, AL 35405
Business: 205-345-0600
Emergency: 800-222-1222
               800-462-0800 (AL)
www.alapoisoncenter.org

ALASKA

JUNEAU

Alaska Poison Control System

Section of Community
Health and EMS
410 Willoughby Ave., Room 109
P.O. Box 110616
Juneau, AK 99811-0616
Business: 907-465-3027
Emergency: 800-222-1222
www.chems.alaska.gov

(PORTLAND, OR)

**Oregon Poison Center (*)
Oregon Health Sciences University**

3181 SW Sam Jackson
Park Rd. CB550
Portland, OR 97239
Business: 503-494-8600
Emergency: 800-222-1222
www.oregonpoison.com

ARIZONA

PHOENIX

**Banner Poison Control Center (*)
Banner Good Samaritan Medical Center**

901 E. Willetta St.
Room 2701
Phoenix, AZ 85006
Business: 602-495-6360
Emergency: 800-222-1222
               800-362-0101 (AZ)
               602-253-3334 (AZ)
www.bannerpoisoncontrol.com

TUCSON

**Arizona Poison and Drug Information Center (*)
Arizona Health Sciences Center**

1501 N. Campbell Ave.
Room 1156
Tucson, AZ 85724
Business: 520-626-7899
Emergency: 800-222-1222

ARKANSAS

LITTLE ROCK

**Arkansas Poison and Drug Information Center
College of Pharmacy - UAMS**

4301 West Markham St.
Mail Slot 522-2
Little Rock, AR 72205-7122
Business: 501-686-5540
Emergency: 800-222-1222
               800-376-4766 (AR)
TDD/TTY: 800-641-3805

ASPCA/ANIMAL POISON CONTROL CENTER

1717 South Philo Rd.
Suite 36
Urbana, IL 61802
Business: 217-337-5030
Emergency: 888-426-4435
               800-548-2423
www.napcc.aspca.org

CALIFORNIA

FRESNO/MADERA

**California Poison Control System-Fresno/Madera Div.(*)
Children's Hospital of Central California**

9300 Valley Children's Place
MB 15
Madera, CA 93638-8762
Business: 559-622-2300
Emergency: 800-222-1222
               800-876-4766 (CA)
TDD/TTY: 800-972-3323
www.calpoison.org

SACRAMENTO

**California Poison Control System-Sacramento Div.(*)
UC Davis Medical Center**

Room HSF 1024
2315 Stockton Blvd.
Sacramento, CA 95817
Business: 916-227-1400
Emergency: 800-222-1222
               800-876-4766 (CA)
TDD/TTY: 800-972-3323
www.calpoison.org

SAN DIEGO

**California Poison Control System-San Diego Div. (*)
UC San Diego Medical Center**

200 West Arbor Dr.
San Diego, CA 92103-8925
Business: 858-715-6300
Emergency: 800-222-1222
               800-876-4766 (CA)
TDD/TTY: 800-972-3323
www.calpoison.org

SAN FRANCISCO

**California Poison Control System-San Francisco Div.(*)
San Francisco General Hospital University of California San Francisco**

P.O. Box 1369
San Francisco, CA 94143-1369
Business: 415-502-6000
Emergency: 800-222-1222
               800-876-4766 (CA)
TDD/TTY: 800-972-3323
www.calpoison.org

COLORADO

DENVER

Rocky Mountain Poison and Drug Center (*)

777 Bannock St.
Mail Code 0180
Denver CO 80204-4507
Business: 303-739-1100
Emergency: 800-222-1222
TDD/TTY: 303-739-1127 (CO)
www.RMPDC.org

CONNECTICUT

FARMINGTON

**Connecticut Regional Poison Control Center (*)
University of Connecticut Health Center**

263 Farmington Ave.
Farmington, CT 06030-5365
Business: 860-679-4540
Emergency: 800-222-1222
TDD/TTY: 866-218-5372
http://poisoncontrol.uchc.edu

DELAWARE

(PHILADELPHIA, PA)

The Poison Control Center (*)
Children's Hospital of
Philadelphia

34th St. & Civic Center Blvd.
Philadelphia, PA 19104-4303
Business: 215-590-2003
Emergency: 800-222-1222
              800-722-7112 (DE)
TDD/TTY: 215-590-8789
www.poisoncontrol.chop.edu

DISTRICT OF COLUMBIA

WASHINGTON, DC

National Capital
Poison Center (*)

3201 New Mexico Ave., NW
Suite 310
Washington, DC 20016
Business: 202-362-3867
Emergency: 800-222-1222
TDD/TTY: 202-362-8563
www.poison.org

FLORIDA

JACKSONVILLE

Florida Poison Information
Center-Jacksonville (*)
SHANDS Hospital

655 West 8th St.
Jacksonville, FL 32209
Business: 904-244-4465
Emergency: 800-222-1222
http://fpicjax.org

MIAMI

Florida Poison Information
Center-Miami (*)
University of Miami–
Department of Pediatrics

P.O. Box 016960 (R-131)
Miami, FL 33101
Business: 305-585-5250
Emergency: 800-222-1222
www.miami.edu/poison-center

TAMPA

Florida Poison
Information Center-Tampa (*)
Tampa General Hospital

P.O. Box 1289
Tampa, FL 33601-1289
Business: 813-844-7044
Emergency: 800-222-1222
www.poisoncentertampa.org

GEORGIA

ATLANTA

Georgia Poison Center (*)
Hughes Spalding Children's
Hospital, Grady Health System

80 Jesse Hill Jr. Dr., SE
P.O. Box 26066
Atlanta, GA 30303-3050
Business: 404-616-9237
Emergency: 800-222-1222
              404-616-9000
              (Atlanta)
TDD: 404-616-9287
www.georgiapoisoncenter.org

HAWAII

(DENVER, CO)

Rocky Mountain Poison
and Drug Center (*)

777 Bannock St.
Mail Code 0180
Denver, CO 80204-4507
Business: 303-739-1100
Emergency: 800-222-1222
www.RMPDC.org

IDAHO

(DENVER, CO)

Rocky Mountain Poison
and Drug Center (*)

777 Bannock St.
Mail Code 0180
Denver, CO 80204-4507
Business: 303-739-1100
Emergency: 800-222-1222
www.RMPDC.org

ILLINOIS

CHICAGO

Illinois Poison Center (*)

222 South Riverside Plaza
Suite 1900
Chicago, IL 60606
Business: 312-906-6136
Emergency: 800-222-1222
TDD/TTY: 312-906-6185
www.illinoispoisoncenter.org

INDIANA

INDIANAPOLIS

Indiana Poison Control Center (*)
Clarian Health Partners
Methodist Hospital

I-65 at 21st St.
Indianapolis, IN 46206-1367
Business: 317-962-2335
Emergency: 800-222-1222
              800-382-9097
              317-962-2323
              (Indianapolis)
TTY: 317-962-2336
www.clarian.org/clinical/
  poisoncontrol

IOWA

SIOUX CITY

Iowa Statewide Poison
Control Center
Iowa Health System and the
University of Iowa Hospitals and
Clinics

2910 Hamilton Blvd., Suite 101
Sioux City, IA 51104
Business: 712-279-3710
Emergency: 800-222-1222
              712-277-2222 (IA)
www.iowapoison.org

KANSAS

KANSAS CITY

Mid-America Poison
Control Center
University of Kansas
Medical Center

3901 Rainbow Blvd.
Room B-400
Kansas City, KS 66160-7231
Business   913-588-6638
Emergency: 800-222-1222
              800-332-6633 (KS)
TDD: 913-588-6639
www.kumc.edu/poison

KENTUCKY

LOUISVILLE

Kentucky Regional
Poison Center (*)

P. O. Box 35070
Louisville, KY 40232-5070
Business: 502-629-7264
Emergency: 800-222-1222
              502-589-8222
              (Louisville)
www.krpc.com

LOUISIANA

MONROE

Louisiana Drug and Poison
Information Center (*)
University of Louisiana at
Monroe

700 University Ave.
Monroe, LA 71209-6430
Business: 318-342-3648
Emergency: 800-222-1222
www.lapcc.org

MAINE

PORTLAND

Northern New England
Poison Center

Maine Medical Center
22 Bramhall St.
Portland, ME 04102
Business: 207-842-7220
Emergency: 800-222-1222
              207-871-2879 (ME)
TDD/TTY: 877-299-4447 (ME)
              207-871-2879 (ME)

MARYLAND

BALTIMORE

Maryland Poison Center (*)
University of Maryland at
Baltimore
School of Pharmacy

20 North Pine St., PH 772
Baltimore, MD 21201
Business: 410-706-7604
Emergency: 800-222-1222
TDD: 410-706-1858
www.mdpoison.com

(WASHINGTON, DC)

National Capital
Poison Center (*)

3201 New Mexico Ave., NW
Suite 310
Washington DC 20016
Business: 202-362-3867
Emergency: 800-222-1222
TDD/TTY: 202-362-8563 (MD)
www.poison.org

MASSACHUSETTS

BOSTON

Regional Center for Poison
Control and Prevention (*)
(Serving Massachusetts and
Rhode Island)

300 Longwood Ave.
Boston, MA 02115
Business: 617-355-6609
Emergency: 800-222-1222
TDD/TTY: 888-244-5313
www.maripoisoncenter.com

MICHIGAN

DETROIT

Regional Poison
Control Center (*)
Children's Hospital of Michigan

4160 John R. Harper
Professional Office Bldg.
Suite 616
Detroit, MI 48201
Business: 313-745-5335
Emergency: 800-222-1222
TDD/TTY: 800-356-3232
www.mitoxic.org/pcc

GRAND RAPIDS

DeVos Children's Hospital Regional Poison Center (*)

100 Michigan St., NE
Grand Rapids, MI 49503
Business: 616-391-3690
Emergency: 800-222-1222
http://poisoncenter.devoschildrens.org

MINNESOTA

MINNEAPOLIS

Minnesota Poison Control System (*) Hennepin County Medical Center

701 Park Ave.
Mail Code 820
Minneapolis, MN 55415
Business: 612-873-6000
Emergency: 800-222-1222
TTY: 612-904-4691
www.mnpoison.org

MISSISSIPPI

JACKSON

Mississippi Regional Poison Control Center, University of Mississippi Medical Center

2500 North State St.
Jackson, MS 39216
Business: 601-984-1675
Emergency: 800-222-1222

MISSOURI

ST. LOUIS

Missouri Regional Poison Center (*) Cardinal Glennon Children's Hospital

7980 Clayton Rd.
Suite 200
St. Louis, MO 63117
Business: 314-772-5200
Emergency: 800-222-1222
TDD/TTY: 314-612-5705
www.cardinalglennon.com

MONTANA

(DENVER, CO)

Rocky Mountain Poison and Drug Center (*)

777 Bannock St.
Mail Code 0180
Denver, CO 80204-4507
Business: 303-739-1100
Emergency: 800-222-1222
TDD/TTY: 303-739-1127
www.RMPDC.org

NEBRASKA

OMAHA

The Poison Center (*) Children's Hospital

8200 Dodge St.
Omaha, NE 68114
Business: 402-955-5555
Emergency: 800-222-1222
www.poison-center.com

NEVADA

(DENVER, CO)

Rocky Mountain Poison and Drug Center (*)

777 Bannock St.
Mail Code 0180
Denver, CO 80204-4507
Business: 303-739-1100
Emergency: 800-222-1222
www.RMPDC.org

(PORTLAND, OR)

Oregon Poison Center (*) Oregon Health Sciences University

3181 SW Sam Jackson Park Rd.
Portland, OR 97201
Business: 503-494-8600
Emergency: 800-222-1222
www.oregonpoison.com

NEW HAMPSHIRE

(PORTLAND, ME)

Northern New England Poison Center

Maine Medical Center
22 Bramhall St.
Portland, ME 04102
Business: 207-842-7220
Emergency: 800-222-1222

NEW JERSEY

NEWARK

New Jersey Poison Information and Education System (*) UMDNJ

65 Bergen St.
Newark, NJ 07101
Business: 973-972-9280
Emergency: 800-222-1222
TDD/TTY: 973-926-8008
www.njpies.org

NEW MEXICO

ALBUQUERQUE

New Mexico Poison and Drug Information Center (*)

MSC09-5080
1 University of New Mexico
Albuquerque, NM 87131-0001
Business: 505-272-4261
Emergency: 800-222-1222
http://HSC.UNM.edu/
     pharmacy/poison

NEW YORK

BUFFALO

Western New York Regional Poison Control Center (*) Children's Hospital of Buffalo

219 Bryant St.
Buffalo, NY 14222
Business: 716-878-7654
Emergency: 800-222-1222
www.fingerlakespoison.org

MINEOLA

Long Island Regional Poison and Drug Information Center (*) Winthrop University Hospital

259 First St.
Mineola, NY 11501
Business: 516-663-2650
Emergency: 800-222-1222
TDD: 516-747-3323
              (Nassau)
              516-924-8811
              (Suffolk)
www.lirpdic.org

NEW YORK CITY

New York City Poison Control Center (*) NYC Dept. of Health

455 First Ave., Room 123
New York, NY 10016
Business: 212-447-8152
Emergency: 800-222-1222
(English)   212-340-4494
              212-POISONS
              (212-764-7667)

Emergency: 212-VENENOS
(Spanish)   (212-836-3667)
TDD: 212-689-9014

ROCHESTER

Finger Lakes Regional Poison and Drug Information Center (*) University of Rochester Medical Center

601 Elmwood Ave.
P.O. Box 321
Rochester, NY 14642
Business: 585-273-4155
Emergency: 800-222-1222
TTY: 585-273-3854

SYRACUSE

Central New York Poison Center (*) SUNY Upstate Medical University

750 East Adams St.
Syracuse, NY 13210
Business: 315-464-7078
Emergency: 800-222-1222
www.cnypoison.org

NORTH CAROLINA

CHARLOTTE

Carolinas Poison Center (*) Carolinas Medical Center

P.O. Box 32861
Charlotte, NC 28232
Business: 704-395-3795
Emergency: 800-222-1222
TDD: 800-735-8262
TTY: 800-735-2962
www.ncpoisoncenter.org

NORTH DAKOTA

(MINNEAPOLIS, MN)

Minnesota Poison Control System (*) Hennepin County Medical Center

701 Park Ave.
Mail Code 820
Minneapolis, MN 55415
Business: 612-873-3144
Emergency: 800-222-1222
www.ndpoison.org

OHIO

CINCINNATI

Cincinnati Drug and Poison Information Center (*) Regional Poison Control System

3333 Burnet Ave.
Vernon Place, 3rd Floor
Cincinnati, OH 45229
Business: 513-636-5111
Emergency: 800-222-1222
TDD/TTY: 800-253-7955
www.cincinnatichildrens.org/dpic

CLEVELAND

Greater Cleveland Poison Control Center

11100 Euclid Ave.
MP 6007
Cleveland, OH 44106-6007
Business: 216-844-1573
Emergency: 800-222-1222
              216-231-4455 (OH)

COLUMBUS

**Central Ohio
Poison Center (*)**

700 Children's Dr.
Room L032
Columbus, OH 43205-2696
Business: 614-722-2635
Emergency: 800-222-1222
           614-228-1323
           937-222-2227
           (Dayton region)
TTY: 614-228-2272
www.bepoisonsmart.com

OKLAHOMA

OKLAHOMA CITY

**Oklahoma Poison
Control Center (*)
Children's Hospital at OU
Medical Center**

940 Northeast 13th St.
Room 3510
Oklahoma City, OK 73104
Business: 405-271-5062
Emergency: 800-222-1222
www.oklahomapoison.org

OREGON

PORTLAND

**Oregon Poison Center (*)
Oregon Health Sciences
University**

3181 S.W. Sam Jackson Park Rd.,
CB550
Portland, OR 97239
Business: 503-494-8600
Emergency: 800-222-1222
www.oregonpoison.com

PENNSYLVANIA

PHILADELPHIA

**The Poison Control Center (*)
Children's Hospital of
Philadelphia**

34th Street & Civic Center Blvd.
Philadelphia, PA 19104-4399
Business: 215-590-2003
Emergency: 800-222-1222
           215-386-2100 (PA)
TDD/TTY: 215-590-8789
www.poisoncontrol.chop.edu

PITTSBURGH

**Pittsburgh Poison Center (*)
Children's Hospital of Pittsburgh**

3705 Fifth Ave.
Pittsburgh, PA 15213
Business: 412-390-3300
Emergency: 800-222-1222
           412-681-6669
www.chp.edu/clinical/03a_
    poison.php

PUERTO RICO

SANTURCE

**San Jorge Children's Hospital
Poison Center**

258 San Jorge St.
Santurce, PR 00912
Business: 787-726-5660
Emergency: 800-222-1222
TTY: 787-641-1934
www.poisoncenter.net

RHODE ISLAND

(BOSTON, MA)

**Regional Center for Poison
Control and Prevention (*)**
(Serving Massachusetts and
Rhode Island)

300 Longwood Ave.
Boston, MA 02115
Business: 617-355-6609
Emergency: 800-222-1222
TDD/TTY: 888-244-5313
www.maripoisoncenter.com

SOUTH CAROLINA

COLUMBIA

**Palmetto Poison Center (*)
College of Pharmacy
University of South Carolina**

Columbia, SC 29208
Business: 803-777-7909
Drug Info: 800-777-7804
Emergency: 800-222-1222
           803-777-1117 (SC)
www.pharm.sc.edu/PPS/pps.htm

SOUTH DAKOTA

(MINNEAPOLIS, MN)

**Hennepin Regional Poison
Center (*) Hennepin County
Medical Center**

701 Park Ave.
Minneapolis, MN 55415
Business: 612-873-6000
Emergency: 800-222-1222
TTY: 612-904-4691
www.mnpoison.org

SIOUX FALLS

**Provides education only—does
not manage exposure cases.**

**Sioux Valley Poison Control
Center (*)**

1305 W. 18th St.
P.O. Box 5039
Sioux Falls, SD 57117-5039
Business: 605-333-6638
www.sdpoison.org

TENNESSEE

NASHVILLE

**Tennessee
Poison Center (*)**

1161 21st Ave. South
501 Oxford House
Nashville, TN 37232-4632
Business: 615-936-0760
Emergency: 800-222-1222
www.poisonlifeline.org

TEXAS

AMARILLO

**Texas Panhandle
Poison Center (*)
Northwest Texas Hospital**

1501 S. Coulter Dr.
Amarillo, TX 79106
Business: 806-354-1630
Emergency: 800-222-1222
www.poisoncontrol.org

DALLAS

**North Texas Poison Center (*)
Texas Poison Center Network
Parkland Health and Hospital
System**

5201 Harry Hines Blvd.
Dallas, TX 75235
Business: 214-589-0911
Emergency: 800-222-1222
www.poisoncontrol.org

EL PASO

**West Texas Regional
Poison Center (*)
Thomason Hospital**

4815 Alameda Ave.
El Paso, TX 79905
Business   915-534-3800
Emergency: 800-222-1222
www.poisoncontrol.org

GALVESTON

**Southeast Texas
Poison Center (*)
The University of Texas
Medical Branch**

3.112 Trauma Bldg.
301 University Ave.
Galveston, TX 77555-1175
Business: 409-766-4403
Emergency: 800-222-1222
www.poisoncontrol.org

SAN ANTONIO

**South Texas
Poison Center (*)
The University of Texas Health
Science Center–San Antonio**

7703 Floyd Curl Dr., MC 7849
San Antonio, TX 78229-3900
Business: 210-567-5762
Emergency: 800-222-1222
www.poisoncontrol.org

TEMPLE

**Central Texas Poison Center (*)
Scott & White Memorial Hospital**

2401 South 31st St.
Temple, TX 76508
Business: 254-724-7401
Emergency: 800-222-1222
www.poisoncontrol.org

UTAH

SALT LAKE CITY

Utah Poison Control Center (*)

585 Komas Dr.
Suite 200
Salt Lake City, UT 84108
Business: 801-581-7504
Emergency: 800-222-1222
           801-587-0600 (UT)
http://uuhsc.utah.edu/poison

VERMONT

(PORTLAND, ME)

**Northern New England
Poison Center**

Maine Medical Center
22 Bramhall St.
Portland, ME 04102
Business: 207-842-7220
Emergency: 800-222-1222

VIRGINIA

CHARLOTTESVILLE

**Blue Ridge Poison Center (*)
University of Virginia Health
System**

P.O. Box 800774
Charlottesville, VA 22908-0774
Business: 434-924-0347
Emergency: 800-222-1222
           800-451-1428 (VA)
www.healthsystem.virginia.edu.
    brpc

RICHMOND

Virginia Poison Center (*)
Virginia Commonwealth
University

P.O. Box 980522
Richmond, VA 23298-0522
Business: 804-828-4780
Emergency: 800-222-1222
                 804-828-9123
TDD/TTY: 804-828-9123

WASHINGTON

SEATTLE

Washington Poison
Center (*)

155 NE 100th St.
Suite 400
Seattle, WA 98125-8011
Business: 206-517-2351
Emergency: 800-222-1222
                 206-526-2121
                 (WA)
TDD: 800-572-0638
                 (WA)
                 206-517-2394
                 (Seattle)
www.wapc.org

WEST VIRGINIA

CHARLESTON

West Virginia
Poison Center (*)

3110 MacCorkle Ave. SE
Charleston, WV 25304
Business: 304-347-1212
Emergency: 800-222-1222
www.wvpoisoncontrol.org

WISCONSIN

MILWAUKEE

Children's Hospital
of Wisconsin Statewide
Poison Center

9000 W. Wisconsin Ave.
P.O. Box 1997, Mail Station 677A
Milwaukee, WI 53226
Business: 414-266-2000
Emergency: 800-222-1222
TDD/TTY: 414-964-3497
www.chw.org

WYOMING

(OMAHA, NE)

The Poison Center (*)
Children's Hospital

8200 Dodge St.
Omaha, NE 68114
Business: 402-955-5555
Emergency: 800-222-1222
www.poison-center.com

DRUG INFORMATION CENTERS

ALABAMA

BIRMINGHAM

Drug Information Service
University of Alabama
UAB Hospital Pharmacy

Drug Information-JT1720
619 S. 19th St.
Birmingham, AL 35249-6860
Mon.-Fri. 8 AM-5 PM
205-934-2162
www.health.uab.edu/pharmacy

Global Drug
Information Service
Samford University
McWhorter School
of Pharmacy

800 Lakeshore Dr.
Birmingham, AL 35229-7027
Mon.-Fri. 8 AM-4:30 PM
205-726-2659
www.samford.edu/schools/
pharmacy/dic/index.html

HUNTSVILLE

Huntsville Hospital Drug
Information Center

101 Sivley Rd.
Huntsville, AL 35801
Mon.-Fri. 7 AM-3:30 PM
256-265-8288

ARIZONA

TUCSON

Arizona Poison and Drug
Information Center
Arizona Health
Sciences Center
University Medical Center

1501 N. Campbell Ave.
Room 1156
Tucson, AZ 85724
7 days/week, 24 hours
520-626-6016
800-222-1222
(Emergency)
www.pharmacy.arizona.edu

ARKANSAS

LITTLE ROCK

Arkansas Poison and Drug
Information Center

4301 W. Markham St.
Slot 522-2
Little Rock, AR 72205
Mon.-Fri. 8:30 AM-5 PM
501-686-5072
(Little Rock area only-
for healthcare
professionals only)
800-228-1233
(AR only - **for**
healthcare
professionals only)

CALIFORNIA

LOS ANGELES

Los Angeles Regional
Drug Information Center
LAC & USC Medical Center

1200 N. State St.
Trailer 25
Los Angeles, CA 90033
Mon.-Fri. 8:30 AM-4 PM
Closed 12 PM to 1 PM
323-226-7741

SAN DIEGO

Drug Information Service
University of California
San Diego Medical Center

200 West Arbor Dr.
MC 8925
San Diego, CA 92103-8925
Mon.-Fri. 9 AM-5 PM
900-226-7536
(for healthcare
professionals only)

SAN FRANCISCO

Drug Information Analysis
Service
University of California,
San Francisco

P.O. Box 1262
521 Parnassus Ave.
Room C152
San Francisco, CA 94143-0622
Mon.-Fri. 8:30 AM-4:30 PM
415-502-9540
(for healthcare
professionals only)

STANFORD

Drug Information Center
University of California
Stanford Hospital and Clinics

300 Pasteur Dr.
Room H-0301
Stanford, CA 94305
Mon.-Fri. 8 AM-4 PM
650-723-6422

COLORADO

DENVER

Rocky Mountain Poison
and Drug Center

990 Bannock St.
(Physical address)
777 Bannock St.
(Mailing address)
Denver, CO 80264
303-739-1123
800-222-1222
(Emergency)
www.rmpdc.org

Drug Information Center
University of Colorado
Health Science Center
School of Pharmacy

4200 E. 9th Ave.,
P.O. Box C239
Denver, CO 80262
Mon.-Fri. 8 AM-5 PM
303-315-8489

CONNECTICUT

FARMINGTON

Drug Information Service
University of Connecticut Health
Center

263 Farmington Ave.
Farmington, CT 06030
Mon.-Fri. 7:30 AM-4 PM
860-679-2783

HARTFORD

Drug Information Center
Hartford Hospital

P.O. Box 5037
80 Seymour St.
Hartford, CT 06102
Mon.-Fri. 8:30 AM-5 PM
860-545-2221
860-545-2961(After
5 PM)
www.hartfordhospital.org

NEW HAVEN

Drug Information Center
Yale-New Haven Hospital

20 York St.
New Haven, CT 06540-3202
Mon.-Fri. 8:30 AM-5 PM
203-688-2248
www.ynhh.org

DISTRICT OF COLUMBIA

Drug Information Service
Howard University Hospital

Room BB06
2041 Georgia Ave. NW
Washington, DC 20060
Mon.-Fri. 8:30 AM-4:30 PM
202-865-1325
800-222-1222
(Emergency)

FLORIDA

FT. LAUDERDALE

Nova Southeastern University
College of Pharmacy
Drug Information Center

3200 S. University Dr.
Ft. Lauderdale, FL 33328
Mon.-Fri. 9 AM-5 PM
954-262-3103
http://pharmacy.nova.edu

GAINESVILLE

Drug Information &
Pharmacy Resource Center
Shands Hospital at
University of Florida

P.O. Box 100316
Gainesville, FL 32610-0316
Mon.-Fri. 9 AM-5 PM
352-265-0408
(for healthcare
professionals only)
http://shands.org/professional/
drugs

JACKSONVILLE

Drug Information Service
Shands Jacksonville

655 W. 8th St.
Jacksonville, FL 32209
Mon.-Fri. 9:30 AM-4 PM
904-244-4185
(for healthcare
professionals only)
904-244-4700
(for consumers,
Mon.-Fri. 9 AM-4 PM)

ORLANDO

Orlando Regional Drug
Information Service
Orlando Regional
Healthcare System

1414 Kuhl Ave., MP 192
Orlando, FL 32806
Mon.-Fri. 8 AM-4 PM
321-841-8717

TALLAHASSEE

Drug Information
Education Center
Florida Agricultural and
Mechanical University
College of Pharmacy and
Pharmaceutical Sciences

Tallahassee, FL 32307
Mon.-Fri. 9 AM-5 PM
850-488-5239

WEST PALM BEACH

Drug Information Center
Nova Southeastern University,
West Palm Beach

3970 RCA Blvd., Suite 7006A
Palm Beach Gardens, FL 33410
Mon.-Fri. 9 AM-5 PM
          561-622-0658
          (for healthcare
          professionals only)

GEORGIA

ATLANTA

Emory University Hospital
Dept. of Pharmaceutical
Services-Drug Information

1364 Clifton Rd. NE
Atlanta, GA 30322
Mon.-Fri. 8:30 AM-5 PM
          404-712-7150
          (for healthcare
          professionals only)

Drug Information Service
Northside Hospital

1000 Johnson Ferry Rd. NE
Atlanta, GA 30342
Mon.-Fri. 9 AM-4 PM
          404-851-8676
          (GA only)

AUGUSTA

Drug Information Center
Medical College of Georgia
Hospital and Clinic

BI2101
1120 15th St.
Augusta, GA 30912
Mon.-Fri. 8:30 AM-5 PM
          706-721-2887

COLUMBUS

Columbus Regional Drug
Information Center

710 Center St.
Columbus, GA 31902
Mon.-Fri. 8 AM-5 PM
          706-571-1934
          (for healthcare
          professionals only)

IDAHO

POCATELLO

Drug Information Center
Idaho State University
School of Pharmacy

970 S. 5th St.
Campus Box 8092
Pocatello, ID 83209
Mon.-Thur. 8:30 AM-5 PM
Fri. 8:30 AM-2:30 PM
Closed 12 PM-1 PM
          208-282-4689
          800-334-7139
          (ID only)
http://pharmacy.isu.edu

ILLINOIS

CHICAGO

Drug Information Center
Northwestern Memorial Hospital

Feinberg Pavilion, LC 700
251 E. Huron St.
Chicago, IL 60611
Mon.-Fri. 8:30 AM-5 PM
          312-926-7573

Drug Information Services
University of Chicago Hospitals

5841 S. Maryland Ave.
MC 0010
Chicago, IL 60637-1470
Mon.-Fri. 9 AM-5 PM
          773-702-1388

Drug Information Center
University of Illinois at Chicago

833 S. Wood St.
MC 886
Chicago, IL 60612-7231
Mon.-Fri. 8 AM-4 PM
          312-996-3681
          (for healthcare
          professionals only)
          312-996-3682
          (for consumers,
          Mon.-Fri. 9
          AM-12 PM)
www.uic.edu/pharmacy/
services/di/index.html

HARVEY

Drug Information Center
Ingalls Memorial Hospital

1 Ingalls Dr.
Harvey, IL 60426
Mon.-Fri. 8 AM-4:30 PM
          708-333-2300

HINES

Drug Information Service
Hines Veterans Administration
Hospital

2100 S. 5th Ave.
Pharmacy Services
MC119
P.O. Box 5000
Hines, IL 60141-5000
Mon.-Fri. 8 AM-4:30 PM
          708-202-8387,
          ext. 23780

PARK RIDGE

Drug Information Center
Advocate Lutheran General
Hospital

1775 Dempster St.
Park Ridge, IL 60068
Mon.-Fri. 7:30 AM-4 PM
          847-723-8128
          (for healthcare
          professionals only)

INDIANA

INDIANAPOLIS

Drug Information Center
St. Vincent Hospital
and Health Services

2001 W. 86th St.
Indianapolis, IN 46260
Mon.-Fri. 8 AM-4 PM
          317-338-3200
          (for healthcare
          professionals only)

Drug Information Service
Clarian Health Partners

Pharmacy Department I-65
at 21st St.
Room CG04
Indianapolis, IN 46202
Mon.-Fri. 8 AM-4:30 PM
          317-962-1750

MUNCIE

Drug Information Center
Ball Memorial Hospital

2401 University Ave.
Muncie, IN 47303
Mon.-Fri. 8 AM-4:30 PM
          765-747-3035

IOWA

DES MOINES

Regional Drug
Information Center
Mercy Medical Center-
Des Moines

1111 Sixth Ave.
Des Moines, IA 50314
Mon.-Fri. 8 AM-4:30 PM
          (regional service;
          in-house service
          answered 7 days/
          week, 24 hours)
          515-247-3286

IOWA CITY

Drug Information Center
University of Iowa
Hospitals and Clinics

200 Hawkins Dr.
Iowa City, IA 52242
Mon.-Fri. 8 AM-4:30 PM
          319-356-2600
          (for healthcare
          professionals only)

KANSAS

KANSAS CITY

Drug Information Center
University of Kansas
Medical Center

3901 Rainbow Blvd.
Kansas City, KS 66160
Mon.-Fri. 8:30 AM-4:30 PM
          913-588-2328
          (for healthcare
          professionals only)

KENTUCKY

LEXINGTON

University of Kentucky
Drug Information Center
Chandler Medical Center

800 Rose St., C-113
Lexington, KY 40536-0293
Mon.-Fri. 8 AM-5 PM
          859-323-5320 or
          859-323-5476

LOUISIANA

MONROE

Louisiana Drug and Poison
Information Center
University of Louisiana at
Monroe College of Pharmacy

Sugar Hall
Monroe, LA 71209-6430
Mon.-Fri. 8 AM-4:30 PM
          318-342-1710

NEW ORLEANS

Xavier University Drug
Information Center
Tulane University
Hospital and Clinic

1440 Canal St.
Suite 808
New Orleans, LA 70112
Mon.-Fri. 9 AM-5 PM
          504-588-5670

MARYLAND

ANDREWS AFB

Drug Information Services

89 MDTS/SGQP
1050 W. Perimeter Rd.
Suite D1-119
Andrews AFB, MD 20762-6660
Mon.-Fri. 7:30 AM-5 PM
          240-857-4565

ANNAPOLIS

The Anne Arundel
Medical Center
Dept. of Pharmacy

2001 Medical Pkwy.
Annapolis, MD 21401
7 days/week, 24 hours
          443-481-4155
www.aahs.org

BALTIMORE

Drug Information Service
Johns Hopkins Hospital

600 N. Wolfe St.
Carnegie 180
Baltimore, MD 21287-6180
Mon.-Fri. 8:30 AM-5 PM
410-955-6348

Drug Information Service
University of Maryland
School of PharmacyPharmacy
Hall

Room 760
20 North Pine St.
Baltimore, MD 21201
Mon.-Fri. 8:30 AM-5 PM
410-706-7568
(consumers only)
410-706-0898
(for healthcare
professionals only)
www.pharmacy.umaryland.
edu/umdi

BETHESDA

Drug Information Service
National Institutes of Health

Building 10, Room 1S-259
10 Center Dr. (MSC1196)
Bethesda, MD 20892-1196
Mon.-Fri. 8:30 AM-5 PM
301-496-2407
www.cc.nih.gov/phar

EASTON

Drug Information
Pharmacy Dept.
Memorial Hospital

219 S. Washington St.
Easton, MD 21601
7 days/week, 7 AM-5:30 PM
410-822-1000,
ext. 5645

MASSACHUSETTS

BOSTON

Drug Information Services
Brigham and Women's Hospital

75 Francis St.
Boston, MA 02115
Mon.-Fri. 7 AM-3 PM
617-732-7166

WORCESTER

Drug Information Pharmacy
UMass Memorial
Medical Center
Healthcare Hospital

55 Lake Ave. North
Worcester, MA 01655
Mon.-Fri. 8:30 AM-5 PM
508-856-3456
508-856-2775
(24-hour)

MICHIGAN

ANN ARBOR

Drug Information Service Dept.
of Pharmacy Services
University of Michigan
Health System

1500 East Medical
Center Dr.
UH B2D301
P.O. Box 0008
Ann Arbor, MI 48109-0008
Mon.-Fri. 8 AM-5 PM
734-936-8200

DETROIT

Drug Information Center
Department of
Pharmacy Services
Detroit Receiving Hospital and
University Health Center

4201 St. Antoine Blvd.
Detroit, MI 48201
Mon.-Fri. 9 AM-5 PM
313-745-4556
www.dmcpharmacy.org

LANSING

Drug Information Services
Sparrow Hospital

1215 East Michigan Ave.
Lansing, MI 48912
7 days/week, 24 hours
517-364-2444

PONTIAC

Drug Information Center
St. Joseph Mercy Oakland

44405 Woodward Ave.
Pontiac, MI 48341
Mon.-Fri. 8 AM-4:30 PM
248-858-3055

ROYAL OAK

Drug Information Services
William Beaumont Hospital

3601 West 13 Mile Rd.
Royal Oak, MI 48073-6769
Mon.-Fri. 8 AM-4:30 PM
248-898-4077

SOUTHFIELD

Drug Information Service
Providence Hospital

16001 West 9 Mile Rd.
Southfield, MI 48075
Mon.-Fri. 8 AM-4 PM
248-849-3125

MISSISSIPPI

JACKSON

Drug Information Center
University of Mississippi
Medical Center

2500 N. State St.
Jackson, MS 39216
Mon.-Fri. 8 AM-4:30 PM
601-984-2060

MISSOURI

KANSAS CITY

University of
Missouri-Kansas City
Drug Information Center

2411 Holmes St., MG-200
Kansas City, MO 64108
Mon.-Fri. 8 AM-5 PM
816-235-5490
http://druginfo.umkc.edu/

SPRINGFIELD

Drug Information Center
St. John's Hospital

1235 E. Cherokee St.
Springfield, MO 65804
Mon.-Fri. 7:30 AM-4:30 PM
417-820-3488

ST. JOSEPH

Regional Medical Center
Pharmacy

5325 Faraon St.
St. Joseph, MO 64506
7 days/week, 24 hours
816-271-6141

MONTANA

MISSOULA

Drug Information Service
University of Montana School of
Pharmacy and Allied Health
Sciences

32 Campus Dr.
Skaggs Bldg. 217
Missoula, MT 59812-1522
Mon.-Fri. 8 AM-5 PM
406-243-5254
800-501-5491
www.umt.edu/druginfo

NEBRASKA

OMAHA

Drug Informatics Service
School of Pharmacy
Creighton University

2500 California Plaza
Omaha, NE 68178
Mon.-Fri. 8:30 AM-4:30 PM
402-280-5101
http://pharmacy.creighton.edu

NEW JERSEY

NEWARK

New Jersey Poison Information
and Education System

65 Bergen St.
Newark, NJ 07107
Mon.-Fri. 8:30 AM- 5 PM
973-972-9280
800-222-1222
(Emergency)
www.njpies.org

NEW BRUNSWICK

Drug Information Service
Robert Wood Johnson
University Hospital

Pharmacy Department
1 Robert Wood Johnson Pl.
New Brunswick, NJ 08901
Mon.-Fri. 8:30 AM-4:30 PM
732-937-8842

NEW MEXICO

ALBUQUERQUE

New Mexico Poison Center
University of New Mexico
Health Sciences Center

MSC09 5080
1 University of New Mexico
Albuquerque, NM 87131
7 days/week, 24 hours
505-272-4261
800-222-1222
(Emergency)
http://hsc.unm.edu/pharmacy/
poison

NEW YORK

BROOKLYN

International Drug
Information Center
Long Island University
Arnold & Marie Schwartz
College of Pharmacy &
Health Sciences

1 University Plaza
RM-HS509
Brooklyn, NY 11201
Mon.-Fri. 9 AM-5 PM
718-780-4184
www.liu.edu

COOPERSTOWN

Drug Information Center
Bassett Healthcare

1 Atwell Rd.
Cooperstown, NY 13326
7 days/week, 24 hours
607-547-3686

NEW HYDE PARK

Drug Information Center
St. John's University at Long Island Jewish Medical Center

270-05 76th Ave.
New Hyde Park, NY 11040
Mon.-Fri. 8 AM-3 PM
718-470-DRUG (3784)

NEW YORK CITY

Drug Information Center
Memorial Sloan-Kettering Cancer Center

1275 York Ave.
RM S-712
New York, NY 10021
Mon.-Fri. 9 AM-5 PM
212-639-7552

Drug Information Center
Mount Sinai Medical Center

1 Gustave Levy Pl.
New York, NY 10029
Mon.-Fri. 9 AM-5 PM
212-241-6619

Drug Information Service
New York Presbyterian Hospital

Room K04
525 E. 68th St.
New York, NY 10021
Mon.-Fri. 9 AM-5 PM
212-746-0741

ROCHESTER

Finger Lakes
Poison and Drug Information Center
University of Rochester

601 Elmwood Ave.
Rochester, NY 14642
Mon.-Fri. 8 AM-5 PM
585-275-3718

ROCKVILLE CENTER

Drug Information Center
Mercy Medical Center

1000 North Village Ave.
Rockville Center, NY 11571-9024
Mon.-Fri. 8 AM-4 PM
516-705-1053

NORTH CAROLINA

BUIES CREEK

Drug Information Center
School of Pharmacy
Campbell University

P.O. Box 1090
Buies Creek, NC 27506
Mon.-Fri. 8:30 AM-4:30 PM
910-893-1200
x2701
800-760-9697
(Toll free) x2701
800-327-5467
(NC only)

CHAPEL HILL

University of North Carolina Hospitals
Drug Information Center
Dept. of Pharmacy

101 Manning Dr.
Chapel Hill, NC 27514
Mon.-Fri. 8 AM-4:30 PM
919-966-2373

DURHAM

Drug Information Center
Duke University Health Systems

DUMC Box 3089
Durham, NC 27710
Mon.-Fri. 8 AM-5 PM
919-684-5125

GREENVILLE

Eastern Carolina Drug Information Center
Pitt County Memorial Hospital
Dept. of Pharmacy Service

P.O. Box 6028
2100 Stantonsburg Rd.
Greenville, NC 27835
Mon.-Fri. 8 AM-5 PM
252-847-4257

WINSTON-SALEM

Drug Information Service Center
Wake-Forest University Baptist Medical Center

Medical Center Blvd.
Winston-Salem, NC 27157
Mon.-Fri. 8 AM-5 PM
336-716-2037
(for healthcare professionals only)

OHIO

ADA

Drug Information Center
Raabe College of Pharmacy
Ohio Northern University

Ada, OH 45810
Mon.-Thurs. 8:30 AM-5 PM, 7-10 PM
Fri. 8:30 AM- 5 PM;
Sun. 2 PM-10 PM
419-772-2307
www.onu.edu/pharmacy/druginfo

CINCINNATI

Drug and Poison Information Center

Children's Hospital Medical Center

3333 Burnet Ave. ML9004
Cincinnati, OH 45229
Mon.-Fri. 9 AM-5 PM
513-636-5054
(Administration)
513-636-5111
(7 days/week, 24 hours)

CLEVELAND

Drug Information Service
Cleveland Clinic Foundation

9500 Euclid Ave.
Cleveland, OH 44195
Mon.-Fri. 8:30 AM-4:30 PM
216-444-6456
(for healthcare professionals only)

COLUMBUS

Drug Information Center
Ohio State University Hospital
Dept. of Pharmacy

Doan Hall 368
410 W. 10th Ave.
Columbus, OH 43210-1228
7 days/week, 24 hours
614-293-8679

Drug Information Center
Riverside Methodist Hospital

3535 Olentangy River Road
Columbus, OH 43214
Mon.-Fri. 8:30 AM-4 PM
614-566-5425

TOLEDO

Drug Information Services
St. Vincent Mercy Medical Center

2213 Cherry St.
Toledo, Ohio 43608-2691
Mon.-Fri. 8 AM-4 PM
419-251-4227
www.rx.medctr.ohio-state.edu

OKLAHOMA

OKLAHOMA CITY

Drug Information Service
Integris Health

3300 Northwest Expressway
Oklahoma City, OK 73112
Mon.-Fri. 8 AM-4:30 PM
405-949-3660

Drug Information Center
OU Medical Center
Presbyterian Tower

700 NE 13th St.
Oklahoma City, OK 73104
Mon.-Fri. 8 AM-4:30 PM
405-271-6226
Fax: 405-271-6281

TULSA

Drug Information Center
Saint Francis Hospital

6161 S. Yale Ave.
Tulsa, OK 74136
Mon.-Fri. 8 AM-4:30 PM
918-494-6339
(for healthcare professionals only)

PENNSYLVANIA

PHILADELPHIA

Drug Information Center
Temple University Hospital
Dept. of Pharmacy

3401 N. Broad St.
Philadelphia, PA 19140
Mon.-Fri. 8 AM-4:30 PM
215-707-4644

Drug Information Service
Tenet Health System
Hahnemann University Hospital
Department of Pharmacy

MS 451
Broad and Vine Streets
Philadelphia, PA 19102
Mon.-Fri. 8 AM-4 PM
215-762-DRUG
(3784)
(for healthcare professionals only)

Drug Information Service
Dept. of Pharmacy
Thomas Jefferson University Hospital

111 S. 11th St.
Philadelphia, PA 19107-5089
Mon.-Fri. 8 AM-5 PM
215-955-8877

University of Pennsylvania Health System Drug Information Service
Hospital of the University of Pennsylvania
Department of Pharmacy

3400 Spruce St.
Philadelphia, PA 19104
Mon.-Fri. 8:30 AM-4 PM
215-662-2903

PITTSBURGH

Pharmaceutical Information Center
Mylan School of Pharmacy
Duquesne University

431 Mellon Hall
Pittsburgh, PA 15282
Mon.-Fri. 8 AM-4 PM
412-396-4600

Drug Information Center
University of Pittsburgh

302 Scaife Hall
200 Lothrop St.
Pittsburgh, PA 15213
Mon.-Fri. 9 AM-3 PM
412-647-3784
(for healthcare professionals only)

UPLAND

Drug Information Center
Crozer-Chester Medical Center
Dept. of Pharmacy

1 Medical Center Blvd.
Upland, PA 19013
Mon.-Fri. 8 AM-4:30 PM
610-447-2851
(for in-house health
care professionals
only)

PUERTO RICO

PONCE

Centro Informacion
Medicamentos
Escuela de Medicina de Ponce

P.O. Box 7004
Ponce, PR 00732-7004
Mon.-Fri. 8 AM-4:30 PM
787-840-2575

SAN JUAN

Centro de Informacion de
Medicamentos-CIM
Escuela de Farmacia-RCM

P.O. Box 365067
San Juan, PR 00936-5067
Mon.-Fri. 8 AM-4:30 PM
787-758-2525,
ext. 1516

SOUTH CAROLINA

CHARLESTON

Drug Information Service
Medical University of
South Carolina

150 Ashley Ave.
Rutledge Tower Annex
Room 604
P.O. Box 250584
Charleston, SC 29425-0810
Mon.-Fri. 9 AM-5:30 PM
843-792-3896
800-922-5250

COLUMBIA

Drug Information Service
University of South Carolina
College of Pharmacy

Columbia, SC 29208
Mon.-Fri. 8 AM-Midnight
803-777-7804
www.pharm.sc.edu

SPARTANBURG

Drug Information Center
Spartanburg Regional
Healthcare System

101 E. Wood St.
Spartanburg, SC 29303
Mon.-Fri. 8 AM-4:30 PM
864-560-6910

TENNESSEE

KNOXVILLE

Drug Information Center
University of Tennessee
Medical Center at Knoxville

1924 Alcoa Highway
Knoxville, TN 37920-6999
Mon.-Fri. 8 AM-4:30 PM
865-544-9124

MEMPHIS

South East Regional Drug
Information Center
VA Medical Center

1030 Jefferson Ave.
Memphis, TN 38104
Mon.-Fri. 6:30 AM-4 PM
901-523-8990, ext.
6720

Drug Information Center
University of Tennessee

875 Monroe Ave.
Suite 116
Memphis, TN 38163
Mon.-Fri. 8 AM-5 PM
901-448-5556

TEXAS

AMARILLO

Drug Information Center
Texas Tech Health
Sciences Center

1300 Coulter Rd.
Amarillo, TX 79106
Mon.-Fri. 8 AM-5 PM
806-356-4008
(for healthcare
professionals only)

GALVESTON

Drug Information Center
University of Texas
Medical Branch

301 University Blvd.
Galveston, TX 77555-0701
Mon.-Fri. 8 AM-5 PM
409-772-2734

HOUSTON

Drug Information Center
Ben Taub General Hospital
Texas Southern
University/HCHD

1504 Taub Loop
Houston, TX 77030
Mon.-Fri. 9 AM-5 PM
713-873-3710

LACKLAND A.F.B.

Drug Information Center
Dept. of Pharmacy
Wilford Hall Medical Center

2200 Bergquist Dr.
Suite 1
Lackland A.F.B., TX 78236
7 days/week, 24 hours
210-292-5414

LUBBOCK

Drug Information and
Consultation Service
Covenant Medical Center

3615 19th St.
Lubbock, TX 79410
Mon.-Fri. 8 AM-5 PM
806-725-0408

SAN ANTONIO

Drug Information Service
University of Texas
Health Science Center
at San Antonio
Department of Pharmacology

7703 Floyd Curl Drive
San Antonio, TX 78229-3900
Mon.-Fri. 8 AM-4 PM
210-567-4280

TEMPLE

Drug Information Center
Scott and White
Memorial Hospital

2401 S. 31st St.
Temple, TX 76508
Mon.-Fri. 8 AM-6 PM
254-724-4636

UTAH

SALT LAKE CITY

Drug Information Service
University of Utah Hospital

421 Wakara Way
Suite 204
Salt Lake City, UT 84108
Mon.-Fri. 8:30 AM-4:30 PM
801-581-2073

VIRGINIA

HAMPTON

Drug Information Center
Hampton University School
of Pharmacy

Kittrell Hall Room 208
Hampton, VA 23668
Mon.-Fri. 9 AM-4 PM
757-728-6693

WEST VIRGINIA

MORGANTOWN

West Virginia Center for
Drug and Health Information
West Virginia University
Robert C. Byrd
Health Sciences Center

1124 HSN,
P.O. Box 9550
Morgantown, WV 26506
Mon.-Fri. 8:30 AM-5 PM
304-293-6640
800-352-2501 (WV)
www.hsc.wvu.edu/SOP

WYOMING

LARAMIE

Drug Information Center
University of Wyoming

P.O. Box 3375
Laramie, WY 82071
Mon.-Fri. 8:30 AM-4:30 PM
307-766-6988

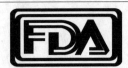

U.S. FOOD AND DRUG ADMINISTRATION

Medical Product Reporting Programs

MedWatch (24-hour service)...800-332-1088
   Reporting of problems with drugs, devices, biologics (except vaccines), medical foods, and dietary supplements.

Vaccine Adverse Event Reporting System (24-hour service) 800-822-7967
   Reporting of vaccine-related problems.

Mandatory Medical Device Reporting 240-276-3000
   Reporting required from user facilities regarding device-related deaths and serious injuries.

Veterinary Adverse Drug Reaction Program 888-332-8387
   Reporting of adverse drug events in animals.

Division of Drug Marketing, Advertising, and Communication (DDMAC) 301-827-2828
   Inquiries from health professionals regarding product promotion.

USP Medication Errors 800-233-7767
   Reporting of medication errors or near-errors to help avoid future problems through improvement in product names and packaging.

Information for Health Professionals

Center for Drug Evaluation and (CDER) Research Drug Information Hotline.........................301-827-4573
   Information on human drugs including hormones.

Center for Biologics Office of Communications..301-827-2000
   Information on biological products including vaccines and blood.

Emergency Operations..301-443-1240
   Emergencies involving FDA-regulated products, tampering reports, and emergency Investigational New Drug requests.

Office of Orphan Products Development 301-827-3666
   Information on products for rare diseases.

General Information

General Consumer Inquiries 888-463-6332
   Consumer information on regulated products/issues.

Freedom of Information..301-827-6500
   Requests for publicly available FDA documents.

Office of Public Affairs..301-827-6250
   Interviews/press inquiries on FDA activities.

Center for Food Safety and Applied Nutrition 888-723-3366
   Information on food safety, seafood, dietary supplements, women's nutrition, and cosmetics.

Consumer Information Service, Center for Devices and Radiological Health 301-443-4190
   Information on medical devices, mammography facilities, and radiation-emitting products.

U.S. FOOD AND DRUG ADMINISTRATION

Medical Product Reporting Programs

MedWatch (24-hour service) 800-332-1088
Reporting of problems with drugs, devices, biologics, and other products and sample alerts.

Vaccine Adverse Event Reporting System (24-hour service) 800-822-7967
Reporting certain vaccine problems.

Mandatory Medical Device Reporting 240-276-3000
Reporting required from user facilities regarding device-related deaths and serious injuries.

Veterinary Adverse Drug Reaction Program 888-332-8387
Reporting of adverse drug events for animals.

Division of Drug Marketing, Advertising and Communication (DDMAC) 301-827-2828
Inquiries from health professionals regarding prescription drug promotion.

USP Medication Errors 800-233-7767
Reporting of medication errors or experiences to avoid future problems through improvements in prescribing, dispensing and packaging.

Information for Health Professionals

Center for Drug Evaluation and (CDER) Research Drug Information Hotline 301-827-4573
Information about human drugs including hormones.

Center for Biologics Office of Communication 301-827-2000
Information on biological products, including vaccines and blood.

Emergency Operations 301-443-1240
Assistance after regular working hours for urgent matters, e.g., recalls and emergency investigational new drug requests.

Office of Orphan Products Development 301-827-3666
Information on products for the treatment of rare diseases.

General Information

Federal Consumer Inquiries 888-463-6332
Questions about health-related medical products issues.

Freedom of Information 301-827-6500
Requests for publicly available information.

Office of Public Affairs 301-827-6250
Interviews, press inquiries, photo services.

Center for Food Safety and Applied Nutrition 888-723-3366
Information on food safety, seafood, dietary supplements, women's nutrition, and cosmetics.

Center for Devices and Radiological Health 301-443-4190
Information on how to report problems with medical devices and radiation-emitting products.